Second Edition

l Guide to the
are of the
Medical Patient

Fred F. Ferri, MD
Chief, Division of
Internal Medicine
St. Joseph's Hospital;
Attending Staff,
Department of Medicine,
Rhode Island Hospital,
Providence, Rhode Island

with 107 illustrations

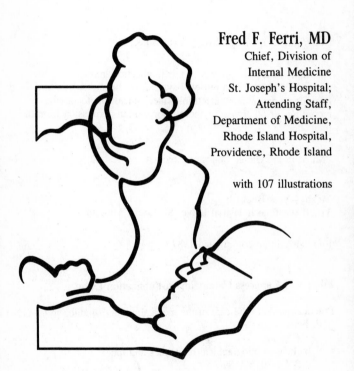

Mosby
Year Book

St. Louis Baltimore Boston Chicago London Philadelphia Sydney Toronto

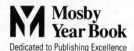
Mosby Year Book
Dedicated to Publishing Excellence

Acquisition Editor: Kimberly Kist
Assistant Editor: Penny Rudolph
Manuscript Editor: George B. Stericker, Jr.
Design: David Zielinski

Printed in the United States of America

Mosby–Year Book, Inc.
11830 Westline Industrial Drive, St. Louis, Missouri

Previous edition copyrighted 1987

Library of Congress Cataloging-in-Publication Data

Practical guide to the care of the medical patient / [edited by] Fred
    F. Ferri.— 2nd ed.
        p. cm.
    Includes bibliographical references and index.
    ISBN 0-8016-1609-3
    1. Internal medicine—Handbooks, manuals, etc.
    2. Diagnosis—Handbooks, manuals, etc.   I. Ferri, Fred F.
    [DNLM: 1. Diagnosis—handbooks. 2. Therapeutics—
handbooks. WB 39 P895]
RC55.P84 1991
616—dc20
DNLM/DLC   90-13664
for Library of Congress   CIP

CL/D/D   9 8 7 6 5 4

Contributors

Robert Burd, M.D., F.A.C.P.,

Section 24.1: Approach to the patient with anemia

Chief, Division of Hematology,
St. Vincent's Medical Center, Bridgeport;
Associate Clinical Professor of Medicine,
Yale University School of Medicine, New Haven, Connecticut

Joseph Di Benedetto, Jr., M.D., F.A.C.P.,

Section 24.13; Breast cancer

Clinical Instructor in Medicine,
Brown University School of Medicine; Rhode Island Hospital and St. Joseph's Hospital, Providence, Rhode Island

Saul Feldman, M.D.,

Section 23.1: Acute gastrointestinal bleeding

Chief, Division of Gastroenterology,
St. Vincent's Medical Center Bridgeport;
Associate Clinical Professor of Medicine,
Yale University School of Medicine, New Haven, Connecticut

Marvin Garrell, M.D., F.A.C.P.,

Chapter 14: Dementia

Director of Medical Education,
St. Vincent's Medical Center, Bridgeport;
Associate Clinical Professor of Medicine,
Yale University School of Medicine, New Haven;
Medical Director,
Jewish Home for the Aged of Fairfield, Fairfield, Connecticut

James Grant, M.D.,

Section 26.1: Renal failure

Chief, Division of Renology,
St. Vincent's Medical Center, Bridgeport;
Associate Clinical Professor of Medicine,
Yale University School of Medicine, New Haven, Connecticut

H. Christina Hanley, M.D.,

Section 22.1: Diabetes mellitus

Chief, Division of
Endocrinology,
St. Vincent's Medical Center,
Bridgeport;
Assistant Clinical Professor of
Medicine,
Yale University School of
Medicine, New Haven,
Connecticut

Joseph Herbin, M.D.,

Section 25.1: Nosocomial infections

Chief, Division of Infectious
Diseases,
St. Vincent's Medical Center,
Bridgeport;
Assistant Clinical Professor of
Medicine,
Yale University School of
Medicine, New Haven,
Connecticut

Powell H. Kazanjian, M.D.,

Section 25.4: AIDS

Associate Physician,
Division of Infectious
Disease, Brigham and
Women's Hospital;
Instructor in Medicine,
Harvard Medical School,
Boston, Massachusetts

George T. Kiss, M.D.,

*Section 28.1: Use and interpretation of
pulmonary function tests*

Chief, Division of Pulmonary
Diseases,
St. Vincent's Medical Center,
Bridgeport;
Associate Clinical Professor of
Medicine,
Yale University School of

Medicine, New Haven,
Connecticut

Iradj Nejad, M.D.

Section 22.4: Hypoglycemia

Endocrinologist,
St. Vincent's Medical Center,
Bridgeport;
Assistant Clinical Professor of
Medicine,
University of Connecticut
School of Medicine,
Farmington, Connecticut

Kenneth Siegel, M.D.

*Section 27.1: Generalized tonic-clonic
seizures*

Chief, Division of Neurology,
St. Vincent's Medical Center,
Bridgeport;
Associate Clinical Professor of
Medicine,
Yale University School of
Medicine, New Haven,
Connecticut

Michael S. Weinstock, M.D.,
F.A.C.E.P.

*Chapter 7: General Management of poisoning
and drug overdose*

Medical Director,
Emergency Department, North
Shore University Hospital,
Manhasset, New York

Preface

This manual is a clear and concise reference for the busy clinican in need of immediate medical information. Its purpose is to provide a fast and efficient way to identify important clinical and laboratory information. It is not intended to substitute for the many excellent medical reference texts that form the cornerstone of one's medical education.

To limit the size of the manual to a pocket reference, less emphasis has been placed on pathophysiology and epidemiology and more emphasis on practical clinical information. A conservative approach to the various medical syndromes is followed throughout the book. Elegant but unnecessary words have been eliminated in favor of simple and accurate expositions of the various subjects. Medical tables have been used extensively throughout the manual to simplify difficult topics and to enhance recollection of principal points.

It is hoped that the concise style of this manual will be of help to the reader, particularly during an active clinical service when time to read is severely limited.

The combination of practical clinical information with drug therapeutics and laboratory medicine makes this manual unique and useful not only to medical residents and medical students but also to practicing physicians and allied health professionals.

Fred F. Ferri

Acknowledgments

I wish to acknowledge the many contributors and consultants for their excellent expositions and sage advice. I am particularly indebted to Everett B. Cooper, M.D., F.A.C.P., Director of Education, Department of Medicine, at St. Vincent's Medical Center, for his scholarly guidance, and to Margaret Robinson, R.Ph., for her assistance on Chapters 32 and 33.

Contents

Appendixes, 741

Key Telephone Numbers

This chapter is a listing of the phone numbers of departments and individuals in the hospital who might be needed for immediate consultation.

Department

Admitting _____

Anesthesia _____

CCU _____

ECG _____

EEG _____

ER _____

ICU _____

Information _____

IV Team _____

Laboratory _____

   Chemistry _____

   Hematology _____

   Microbiology _____

   Other _____

Medical Records _____

Nuclear Medicine _____

Paging _____

Pathology _____

Pharmacy _____

Physical Therapy _____

Pulmonary Function _____

Radiology _____

Recovery Room _____

Respiratory Therapy _____

Security _____

Social Service _____

Sonography _____

Other _____

Nursing Stations

House Staff

Attending Staff

Medical Record
Abbreviations

a arterial
Aa alveolar/arterial
A₂ aortic second sound
āā of each
AB apical beat
abd abdomen
ABG arterial blood gas
abn abnormal
ABVD doxorubicin (Adriamycin), bleomycin, vinblastine, dacarbazine (DTIC)
ac before meals
A/C assist control
ACE angiotension-converting enzyme, adrenocortical extract
acet acetone
aCL anticardiolipin (antibody)
ACLS advanced cardiovascular life support
ACT activated clotting time
ACTH adrenocorticotropic hormone
A.D.A. American Dental Association, American Diabetic Association, American Dietetic Association
ADH antidiuretic hormone
ADL activities of daily living
ad lib as desired, freely
adm admission
AF atrial fibrillation
AFB acid-fast bacilli
A/G albumin/globulin ratio
AG anion gap
AIDS acquired immune deficiency syndrome
AJ ankle jerk
AKA above-knee amputation
AL arterial line
alb albumin
alk phos alkaline phosphatase
ALL acute lymphoblastic leukemia

ALS amyotrophic lateral sclerosis
ALT alanine aminotransferase
AM morning
AMA against medical advice
AMI acute myocardial infarction
AML acute myelogenous leukemia
amp ampule
AMP adenosine monophosphate
amt amount
amy amylase
ANA antinuclear antibody
ANCA antineutrophil cytoplasmic antibody
ANLL acute nonlymphocytic leukemia
AODM adult-onset diabetes mellitus
AOP aortic pressure
A&P auscultation and percussion
AP anteroposterior
APAG antipseudomonal aminoglycosidic penicillin
appt appointment
APSAC anisoylated plasminogen/streptokinase activator complex
APTT activated partial thromboplastin time
APUD amine precursor uptake decarboxylase
aq water
AR aortic regurgitation
ARC AIDS-related complex
ARDS acute respiratory distress syndrome
ARF acute renal failure
ARM arterial rupture of membranes
ART assessment, review, and treatment
AS atriosystolic, aortic stenosis
asa aspirin

3

A.S.A. American Society of Anesthesiologists
ASH asymmetric septal hypertrophy
ASHD arteriosclerotic heart disease
ASLO anti–streptolysin O
AST aspartate aminotransferase
at fib atrial fibrillation
ATC around the clock
ATG antithymocyte globulin
ATN acute tubular necrosis
AV arteriovenous, atrioventricular
AVM arteriovenous malformation
AVP arginine vasopressin
AZT zidovudine
B black
ba barium
BACOD bleomycin, doxorubicin (Adriamycin), cyclophosphamide, vincristine (Oncovin), dexamethasone
BACOP bleomycin, doxorubicin (Adriamycin), cyclophosphamide, vincristine (Oncovin), prednisone
BAL British anti-Lewisite (dimercaprol)
BBB bundle branch block
BC blood culture
BCG bacillus Calmette-Guérin
BCNU carmustine
BCP birth control pill
BE barium enema
BEE basal energy expenditure
bid two times a day
bilat bilateral
bili bilirubin
BKA below-knee amputation
Bl s blood sugar
BM bowel movement
BMR basal metabolic rate
BP blood pressure
BPH benign prostatic hypertrophy
bpm beats per minute
BR bed rest
BRP bathroom privileges
BS or bs breath sounds
BSA body surface area
BSO bilateral salpingo-oophorectomy
BTL bilateral tubal ligation
BUN blood urea nitrogen
BW body weight
Bx biopsy
c̄ with
C centigrade

C3 to C9 protein components of complement system
Ca cancer
Ca^{+2} calcium
C/A Clinitest and acetone
CAB coronary artery bypass
CABG coronary artery bypass graft
CAD coronary artery disease
CAF cyclophosphamide, doxorubicin (Adriamycin), 5-fluorouracil
cal calorie
cap capsule
CAT computerized axial tomography
cath catheterization
CAV cyclophosphamide, doxorubicin (Adriamycin), vincristine
CBC complete blood cell count
CBD common bile duct
cc cubic centimeter
CC chief complaint
CCr creatine clearance
CCU coronary care unit
CD4 helper-inducer T cells
CD8 suppressor-cytotoxic T cells
CEA carcinoembryonic antigen
CF complement fixation, conversion factor
CGL chronic granulocytic (myelogenous) leukemia
CHD congenital heart disease
CHF congestive heart failure
cho carbohydrate
CHOP cyclophosphamide, doxorubicin, vincristine (Oncovin), prednisone
CI cardiac index
CIE counterimmunoelectrophoresis
CK creatine kinase
CK-MB creatine kinase, myocardial band
cl clear
Cl$^-$ chloride
CLL chronic lymphocytic leukemia
cm centimeter
CM costal margin
CMF cyclophosphamide, methotrexate, 5-fluorouracil
CML chronic myelogenous leukemia
CMV cytomegalovirus, continuous mechanical ventilation
CNS central nervous system
CO cardiac output, carbon monoxide
c/o complains of
CO$_2$ carbon dioxide
CoA coenzyme A

COMLA cyclophosphamide, vincristine (Oncovin), methotrexate, leucovorin, cytosine arabinoside

conc concentrate

COPD chronic obstructive pulmonary disease

CPAP continuous positive airway pressure

CPK creatine phosphokinase

CPR cardiopulmonary resuscitation

Cr creatinine

CR cardiorespiratory

CRH corticotropin releasing hormone

C/S culture and sensitivity

CSF cerebrospinal fluid

C/sec cesarean section

CT computed tomography

Cu copper

CV cardiovascular

cva costovertebral angle

CVA cerebrovascular accident

CVP central venous pressure

CXR chest x-ray

cysto cystoscopy

D&C dilation and curettage

D/C discontinue

D&S dilation and suction

DAT diet as tolerated

DBIL direct bilirubin

DCF 2′ deoxycoformycin

DDAVP desmopressin

ddI dideoxyinosine

DFA direct fluorescent antibody

DGI disseminated gonococcal infection

DHPG ganciclovir

Dial dialysis

DIC disseminated intravascular coagulation

dil dilute

DIP distal interphalangeal, desquamative interstitial pneumonitis

DKA diabetic ketoacidosis

DL_{CO} diffusing capacity of lung for carbon monoxide

dl deciliter

DLE drug related lupus erythematosus

DM diabetes mellitus

DNA deoxyribonucleic acid

DOA dead on arrival

DP dorsalis pedis

DPT diphtheria, pertussis, tetanus

DR delivery room

ds double strand

DSD dry sterile dressing

DTIC dacarbazine

DTR deep tendon reflex

DTs delirium tremens

DU duodenal ulcer

DUB dysfunctional uterine bleeding

DVT deep venous thrombosis

D_5W dextrose (5%) in water

Dx diagnosis

EBL estimated blood loss

EBV Epstein-Barr virus

ECF extended care facility, extracellular fluid

ECG electrocardiogram

ECM erythema chronicum migrans

EDC estimated date of confinement

EDTA ethylene diamine tetraacetate

EEG electroencephalogram

EENT eyes, ears, nose, and throat

EF ejection fraction

EIA electroimmunoassay

EKG electrocardiogram

elect electrolyte

ELISA enzyme-linked immunoassay

elix elixir

EMD electromechanical dissociation

EMG electromyogram

ENT ear, nose, and throat

EOM extraocular movements

EPO erythropoietin

EPS extrapyramidal symptoms

ER emergency room, estrogen receptor

ERCP endoscopic retrograde cholangiopancreatography

ERS evacuation retained secundines

ESR erythrocyte sedimentation rate

ESRD end-stage renal disease

EST, ECT electroshock therapy

EUA examination under anesthesia

et al and others

ext extract, extremities

F Fahrenheit

FABM3 acute promyelocytic leukemia

FBS fasting blood sugar

FDP fibrin degradation product

Fe Iron

FE fractional excretion

FEV forced expiratory volume

FF force fluids

FFP fresh frozen plasma

FH family history

FHC family health center

FHM fetal heart monitor

FHR fetal heart rate

FIo_2 fraction of inspired oxygen

fl fluid, femtoliter
fL femtoliter
FMF familial Mediterranean fever
FNA fine needle aspiration
FS frozen section
FSH follicle stimulating hormone
FTA-ABS fluorescent treponemal antibody absorbed
FTI free thyroxine index
5-FU 5-fluorouracil
FUO fever of undetermined origin
FVC forced vital capacity
FWB full weight bearing
fx fracture
g gram
Ga gallium
GA general anesthesia
GB gallbladder
Gc gonococcus
GERD gastroesophageal reflux disease
GFR glomerular filtration rate
GGT γ-glutamyltransferase
GGTP γ-glutamyltranspeptidase
GI gastrointestinal
GIP gastric inhibitory polypeptide
GITS gastrointestinal therapeutic system
glu glucose
GN graduate nurse, glomerulonephritis
G_6PD glucose-6-phosphate dehydrogenase
gr grain
GSW gun shot wound
gtt drop
GTT glucose tolerance test
GU genitourinary
GVHD graft versus host disease
G/W enema glycerine and water enema
Gyn gynecology
H_2 histamine$_2$
H/A headache
HA hyperalimentation
HAV hepatitis A virus
Hb hemoglobin
HB_cAg hepatitis B core antigen
HB_sAg hepatitis B surface antigen
HBIG hepatitis B immune globulin
HBP high blood pressure
HBV hepatitis B virus
HCO_3^- bicarbonate
hct hematocrit
HCV hepatitis C virus
HD hospital discharge

HDL high-density lipoprotein
HDV hepatitis D virus
HEENT head, eyes, ears, nose, and throat
HEMPAS hereditary erythroblastic multinuclearity associated with positive acidified serum
Hg hemoglobin
H/H hemoglobin/hematocrit
5-HIAA 5-hydroxyindoleacetic acid
HIV human immunodeficiency virus
H&L heart and lungs
HLA human leukocyte antigen
HMG-CoA 3-hydroxy-3-methylglutaryl coenzyme A
HNP herniated nucleus pulposus
H_2O water
H_2O_2 hydrogen peroxide
HOCM hypertrophic obstructive cardiomyopathy
HORF high-output renal failure
H&P history and physical exam
HPI history of present illness
HR heart rate
HRS hepatorenal syndrome
hs hour of sleep (at bedtime)
HSV herpes simplex virus
ht height
HTN hypertension
hx history
I&D incision and drainage
IABP intraaortic balloon pump
IBC iron-binding capacity
IBD inflammatory bowel disease
IBS irritable bowel syndrome
ICP intracranial pressure
ICU intensive care unit
ID intradermal
IDDM insulin dependent diabetes mellitus
IF idiopathic flushing
IFA immunofluorescent assay
IHSS idiopathic hypertrophic subaortic stenosis
Ig immunoglobulin
ILD interstitial lung disease
IM intramuscular
Imp impression
IMV intermittent mandatory ventilation
inf infusion
inh inhalation
inj injection
I&O intake and output

IOP intraocular pressure
IPG impedance plethysmography
iPLP parathyroid hormone–like protein by radioimmunoassay
IPPB intermittent positive pressure breathing
iPTH parathyroid hormone by radioimmunoassay
IQ intelligence quotient
ISG immune serum globulin
ITP idiopathic thrombocytopenic purpura
IUD intrauterine device
IV intravenous
IVC inferior vena cava
IVP intravenous pyelogram
J joule
JG juxtaglomerular
JVD jugular venous distention
JVP jugular vein pulse
kat katal (mole/sec)
K⁺ potassium
KJ knee jerk
kg kilogram
17-KS 17-ketosteroid
KUB kidney, ureter, and bladder
l left
L liter
LA left atrium
lab laboratory
lac laceration
LAD left axis deviation
LAHB left anterior hemiblock
lap laparotomy
LAP leukocyte alkaline phosphatase
LAV lymphadenopathy-associated virus (same as HIV)
lb pound
LBP low back pain
LBBB left bundle branch block
LDH lactate dehydrogenase
LDL low density lipoprotein
LES lower esophageal sphincter
LFT liver function test
LGV lymphogranuloma venereum
LH luteinizing hormone
LHRH luteinizing hormone–releasing hormone
Li lithium
Lip lipid
liq liquid
LLL left lower lobe
LLQ left lower quadrant
LMD local medical doctor
LMP last menstrual period

LNMP last normal menstrual period
LOC level of consciousness
LP lumbar puncture
LPHB left posterior hemiblock
LPN licensed practical nurse
LSB left sternal border
LSK liver, spleen, and kidney
LUL left upper lobe
LUQ left upper quadrant
LVEDP left ventricular end diastolic pressure
LVH left ventricular hypertrophy
L & W living and well
m murmur
M midnight, monoclonal
M1 to M7 categories of ANLL
MACE methotrexate, doxorubicin (Adriamycin), cyclophosphamide, epipodophyllotoxin
MAO monoamine oxidase
MAP mean arterial pressure
MAT multi-focal atrial tachycardia
max maximum
MB izoenzyme of cardiac origin
MBC minimum bactericidal concentration
MCA middle cerebral artery
MCL midclavicular line
MCP metacarpophalangeal
MCTD mixed connective tissue disease
MCV mean cell volume
med medication
MED medical
MEN multiple endocrine neoplasia
mEq milliequivalent
MERSA methicillin-resistant *Staphylococcus aureus*
mets metastases
MF maturation factor
mg milligram
Mg²⁺ magnesium
MH malignant hyperthermia
MHTAP microhemagglutination assay for antibody to *Treponema pallidum*
MI myocardial infarction
MIA *Mycobacterium intracellulare avium*
MIBG meta-iodobenzyl guanidine
MIC minimum inhibitory concentration
min minute
mixt mixture
µkat microkatal (micromole/sec)
ml milliliter

ML malignant lymphoma

μmol micromole

mm millimeter

mM, mmol millimole

mod moderate

MOM milk of magnesia

MOPP mechlorethamine, vincristine (Oncovin), procarbazine, prednisone

mOsm milliosmol

MP metacarpophalangeal

MPGN membrane proliferative glomerulonephritis

MPTP analog of meperidine (used by drug addicts)

MR mitral regurgitation

MRI magnetic resonance imaging

MS mitral stenosis, mental status

MSU monosodium urate

MTC medullary thyroid carcinoma

MTP metatarsophalangeal

MUGA multiple gated (image) acquisition (analysis)

MVA motor vehicle accident

MVP mitral valve prolapse; mitomycin, vinblastine, cisplatin (Platinol)

MVV maximum voluntary ventilation

N normal

NA not applicable

Na⁺ sodium

NaHCO₃ sodium bicarbonate

NAPA N-acetyl-procainamide, N-acetyl-paraaminophenol

NAS no added sodium

NB newborn

NCP nursing care plan

neg negative

NETT nasal endotracheal tube

Neuro neurology

ng nanogram

NG nasogastric

NGU nongonococcal urethritis

NH₃ ammonia

NHL non-Hodgkin's lymphoma

NIDDM non–insulin dependent diabetes mellitus

NIH National Institutes of Health

NKA no known allergy

nkat nanokatal (nanomole/sec)

NKDA no known drug allergy

NM neuromuscular

no number

noc night

NPH normal pressure hydrocephalus, neutral protamine Hagedorn (insulin)

NPO nothing by mouth

NS normal saline

NSAID nonsteroidal antiinflammatory drug

NSILA nonsuppressable insulin-like activity

NSR normal sinus rhythm

NTG nitroglycerin

NYHA New York Heart Association

OA oral airway

OAF osteoclast activating factor

OB obstetrics

OD overdose

OD right eye

OETT oral endotracheal tube

17-OHCS 17-hydroxycorticosteroid

25-OHD 1,25-dihydroxyvitamin D

oint ointment

OOB out of bed

OOP out on pass

OPD outpatient department

opt optimum

ophth ophthalmology

OR operating room

Oral oral surgery

Orth or ortho orthopedics

OS left eye

osm osmolality

OT occupational therapy

OU each eye

oz ounce

p after

p̄ pulse

P wave part of the electrocardiographic cycle representing atrial depolarization (stimulation)

P₂ pulmonic second sound

Paco₂ partial pressure of CO_2 in arterial blood

Pao₂ partial pressure of O_2 in arterial blood

P&A percussion and auscultation

PA posteroanterior, pulmonary artery

PADP pulmonary artery diastolic pressure

PAM pulse amplitude modulation

pap Papanicolaou

PAP pulmonary artery pressure

para number of pregnancies

PAS paraaminosalicylic acid

PASP pulmonary artery systolic pressure

PAT paroxysmal atrial tachycardia

PAWP pulmonary artery wedge pressure

pc after meals

Pco$_2$ carbon dioxide tension

PCP *Pneumocystis carinii* pneumonia, phencyclidine

PCWP pulmonary capillary wedge pressure

PE physical exam, pulmonary embolism

PEARL pupils equal and reactive to light

ped pediatric

PEEP positive end-expiratory pressure

PEFR peak expiratory flow rate

per by

PERRLA pupils equal, round, reactive to light and accommodation

PFT pulmonary function test

pg picogram

PGE prostaglandin E

PH past history

phos phosphorus

PHP pseudohypoparathyroidism

PHR peak heart rate

PI present illness

PID pelvic inflammatory disease

PIP proximal interphalangeal

PKU phenylketonuria

PLA plasminogen activator

PLP parathyroid hormone–like protein

PM afternoon

PMI point of maximum impulse

PMN polymorphonuclear leukocyte

PMP previous menstrual period

PM & R physical medicine and rehabilitation

PMR polymyalgia rheumatica

PND paroxysmal nocturnal dyspnea

PNH paroxysmal nocturnal hemoglobinuria

PO by mouth

PO$_4$$^{-3}$ phosphate

postop postoperative

Po$_2$ oxygen tension

PP postpartum

PPD purified protein derivative

PPNG penicillinase-producing *Neisseria gonorrhoeae*

PR per rectum, pulmonic regurgitation, progesterone receptor

PR interval part of electrocardiographic cycle from onset of atrial depolarization to onset of ventricular depolarization

preop preoperative

prep preparation

PROM premature rupture of membranes

prn as needed

PRSP penicillinase-resistant synthetic penicillin

PS pulmonic stenosis

PSGN post-streptococcal glomerulonephritis

psi pounds per square inch

PSVT paroxysmal supraventricular tachycardia

Psych or psych psychiatry

pt patient

PT prothrombin time, physical therapy, posterior tibia

PTA prior to admission

PTC percutaneous transhepatic cholangiography

PTCA percutaneous transluminal coronary angioplasty

Pth pathology

PTH parathormone

PTRA percutaneous transluminal renal angioplasty

PTT partial thromboplastin time

PTU propylthiouracil

PUD peptic ulcer disease

PWP pulmonary wedge pressure

PVC premature ventricular contraction

PVR pulmonary vascular resistance

PX physical

q every

qd every day

qh every hour

qhs every bed time

qid four times a day

qns quantity not sufficient

qod every other day

qs quantity sufficient

QRS part of electrocardiographic wave representing ventricular depolarization (stimulation)

r right

R respiratory rate (per min)

RA rheumatoid arthritis, right atrium

RAI radioactive iodine

RAN resident's admission note

RAP right atrial pressure

RBBB right bundle branch block

RBC red blood cells

RDS respiratory distress syndrome

RDW red cell distribution width

R&E round and equal
readm readmission
REM rapid eye movement
RF rheumatoid factor
Rh Rhesus blood factor
RIA radio immunoassay
RL Ringer's lactate
RIND reversible ischemic neurologic deficit
RLL right lower lobe
RLQ right lower quadrant
RML right middle lobe
RN registered nurse
RNA ribonucleic acid
R/O rule out
ROM range of motion
ROS review of systems
RPGN rapidly progressive glomerulonephritis
RPI reticulocyte production index
RPR rapid plasma reagin
rpt repeat
RPT registered physical therapist
RR recovery room
RSR regular sinus rhythm
rt-PA recombinant tissue plasminogen activator
R/T related to
rT$_3$ reverse triiodothyronine
RTA renal tubular acidosis
RTC return to clinic
RUL right upper lobe
RUQ right upper quadrant
RV right ventricle, residual volume
RVH renovascular hypertension, right ventricular hypertrophy
Rx therapy, treatment, prescription
S$_1$ first heart sound
S$_2$ second heart sound
S$_3$ third heart sound
S$_4$ fourth heart sound
s̄ without
S/A sugar and acetone
SA sinoatrial
SAH subarachnoid hemorrhage
sat saturated
SB stillbirth
SBE subacute bacterial (infective) endocarditis
SBP spontaneous bacterial peritonitis
SBT serum bactericidal titer
SC subcutaneous
SCP standard care plan

SGA small for gestational age
SGOT serum glutamic oxalaoacetic transaminase (aspartate aminotransferase, AST)
SI Système Internationale
SIADH syndrome of inappropriate secretion of antidiuretic hormone
SGPT serum glutamic pyruvate transaminase (alanine aminotransferase, ALT)
SL sublingual
SLE systemic lupus erythematosus
SLR straight leg raising
SMI suggested minimum increment
SMS somatostatin
SNF skilled nursing facility
SO$_2$ oxygen saturation
SOB short of breath
SOC state of consciousness
sol solution
S/P status post
SQ subcutaneous
SR slow release
SRM spontaneous rupture membranes
s̄s̄ half
S/S signs and symptoms
SS Sjögren's syndrome
SSE soap suds enema
SSKI saturated solution potassium iodide
SSS sick sinus syndrome
ST segment part of electrocardiographic cycle representing the beginning of ventricular repolarization (recovery)
stat immediately
STD sexually transmitted disease
STS serologic test for syphilis
subcu, SC subcutaneous
supp suppository
Surg surgery
susp suspension
SVC superior vena cava
SVR systemic vascular resistance
SVT supraventricular tachycardia
Sx symptoms
syr syrup
T wave part of the ECG cycle, representing a portion of ventricular repolarization (recovery)
T$_3$ triiodothyronine

T_4 thyroxine
T&A tonsillectomy and adenoidectomy
tab tablet
TAH total abdominal hysterectomy
TB tuberculosis
TBG thyroxine binding globulin, total blood gases
TBIL total bilirubin
TBNa total body sodium
Tbsp tablespoon
TBW total body water
T/C throat culture
temp temperature
TENS transcutaneous electrical nerve stimulation
Tg thyroglobulin
THBR thyroid hormone–binding ratio
TIA transient ischemic attack
TIBC total iron-binding capacity
tid three times daily
tinc tincture
TLC total lung capacity
TM tympanic membrane
TMP-SMX trimethoprim/sulfamethoxazole
TNM tumor-nodes-metastases
TO telephone order
top topical
tPA tissue plasminogen activator
TP total protein
TPI *Treponema pallidum* immobilization
TPN total parenteral nutrition
TPR temperature, pulse, and respiration
TR tricuspid regurgitation
TRAP tartrate-resistant acid phosphatase
TRF thyrotropin releasing factor
T_3RIA triiodothyronine level by radioimmunoassay
T_3RU T_3 resin uptake
TRH thyrotropin releasing hormone
TRIG triglycerides
TS tricuspid stenosis
TSAb thyroid stimulating antibodies
TSH thyroid stimulating hormone
tsp teaspoon
TT thrombin time
TTP thrombotic thrombocytopenic purpura, ribothymidine 5′triphosphate
TTS transdermal therapeutic system
TUR transurethral resection
TURP transurethral resection prostate
TU tuberculin unit
TV tidal volume
TWAR *Chlamydia psittaci*
Tx therapy
U unit
UA umbilical artery
U/A urinalysis
UGI upper gastrointestinal
ung ointment
U/P urine/plasma ratio (concentration)
URAC uric acid
URI upper respiratory tract infection
USP United States Pharmacopeia
UTI urinary tract infection
UV ultraviolet
v mixed venous
V volume
vag hyst vaginal hysterectomy
VAMP vincristine, doxorubicin (Adriamycin), methylprednisolone
VAT ventricular activation time
VD veneral disease
VDRL Venereal Disease Research Laboratories (test for syphilis)
VC vital capacity
VER visual evoked response
VF ventricular fibrillation
VIP vasoactive intestinal polypeptide
VLDL very low density lipoprotein
VMA vanillylmandelic acid
VPC ventricular premature contraction
VO verbal order
VP-16 epipodophyllotoxin
vs visit
VS vital signs
VSD ventricular septal defect
VT/VF ventricular tachycardia/fibrillation
W white
WBC white blood (cell) count
w/c wheel chair
WD well developed
WF white female
WHO World Health Organization
WN well nourished
WNL within normal limits
WPW Wolff Parkinson White
wt weight
y/o years old
X times
ZDV zidovudine
Z-E Zollinger-Ellison (syndrome)

SYMBOLS

@	at
+ +	moderate amount
+ + +	large amount
0	zero, none
°	degree
♀	female
♂	male
#	number
↑	increased
↓	decreased

>	greater than
<	less than
μ or μm	micron (micrometer)
+	positive, presence
"	minute
'	second
ø	absence of
✔	check
−	negative, absence
△	changes

NOTICE: The science of medicine is constantly evolving. Every attempt has been made by the author and consultants to ensure that this manual includes the latest recommendations from the medical literature. Doses of drugs and treatment recommendations have been carefully reviewed. **However, it is strongly recommended that the reader become completely familiar with the manufacturer's product information when prescribing any of the drugs described in this manual.** This recommendation is especially important with new or infrequently used drugs. As new information becomes available, changes in treatment modalities invariably follow; therefore when choosing a particular treatment, the reader should consider not only the information provided in this manual but also any recently published medical literature on the subject.

Approach to the Medical Patient

3

HISTORY AND PHYSICAL EXAM[1,2,4]

1. Chief complaint: reason for seeking medical attention; when possible it should be stated in the patient's own words.
2. Present illness: chronologic narrative of the patient's medical problems. The description of the symptoms should include the following: location, quality (deep, sharp, stinging), quantity or severity, timing (onset, duration, frequency), aggravating or relieving factors, associated manifestations, prior investigations, prior treatment, and radiation to another site.
3. Past medical history: general state of health, significant childhood illnesses, prior hospitalizations (medical, surgical), blood transfusions, and traumas.
4. Allergies: foods, drugs; describe the type of allergic reaction.
5. Current medications: dose, frequency, and duration of present drug regimen; include all nonprescription drugs.
6. Family history: age and health status or age and cause of death of each immediate family member. Inquire about a family history of diabetes, heart disease, hypertension, cancer, arthritis, mental disorders, or any hereditary conditions.
7. Social history
   a. Life style, home situation, significant others
   b. Cigarette smoking (quantity in pack years), alcohol usage (see Table 3-1)
   c. Occupational history
   d. Religious beliefs relevant to health
8. Review of systems
   a. General: overall state of health, usual weight, recent weight change, fever, night sweats, sleeping habits, appetite
   b. Skin: rashes, pruritus, color change, pigmentation
   c. Head: headaches, trauma
   d. Eyes: vision, visual disturbances, last eye exam
   e. Ears: hearing, tinnitus, vertigo, infections, discharge
   f. Nose and sinuses: epistaxis, nasal stuffiness, sinusitis, sense of smell

Table 3-1   CAGE questionnaire for screening of alcohol abuse[3]

C:	"Have you ever felt you ought to Cut down on drinking?"
A:	"Have people Annoyed you by criticizing your drinking?"
G:	"Have you ever felt bad or Guilty about your drinking?"
E:	"Have you ever had a drink first thing in the morning to steady your nerves or get rid of a hangover (Eye-opener)?"

From Ewing JA: JAMA 252:1905, 1984.

g. Mouth and throat: condition of teeth, last dental exam, presence of sore throat or mouth lesions
h. Neck: lumps, "swollen glands," pain in neck region
i. Breasts: pain, history of lumps, bleeding, nipple discharge; if female, inquire if she performs self-exam
j. Respiratory: cough, wheezing, sputum (quantity, color), shortness of breath, pain associated with breathing
k. Cardiac: chest pain, palpitations, orthopnea, edema, heart murmurs, history of high blood pressure
l. Gastrointestinal: nausea, vomiting, change in bowel habits, GI bleeding, constipation, diarrhea, abdominal pain, increased girth
m. Genitourinary: dysuria, frequency, urgency, nocturia, discharges, venereal diseases, libido, sexual problems, bleeding
n. Gynecologic/reproductive: age at menarche, last menstrual period, frequency and duration of periods, number and complications of pregnancies, age at menopause, contraception
o. Musculoskeletal: weakness, arthritis, gout, joint pains, swelling or stiffness, muscle cramps
p. Peripheral vascular: varicose veins, thrombophlebitis, claudication, Raynaud's phenomenon
q. Neuropsychiatric: seizures, syncope, weakness, paralysis/paresis, extreme mood changes, insomnia, anxiety, psychiatric care, suicidal ideation
r. Endocrine: heat or cold intolerance, polydypsia, polyuria, polyphagia
s. Hematologic: easy bruising, transfusion reactions, excessive bleeding, history of anemia
9. Physical exam (see box on pp. 25 and 26 for a sample).
a. Vital signs: record pulse, respiration, temperature, and blood pressure (position, measured in both arms)
b. General description: observe state of health, general appearance, nutritional status, body development, personal hygiene, posture, signs of anxiety, and apparent age
c. Skin
(1) Observe texture, color, temperature, turgor, color, and note any lesions
(2) Note distribution, amount, and texture of hair
(3) Note color of nail beds and shape of nails
d. Lymph nodes: note size, consistency, mobility, and tenderness of lymph nodes

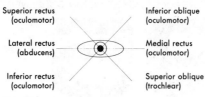

Figure 3-1
Muscles that control eye movements.

e. Head: note size, shape, symmetry, and any unusual lesions
f. Eyes: note position and alignment of eyes; inspect lacrimal glands, eyelids, cornea, sclera, and pupils; test visual fields and pupillary reactions; closely examine the fundi; observe range of eye movements (Fig. 3-1); assess near vision with the Rosenbaum chart (Fig. 3-2)

Of interest is the Argyll Robertson pupil, which constricts with light but not with convergence. Classically associated with neurosyphilis, it can be seen with sarcoidosis, multiple sclerosis, diabetes mellitus, Lyme disease, CNS tumors or hemorrhage, Wernicke's encephalopathy, and other conditions associated with lesions in the area of the Edinger-Westphal nucleus.

g. Ears: inspect auricles, canals, and tympanic membranes; check auditory acuity by whispering in the patient's ear or by placing watch against the patient's ear
h. Nose and sinuses: inspect the external nose, nasal mucosa, and septum; palpate frontal and maxillary sinuses for evidence of tenderness
i. Mouth and throat: inspect lips, gums, teeth, tongue, palate, and pharynx
j. Neck
    (1) Palpate thyroid gland, inspect and palpate cervical nodes, and examine trachea

    When palpating the carotid arteries, never do both sides simultaneously (may cause syncope).
    (2) Auscultate carotids for pulses, upstroke, and presence of bruits
    (3) Note presence of jugular venous distention and angle of distention
    (4) Note range of neck movements and any nuchal rigidity
k. Back: Inspect and palpate spine and muscles of back; note any kyphosis or scoliosis
l. Chest
    (1) Inspect, palpate, and percuss lungs and heart
    (2) Observe respiratory movements and use of respiratory muscles
    (3) Listen to quality and intensity of breath sounds
    (4) Listen for e to a change, whispered pectoriloquy ("ninety-nine")

ROSENBAUM POCKET VISION SCREENER

95

874

2843

6 3 8   E Ш Ǝ   X O O

8 7 4 5   Ǝ M Ш   O X O

6 3 9 2 5   M E Ǝ   X O X

4 2 8 3 6 5   Ш E M   O X O

3 7 4 2 5 8   Ǝ Ш Ǝ   X X O

9 3 7 8 2 6   Ш M E   X O O

4 2 8 7 3 9   E Ш M   O O X

	distance equivalent
	$\frac{20}{800}$

Point	Jaeger	
		$\frac{20}{400}$
26	16	$\frac{20}{200}$
14	10	$\frac{20}{100}$
10	7	$\frac{20}{70}$
8	5	$\frac{20}{50}$
6	3	$\frac{20}{40}$
5	2	$\frac{20}{30}$
4	1	$\frac{20}{25}$
3	1+	$\frac{20}{20}$

Card is held in good light 14 inches from eye. Record vision for each eye separately with and without glasses. Presbyopic patients should read thru bifocal segment. Check myopes with glasses only.

DESIGN COURTESY J. G. ROSENBAUM, M.D.

PUPIL GAUGE (mm.)

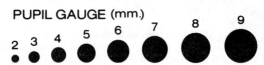

2   3   4   5   6   7   8   9

Figure 3-2
Rosenbaum chart for testing near vision.

Table 3-2   Response of selected murmurs to physiologic intervention

Cardiac Murmur	Accentuation	Decrease
Systolic		
Aortic stenosis (AS)	Valsalva release	Handgrip
	Sudden squatting	Valsalva
	Passive leg raising	Standing
Idiopathic hypertrophic subaortic stenosis (IHSS)	Valsalva strain	Handgrip
	Standing	Squatting
		Leg elevation
Mitral regurgitation	Sudden squatting	Valsalva
	Isometric handgrip	Standing
Pulmonic stenosis	Valsalva release	Expiration
Tricuspid regurgitation	Inspiration	Expiration
	Passive leg raising	
Diastolic		
Aortic regurgitation	Sudden squatting	
	Isometric handgrip	
Mitral stenosis	Exercise	
	Left lateral position	
	Isometric handgrip	
	Coughing	
Tricuspid stenosis	Inspiration	Expiration
	Passive leg raising	

  m. Heart
     (1) Inspect and palpate precordium; locate apical impulse
     (2) Using both bell and diaphragm, auscultate for S_1, S_2 (intensity, splitting), abnormal heart sounds (S_3, S_4 clicks, rubs, hums, snaps), murmurs (note timing, intensity, pitch, location, radiation, quality)
     (3) Use special maneuvers or positions to accentuate abnormal heart sounds (Table 3-2); refer to Table 3-3 for grading of murmurs and to Fig. 3-3 for description of murmurs
  n. Breast
     (1) Inspect breasts with patient's arms relaxed, elevated, and then with patient's hands pressed against hips
     (2) Note symmetry, contour, abnormal shapes, skin color, retraction, thickening, edema, venous pattern

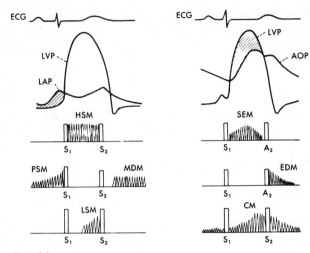

Figure 3-3
Simultaneous recording of ECG, aortic pressure (AOP), left ventricular pressure (LVP), and left atrial pressure (LAP). *HSM,* Holosystolic murmur; *PSM,* presystolic murmur; *MDM,* middiastolic murmur; *MSM,* midsystolic murmur; *EDM,* early diastolic murmur; *LSM,* late systolic murmur; *CM,* continuous murmur. (From O'Rourke RA, Braunwald E: In Petersdorf RG, et al: Harrison's Principles of internal medicine, ed 10, New York, 1983, McGraw-Hill Book Co.)

Table 3-3   Grading of cardiac murmurs

Grade	Description
I	Faintest audible
	Can be heard only with special effort
II	Faint, but easily audible
III	Moderately loud
IV	Loud; associated with a thrill
V	Very loud; associated with a thrill
	May be heard with a stethoscope off chest
VI	Maximum loudness; associated with a thrill; heard without a stethoscope

     (3) Inspect nipples for size, shape, inversion, rashes, ulceration, discharge

     (4) Palpate for presence of masses and tenderness; feel for the presence of axillary adenopathy

o. Abdomen

     (1) Observe skin color, contour, scars, masses, obesity, rigidity, ascites, venous pattern, and pulsatile masses

     (2) Auscultate for bowel sounds and abdominal bruits

     (3) Percuss abdomen and note tympany, shifting dullness, and size of liver and spleen

     (4) Note size, shape, consistency, and tenderness

p. Rectal examination

     (1) Examine anus and rectal wall for lesions, inflammation, and sphincter tone; note any nodules or other abnormalities

     (2) Test any fecal material for occult blood

     (3) In male patients, palpate prostate and identify lateral lobes (note size, shape, and consistency of prostate)

q. Genitalia

     (1) Male

        (a) Inspect distribution of pubic hair

        (b) Examine penis (note any ulcers, nodules, scars, signs of inflammation); gently compress glans and note any discharge or tenderness

        (c) Inspect scrotum (note any lumps, swelling, nodules, ulcers, size and shape of both testicles); transilluminate any swelling

        (d) Inspect inguinal and femoral areas for bulges; examine patient for presence of hernias

     (2) Female

        (a) Inspect external genitalia (labia, clitoris, urethral orifice, vaginal opening) and note distribution of pubic hair; note any nodules, discharges, bulges, and swelling

        (b) Perform internal examination (if indicated): insert speculum and note vaginal wall and cervical os; obtain specimen for cervical cytology; perform bimanual exam with index and middle finger (placing the other hand above abdomen); identify position and mobility of cervix; note any uterine and ovarian masses, enlargement, or tenderness

        (c) Perform rectovaginal exam; note any nodules or other lesions

r. Inguinal area: palpate for inguinal nodes; palpate femoral arteries (describe pulses, note any bruits)

s. Neurologic

     (1) Mental status and speech: check orientation, memory, expression, quality, quantity, and organization of speech (see Table 3-4 for description of Glasgow coma scale, useful in patients with neurologic abnormalities)

     (2) Cranial nerves: see Table 3-5 for testing of cranial nerves

Table 3-4 Glasgow coma scale*

Eye Opening	Best Motor Response	Best Verbal Response	Score
No response	None	None	1
Opens with painful stimulus	Extension (decerebrate rigidity) with painful stimulus	Unintelligible sounds	2
Opens with verbal command	Flexion (decorticate rigidity) with painful stimulus	Use of inappropriate words	3
	Withdrawal from noxious stimulus	Confused, disoriented conversation	4
Opens spontaneously	Localization of pain, pushes away noxious stimulus	Oriented, able to converse	5
	Obeys simple verbal commands	Alert and oriented	6

*Total score is determined by adding the best score from each category (eye opening, best motor response, best verbal response).

For example, a patient may

Open eyes with verbal command	3
Obey simple verbal commands	6
Use inappropriate words	3
Total score	12

Table 3-5 Testing of cranial nerves

I Olfactory	Sense of smell
II Optic	Vision (visual acuity, visual fields, color)
III Oculomotor ⎫ IV Trochlear ⎬ VI Abducens ⎭	Extraocular movements (Fig. 3-1), pupillary constriction (oculomotor), elevation of upper lids
V Trigeminal	Mastication, sensory of forehead, face, and jaw
VII Facial	Facial expression, taste in anterior two thirds of tongue
VIII Acoustic	Hearing and balance
IX Glossopharyngeal ⎱ X Vagus ⎰	Sensory and motor functions of pharynx and larynx (gag reflex, position of uvula, swallowing)
XI Accessory	Shrugging of shoulders, movement of head
XII Hypoglossal	Motor control of tongue

    (3) Sensory: pinprick, light touch, joint position, temperature, vibration (see Figs. 3-4 and 3-5 for peripheral nerve distribution in the skin)

    (4) Cerebellar functions: evaluate rapid alternating hand movements, heel-to-shin, finger-to-nose, and gait

    (5) Motor: check muscle strength (see Table 3-6 for grading muscle strength), muscle tone, coordination; check Romberg's sign, reflexes (see Table 3-7 for grading of deep tendon reflexes), plantar responses, note any abnormal reflexes

3.2 ADMISSION ORDERS

Use the mnemonic: ABC-DAVID

A (admit to): indicate ward where patient is being admitted and attending physician (e.g., CCU, Dr. Smith's service)

B (because): indicate admitting diagnosis (e.g., R/O MI)

C (condition): patient's general condition (stable, fair, poor, critical)

D (diet) specify whether regular, clear liquids, no added sodium (see box on pp. 27 and 28 for various diets)

A (allergies): indicate medications and specific food products to which the patient has experienced an allergic reaction

(activity): specify bed rest, ad lib, bathroom privileges

V (vital signs): specify frequency (e.g., qid, q4h); also indicate any special nursing orders (e.g., vital signs and neurologic signs qh × 24h, then q4h if stable)

I (IV fluids): specify any IV solutions and rate of infusion (refer to Table 3-8 for commonly used IV solutions)

D (diagnostic tests): laboratory tests, x-rays, ECG, special tests

(drugs): indicate medication, dose, frequency, special restrictions (e.g., digoxin 0.25 mg PO qd; if heart rate <55 bpm, hold digoxin and notify house officer)

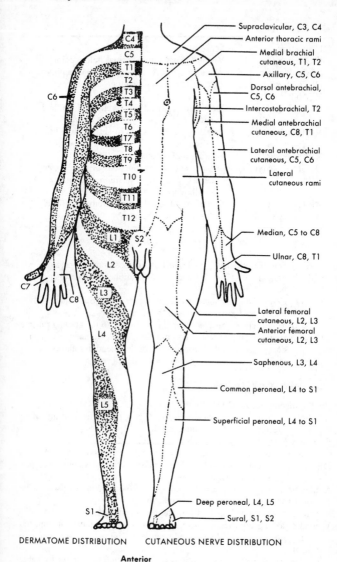

DERMATOME DISTRIBUTION   CUTANEOUS NERVE DISTRIBUTION

Anterior

Figure 3-4
Cutaneous sensation on the anterior aspect of the body. (From DeGowin EL, DeGowin RL: Bedside diagnostic examination, ed 4, New York, 1981, MacMillan Publishing Co.)

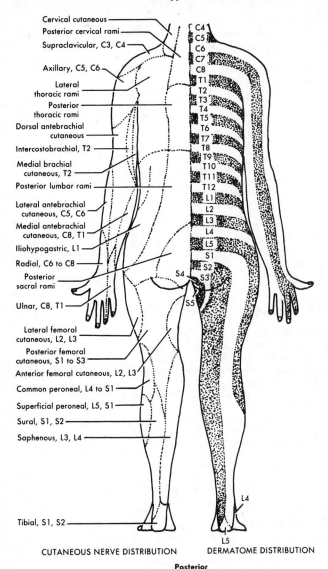

CUTANEOUS NERVE DISTRIBUTION   DERMATOME DISTRIBUTION

Posterior

Figure 3-5

Cutaneous sensation on the posterior aspect of the body. (From DeGowin, EL, DeGowin RL: Bedside diagnostic examination, ed 4, New York, 1981, MacMillan Publishing Co.)

Table 3-6   Grading of muscle strength

0	Absent muscular contraction
1	Minimal contraction
2	Active movement with gravity eliminated
3	Active movement against gravity only
4	Active movement against gravity and some resistance
5	Normal muscle strength

Table 3-7   Grading of deep tendon reflexes

0	Absent
+	Hypoactive
+ +	Normal
+ + +	Brisker than average
+ + + +	Hyperactive, often indicative of disease

3.3   PROGRESS NOTES

Use the "SOAP" mnemonic:

S (subjective): observations, patient complaints

"My chest hurts when I take a deep breath"

O (objective): description of physical findings and recording of lab, x-ray, or ECG data

Blood pressure: 140/90; pulse: 84; respirations: 20; temperature: 38° C

Skin: warm, dry, no petechiae

HEENT: pharyngeal erythema

Lungs: ↓ BS in rt base, no rubs, rales, or wheezing

Heart: S_1, S_2, tachycardic, s̄ murmurs

Abd: soft, bowel sounds active, s̄ tenderness

Ext: no clubbing, cyanosis, or edema

Lab

WBC: 15,900 c̄ shift to left (12 stabs, 65 segs)

ABG: Po_2—55, Pco_2—30, pH—7.50

CXR: RLL infiltrate

ECG: normal sinus rhythm without evidence of ischemia

A (assessment): analysis of data and tentative diagnosis

RLL pneumonia

P (plan): diagnostic studies and therapeutic regimen

1. Nasal O_2—2L
2. Sputum Gram stain and cultures, blood cultures
3. Antibiotic therapy based on results of Gram stain

Sample Physical Exam

1. Vital signs
   a. Blood pressure: 124/70
   b. Pulse: 74
   c. Respirations: 16
   d. Temperature: 37° C
2. General description: the patient is a 45 yr old white female who looks her stated age; she is pleasant, appears to be well nourished, and seems in a good state of health.
3. Skin: the skin is warm and dry; turgor is adequate; color is normal. There is no icterus, purpura, rash, or unusual pigmentation noted. Hair is normal in appearance, distribution, and texture.
4. Lymph nodes: there is no cervical, supraclavicular, axillary, epitrochlear, or inguinal adenopathy.
5. HEENT:
   a. Head: normocephalic and atraumatic; no lesions noted.
   b. Eyes: cornea is without lesions, conjunctiva is clear, sclera is white. Pupils are equal, measuring approximately 3 mm in diameter, round, and reactive to light and accommodation. Extraocular movements are within normal limits without any nystagmus or strabismus. Fundi appear benign. Disks are well delineated. There are no hemorrhages or exudates. Visual acuity is 20/20 bilaterally, and visual fields are within normal limits.
   c. Ears: normal in appearance. Auditory canal appears clean and without lesions. The tympanic membranes are intact. Hearing is adequate.
   d. Nose: septum appears to be within normal limits and without deviation. Nasal mucosa appears pink and without any abnormal discharge. No nasal polyps or other lesions are noted. Frontal and maxillary sinuses are nontender.
   e. Mouth and throat: lips are without cyanosis or pallor. Buccal mucosa is normal in appearance. Teeth appear to be in good condition. Tongue shows no lesions or tremor. Pharyngeal mucosa is pink and does not reveal any lesions, exudates, erythema, or evidence of inflammation. Gag reflex is intact.
6. Neck: neck is supple. Full range of motion is present. There is no evidence of tracheal deviation, jugular venous distention, or lymphadenopathy. Carotid pulses are 2+, equal bilaterally, and without any bruits. Carotid upstroke is within normal limits. Thyroid gland is normal in size; its palpation does not reveal any nodules or masses.
7. Back: spinal curvature is normal; there is no scoliosis or kyphosis present.
8. Chest: thorax is symmetric. Full expansion is noted bilaterally. AP diameter is within normal limits.
9. Lungs: fremitus is equal bilaterally. Lung fields are resonant throughout. Breath sounds and voice sounds are normal. There are no rales or rhonchi.

Continued.

10. Heart: palpation reveals no heaves or thrills. The point of maximum impuse (PMI) is medial to the midclavicular line, fourth intercostal space. Auscultation reveals S_1, S_2 of normal intensity. There are no S_3, S_4 rubs, clicks, or other abnormal heart sounds. Heart rate is approximately 70 beats/min and rhythm is regular.

11. Breasts: breasts are symmetric and have a normal contour. Skin is of normal color and appearance; there is no edema, ulceration, or erythema. Nipples are of normal size and shape; there is no nipple retraction, ulceration, or discharge. Palpation does not reveal any tenderness or masses.

12. Abdomen: abdomen is of normal size and contour. There are no capillary dilatations, skin lesions, or surgical scars noted. Auscultation reveals normoactive bowel sounds and no abdominal bruits. Palpation reveals no abdominal tenderness, guarding, or masses. The liver edge is felt approximately 1 inch below the right costal margin; it is firm, sharp, and smooth. The liver percusses to approximately 8 to 10 cm in total span. The spleen is not palpable.

13. Rectal exam: rectal exam reveals no external anal lesions. Sphincter tone is normal. There are no internal or external hemorrhoids. Rectal mucosa appears normal, and there are no nodules or masses present. Stool is brown and negative for occult blood.

14. Genitalia: inspection reveals normal distribution of pubic hair. Clitoris and labia are without lesions. Internal examination with speculum reveals normal vaginal wall. The cervical os is well visualized. No lesions or discharges are noted. A specimen was obtained for cervical cytology. Bimanual exam reveals no cervical tenderness or masses. Uterus and ovaries are nontender and of normal size.

15. Inguinal area: there is no lymphadenopathy noted. Femoral pulses are 2+ and equal bilaterally. Auscultation reveals no femoral bruits.

16. Extremities: there is no clubbing, cyanosis, or edema. Brachial, radial, popliteal, dorsalis pedis, and posterior tibialis pulses are 2+ and equal bilaterally. Musculoskeletal exam reveals no joint deformities and full range of motion. There is no bone, joint, or muscle tenderness noted.

17. Neurologic: patient is alert and oriented to time, person, and place. Cranial nerves 2 to 12 are within normal limits. Speech, memory, and expression are within normal limits. Muscle strength is 5/5 in both upper and lower extremities. There is no muscle atrophy or involuntary movement noted. Testing of cerebellar function reveals normal gait, negative Romberg test, and good coordination in finger-to-nose, heel-to-shin, and alternate motion testing. Sensory is intact to light touch, pain, and vibratory stimuli. There are no focal motor/sensory deficits present. Deep tendon reflexes are 2+ and equal bilaterally.

Common Hospital Diets

Bland: eliminates gastric irritants such as pepper, alcohol, caffeine, coffee, tea, soda, cocoa, and foods not tolerated by patient

Calorie control: physician determines calorie level; sugar and sweets are generally eliminated

Low-cholesterol: restricts food high in cholesterol, decreases saturated fat, provides approximately 300 mg of cholesterol daily

Diabetic (A.D.A.): physician indicates calorie level

Low-fat: eliminates high-fat foods, fried foods, and whole milk; designed to limit total amount of fat to 40-45 g/day

Gluten-free: eliminates products and by-products of wheat, oats, rye, and barley

High-fiber: increases volume of indigestible carbohydrates

High-protein, high-calorie: no restriction, 3000+ calories, 120 g protein

Hypoglycemic: no sugar or sweets; six small meals containing protein

Lactose-free: eliminates milk, milk products, and foods containing lactose, milk, or milk solids

Lactose-restricted: provides foods that contain only minimum lactose, based on the individual's tolerance

Low-residue: limits volume of indigestible carbohydrates, milk, and dairy products

Clear liquid: clear broth and juice, gelatin, water, ice, coffee, tea, soda, sugar, and salt; 600 calories, 10 g protein

Sodium restriction: 4 g NAS (no added salt)—no salt or highly salted foods; 2 g—no salt or highly salted foods, limited milk, meat, bread, butter; 1 g—more limited milk, meat, bread, butter; 500 mg—no salt or salty foods, extremely limited milk, meat, bread and butter (unpalatable for most)

Full liquid: clear liquid items plus strained cream soups, juices, cooked cereal, ice cream, sherbet, custard, pudding, milk, and milk beverages; calorie and protein content adequate

High-protein clear liquid: clear liquid items, Citrotein, and high-protein gelatin supplements; 1500 calories; 75 g protein

Mechanical soft: minimizes the amount of chewing necessary for ingestion of food; ground meats are provided along with a soft diet

Potassium-restricted: physician should specify level: 2 g—moderate restriction, eliminates high-potassium foods; 1.5 g or less—greater restriction, eliminates high-potassium foods, limits quantity of acceptable foods; achieving adequate calories may be a problem

Continued.

Common Hospital Diets—cont'd

Postgastrectomy: six small feedings, simple sugars kept to a minimum, no fluids served with meals

Protein-restricted: physician should specify level: *60 g*—liberal, approaches regular diet with some limit on quantities; *40 g*—moderate restriction, severely limits quantity of milk, meat or substitute, and egg; *20 g*—severe restriction, eliminates milk, limits meat, egg, or substitute to 2 oz daily and starch to 3 servings daily; fruit, sugars, and fat are given ad lib; caloric intake is inadequate (very unpalatable)

Regular: no restriction

Soft: texture of food is soft; NOTE: if modification of texture is desired, physician should order mechanical soft (ground)

3.4   DISCHARGE SUMMARY

The discharge summary should contain only essential information regarding the investigation and treatment of the patient's illness. It should briefly describe the following:

1. Why the patient entered the hospital: a brief statement of the chief complaint, admission diagnosis, and history of the present illness
2. The pertinent laboratory, x-ray, and physical findings; negative findings may be as pertinent as positive ones
3. The medical and/or surgical treatment, including the patient's response, any complications, and consultations; give a rationale for what was or was not done
4. The patient's condition when discharged (ambulation, self-care, ability to work)
5. Instructions given on continuing care, such as medication by name and specific dosage, diet, type and amount of physical activity, other therapeutic measures, referrals, and appointments
6. The principal diagnosis and additional or secondary diagnoses

Definitions

Principal diagnosis: the diagnosis that best explains the reason for admission to the hospital; this may not be the same as the most serious event.

Complication: a significant event that either prolongs the stay or requires alteration of treatment, such as a pulmonary embolus after a hip fracture.

Table 3-8 Composition of selected IV solutions

IV Solution	Na (mEq/L)	K (mEq/L)	Cl (mEq/L)	Lactate (mEq/L)	Ca (mEq/L)	Calories/L
0.9% NaCl (NS)	154	0	154	0	0	0
5% Dextrose (D₅W)	0	0	0	0	0	170
5% Dextrose + 0.9% NaCl (D₅NS)	154	0	154	0	0	170
5% Dextrose + 0.45% NaCl (D₅½NS)	77	0	77	0	0	170
5% Dextrose + 0.33% NaCl (D₅⅓NS)	56	0	77	0	0	170
Lactated Ringer's solution	130	4	109	28	3	9
3% NaCl	513	0	513	0	0	0
5% NaCl	855	0	855	0	0	0
0.45% NaCl	77	0	77	0	0	0
10% Dextrose (D₁₀W)	0	0	0	0	0	340

References

1. Bates B: A guide to physical examination, ed 3, Philadelphia, 1983, JB Lippincott Co.
2. DeGowin EL, DeGowin RL: Bedside diagnostic examination, ed 4, New York, 1981, Macmillan Publishing Co Inc.
3. Ewing JA: Detecting alcoholism; the CAGE questionnaire, JAMA 252:1905, 1984.
4. Sherman JL, Fields SK: Guide to patient evaluation, ed 3, New York, 1978, Medical Examination Publishing Co Inc.

Preventive Medicine

4.1 BREAST CANCER SCREENING IN ASYMPTOMATIC WOMEN

1. Monthly breast self-examination for women over 40 yr of age
2. Clinical breast exam every 3 yr for women 20-40 yr of age, annually thereafter
3. Mammography*
   a. Baseline mammogram between 35 and 40 yr of age†
   b. Mammogram every 1 or 2 yr from age 40 to 50
   c. Mammogram yearly from age 50

4.2 COLON CANCER SCREENING IN THE GENERAL POPULATION

1. Yearly digital rectal exam is indicated starting at age 40-50
2. Fecal occult blood testing with guaiac-impregnated paper (Hemoccult)
   a. Should be done yearly starting at age 40-50
   b. Test at least three specimens from consecutive bowel movements
   c. Patients should be instructed to avoid red meat, iron, and high-peroxidase foods (e.g., horseradish, turnips) to avoid false-positives
   d. Women should not be tested during or immediately following a menstrual period (false-positives)
   e. Aspirin and nonsteroidal antiinflammatory drugs (NSAIDs) should be avoided during testing (may cause occult blood from UGI bleed)
   f. Ascorbic acid may cause false-negative results
   g. Positive results are seen in 2-6% of patients tested; within this positive group, carcinoma is detected in 5-10% and adenomas in 20-40%[2]
3. Flexible sigmoidoscopy to 65 mm is recommended in all individuals between 50 and 75 yr of age every 3 to 5 yr[1] *

---

*There is considerable controversy regarding these screening guidelines.
†If there is a first degree familial history of breast carcinoma, a baseline mammogram is advisable 10 yr before the age of familial diagnosis (e.g., annual mammogram from age 32 if mother developed breast cancer at age 42).

| 4.3 | **CERVICAL CYTOLOGIC SCREENING**

1. Initial Papanicolau test (Pap smear) should be done at age 18-20 or when a woman becomes sexually active, whichever comes first
2. After two normal exams, repeat smears after 3 yr
3. Duration of testing is controversial; the American College of Obstetricians and Gynecologists recommends indefinite testing, whereas the American Cancer Society advocates testing only until age 65
4. Continued testing is not advocated in women who have had a hysterectomy with removal of the cervix
5. More frequent testing is advocated in women at high risk for carcinoma of the cervix:
   a. Early onset of sexual activity
   b. Multiple partners in a lifetime or intercourse with a male who has had multiple partners
   c. History of condyloma acuminata or genital herpes
   d. Cigarette smoking
   e. Use of oral contraceptives or exposure to estrogens in utero

Reference

1. Eddy DM: Screening for colorectal cancer, Ann Intern Med 113:373, 1990.
2. Fleischer DE, et al: Detection and surveillance of colorectal cancer, JAMA 261:580, 1989.

Data Evaluation

5.1 GRAM STAIN PROCEDURE

1. Briefly heat-fix air-dried smear by passing it gently through a Bunsen flame
2. Flood slide with crystal violet for 1 min
3. Wash off slide lightly with water and then flood with Gram's iodine for 1 min
4. Wash off slide and add 95% ethyl alcohol to decolorize for 15 sec
5. Wash off slide and add counterstain (safranin) for 1 min
6. Wash off safranin and blot slide dry
7. Examine smear under oil immersion (a properly stained area will show pink PMN nuclei):

> Gm + organism: (purple)
>
> Gm − organism: (red)

5.2 ACID-FAST STAIN PROCEDURE

1. Briefly heat-fix air-dried smear by passing it gently through a Bunsen flame
2. Flood slide with carbol-fuchsin for 2½ min
3. Wash off slide with water and completely decolorize the slide with acid alcohol
4. Wash off slide and flood it with methylene blue for 30 sec
5. Wash off methylene blue and blot slide dry
6. Examine smear under oil immersion:

> Acid-fast organisms (red)
>
> Non−acid-fast organisms (blue)

5.3 EVALUATION OF URINE SEDIMENT

Fig. 5-1 illustrates abnormalities frequently observed in urinary sediment.

5.4 EVALUATION OF CHEST X-RAY

Fig. 5-2 illustrates the location of various pulmonary and cardiac structures seen on a chest x-ray film (posteroanterior view).

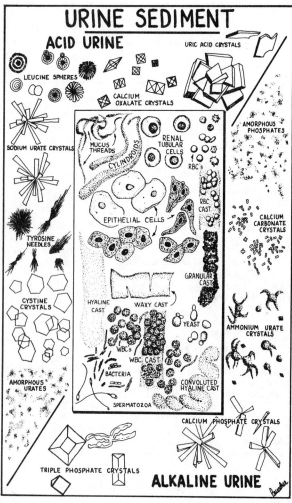

Figure 5-1
Microscopic examination of urine sediment. (From Biller JA, Yeager AM [editors]: The Harriet Lane handbook: a manual for pediatric house officers, ed 9, Chicago, 1981, Year Book Medical Publishers Inc. Reproduced with permission from Johns Hopkins Hospital and Year Book Medical Publishers Inc.)

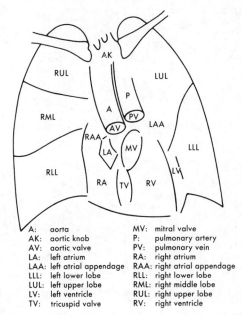

A:	aorta	MV:	mitral valve
AK:	aortic knob	P:	pulmonary artery
AV:	aortic valve	PV:	pulmonary vein
LA:	left atrium	RA:	right atrium
LAA:	left atrial appendage	RAA:	right atrial appendage
LLL:	left lower lobe	RLL:	right lower lobe
LUL:	left upper lobe	RML:	right middle lobe
LV:	left ventricle	RUL:	right upper lobe
TV:	tricuspid valve	RV:	right ventricle

Figure 5-2
Schematic chest x-ray showing the pulmonary lobes, heart chambers, and heart valves (posteroanterior view).

5.5 ELECTROCARDIOGRAM

Fig. 5-3 illustrates a normal 12-lead ECG. Note the normal QRS configuration in the various leads and the R wave progression in the precordial leads. Fig. 5-4 illustrates selected ECG abnormalities.

5.6 USE AND INTERPRETATION OF SWAN-GANZ CATHETER DATA

1. Description: the Swan-Ganz catheter is a flexible quadruple-lumen tube 110 cm long and scored in 10 cm increments (Fig. 5-5). Its four lumens are as follows:
   a. Distal (PA) lumen: used to record PAP, PCWP, and to obtain mixed venous blood for oxygen content analysis
   b. Proximal (RA) lumen: used to record RAP or CVP
   c. Balloon lumen: terminates 1 cm from the tip of the catheter. When the balloon is inflated, it moves in the direction of the blood flow, guiding the catheter through the right atrium, right ventricle, and into the pulmonary artery wedging into one of the smaller vessels. In

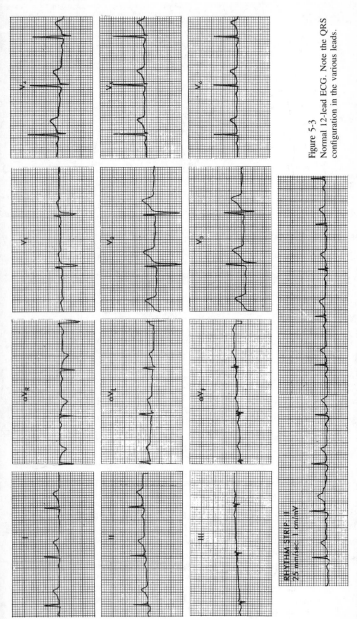

Figure 5-3
Normal 12-lead ECG. Note the QRS configuration in the various leads.

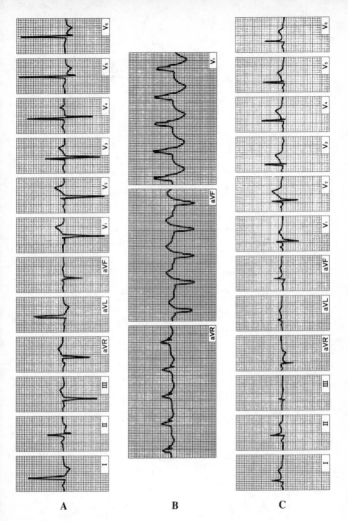

A   B   C

Figure 5-4

A, *Left ventricular hypertrophy.* Tall R wave in aVL (>11 mm); voltage of the S wave in V_1 plus the R in V_5 or V_6 >35 mm; the R voltage in V_5 or V_6 >27 mm; T wave inversion and ST segment depression common in the lateral leads (I, aVL, V_{5-6}); poor R wave progression in the V leads; the R in lead I plus the S in lead III >25 mm. (NOTE: These voltage criteria pertain to adults older than 35 yr.) **B,** *Quinidine toxicity.* Both quinidine and procainamide can produce first-, second-, or third-degree AV block, AV dissociation, AV nodal rhythm, idioventricular rhythm, VPCs, VT/VF, and cardiac arrest; this strip shows idioventricular rhythm with widened and bizarre QRS complexes; P waves cannot be identified; there is QT prolongation with the development of torsade de pointes; VT can be seen (also occurs with other Class IA antiarrhythmic agents). **C,** *Pericarditis.* ST segment elevation in leads I, II, aVL, aVF, and V_{2-6}; ST segment changes usually occur in leads overlying an area of pericardial inflammation. (Strips **A** to **G** courtesy Merck, Sharp & Dohme.)

Continued.

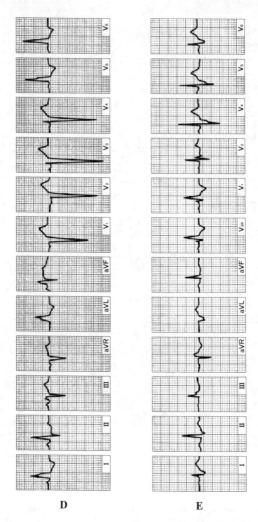

D   E

Figure 5-4, cont'd

D, *Complete left bundle branch block.* Horizontal heart; the patterns vary with the position of the heart; the following may be seen: wide slurred R in V_{5-6}, a QRS prolonged ≥0.12 sec, lengthened VAT or intrinsicoid deflection, aVL similar to V_{5-6}, lead I similar to aVL and V_{5-6} (with depression of the ST segments and inversion of the T waves). **E,** *Complete right bundle branch block.* QRS ≥0.12 sec; wide slurred S waves in V_{5-6}; rsR' complexes in V_{3R} and V_{1-2}, with absent Q waves; VAT prolonged in V_{3R} and V_{1-2}; a wide S wave in lead I.

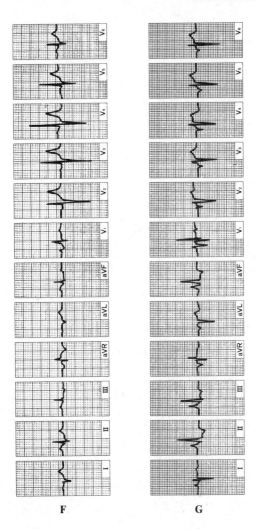

Figure 5-4, cont'd

F, *Left atrial hypertrophy (mitral stenosis).* Wide notched P in leads II, III, aVF, and V_{4-6}; duration of the P wave ≥ 0.12 sec; diphasic P in V_1 with a broad negative phase; P terminal force at least "a small box wide and a small box deep." **G,** *Right atrial hypertrophy (chronic pulmonary disease).* Tall peaked P wave in II, III, and aVF (>2.5 mm); large diphasic or inverted P in V_1.

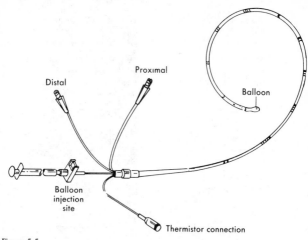

Figure 5-5
Swan-Ganz catheter. (From Quaal SJ: Comprehensive intraaortic balloon pumping, St Louis, 1984, The CV Mosby Co.)

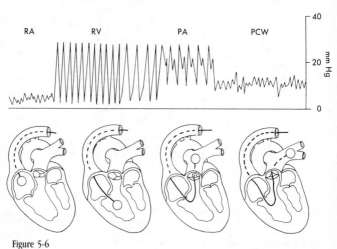

Figure 5-6
Swan-Ganz pressure waveforms in relation to catheter position. (From Rosen P, et al [editors]: Emergency medicine: concepts and clinical practice, St Louis, 1983, The CV Mosby Co.)

this position it records downstream pressure (PCWP), which is normally about equal to left atrial pressure.

  d. Thermistor lumen: contains temperature-sensitive wires. It is used to calculate cardiac output by thermodilution technique.

2. Catheter insertion: percutaneous insertion via the internal jugular (central or anterior) approach appears to be the safest. Complications (sepsis, thrombophlebitis, deep venous thrombosis) occur more often when the catheter is placed through antecubital cutdown.[4]

3. Verification of catheter tip location: the location of the catheter tip is determined by recognition of the characteristic pressure waveform morphology of each heart chamber (Fig. 5-6)

4. Risks of right heart catheterization[3]:
  a. Cardiac dysrhythmias—77.5%
  b. Thrombosis—2.6%
  c. Sepsis—1.7%
  d. Pulmonary infarction—1.7%
  e. Pulmonary valve perforation—0.8%

5. Indications for hemodynamic monitoring: pulmonary artery flow-directed catheters should be used only in situations where there is a high probability that the data collected will result in more effective patient management.[5] It is generally agreed that Swan-Ganz catheterization is indicated in severely ill, hemodynamically unstable patients who do not respond to therapy that is deemed appropriate after a careful clinical evaluation.[2] Additional indications for hemodynamic monitoring in the medical setting are as follows[5]:
  a. Acute cardiac conditions (complicated MI, right ventricular infarction, perforated ventricular septum, and mitral regurgitation)
  b. Chronic cardiac insufficiency (constrictive pericarditis, congestive cardiomyopathy, and therapy of end-stage cardiac failure)
  c. Miscellaneous (acute non–myocardial infarction pulmonary edema, severe noncardiac hypotension)

6. Data interpretation: see Tables 5-1, 5-2, and 5-3.

Table 5-1 Effects of therapeutic measures on hemodynamic measurements

Therapeutic Measure	CO	SVR	PCWP
IV fluids	N/↑	N/↑	↑
Diuretics	N/↓ ↓	↓ /Secondary ↑	↓
Nitrates	N/↑/↓	↓	↓
Nitroprusside	↑	↓ ↓	N/↓
Catecholamines	N/↑ ↑	↑ ↑ ↑	N/↑
Dopamine	N/↑	↑ ↑	N/↑ ↑
Dobutamine	↑ ↑	↓	N/↓

KEY: N, no effect; ↑, increases; ↓, decreases.

Table 5-2 Hemodynamic measurements in specific disease states

Septic shock
   Early: ↓ PCWP, ↓ SVR, ↑ CO
   Late: ↓ PCWP, ↑ SVR, ↓ CO
Neurogenic shock: ↓ PCWP, ↓ SVR, N/↓ CO
Cardiac tamponade: ↑ PCWP, ↑ SVR, ↓ CO, ↓ CI
   CVP = PADP = PCWP
Pulmonary embolism: Normal PCWP, ↑ PADP, ↓ CI
Cardiogenic shock: ↑ PCWP, ↑ PADP, ↓ CO, ↓ CI, ↑ SVR
Hypovolemic shock: ↓ PCWP, ↓ CO, ↑ SVR, ↓ CI
Right ventricular infarct: RAP/PCWP ≥ 0.8

KEY: ↑, Increases; ↓, decreases.

5.7 **INTRAAORTIC BALLOON PUMP**

1. Description: the intraaortic balloon pump (IABP) is a polyurethane balloon inserted percutaneously in the femoral artery and positioned in the descending aorta.
2. Mechanism of action: it provides left ventricular support using the following mechanisms[1]:
   a. Systolic unloading: its deflation immediately before the onset of systole creates a low pressure which results in:
     (1) ↓ Left ventricular work for ejection
     (2) ↓ Myocardial O_2 requirements
     (3) ↓ LVEDP
     (4) ↑ Stroke volume
   b. Diastolic augmentation: its inflation at end of systole results in:
     (1) ↑ Diastolic pressure
     (2) ↑ Coronary perfusion pressure
     (3) Potential ↑ in coronary blood flow
3. Major indications:
   a. Low-output state (cardiogenic shock, gram-negative septic shock)
   b. Angina refractory to medical management
   c. Postinfarction VSD and MR
   d. Surgery in high-risk cardiac patients
4. Major contraindications:
   a. Dissecting aortic aneurysm
   b. Severe aortic regurgitation
   c. Severe peripheral vascular disease

Table 5-3 Data collection and interpretation

Hemodynamic Measurement	Normal Value	Clinical Significance	Abnormalities
Right atrial pressure (RAP)	0-8 mm Hg	Equivalent to central venous pressure (CVP)	↑ Right ventricular failure, pulmonary embolism, tricuspid valve abnormalities, pericardial tamponade, right ventricular infarction ↓ Hypovolemia
Pulmonary artery pressure (PAP)	Systolic 15-30 mm Hg Diastolic 5-12 mm Hg Mean 10-20 mm Hg	PAP is equal to RV pressure during systole while the pulmonary valve is open. If the pulmonary vascular resistance is normal, the pulmonary artery diastolic pressure (PADP) is 1-4 mm Hg greater than PCWP and can be substituted for it in following the patient's hemodynamic measurements.	↑ Pulmonary embolism, chronic lung disease, VSD, cardiogenic shock, right ventricular infarction If the PADP is 5mm Hg > PCWP, consider: ARDS, pulmonary emboli, or COPD
Pulmonary capillary wedge pressure (PCWP)	5-12 mm Hg	PCWP is normally equal to left atrial pressure; it is therefore a sensitive indicator of the presence of pulmonary congestion and left-sided CHF. PCWP is not equal to left	↑ Left ventricular failure with resultant pulmonary congestion, acute mitral insufficiency, tamponade, decreased left ventricular compliance (hypertrophy, infarction)

Continued.

Table 5-3 Data collection and interpretation—cont'd

Hemodynamic Measurement	Normal Value	Clinical Significance	Abnormalities
		ventricular end diastolic pressure (LVEDP) in the following situations: PCWP > LVEDP: Mitral stenosis Patient receiving PEEP Left atrial myxoma Pulmonary venous obstruction PCWP < LVEDP: "Stiff" left ventricle ↑ LVEDP (>25 mm Hg)	
Cardiac output (CO)	3.5-7 L/min	CO = stroke volume multiplied by heart rate	↓ Cardiac dysrhythmias, ↓ contracting muscle mass (myocardial ischemia, MI), mitral insufficiency, VSD

Parameter	Normal value	Definition/formula	Clinical implications
Cardiac index (CI)	2.5-4.0 L/min^2	CI relates CO to body surface area (BSA), CI = CO/BSA	↑ High output failure secondary to fluid overload, hepatocellular failure, renal disease, septic shock → Hypovolemia, cardiogenic shock, pulmonary embolism, hypothyroidism, CHF with failing ventricle
Systemic vascular resistance (SVR)	900-1300 dyne/sec/cm^{-5}	Resistance against which the left ventricle must work to eject its stroke volume. SVR = ($\overline{\text{MAP}}$ − RAP) × 80/CO	↑ Hypervolemic vasoconstrictive states (hypertension, cardiogenic shock, traumatic shock) → Septic shock, acute renal failure, pregnancy
Pulmonary vascular resistance (PVR)	155-255 dyne/sec/cm^{-5}	PVR = ($\overline{\text{PAP}}$ − PAWP) × 80/CO	↑ Cor pulmonale, pulmonary embolism, valvular heart disease, CHF → Hypervolemic states, pregnancy

References

1. Chatterjee K, Don H (editors): Intraaortic balloon pump. In Don H: Decisions in critical care (Toronto, BC Decker Inc), St Louis, 1985, The CV Mosby Co.
2. Connors AF, et al: Evaluation of right heart catheterization in the critically ill patient without acute myocardial infarction, N Engl J Med 308:263, 1983.
3. Elliot CG, et al: Complications of pulmonary artery catheterization in the care of critically ill patients: a prospective study, Chest 76:647, 1979.
4. Moza SK, DelGuercio LRM: The Swan-Ganz catheter: its clinical versatility, Hosp Pract 18:239, 1983.
5. Robin ED: The cult of the Swan-Ganz catheter, Ann Intern Med 103:445, 1985.
6. Swan HJC, Ganz W: Measurement of right atrial and pulmonary arterial pressures and cardiac output: clinical applications of hemodynamic monitoring. In Stollerman GH, et al (editors): Advances in internal medicine, vol 27, Chicago, 1982, Year Book Medical Publishers Inc.

Differential Diagnosis

This chapter covers the differential diagnoses of the following disorders:

Abdominal pain
Amenorrhea
Ascites
Ataxia
Back pain
Cardiac murmurs
Chest pain (nonpleuritic)
Chest pain (pleuritic)
Coma
Constipation
Dysphagia
Edema of lower extremities
Fever and rash
GI bleeding
Headache
Hematuria
Hemoptysis

Hepatomegaly
Hirsutism
Jaundice
Lymphadenopathy
Mediastinal masses or widening
Metastatic neoplasms
Paraplegia
Pleural effusions
Polyuria
Popliteal swelling
Proteinuria
Pruritus
Purpura
Shoulder pain
Splenomegaly
Vertigo
Vomiting

The differential diagnoses of many other medical conditions (e.g., delirium, dementia, diarrhea, hypoglycemia, hypocalcemia/hypercalcemia, hyponatremia/hypernatremia, syncope) are discussed in more detail in other chapters.

6.1 ABDOMINAL PAIN

Diffuse

Early appendicitis
Aortic aneurysm
Gastroenteritis
Intestinal obstruction
Diverticulitis
Peritonitis
Mesenteric insufficiency or infarction
Pancreatitis

Inflammatory bowel disease
Irritable bowel
Mesenteric adenitis
Metabolic: toxins, lead poisoning, uremia, drug overdose, DKA, heavy metal poisoning
Sickle cell crisis
Pneumonia (rare)
Trauma

47

Urinary tract infection, PID
Other: Acute intermittent porphyria, tabes dorsalis, periarteritis nodosa, Henoch-Schönlein purpura, adrenal insufficiency

Epigastric

Gastric: PUD, gastric outlet obstruction, gastric ulcer
Duodenal: PUD, duodenitis
Biliary: cholecystitis, cholangitis
Hepatic: hepatitis
Pancreatic: pancreatitis
Intestinal: high small bowel obstruction, early appendicitis
Cardiac: angina, MI, pericarditis
Pulmonary: pneumonia, pleurisy, pneumothorax
Subphrenic abscess

Suprapubic

Intestinal: colon obstruction or gangrene, diverticulitis, appendicitis
Reproductive system: ectopic pregnancy, mittelschmerz, torsion of ovarian cyst, PID, salpingitis, endometriosis
Cystitis

Right upper quadrant (RUQ)

Biliary: calculi, infection, inflammation, neoplasm
Hepatic: hepatitis, abscess, hepatic congestion, neoplasm, trauma
Gastric: PUD, pyloric stenosis, neoplasm, alcoholic gastritis, hiatal hernia
Pancreatic: pancreatitis, neoplasm, stone in pancreatic duct or ampulla
Renal: calculi, infection, inflammation, neoplasm
Pulmonary: pneumonia, pulmonary infarction
Intestinal: retrocecal appendicitis, intestinal obstruction, high fecal impaction

Cardiac: myocardial ischemia (particularly involving the inferior wall), pericarditis
Cutaneous: herpes zoster
Trauma
Fitz-Hugh-Curtis syndrome (perihepatitis)

Left upper quadrant (LUQ)

Gastric: PUD, gastritis, pyloric stenosis, hiatal hernia
Pancreatic: pancreatitis, neoplasm, stone in pancreatic duct or ampulla
Cardiac: MI, angina pectoris
Splenic: splenomegaly, ruptured spleen, splenic abscess, splenic infarction
Renal: calculi, pyelonephritis, neoplasm
Pulmonary: pneumonia, empyema, pulmonary infarction
Vascular: ruptured aortic aneurysm
Cutaneous: herpes zoster
Trauma
Intestinal: high fecal impaction, perforated colon

Periumbilical

Intestinal: small bowel obstruction or gangrene, early appendicitis
Vascular: mesenteric thrombosis, dissecting aortic aneurysm
Pancreatic: pancreatitis
Metabolic: uremia, DKA
Trauma

Right lower quadrant (RLQ)

Intestinal: acute appendicitis, regional enteritis, incarcerated hernia, cecal diverticulitis, intestinal obstruction, perforated ulcer, perforated cecum, Meckel's diverticulitis
Reproductive: ectopic pregnancy, ovarian cyst, torsion of ovarian cyst, salpingitis, tuboovarian

abscess, mittelschmerz, endometriosis, seminal vesiculitis
Renal: renal and ureteral calculi, neoplasms, pyelonephritis
Vascular: leaking aortic aneurysm
Psoas abscess
Trauma
Cholecystitis

Left lower quadrant (LLQ)

Intestinal: diverticulitis, intestinal obstruction, perforated ulcer, inflammatory bowel disease, perforated descending colon, inguinal hernia, neoplasm, appendicitis
Reproductive: ectopic pregnancy, ovarian cyst, torsion of ovarian cyst, tuboovarian abscess, mittelschmerz, endometriosis; seminal vesiculitis
Renal: renal or ureteral calculi, pyelonephritis, neoplasm
Vascular: leaking aortic aneurysm
Psoas abscess
Trauma

6.2 AMENORRHEA

Pregnancy, early menopause
Hypothalamic dysfunction: defective synthesis or release of LHRH, anorexia nervosa, stress, exercise
Pituitary dysfunction: neoplasm, postpartum hemorrhage, surgery, radiotherapy
Ovarian dysfunction: gonadal dysgenesis, 17-α-hydroxylase deficiency, premature ovarian failure, polycystic ovarian disease, gonadal stromal tumors
Uterovaginal abnormalities
  • Congenital: imperforate hymen, imperforate cervix, imperforate or absent vagina, müllerian agenesis
  • Acquired: destruction of endometrium with curettage (Asherman's syndrome), closure of cervix or vagina caused by traumatic injury, hysterectomy
Other: metabolic diseases (liver, kidney), malnutrition, rapid weight loss, exogenous obesity, endocrine abnormalities (Cushing's syndrome, Graves' disease, hypothyroidism)

6.3 ASCITES

Hypoalbuminemia: nephrotic syndrome, protein-losing gastroenteropathy, starvation
Cirrhosis
Hepatic congestion: CHF, constrictive pericarditis, tricuspid insufficiency, hepatic vein obstruction (Budd-Chiari syndrome), inferior vena cava or portal vein obstruction
Peritoneal infections: TB and other bacterial infections, fungal diseases, parasites
Neoplasms: primary hepatic neoplasms, metastases to liver or peritoneum, lymphomas, leukemias, myeloid metaplasia
Lymphatic obstruction: mediastinal tumors, trauma to the thoracic duct, filariasis
Ovarian disease: Meigs' syndrome, struma ovarii
Chronic pancreatitis or pseudocyst: pancreatic ascites

Leakage of bile: bile ascites
Urinary obstruction or trauma: urine ascites
Myxedema
Chylous ascites

6.4   ATAXIA

Vertebral-basilar artery ischemia
Diabetic neuropathy
Tabes dorsalis
Vitamin B_{12} deficiency
Multiple sclerosis and other demyelinating diseases
Meningomyelopathy
Cerebellar neoplasms, hemorrhage, abscess, infarct
Nutritional (Wernicke's encephalopathy)
Paraneoplastic syndromes
Parainfectious: Guillain-Barré syndrome, acute ataxia of childhood and
   young adults
Toxins: phenytoin, alcohol, sedatives, organophosphates
Wilson's disease (hepatolenticular degeneration)
Hypothyroidism
Myopathy
Cerebellar and spinocerebellar degeneration: ataxia, telangiectasia, Fried-
   reich's ataxia
Frontal lobe lesions: tumors, thrombosis of anterior cerebral artery, hydro-
   cephalus
Labyrinthine destruction: neoplasm, injury, inflammation, compression
Hysteria
AIDS

6.5   BACK PAIN

Trauma: injury to bone, joint, or ligament
Mechanical: pregnancy, obesity, fatigue, scoliosis
Degenerative: osteoarthritis
Infections: osteomyelitis, subarachnoid or spinal abscess, TB, meningitis
Metabolic: osteoporosis, osteomalacia
Vascular: leaking aortic aneurysm, subarachnoid or spinal hemorrhage/in-
   farction
Neoplastic: myeloma, Hodgkin's disease, carcinoma of pancreas, meta-
   static neoplasm from breast, prostate, lung
GI: penetrating ulcer, pancreatitis, cholelithiasis, inflammatory bowel dis-
   ease
Renal: hydronephrosis, calculus, neoplasm
Hematologic: sickle cell crisis, acute hemolysis
Gynecologic: neoplasm of uterus, ovary, dysmenorrhea, salpingitis, uterine
   prolapse
Inflammatory: ankylosing spondylitis, psoriatic arthritis, Reiter's syndrome
Lumbosacral strain
Psychogenic: malingering, hysteria, anxiety

6.6   CARDIAC MURMURS

Systolic

Mitral regurgitation (MR)
Tricuspid regurgitation (TR)
Ventricular septal defect (VSD)
Aortic stenosis (AS)
Idiopathic hypertrophic subaortic stenosis (IHSS)
Pulmonic stenosis (PS)
Innocent murmur of childhood
Coarctation of aorta

Diastolic

Aortic regurgitation (AR)
Atrial myxoma
Mitral stenosis (MS)
Pulmonary artery branch stenosis
Tricuspid stenosis (TS)
Graham-Steell murmur (diastolic decrescendo murmur heard in severe pulmonary hypertension)
Pulmonic regurgitation (PR)
Severe mitral regurgitation (MR)
Austin Flint murmur (diastolic rumble heard in severe AR)
Severe VSD and patent ductus arteriosus

Continuous

Patent ductus arteriosus
Pulmonary AV fistula

6.7   CHEST PAIN (NONPLEURITIC)

Cardiac: myocardial ischemia/infarction, myocarditis
Esophageal: spasm, rupture, esophagitis, ulceration, neoplasm, achalasia, diverticula, foreign body
Referred pain from subdiaphragmatic GI structures
   • Gastric and duodenal: hiatal hernia, alcoholic gastritis, neoplasm, PUD
   • Gallbladder and biliary: cholecystitis, cholelithiasis, impacted stone, neoplasm
   • Pancreatic: pancreatitis, neoplasm
Dissecting aortic aneurysm
Pain originating from skin, breasts, and musculoskeletal structures: herpes zoster, mastitis, cervical spondylosis
Mediastinal tumors: lymphoma, thymoma
Pulmonary: neoplasm, pneumonia, pulmonary embolism/infarction
Psychoneurosis
Chest pain associated with mitral valve prolapse

6.8 CHEST PAIN (PLEURITIC)

Cardiac: pericarditis, postpericardiotomy/Dressler syndrome
Pulmonary: pneumothorax, hemothorax, embolism/infarction, pneumonia,
  empyema, neoplasm, bronchiectasis, TB, carcinomatous effusion
GI: liver abscess, pancreatitis, Whipple's disease with associated pericardi-
  tis
Subdiaphragmatic abscess
Pain originating from skin and musculoskeletal tissues: costochondritis,
  chest wall trauma, fractured rib, interstitial fibrositis, myositis, strain of
  pectoralis muscle, herpes zoster, soft tissue and bone tumors
Collagen-vascular diseases with pleuritis
Psychoneurosis
Familial Mediterranean fever (FMF)

6.9 COMA

Vascular: hemorrhage, thrombosis, embolism
CNS infections: meningitis, encephalitis, cerebral abscess
Cerebral neoplasms with herniation
Head injury: subdural hematoma, cerebral concussion, cerebral contusion
Drugs: narcotics, sedatives, hypnotics
Ingestion or inhalation of toxins: CO, alcohol, lead
Metabolic disturbances:
  - Hypoxia
  - Hypoglycemia, hyperglyce-
    mia
  - Electrolyte disorders
  - Acid-base disorders
  - Hepatic failure
  - Uremia
Hypothyroidism
Hypothermia, hyperthermia
Hypotension, malignant hypertension
Postictal

6.10 CONSTIPATION

Intestinal obstruction
  - Fecal impaction
  - GI neoplasm
  - Gallstone ileus
  - Adhesions
  - Volvulus
  - Intussusception
  - Inflammatory bowel disease
  - Diverticular disease
  - Strangulated femoral hernia
  - Tuberculous stricture
  - Ameboma
  - Hematoma of bowel wall
    secondary to trauma or
    anticoagulants
Poor dietary habits: insufficient bulk in diet, inadequate fluid intake
Change from daily routine: travel, hospital admission, physical inactivity
Acute abdominal conditions: renal colic, salpingitis, biliary colic, appendi-
  citis
Hypercalcemia or hypokalemia, uremia
Irritable bowel syndrome, pregnancy, anorexia nervosa, depression
Painful anal conditions: hemorrhoids, fissure, stricture

Decreased intestinal peristalsis: old age, spinal cord injuries, myxedema, diabetes, multiple sclerosis, parkinsonism, and other neurologic diseases
Drugs: codeine, morphine, antacids with aluminum, verapamil, anticonvulsants, anticholinergics, disopyramide
Hirschsprung's disease, meconium ileus, congenital atresia in infants

6.11 DYSPHAGIA

Esophageal obstruction: neoplasm, foreign body, achalasia, stricture, spasm, esophageal web, diverticulum, *Schatzkiring*
Peptic esophagitis with stricture, Barrett's stricture
External esophageal compression: neoplasms (thyroid neoplasm, lymphoma, mediastinal tumors), aortic aneurysm, vertebral spurs, aberrant right subclavian artery (dysphagia lusoria)
Hiatal hernia
Oropharyngeal lesions: pharyngitis, glossitis, stomatitis, neoplasms
Hysteria: globus hystericus
Neurologic and/or neuromuscular disturbances: bulbar paralysis, myasthenia gravis, ALS, multiple sclerosis, parkinsonism, CVA, diabetic neuropathy
Toxins: poisoning, botulism, tetanus, postdiphtheric dysphagia
Systemic diseases: scleroderma, amyloidosis, dermatomyositis
Candida and herpes esophagitis
Presbyesophagus

6.12 DYSPNEA

Upper airway obstruction: trauma, neoplasm, epiglottitis, laryngeal edema, tongue retraction, laryngospasm, abductor paralysis of vocal cords, aspiration of foreign body
Lower airway obstruction: neoplasm, COPD, asthma, aspiration of foreign body
Pulmonary infection: pneumonia, abscess, empyema, TB, bronchiectasis
Pulmonary hypertension
Pulmonary embolism/infarction
Parenchymal lung disease
Pulmonary vascular congestion
Cardiac disease: ASHD, valvular lesions, cardiac dysrhythmias, cardiomyopathy, pericardial effusion, cardial shunts
Space-occupying lesions: neoplasm, large hiatal hernia, pleural effusions
Disease of chest wall: severe kyphoscoliosis, fractured ribs, sternal compression, morbid obesity
Neurologic dysfunction: Guillain-Barré syndrome, botulism, polio, spinal cord injury
Interstitial pulmonary disease: sarcoidosis, collagen vascular diseases, DIP, Hamman-Rich pneumonitis, etc.
Pneumoconioses: silicosis, berylliosis, etc.
Mesothelioma
Pneumothorax, hemothorax, pleural effusion
Inhalation of toxins

Cholinergic drug intoxication
Carcinoid syndrome
Hematologic: anemia, polycythemia, hemoglobinopathies
Thyrotoxicosis, myxedema
Diaphragmatic compression caused by abdominal distention, subphrenic
    abscess
Lung resection
Metabolic abnormalities: uremia, hepatic coma, DKA
Sepsis
Atelectasis
Psychoneurosis
Diaphragmatic paralysis
Pregnancy

6.13   EDEMA OF LOWER EXTREMITIES

CHF (right-sided)
Hepatic cirrhosis
Nephrosis
Myxedema
Lymphedema
Pregnancy
Abdominal mass: neoplasm, cyst
Venous compression from abdominal aneurysm
Varicose veins
Bilateral cellulitis
Bilateral thrombophlebitis
Venous thrombosis
Retroperitoneal fibrosis

6.14   FEVER AND RASH

Drug hypersensitivity: penicillin, sulfonamides, thiazides, anticonvulsants,
    allopurinol
Viral infection: measles, rubella, varicella, erythema infectiosum, roseola,
    enterovirus infection, viral hepatitis, infectious mononucleosis
Other infections: meningococcemia, staphylococcemia, scarlet fever, ty-
    phoid fever, *Pseudomonas* bacteremia, Rocky Mountain spotted fever,
    Lyme disease, secondary syphilis, bacterial endocarditis, babesiosis,
    brucellosis, listeriosis
Serum sickness
Erythema multiforme
Erythema marginatum
Erythema nodosum
SLE
Dermatomyositis
Allergic vasculitis
Pityriasis rosea
Herpes zoster

6.15   GASTROINTESTINAL BLEEDING

Upper GI bleeding (originating above the ligament of Treitz)

Oral or pharyngeal lesions: swallowed blood from nose or oropharynx

Swallowed hemoptysis

Esophageal: varices, ulceration, esophagitis, Mallory-Weiss tear, carcinoma, trauma

Gastric: peptic ulcer (including Cushing and Curling's, ulcers), gastritis, angiodysplasia, gastric neoplasms, hiatal hernia, gastric diverticulum, pseudoxanthoma elasticum, Rendu-Osler-Weber syndrome

Duodenal: peptic ulcer, duodenitis, angiodysplasia, aortoduodenal fistula, duodenal diverticulum, duodenal tumors, carcinoma of ampulla of Vater, parasites (e.g., hookworm), Crohn's disease

Biliary: hematobilia (e.g., penetrating injury to liver, hepatobiliary malignancy, endoscopic papillotomy)

Lower GI bleeding (originating below the ligament of Treitz)

Small intestine

Ischemic bowel disease (mesenteric thrombosis, embolism, vasculitis, trauma)

Small bowel neoplasm: leiomyomas, carcinoids

Hereditary hemorrhagic telangiectasia (Rendu-Osler-Weber syndrome)

Meckel's diverticulum and other small intestine diverticula

Aortoenteric fistula

Intestinal hemangiomas: blue rubber-bleb nevi, intestinal hemangiomas, cutaneous vascular nevi

Hamartomatous polyps: Peutz-Jeghers syndrome (intestinal polyps, mucocutaneous pigmentation)

Infections of small bowel: tuberculous enteritis, enteritis necroticans

Volvulus

Intussusception

Lymphoma of small bowel, sarcoma, Kaposi's sarcoma

Irradiation ileitis

AV malformation of small intestine

Inflammatory bowel disease

Polyarteritis nodosa

Other: Pancreatoenteric fistulas, Schöenlein-Henoch purpura, Ehler-Danlos syndrome, SLE, amyloidosis, metastic melanoma

Colon

Carcinoma (particularly left colon)

Diverticular disease

Inflammatory bowel disease

Ischemic colitis

Colonic polyps

Vascular abnormalities: angiodysplasia, vascular ectasia

Radiation colitis

Infectious colitis
Uremic colitis
Aortoenteric fistula
Lymphoma of large bowel
Hemorrhoids
Anal fissure
Trauma, foreign body
Solitary rectal/cecal ulcers
Long-distance running

6.16 HEADACHE

Vascular: migraine, cluster headaches, temporal arteritis, hypertension, cavernous sinus thrombosis

Musculoskeletal: neck and shoulder muscle contraction, strain of extraocular and/or intraocular muscles, cervical spondylosis, temporomandibular arthritis

Infections: meningitis, encephalitis, brain abscess, sepsis, sinusitis, osteomyelitis, parotitis

Cerebral neoplasm

Subdural hematoma

Cerebral hemorrhage/infarct

Pseudotumor cerebri

Normal pressure hydrocephalus (NPH)

Postlumbar puncture

Cerebral aneurysm, arteriovenous malformations

Posttrauma

Dental problems: abscess, periodontitis, poorly fitting dentures

Trigeminal neuralgia, glossopharyngeal neuralgia

Otitis and other ear diseases

Glaucoma and other eye diseases

Metabolic: uremia, carbon monoxide inhalation, hypoxia

Pheochromocytoma, hypoglycemia, hypothyroidism

Effort induced: benign exertional headache, cough headache, coital cephalalgia

Drugs: alcohol, nitrates, histamine antagonists

Paget's disease of skull

Emotional, psychiatric

6.17 HEMATURIA

Use the mnemonic TICS

T (trauma): blow to kidney, insertion of Foley catheter or foreign body in urethra, prolonged and severe exercise, very rapid emptying of overdistended bladder

(tumor): hypernephroma, Wilms' tumor, papillary carcinoma of the bladder, prostatic and urethral neoplasms

(toxins): turpentine, phenols, sulfonamides and other antibiotics, cyclophosphamide, NSAIDs

I (infections): glomerulonephritis, TB, cystitis, prostatitis, urethritis, *Schistosoma haematobium*, yellow fever, blackwater fever

(inflammatory processes): Goodpasture's syndrome, periarteritis, postir-
radiation
C (calculi): renal, ureteral, bladder, urethra
(cysts): simple cysts, polycystic disease
(congenital anomalies): hemangiomas, aneurysms, AVM
S (surgery): invasive procedures, prostatic resection, cystoscopy
(sickle cell disease and other hematologic disturbances): hemophilia,
thrombocytopenia, anticoagulants
(somewhere else): bleeding genitals, factitious (drug addicts)

6.18 HEMOPTYSIS

Cardiovascular

Pulmonary embolism/infarction
Left ventricular failure
Mitral stenosis
AV fistula
Severe hypertension
Erosion of aortic aneurysm

Pulmonary

Neoplasm (primary or metastatic)
Infection
- Pneumonia: *Streptococcus pneumoniae, Klebsiella pneumoniae,
  Staphylococcus aureus, Legionella pneumophila*
- Bronchiectasis
- Abscess
- TB
- Bronchitis
- Fungal infections (aspergillosis, coccidiodomycosis)

Parasitic infections (amebiasis, ascariasis, paragonimiasis)
Vasculitis: Wegener's granulomatosis, Churg-Strauss syndrome, Henoch-
Schönlein purpura
Goodpasture's syndrome
Trauma (needle biopsy, foreign body, right heart catheterization, prolonged
and severe cough)
Cystic fibrosis, bullous emphysema
Pulmonary sequestration
Pulmonary AV fistula
SLE
Idiopathic pulmonary hemosiderosis
Drugs: aspirin, anticoagulants, penicillamine
Pulmonary hypertension
Mediastinal fibrosis

Other

Epistaxis
Laryngeal bleeding (laryngitis, laryngeal neoplasm)
Hematologic disorders (clotting abnormalities, DIC, thrombocytopenia)

HEPATOMEGALY

Frequent jaundice

Infectious hepatitis
Toxic hepatitis
Carcinoma: liver, pancreas, bile ducts, metastatic neoplasm to liver
Cirrhosis
Obstruction of common bile duct
Alcoholic hepatitis
Biliary cirrhosis
Cholangitis
Hemochromatosis with cirrhosis

Infrequent jaundice

CHF
Amyloidosis
Liver abscess
Sarcoidosis
Infectious mononucleosis
Alcoholic fatty infiltration
Lymphoma
Leukemia
Budd-Chiari syndrome
Myelofibrosis with myeloid metaplasia
Familial hyperlipoproteinemia type 1
Other: amebiasis, hydatid disease of liver, schistosomiasis, kala-azar
    (*Leishmania donovani*), Hurler's syndrome, Gaucher's disease, kwash-
    iorkor

 HIRSUTISM

Idiopathic: familial, possibly increased sensitivity to androgens
Menopause
Polycystic ovarian syndrome
Drugs: androgens, anabolic steroids, methyltestosterone, minoxidil, diaz-
    oxide, phenytoin, glucocorticoids, cyclosporine
Congenital adrenal hyperplasia
Adrenal virilizing tumor
Ovarian virilizing tumor: arrhenoblastoma, hilus cell tumor
Pituitary adenoma
Cushing's syndrome
Hypothyroidism (congenital and juvenile)
Acromegaly
Testicular feminization

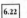 **JAUNDICE**

Predominance of direct (conjugated) bilirubin

Extrahepatic obstruction:
- Common duct abnormalities: calculi, neoplasm, stricture, cyst, sclerosing cholangitis
- Metastatic carcinoma
- Pancreatic carcinoma, pseudocyst
- Ampullary carcinoma

Hepatocellular disease: hepatitis, cirrhosis
Drugs: estrogens, phenothiazines, captopril, methyltestosterone, labetalol
Cholestatic jaundice of pregnancy
Hereditary disorders: Dubin-Johnson syndrome, Rotor's syndrome
Recurrent benign intrahepatic cholestasis

Predominance of indirect (unconjugated) bilirubin

Hemolysis: hereditary and acquired hemolytic anemias
Inefficient marrow production
Impaired hepatic conjugation: chloramphenicol, pregnanediol
Neonatal jaundice
Hereditary disorders: Gilbert's syndrome, Crigler-Najjar syndrome

6.22 **LYMPHADENOPATHY**

Generalized

AIDS, ARC
Lymphoma: Hodgkin's disease, non-Hodgkin's lymphoma
Leukemias
Infectious mononucleosis, CMV
Rheumatoid arthritis (more common in chronic juvenile arthritis)
Diffuse skin infection: generalized furunculosis, multiple thick bites
Parasitic infections: toxoplasmosis, filariasis, leishmaniasis
Serum sickness
Collagen vascular diseases
Dengue (arbovirus infection)
Sarcoidosis
Drugs: isoniazid, hydantoin derivatives, antithyroid and antileprosy drugs
Secondary syphilis

Localized

Any of the causes of generalized lymphadenopathy
Draining lymphatics from local infection: infected furuncle, throat infection, dental abscess, lymphogranuloma venereum, brucellosis, parasitic infections, cat-scratch disease
Neoplasm
TB (scrofula)

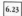 **MEDIASTINAL MASSES OR WIDENING ON CHEST X-RAY**

Lymphoma: Hodgkin's disease and non-Hodgkin's lymphoma
Sarcoidosis
Vascular: aortic aneurysm, ectasia or tortuosity of aorta or bronchocephalic
  vessels
Carcinoma: lungs, esophagus
Esophageal diverticula
Hiatal hernia
Prominent pulmonary outflow tract: pulmonary hypertension, pulmonary
  embolism, right-to-left shunts
Trauma: mediastinal hemorrhage
Pneumomediastinum
Lymphadenopathy caused by silicosis and other pneumoconioses
Leukemias
Infections: TB, viral (rare), *Mycoplasma* (rare), fungal, tularemia
Substernal thyroid
Thymoma
Teratoma
Bronchogenic cyst
Pericardial cyst
Neurofibroma, neurosarcoma, ganglioneuroma

 METASTATIC NEOPLASMS

Bone	Brain	Liver	Lung
Breast	Lung	Colon	Breast
Lung	Breast	Stomach	Colon
Prostate	Melanoma	Pancreas	Kidney
Thyroid	GU tract	Breast	Testis
Kidney	Colon	Lymphomas	Stomach
Bladder	Sinuses	Bronchus	Thyroid
Endometrium	Sarcoma	Lung	Melanoma
Cervix	Skin		Sarcoma
	Thyroid		

6.25 **PARAPLEGIA**

Trauma: penetrating wounds to motor cortex, fracture-dislocation of vertebral column with compression of spinal cord or cauda equina, prolapsed
  disk, electrical injuries
Neoplasm: parasagittal region, vertebrae, meninges, spinal cord, cauda
  equina, Hodgkin's disease, NHL, leukemic deposits, pelvic neoplasms
Multiple sclerosis and other demyelinating disorders
Mechanical compression of spinal cord, cauda equina, or lumbosacral
  plexus: Paget's disease, kyphoscoliosis, herniation of intervertebral disc,
  spondylosis, ankylosing spondylitis, rheumatoid arthritis, aortic aneurysm

Infections: spinal abscess, syphilis, TB, poliomyelitis, leprosy
Thrombosis of superior sagittal sinus
Polyneuritis: Gullain-Barré syndrome, diabetes, alcohol, beri-beri, heavy
    metals
Heredofamilial muscular dystrophies
ALS
Congenital and familial conditions: syringomyelia, myelomeningocele, my-
    elodysplasia
Hysteria

 PLEURAL EFFUSIONS

Exudative (refer to Section 30.2 for diagnosis)
Neoplasm: bronchogenic carcinoma, breast carcinoma, mesothelioma, lym-
    phoma, ovarian carcinoma, multiple myeloma, leukemia, Meigs' syn-
    drome
Infections: viral pneumonia, bacterial pneumonia, *Mycoplasma*, TB, fungal
    and parasitic diseases
Trauma
Collagen-vascular diseases: SLE, RA, scleroderma, polyarteritis, Wegen-
    er's granulomatosis
Pulmonary infarction
Pancreatitis
Postcardiotomy/Dressler's syndrome
Drug-induced lupus erythematosus (hydralazine, procainamide)
Postabdominal surgery
Ruptured esophagus
Chronic effusion secondary to congestive failure

Transudative (refer to Section 30.2 for diagnosis)
CHF
Hepatic cirrhosis
Nephrotic syndrome
Hypoproteinemia from any cause
Meigs' syndrome

6.27 **POLYURIA**

Diabetes mellitus
Diabetes insipidus
Primary polydipsia (compulsive water drinking)
Hypercalcemia
Hypokalemia
Postobstructive uropathy
Diuretic phase of renal failure
Drugs: diuretics, caffeine, lithium
Sickle cell trait or disease, chronic pyelonephritis (failure to concentrate
    urine)
Anxiety, cold weather

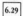 POPLITEAL SWELLING

Phlebitis (superficial)
Lymphadenitis
Trauma: fractured tibia or fibula, contusion, traumatic neuroma
Deep vein thrombosis
Ruptured varicose vein
Baker's cyst
Popliteal abscess
Osteomyelitis
Ruptured tendon
Aneurysm of popliteal artery
Neoplasm: lipoma, osteogenic sarcoma, neurofibroma, fibrosarcoma

6.29 PROTEINURIA

Nephrotic syndrome as a result of primary renal diseases
Malignant hypertension
Malignancies: multiple myeloma, leukemias, Hodgkin's disease
CHF
Diabetes mellitus
SLE, rheumatoid arthritis
Sickle cell disease
Goodpasture's syndrome
Malaria
Amyloidosis, sarcoidosis
Tubular lesions: cystinosis
Functional (after heavy exercise)
Pyelonephritis
Pregnancy
Constrictive pericarditis
Renal vein thrombosis
Toxic nephropathies: heavy metals, drugs
Radiation nephritis
Orthostatic (postural) proteinuria
Benign proteinuria: fever, heat or cold exposure

PRURITUS

Dry skin
Drug eruption
Scabies
Skin diseases
Myeloproliferative disorders: mycosis fungoides, Hodgkin's lymphoma,
    multiple myeloma, polycythemia vera
Cholestatic liver disease
Endocrine disorders: diabetes mellitus, thyroid disease, carcinoid
Carcinoma: breast, lung, gastric
Chronic renal failure

Iron deficiency
AIDS
Neurosis

6.31   PURPURA

Trauma
Septic emboli, atheromatous emboli
DIC
Thrombocytopenia
Meningococcemia
Rocky Mountain spotted fever
Hemolytic-uremic syndrome
Viral infection: echo, coxsackie
Scurvy
Other: left atrial myxoma, cryoglobulinemia, vasculitis, hyperglobulinemic
     purpura

6.32   SHOULDER PAIN

With local findings in shoulder

Trauma: contusion, fracture, muscle strain, trauma to spinal cord
Arthrosis, arthritis, rheumatoid arthritis, ankylosing spondylitis
Bursitis, synovitis, tendinitis, tenosynovitis
Aseptic (avascular) necrosis
Local infection: septic arthritis, osteomyelitis, abscess, herpes zoster, TB

Without local findings in shoulder

Cardiovascular disorders: ischemic heart disease, pericarditis, aortic aneu-
     rysm
Subdiaphragmatic abscess, liver abscess
Cholelithiasis, cholecystitis
Pulmonary lesions: apical bronchial carcinoma, pleurisy, pneumothorax,
     pneumonia
GI lesions: PUD, gastric neoplasm, peptic esophagitis
Pancreatic lesions: carcinoma, calculi, pancreatitis
CNS abnormalities: neoplasm, vascular abnormalities
Multiple sclerosis
Syringomyelia
Polymyositis/dermatomyositis
Psychogenic
Polymyalgia rheumatica
Ectopic pregnancy

6.33   SPLENOMEGALY

Hepatic cirrhosis
Neoplastic involvement: CML, CLL, lymphoma, polycythemia vera, my-
     eloid metaplasia, multiple myeloma
Bacterial infections: TB, infectious endocarditis, typhoid fever, splenic ab-
     scess

Viral infections: infectious mononucleosis, viral hepatitis
Gaucher disease and other lipid storage diseases
Sarcoidosis
Parasitic infections (malaria, kala-azar, histoplasmosis)
Hereditary and acquired hemolytic anemias
Idiopathic thrombocytopenic purpura (ITP)
Collagen-vascular disorders: SLE, rheumatoid arthritis (Felty's syndrome),
    polyarteritis nodosa
Serum sickness, drug hypersensitivity reaction
Splenic cysts and benign tumors: hemangioma, lymphangioma
Thrombosis of splenic or portal vein

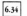 **VERTIGO**

Peripheral

Otitis media
Acute labyrinthitis
Vestibular neuronitis
Benign positional vertigo
Meniere's disease
Ototoxic drugs: streptomycin, gentamycin
Lesions of the eighth nerve: acoustic neuroma, meningioma, mononeurop-
    athy, metastatic carcinoma
Mastoiditis

CNS or systemic

Vertebrobasilar artery insufficiency
Posterior fossa tumor or other brain tumors
Infarction/hemorrhage of cerebral cortex, cerebellum, or brainstem
Basilar migraine
Metabolic: drugs, hypoxia, anemia, fever
Hypotension/severe hypertension
Multiple sclerosis
CNS infections: viral, bacterial
Temporal lobe epilepsy
Arnold-Chiari malformation, syringobulbia
Psychogenic: ventilation, hysteria

6.35   **VOMITING**

GI disturbances:
- Obstruction: esophageal, pyloric, intestinal
- Infections: viral or bacterial enteritis, viral hepatitis, food poisoning
- Pancreatitis
- Appendicitis
- Biliary colic
- Peritonitis
- Perforated bowel
- Diabetic gastroparesis
- Other: Gastritis, PUD, IBD, GI tract neoplasms

Drugs: morphine, digitalis, cytotoxic agents, bromocriptine
Severe pain: MI, renal colic
Metabolic disorders: uremia, acidosis/alkalosis, hyperglycemia, DKA, thyrotoxicosis
Trauma: blows to the testicles, epigastrium
Vertigo
Reye's syndrome
Increased intracranial pressure
CNS disturbances: trauma, hemorrhage, infarction, neoplasm, infection, hypertensive encephalopathy, migraine
Radiation sickness
Vomiting associated with pregnancy
Motion sickness
Bulimia, anorexia nervosa
Psychogenic: emotional disturbances, offensive sights or smells
Irritation of the fauces
Severe coughing
Pyelonephritis

7 General Management of Poisoning and Drug Overdose

Michael S. Weinstock

Over the last two decades there has been an alarming increase in drug overdose and poisoning throughout the United States. Patients who come to the emergency department as victims of poisoning or overdose, whether accidental or intentional, can be diagnostic dilemmas for the clinician. The physician should consider the possibility of poisoning in patients who are comatose or have psychotic/combative behavior, unusual cardiac dysrhythmias, unexplained acidosis, or after traumatic suicide attempts. Individuals who use street drugs may not be aware of the ingredients or adulteration of such substances and may have a confusing presentation as a result of polydrug ingestion.

For the purpose of this chapter, the terms poisoning and drug overdose are used interchangeably.

According to Haddad and Winchester,[2] the general management of poisoned patients can be divided into the following phases:

1. Emergency management and stabilization
2. History and physical examination
3. Clinical evaluation of major toxic signs
4. Elimination of the poison from the GI tract, skin, and eyes
5. Administration of an antidote, if available
6. Elimination of absorbed substances
7. Supportive therapy

7.1   GENERAL APPROACH TO MANAGEMENT

1. Emergency stabilization
   a. Ensure adequate ventilation and examine the airway for patency and intact gag reflex. In comatose patients, suction excessive secretions and provide an oral airway. Patients who are obtunded, comatose, or who have a depressed respiratory effort should be ventilated by endotracheal intubation. If the patient is awake and resistance is too great, proceed with treatment. Oxygen therapy should be liberal (100% in "young lungs") in the initial phases of management. After intubation, listen to the chest to ensure adequate and symmetric ventilation.
   b. Establish intravenous access using a large-bore angiocatheter, and

simultaneously draw adequate samples for appropriate lab studies, including electrolytes, glucose, PT, PTT, and toxicologic screening; evaluation of arterial blood gases may also be indicated at this time. CAUTION: Carbon monoxide levels may require a separate order. A balanced salt solution is preferred for initial resuscitation. If the patient is hypotensive, a fluid challenge based on weight should be administered. Ensure adequate perfusion. Note that some poisons can enhance or promote pulmonary edema, and large volumes of fluids are to be administered with caution.

  c. All comatose patients should receive an intravenous bolus of 50 g of glucose followed by 1 to 2 mg of naloxone (Narcan) intravenously. The patient is then reevaluated for response.

  d. Foley catheterization should be considered in patients who are comatose. Urine should be sent for toxicologic studies.

  e. If the patient has generalized seizures, these should be controlled with appropriate dosages of diazepam. NOTE: Withdrawal may be heralded by seizures, and the clinician should be alert to that possibility.

2. History and physical exam

  a. When the patient is unable to communicate, identification of the poison or any antecedent medical history is sometimes available from police, emergency medical service personnel, family, or friends. Good detective work can save time and decrease morbidity and mortality.

  b. Careful examination can provide reliable information as to the type of poisoning (Table 7-1). Unusual odors on the patient's breath should be noted along with any bruising (suspect trauma), skin markings, diaphoresis, variation in pupil size, or dysrhythmias, especially in young patients.

3. Clinical evaluation

  a. A 12-lead ECG should be taken. Even in the absence of any dysrhythmia, the ECG can provide clues as to what was ingested, such as a prolonged QT interval in phenothiazine overdose or a widened QRS complex in tricyclic overdose. Several substances may cause dysrhythmias (Table 7-2).

  b. Laboratory evaluation can help identify toxic agents or an underlying disease. The many causes of high anion gap metabolic acidosis are summarized in the following list:*

Uremia	Methanol poisoning
Diabetic ketoacidosis	Ethylene glycol poisoning
Lactic acidosis	Nondiabetic alcoholic ketoacidosis
Salicylate toxicity	Paraldehyde toxicity

4. Elimination of ingested poisons from the GI tract: In patients presenting to the emergency room more than 1 hr postingestion, gastric emptying may have little benefit. In an extensive study of 592 patients to evaluate the efficacy of gastric emptying procedures in

*From Haddad LM, Winchester J (editors): Clinical management of poisoning and drug overdose. Philadelphia, 1983, WB Saunders Co.

Table 7-1 Examples of symptom complexes or toxidromes

Level of Consciousness	Respirations	Pupils	Other	Possible Toxic Agent
Coma	↓ ↑	Pinpoint	Fasciculations	Organophosphate insecticides
Coma	→	Pinpoint	Tracks	Opiates
Coma	Apneustic	Pinpoint	Decerebrate posturing	Pontine (brainstem) structural lesion
Awake			Torsion (head/neck)	Phenothiazines, haloperidol
Coma	→	Pinpoint	Cardiac dysrhythmia	Phenothiazines
Coma	→	Dilated	Cardiac dysrhythmia	Tricyclic antidepressants
			Convulsions	
Coma	← →		Uremic frost	Uremia
Coma	← →	Dilated	Hypothermia	Sedatives, barbiturates
Semicoma	←		Diaphoresis	Salicylates
			Tinnitus	
			Fever	
Agitated, hallucinating	↑	Dilated	Fever	Anticholinergics
			Flushing	
			Dry skin and mucous membranes	

From Haddad LM, Winchester J (editors): Clinical management of poisoning and drug overdose, Philadelphia, 1983, WB Saunders Co.

Table 7-2 Examples of cardiac dysrhythmias secondary to drug toxicity

Drug	Common Dysrhythmias
Amphetamines	Sinus tachycardia, SVT
β-Blockers	Bradycardia, AV block
Digitalis	Bradycardia, AV block, PAT with block, PVC, junctional tachycardia
Ethylene glycol	Narrow QRS (from hypocalcemia)
Phencyclidine (PCP)	Tachycardia, PVC
Phenothiazines	Q and T wave distortions
Quinidine	Prolonged QT, AV block, widened QRS (see Fig. 5-4,*B*)
Sympathomimetics	Tachycardia, ventricular dysrhythmias
Theophylline	Tachycardia, MAT, ventricular dysrhythmias
Tricyclic antidepressants	SVT, wide QRS

altering clinical outcome, Kulig et al.[4] reached the following conclusions:

a. A satisfactory clinical outcome can be achieved in drug overdose patients without gastric emptying procedures being performed routinely.

b. The use of syrup of ipecac in the ER is not of benefit in patients who present hours after an oral drug overdose.

c. Gastric lavage in obtunded patients is of questionable value if the ingestion occurred more than 1 hr before ER presentation.

d. Mandatory gastric emptying as initial treatment of all drug overdose patients should not be the accepted standard of care; in most cases the administration of activated charcoal and vigorous supportive measures are sufficient treatment.

If the patient is evaluated within 1 hr or less an attempt should be made to remove the substances from the GI tract in either antegrade or retrograde fashion. Whether vomiting should be induced with syrup of ipecac or the gastric contents emptied with a large-bore tube and irrigation depends on what was ingested and the level of consciousness.

a. Syrup of ipecac: for an awake child or adult, 15 ml or 30 ml is given PO and followed by large amounts of fluids such as water. Exceptions to this include: patients who are comatose or obtunded, and those who have ingested caustics, petroleum products of low volatility and surface tension, or phenothiazines. Haddad and Winchester[2] note that most authorities agree that the use of syrup of ipecac with petroleum distillates is justified when this product is a carrier for a more toxic substance.

b. Gastric lavage: to recover pill fragments, a large-bore no. 36 French Ewald tube should be used, keeping in mind that the airway should

be cautiously guarded. Intubation is especially appropriate in the obtunded patient or when removing petroleum distillates.
   c. Activated charcoal is a standard treatment for poisoned patients. Adults should receive 50 to 100 g of activated charcoal in a slurry or instilled down a gastric or nasogastric tube. The pediatric dose is 30 to 50 g. This dose may be repeated 3 or 4 times in the initial 24 hr of management. Following is a partial list of common substances known to be absorbed by activated charcoal:

Atropine	Morphine
Barbiturates	Phenytoin
Chlorpromazine	Quinidine
Cocaine	Salicylates
Colchicine	Theophylline
Dextroamphetamine	Tolbutamide
Digitalis	Tricyclic antidepressants
Meprobamate	

   d. Cathartics increase transit time and therefore hasten elimination of the bound toxic substance. Either magnesium sulfate or magnesium citrate is usually employed. However, Krenzelok et al.[3] demonstrated a mean transient time of 0.9 hr using sorbitol in a slurry with activated charcoal (50 g of charcoal in a 70% sorbitol solution), compared with 4.4 hr with magnesium citrate. Sorbitol should not be employed with small children since the risk of significant diarrhea with dehydration is high.
5. Elimination of adsorbed substances: the clinician essentially has four modalities, depending on the type of poisoning.[2]
   a. Forced diuresis (caution: some poisons enhance pulmonary edema)
   b. Alkalinization by adding sodium bicarbonate to the solution (e.g., 0.5-1 mEq/kg/L)

   (1) Dysrhythmias secondary to tricyclic poisoning
   (2) Salicylates
   (3) Barbiturates
   (4) Phenylbutazone
   (5) Isoniazid

   c. Acidification by administering ammonium chloride or ascorbic acid
   (1) Phencyclidine
   (2) Amphetamines
   (3) Quinine
   (4) Fenfluramine
   d. Sorbent hemoperfusion and dialysis
6. The pharmacokinetics of salicylates[1] and acetaminophen[6] has been well studied. Using standardized nomograms, the clinician can predict toxicity (Figs. 7-1 and 7-2). It is emphasized that the time from ingestion to the time of serum sample is critical in the interpretation of the nomogram.
   a. Management of salicylate overdose should include the following[5]:
      (1) Gastric lavage

(2) Administration of activated charcoal

(3) Forced alkaline diuresis (e.g., $D_5\frac{1}{2}NS$ IV with 44 mEq bicarbonate/L at 300 ml/hr)

(4) Consider dialysis if serum salicylate level is greater than 70 mg/dl

(5) Vitamin K 10 mg IM or IV (salicylate inhibition of vitamin K may lead to GI bleeding)

(6) Monitor ABG (respiratory alkalosis initially, followed by metabolic acidosis)

(7) Monitor serum K^+ (tendency to hypokalemia)

b. Acetaminophen overdose requires the following[5]:

(1) Gastric lavage (activated charcoal should not be used since it may impair absorption)

(2) Determine blood level; if in toxic range, start N-acetylcysteine (Mucomyst) 140 mg/kg PO loading dose followed by 70 mg/kg PO q4h for 68 hr (N-acetylcysteine therapy must be started within 16 hours of acetaminophen overdose)

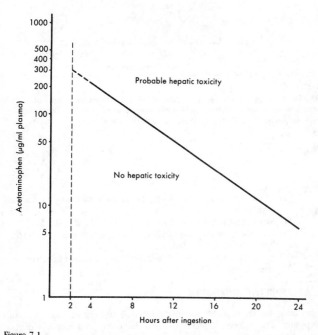

Figure 7-1

Semialgorithmic plot of plasma acetaminophen levels versus time. (Reproduced with permission from Rumack BH, Matthew H: Pediatrics 55:871, 1975.)

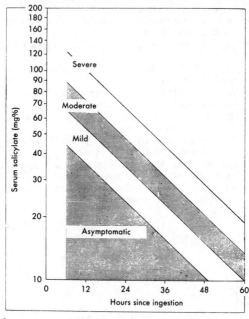

Figure 7-2
The Done nomogram correlates the serum salicylate level with the severity of ingestion at a given time after ingestion of a single dose of salicylate. (Reproduced with permission from Done AK: Pediatrics 26:800, 1960.)

    (3) Monitor acetaminophen level, use graph to plot possible hepatic toxicity
    (4) Provide adequate IV hydration (e.g., D₅½NS at 150 ml/hr)
    (5) Monitor liver function studies, ABGs, serum glucose, electrolytes, BUN, and creatinine
    (6) If acetaminophen level is nontoxic may discontinue acetylcysteine therapy

7.2   SPECIFIC ANTIDOTES

Few antidotes are available for specific therapy of drug overdose or toxic exposure. The number of pharmaceutical, industrial, and naturally occurring products or substances that are potentially lethal is almost infinite. Examples of specific antidotes appear in Table 7-3.

Table 7-3 Emergency antidotes

Poison	Antidote	Adult Dosage*	Comments
Acetaminophen	N-Acetylcysteine	140 mg/kg initial dose	Most effective within 16 hr
Arsenic	see Mercury		
Atropine	Physostigmine	Initial dose 0.5-2 mg IV	Can produce convulsions or bradycardia
Benzodiazepines	Flumazenil†	1 mg IV	Patient should rapidly awaken if benzodiazepines are responsible for obtunded state
Carbon monoxide	Oxygen		
Cyanide	Amyl nitrite	Pearls every 2 min	Methemoglobin-cyanide complex
	then		
	Sodium nitrite	10 ml of 3% sol over 3 min IV 0.33 ml (10 mg of 3% sol) kg initially for children	Causes hypotension; dosage assumes normal hemoglobin
	Sodium thiosulfate	25% sol: 50 ml IV over 10 min; 1.65 ml/kg for children	Forms harmless sodium thiocyanate
Ethylene glycol	see Methyl alcohol		
Gold	see Mercury		
Iron	Deferoxamine	Initial dose: 40-90 mg/kg IM not to exceed 1 g	Deferoxamine mesylate—forms excretable ferrioxamine complex

Adapted from an American College of Emergency Physicians poster on poisoning (Dallas Tex, 1980). From Haddad LM, Winchester J (editors): Clinical management of poisoning and drug overdose, Philadelphia, 1983, WB Saunders Co.

*Dosages listed may require modification according to specific clinical conditions.

†Pending FDA approval.

Table 7-3 Emergency antidotes—cont'd

Poison	Antidote	Adult Dosage*	Comments
Beta blockers	Glucagon	5 mg/hr infusion	
Calcium channel blockers	Calcium chloride	Bolus of 60 mmol over 30 min followed by an infusion of 50 mmol/hr	10% CaCl₂ contains 2 mmol/ml
Lead	Calcium disodium versenate	1 amp/250 ml D₅W over 1 hr	5 ml amp IV 20% sol; dilute to less than 3% sol—calcium displaced by lead
Mercury (arsenic, gold)	BAL (British anti-Lewisite)	5 mg/kg IM as soon as possible	Each ml BAL in oil has dimercaprol, 100 mg in 210 mg (21%) benzyl benzoate and 680 mg peanut oil—forms stable nontoxic excretable cyclic compound
Methyl alcohol (ethylene glycol)	Ethyl alcohol In conjunction with dialysis	1 ml/kg of 100% ethanol initially in glucose sol; maintain blood level of 100 mg/dl	Competes for alcohol dehydrogenase; prevents formation of formic acid, oxalates

Nitrites	Methylene blue	0.2 ml/kg of 1% solution IV over 5 min	Often exchange transfusion is needed for severe methemoglobinemia
Opiates, Darvon, Lomotil	Naloxone	0.4-0.8 mg IV 0.01 mg/kg IV for children	Naloxone—no respiratory depression (0.4 mg/1 ml amp)
Organophosphates	Atropine	Initial dose: 0.5-2 mg IV 0.05 mg/kg IV initially for children	Physiologically blocks acetylcholine; up to 5 mg IV every 15 min may be necessary in the critical adult patient
	Pralidoxime (Protopam)	Initial dose: 1 g IV children: 25-50 mg/kg IV	Specific: breaks alkyl phosphate-cholinesterase bond; up to 500 mg every hr may be necessary in the critical adult patient

| 7.3 | **SUPPORTIVE THERAPY**

Throughout the treatment process, supportive therapy is the mainstay of patient care. Continual monitoring, maintaining the airway, and ensuring adequate ventilation and perfusion will influence patient outcome.

References

1. Done AK: Salicylate intoxication, Pediatrics 26:800, 1960.
2. Haddad LM: General approach to the emergency management of poisoning. In Haddad LM, Winchester JF (editors): Clinical management of poisoning and drug overdose, Philadelphia, 1983, WB Saunders Co.
3. Krenzelok EP, Keller R, Stewart RD: Gastrointestinal transit times of cathartics combined with charcoal, Ann Emerg Med 14:1152, 1985.
4. Kulig K, Bar-Or D, Cantrill S, et al: Management of acutely poisoned patients without gastric emptying, Ann Emerg Med 14:562, 1985.
5. Nicholson DP: The immediate management of overdose, Med Clin North Am 67:1285, 1983.
6. Rumac BH, Peterson RG: Acetaminophen overdose: incidence, diagnosis, and management in 416 patients, Pediatrics 62(suppl):898, 1978.

Hypertension

Definition[7]
Table 8-1 describes the classification of blood pressure in adults.

Etiology
1. Essential (primary) hypertension (90%)
2. Renal hypertension (5%)
   a. Renal parenchymal disease (3%)
   b. Renovascular hypertension (<2%)
3. Endocrine (4-5%)
   a. Oral contraceptives (4%)
   b. Primary aldosteronism (0.5%)
   c. Pheochromocytoma (0.2%)
   d. Cushing's syndrome (0.2%)
4. Coarctation of aorta (0.2%)

8.1 APPROACH TO THE HYPERTENSIVE PATIENT

1. Obtain pertinent history
   a. Age of onset of hypertension, previous antihypertensive therapy
   b. Family history of hypertension and cardiovascular disease
   c. Diet and salt intake, alcohol, drugs (e.g., oral contraceptives, NSAIDs, decongestants, steroids, cyclosporine)
   d. Occupation and life-style, socioeconomic status, psychological factors
   e. Other cardiovascular risk factors: hyperlipidemia, obesity, diabetes mellitus, carbohydrate intolerance
   f. Symptoms of secondary hypertension
      (1) Headache, palpitations, excessive perspiration (possible pheochromocytoma)
      (2) Weakness, polyuria (consider hyperaldosteronism)
      (3) Claudication of lower extremities (seen with coarctation of aorta)
2. Physical exam
   a. Evaluate skin for presence of café au lait spots (neurofibromatosis), uremic appearance (chronic renal failure), striae (Cushing's syndrome)

77

Table 8-1 Classification of blood pressure (mm Hg, or torr) in adults aged 18 yr or older*

BP Range (mm Hg)	Category†
DBP	
<85	Normal BP
85-89	High-normal BP
90-104	Mild hypertension
105-114	Moderate hypertension
≥115	Severe hypertension
SBP when DBP <90 mm Hg	
<140	Normal BP
140-159	Borderline isolated systolic hypertension
≥160	Isolated systolic hypertension

*Classification based on the average of two or more readings on two or more occasions. BP indicates blood pressure; DBP, diastolic blood pressure; and SBP, systolic blood pressure.
†A classification of borderline isolated systolic hypertension (SBP, 140 to 159 mm Hg) or isolated systolic hypertension (SBP, ≥ 160 mm Hg) takes precedence over high-normal BP (DBP, 85 to 89 mm Hg) when both occur in the same person. High-normal BP (DBP, 85 to 89 mm Hg) takes precedence over a classification of normal BP (SBP, <140 mm Hg) when both occur in the same person.
From 1988 Report of the Joint National Committee on Detection, Evaluation, and Treatment of High Blood Pressure, Arch Intern Med 148:1023, 1988.

    b. Perform careful funduscopic exam: check for papilledema, retinal exudates, hemorrhages, arterial narrowing, AV compression
    c. Perform extensive cardiopulmonary exam: check for loud aortic component of S_2, S_4, ventricular lift
    d. Check abdomen for masses (pheochromocytoma), polycystic kidneys, presence of bruits over the renal arteries (renal artery stenosis), dilation of the aorta
    e. Measure blood pressure in both upper extremities (if values are discrepant, use the higher value)
    f. Examine arterial pulses (dilated or absent femoral pulses and blood pressure greater in upper extremities than lower extremities suggests aortic coarctation).
    g. Note the presence of truncal obesity (Cushing's syndrome) and pedal edema (CHF, nephrosis)
3. Lab evaluation
    a. Urinalysis: examine sediment for evidence of renal disease
    b. BUN, creatinine: to rule out renal disease
    c. Serum potassium level: low potassium is suggestive of primary aldosteronism
    d. CBC: for a baseline value before starting therapy
    e. Screen for coexisting diseases that may adversely effect prognosis
      (1) Fasting serum glucose
      (2) Serum cholesterol

(3) Serum triglycerides, HDL, and LDL (only if hypercholesterolemia is detected)
4. ECG: check for presence of left ventricular hypertrophy (LVH) with strain pattern
5. Chest x-ray film is not routinely advocated; may be useful to evaluate cardiac size, presence of LVH, and rib notching (aortic coarctation)
6. Additional tests if particular causes of hypertension are suspected
   a. If pheochromocytoma or Cushing's disease are suspected, refer to Chapter 22 for diagnostic evaluation
   b. Renovascular hypertension[10] (RVH): The two major causes are atherosclerotic lesions (60-70%) and fibromuscular dysplasias
      (1) Renal arteriography is the "gold standard" if renal artery stenosis is suspected; findings diagnostic of renal artery stenosis are: stenosis >70%, presence of collateral renal arteries, or poststenotic dilation
      (2) Renal ultrasound (unilateral small kidney) and enalapril renography are often used as screening tests in RVH
      (3) Measurement of plasma renin activity from each renal vein can also provide valuable diagnostic information:
         • A ratio >1.6:1 of affected to unaffected side is suggestive of renovascular hypertension
         • Renin response to captopril is useful for identifying patients with renovascular disease; these patients exhibit greater depressor responses to captopril and also greater reactive increases in plasma renin[6]
7. Factors adversely affecting prognosis
   a. Preventable factors: smoking, obesity, hypercholesterolemia, poorly controlled DM
   b. Uncontrollable factors: early age of onset, male sex, black race
   c. Evidence of end organ damage
      (1) Heart (LVH, MI, CHF)
      (2) Eyes (exudates, papilledema, hemorrhages)
      (3) Kidney (renal insufficiency)
      (4) CNS (CVA)

8.2 MEDICAL THERAPY

1. Initial treatment of patients with high normal or mild hypertension is nonpharmacological, aimed at reduction of blood pressure and other cardiovascular risk factors:
   a. Sodium restriction
   b. Weight loss if the patient is obese
   c. Regular aerobic exercise
   d. Behavior modification to decrease stress
   e. Restriction of alcohol, avoidance of tobacco
2. Reevaluate patient after 4-6 wk; if the patient is still hypertensive, drug therapy is appropriate (Fig. 8-1)
3. In patients with mild-moderate hypertension and/or significant risk factors for cardiovascular disease, initial pharmacologic treatment may be

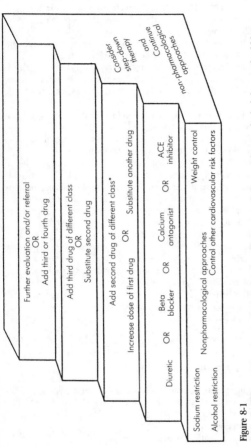

Figure 8-1

Individualized step-care therapy for hypertension. For some patients, nonpharmacological therapy should be tried first. If the blood pressure goal is not achieved, add pharmacological therapy. Other patients may require pharmacological therapy initially. In these instances nonpharmacological measures may be a helpful adjunct. ACE denotes angiotensin-converting enzyme; asterisk (*), drugs such as diuretics, β-blockers, calcium antagonists, ACE inhibitors, α-blockers, centrally acting α_2-agonists, *Rauwolfia serpentina*, and vasodilators. (From 1988 Report of the Joint National Committee on Detection, Evaluation, and Treatment of High Blood Pressure, Arch Intern Med 148:1023, 1988.)

appropriate. The 1988 Joint National Committee on Hypertension recommends one of four major classes of antihypertensives as initial drug therapy: diuretics, beta blockers, calcium antagonists, or ACE inhibitors. Therapy is individualized after consideration of concomitant diseases (Table 8-2), age, race, and life-style. In addition to being effective, the antihypertensive agent should improve the cardiovascular risk factors, with the least interference in quality of life. The advantages and limitations of each of these four classes of drugs are described below:

a. Diuretics: Table 33-24 describes the commonly used diuretics
    (1) Advantages
        - Inexpensive, once/day dosing
        - Useful in blacks, edema states, CHF, chronic renal disease (loop diuretics are more effective than thiazides), elderly patients (use only very low doses)
        - Decreased incidence of hip fractures in elderly patients[5]
    (2) Disadvantages
        - Significant adverse metabolic effects (Table 8-3). Indapamide (an indoline diuretic), unlike thiazides, has a neutral effect on lipids
        - Increased risk of cardiac dysrhythmias, sexual dysfunction

b. Beta blockers: Table 33-18 describes the various beta blockers. These agents differ significantly from one another in terms of differential blockade of beta$_1$ and beta$_2$ receptors, lipid solubility, intrinsic sympathomimetic activity, and metabolic clearance rate. The use of beta$_2$ selective agents ameliorates some of the disadvantages of the beta blockers. Labetalol also has alpha-blocking activity and no deleterious effect on peripheral blood flow or concomitant renal disease.
    (1) Advantages
        - Ideal in hypertensive patients with ischemic heart disease or post-MI
        - Favored in hyperkinetic young patients (resting tachycardia, wide pulse pressure, and hyperdynamic chest walls)
    (2) Disadvantages
        - Adverse effect on quality of life (increased incidence of fatigue, depression, impotence)
        - Aggravation of CHF, bronchospasm, hyperglycemia, peripheral vascular disease; adverse effects on lipids (Table 8-3), masking of signs and symptoms of hypoglycemia in diabetics

c. Calcium antagonists: Table 33-19 compares the various calcium antagonists. They represent a heterogeneous group of compounds with different mechanism of action and side effects. Dihydropyridine agents (e.g., nifedipine, nicardipine) are primarily potent vasodilators. Their major side effects are peripheral edema, flushing, and dizziness. Non-dihydropyridine agents (e.g., verapamil, diltiazem) produce coronary vasodilation and decrease heart rate. Constipation and conduction abnormalities are notable side effects.
    (1) Advantages
        - Helpful in hypertensive patients with ischemic heart disease
        - Generally favorable effect on quality of life

Table 8-2 Effect of coexisting morbidity on the selection of antihypertensive agents

Condition	Preferred Drugs	Drugs to be Avoided
Diabetes mellitus	ACE inhibitors Alpha$_1$ blockers (e.g., prazosin) Calcium antagonists	Beta blockers Diuretics
CHF	ACE inhibitors Diuretics	Beta blockers Selected calcium antagonists (verapamil, diltiazem)
Ischemic heart disease	Alpha$_1$ blockers Beta blockers Calcium antagonists	Diuretics Hydralazine Alpha$_1$ blockers
COPD/bronchospasm	Calcium antagonists ACE inhibitors Diuretics	Beta blockers
Peripheral vascular disease	Calcium antagonists ACE inhibitors Diuretics	Beta blockers
Sexual dysfunction	ACE inhibitors Calcium antagonists	Beta blockers Centrally acting alpha blockers (e.g., methyldopa) Diuretics
Hyperlipidemia	Alpha$_1$ blockers Calcium antagonists ACE inhibitors	Diuretics (except indapamide) Beta blockers
Chronic renal failure	Loop diuretics ACE inhibitors* Calcium antagonists	Beta blockers Potassium sparing diuretics

*Use with caution; monitor renal function frequently.

Table 8-3 Effects of antihypertensive agents on lipid profile, blood pH, serum electrolytes

Agent	Total Cholesterol	LDL Cholesterol	HDL Cholesterol	Triglycerides	pH	Uric Acid	K$^+$	Mg^{2+}	Ca^{2+}	Na$^+$
Thiazide diuretics	—/↑	↑/↑	↑/↑	↑	Alkalosis	↑	↓	↓	↑	↓
Beta blockers	—	—	↓/↑	↑	Acidosis	—	—/↑	—	—	↑/↓
Calcium antagonists	—	↓/↑	—	—	? Acidosis	—	↓	↑	↓	↑/↓
ACE inhibitors	—	↓/↑	—	—	Acidosis	—	—	—	—	→
Alpha$_1$ adrenergic blockers	↓	↓/↑	—/↑	—/↓		—	—	—	—	—

Key: ↑, increased; ↓, decreased; —, no change; K$^+$, potassium; Mg^{2+}, magnesium; Ca^{2+}, calcium; Na$^+$, sodium

- Can be used in bronchospastic disorders, renal disease, peripheral vascular disease, metabolic disorders (gout, diabetes, hyperlipidemias), and salt-sensitive hypertensives (in whom diuretics are not desirable)

  (2) Disadvantages
  - Excessive cost
  - Verapamil and diltiazem should be avoided in CHF because of their chronotropic and inotropic effects
  - Pedal edema often seen with nifedipine; constipation can be severe in elderly patients on verapamil

  d. ACE inhibitors: These agents have similar efficacy and mechanism of action. Their major differences are in their duration of action (enalapril, lisinopril are longer acting than captopril) and side effects (coughing is most common with enalapril, rash and taste disturbances occur more frequently with captopril). Table 33-1 describes the characteristics of the various ACE inhibitors.

  (1) Advantages
  - Well tolerated, favorable impact on quality of life
  - Useful in hypertension complicated by CHF
  - Helpful in prevention of diabetic renal disease
  - Effective in decreasing LVH

  (2) Disadvantages
  - Excessive cost
  - Hyperkalemia may occur in patients with diabetes or severe renal insufficiency
  - Less effective in black patients
  - Hypotension may occur in volume depleted patients
  - May worsen renal insufficiency

4. Subsequent therapy[7]: If the initial drug is inadequate to control the hypertension, there are three therapeutic options:
   a. Titrate the dose of the initial drug to the maximum recommended
   b. Add an agent from another class
   c. Discontinue the initial choice, and substitute a drug from another class

5. Treatment of renovascular hypertension (RVH)[10]: The therapeutic approach varies with the etiology of RVH
   a. Young patients with fibromuscular dysplasia are best treated with percutaneous transluminal renal angioplasty (PTRA).
   b. Medical therapy is advisable in elderly patients with atheromatous renovascular hypertension. Useful agents are
      (1) Beta blockers (very effective in beta with elevated plasma renin)
      (2) ACE inhibitors (very effective; however, should be avoided in patients with bilateral renal artery stenosis or in patients with a solitary kidney and renal stenosis)
      (3) Minoxidil (combined with a beta blocker to attenuate reflex tachycardia) is useful in RVH resistant to other agents
      (4) Diuretics are often used in combination with beta blockers, ACE inhibitors, or minoxidil because of the significant sodium and water retention associated with RVH

c. Surgical revascularization is generally reserved for atheromatous RVH in patients responding poorly to medical therapy (uncontrolled hypertension, deteriorating renal function).

6. Drug therapy in the hypertensive pregnant patient
   a. The American Obstetrical Committee defines 130/80 mm Hg as the upper limit of normal at any time during pregnancy.
   b. A rise of 30 mm Hg systolic or 15 mm Hg diastolic is also considered abnormal regardless of the absolute values obtained.
   c. When the blood pressure does not respond to bed rest and proper diet, antihypertensive drug therapy is started with one of the following agents: methyldopa, hydralazine, or beta adrenergic blockers.

 HYPERTENSIVE EMERGENCIES

Definition

Hypertensive emergencies are potentially life-threatening situations that are secondary to elevated blood pressure. The rate of blood pressure rise is a critical factor. Clinical manifestations consist of grade IV hypertensive retinopathy (exudates, hemorrhages, and papilledema) and/or cardiovascular compromise.

Therapy

Hypertensive emergencies should be treated immediately. The choice of therapeutic agent varies with the cause of the hypertensive crisis. Table 8-4 lists medications commonly used in hypertensive emergencies. All of the drugs require close monitoring of the patient's blood pressure (preferably with an arterial line in an ICU).

Two newer antihypertensives with potential use in hypertensive emergencies are

1. Dilevatol, an isomer of labetalol. It lowers blood pressure through reduction of peripheral vascular resistance. It has the advantage of producing gradual, controlled lowering of both systolic and diastolic blood pressure without need for intraarterial monitoring[8].
2. Nicardipine, a water-soluble dihydropyridine calcium antagonist. It is effective when administered IV to patients with severe hypertension[9] (Table 8-4).

Both these agents can be used orally following adequate blood pressure control with the intravenous doses.

The following are three important points to consider when treating hypertensive emergencies:

1. A plan for long-term therapy should be introduced at the time of the initial emergency treatment.
2. Agents that reduce arterial pressure can cause the kidneys to retain sodium and water; therefore, the judicious administration of diuretics should accompany their use.[2]
3. Cerebral hypoperfusion may occur if the mean blood pressure is lowered >40% in the initial 24 hr.[1]

Table 8-4 Drug therapy of hypertensive emergencies[3,4]

Drug	Onset of Action	Duration	Dosage	Mechanism of Action
Nitroprusside (Nipride)	Immediate	<3 min	IV infusion 50 mg/500 ml of D_5W at a rate of 0.5-0.8 $\mu g/kg/min$ Titrate to blood pressure Maximum dosage is 10 $\mu g/kg/min$ (refer to Chapter 32 for additional information on nitroprusside)	Vasodilation
Diazoxide (Hyperstat)	1-5 min	6-12 hr	IV injection 25-150 mg over 5 min or IV infusion at 30 mg/min until desired effect	Vasodilation
Hydralazine (Apresoline)	15-20 min	3-6 hr	IM/IV 10-40 mg q4-6h prn	Vasodilation
Trimethaphan (Arfonad)	Immediate	10-15 min	IV infusion 500 mg/500 ml D_5W at 1 mg/ml Titrate to blood pressure	Ganglionic blockade
Nifedipine (Procardia)	1-5 min	3-5 hr	10 mg capsule SL*	Vasodilation
Labetalol (Trandate)	5-10 min	3-6 hr	20 mg by slow IV injection over 2 min (may repeat with 40-80 mg q10 min, do not exceed 300 mg total)	β-Blocker, α-1-vasodilator
Nicardipine†	1-5 min	3-6 hr	5 mg/hr, increase by 2 mg/hr every 15 min; maximum dosage is 15 mg/hr	Vasodilation

*Perforate capsule (5-10 holes with small needle) and ask patient to chew the capsule and expel material contained within.[4]
†Pending FDA approval.

Indications	Contraindications	Side Effects
Drug of choice in: Hypertensive encephalopathy Hypertension and intracranial bleed Malignant hypertension Hypertension and heart failure Dissecting aortic aneurysm (used in combination with propranolol)	Hypersensitivity to nitroprusside	Nausea, apprehension, thiocyanate toxicity
Second drug of choice in: Hypertensive encephalopathy Malignant hypertension	Ischemic heart disease Intracranial hemorrhage	Tachycardia, nausea, hyperglycemia, sodium retention, cardiac ischemia
Drug of choice in eclampsia	Hypertension with heart failure	Tachycardia, cardiac ischemia
Drug of choice in dissecting aortic aneurysm (if propranolol cannot be used with nitroprusside)	Hypertension and renal failure	Urinary retention, paralytic ileus, tachyphylaxis
Severe hypertension	Hypersensitivity to nifedipine	Headache, palpitations, fluid retention
Severe hypertension	Bronchial asthma, CHF, bradycardia, second- or third-degree heart block, cardiogenic shock	Postural hypotension, dizziness, fatigue, nausea, bronchoconstriction
Treatment of hypertensive crisis	Hypersensitivity to nicardipine	Headache, nausea, vomiting, hypotension

References

1. Dinsdale HB: Hypertensive encephalopathy, Neurol Clin 1:3, 1983.
2. Frolich ED: Practical management of hypertension, Curr Probl Cardiol 10(7):1, 1985.
3. Goldberger E: Treatment of cardiac emergencies, ed 4, St Louis, 1985, The CV Mosby Co.
4. Haft JI, Litterer WG III: Chewing nifedipine to rapidly treat hypertension, Arch Intern Med 144:2357, 1984.
5. LaCroix AZ, et al: Thiazide diuretic agents and the incidence of hip fracture, N Engl J Med 322:286, 1990.
6. Muller RB, et al: The captopril test for identifying renovascular disease in hypertensive patients, Am J Med 80:633, 1986.
7. Report of the Joint National Committee on Detection, Evaluation, and Treatment of High Blood Pressure, Arch Intern Med 148:1023, 1988.
8. Wallin JD, Cook E, et al: Dilevatol in severe hypertension: a multicenter trial of bolus intravenous dosing, Arch Intern Med 149:2655, 1989.
9. Wallin JD, Fletcher E, et al: Intravenous nicardipine for the treatment of severe hypertension, Arch Intern Med 149:2662, 1989.
10. Working Group on Renovascular Hypertension: Detection, evaluation, and treatment of renovascular hypertension, Arch Intern Med 147:820, 1987.

Dyslipoproteinemias

Definition
A dyslipoproteinemia is an abnormality of lipid metabolism or transport manifested by elevation of cholesterol and/or triglyceride levels.

Relationship to coronary artery disease
Increased levels of LDL cholesterol, low levels of HDL cholesterol, or cholesterol/HDL ratio >4.5 are associated with increased risk of coronary artery disease.

Classification of lipoprotein abnormalities
Table 9-1 describes the classification and clinical manifestations of the various lipoprotein abnormalities.

Diagnostic approach[1]
1. The total blood cholesterol level is the basis for the initial classification:

   <200 mg/dl—desirable
   200-239 mg/dl—borderline-high
   ≥240 mg/dl—high

2. All blood cholesterol levels above 200 mg/dl should be confirmed by repeat measurement, with the average used to guide clinical decisions.
3. Lipoprotein analysis (HDL-cholesterol and triglycerides) should be performed in patients with high or borderline-high cholesterol, particularly if the patient has any of the following coronary heart disease (CHD) factors:
   a. Male sex
   b. Family history of premature CHD (definite myocardial infarction or sudden death before age 55 in a parent or sibling)
   c. Cigarette smoking (currently more than ten/day)
   d. Hypertension
   e. Low HDL-cholesterol (below 35 mg/dl confirmed by repeat measurement)
   f. Diabetes mellitus
   g. History of definite cerebrovascular or occlusive peripheral vascular disease

Table 9-1 Classification and clinical manifestations of dyslipoproteinemias

Type	I	IIa	IIb	III	IV	V
Plasma lipoprotein pattern	↑ Chylomicrons	↑ LDL	↑ LDL, ↑ VLDL	↑ Abnormal ILDL	↑ VLDL	↑ VLDL, ↑ chylomicrons
Cholesterol	N	↑	↑	↑	N	N/↑
Triglyceride	↑	N	↑	↑	↑	↑
Prevalence	Very rare	Common	Common	Uncommon	Common	Uncommon
Risk of atherogenesis	No increase	↑↑	↑↑	↑↑	No increase/mild	No increase
Clinical signs and symptoms	Eruptive xanthomas Pancreatitis Lipemia retinalis Hepatosplenomegaly	Xanthelasma Tuberous xanthomas Tendinous xanthomas Arcus corneae	Xanthelasma Tuberous xanthomas Tendinous xanthomas Arcus corneae	Tuberous xanthomas Tendinous xanthomas Peripheral vascular disease ↑ Incidence of diabetes mellitus Hyperuricemia	↑ Incidence of diabetes mellitus Hyperuricemia Infrequent eruptive and tuberous xanthomas	Eruptive xanthomas Pancreatitis ↑ Incidence of diabetes mellitus Lipemia retinalis Arthritis Emotional lability

KEY: ↑, increased; N, normal; ILDL, intermediate low density lipoprotein; LDL, low density lipoprotein; VLDL, very low density lipoprotein

  h. Severe obesity (≥30% of overweight)
4. If triglycerides are <400 mg/dl, LDL cholesterol can be calculated us-
    ing the following formula:

$$\text{LDL cholesterol} = \text{Total cholesterol} - \text{HDL cholesterol} - (\text{Triglycerides}/5)$$

5. Further treatment is based on the LDL cholesterol levels (Fig. 9-1).

Medical management[1]

1. Dietary treatment is the cornerstone of therapy to reduce blood choles-
    terol levels and to promote weight loss in the overweight patient.
    a. Step One: Saturated fat intake <10% of calories; total fat intake
        <30% of calories; dietary cholesterol intake <300 mg/day
    b. Step Two: Further reduction in saturated fat intake to <7% of calo-
        ries, and in dietary cholesterol to <200 mg/day
2. For most patients dietary therapy should be continued for at least 6 mo
    before deciding whether to add drug treatment.
3. The therapeutic goals recommended, like the cholesterol levels for initi-
    ating therapy, are influenced by the presence of definite CHD or other
    CHD-risk factors. Patients with neither CHD nor two other risk factors
    should reduce LDL-cholesterol to below 160 mg/dl. Patients with defi-
    nite CHD or two other CHD-risk factors should have a goal of reducing
    LDL-cholesterol to below 130 mg/dl.
4. The recommended goals are minimal. If lower ones can be achieved,
    risk may be further reduced.
5. Although the goal of therapy is to lower LDL-cholesterol concentration,
    total cholesterol can be used to monitor response to diet for conve-
    nience.
6. Fig. 9-2 illustrates the approach to dietary management.
7. Drug therapy is indicated (following appropriate dietary treatment) in
    patients with LDL-cholesterol of ≥190 mg/dl and those with LDL-cho-
    lesterol 169-189 mg/dl who also have definite CHD or two other risk
    factors.
8. Fig. 9-3 illustrates the approach to drug treatment.
9. Table 33-21 compares the various cholesterol-lowering agents.

Reference

1. Report of the National Cholesterol Education Program Expert Panel on Detection,
   Evaluation, and Treatment of High Blood Cholesterol in Adults, Arch Intern Med
   148:36, 1988.

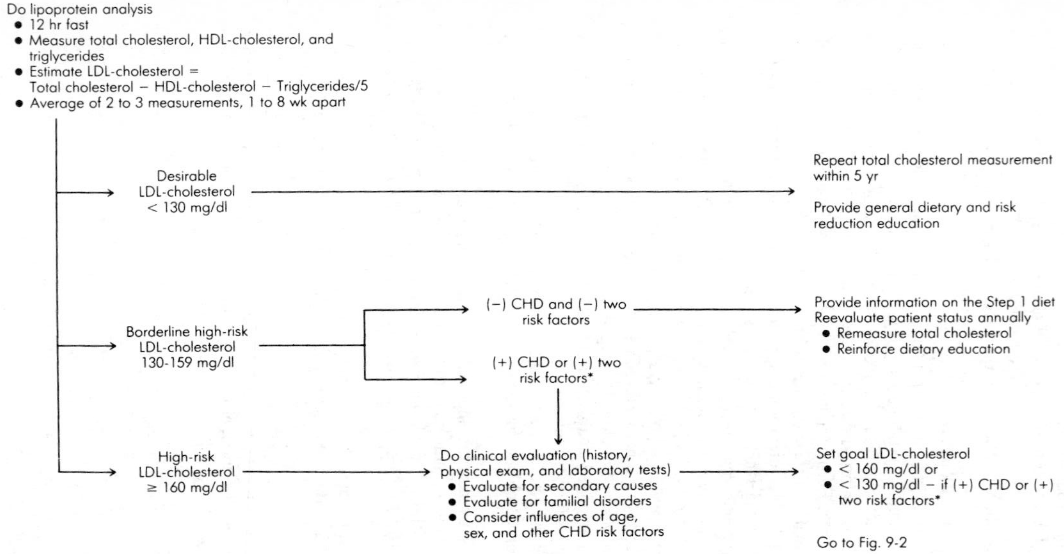

Do lipoprotein analysis
● 12 hr fast
● Measure total cholesterol, HDL-cholesterol, and triglycerides
● Estimate LDL-cholesterol =
  Total cholesterol – HDL-cholesterol – Triglycerides/5
● Average of 2 to 3 measurements, 1 to 8 wk apart

Desirable
LDL-cholesterol
< 130 mg/dl

→ Repeat total cholesterol measurement within 5 yr

Provide general dietary and risk reduction education

Borderline high-risk
LDL-cholesterol
130-159 mg/dl

High-risk
LDL-cholesterol
≥ 160 mg/dl

(–) CHD and (–) two risk factors

→ Provide information on the Step 1 diet
Reevaluate patient status annually
● Remeasure total cholesterol
● Reinforce dietary education

(+) CHD or (+) two risk factors*

→ Do clinical evaluation (history, physical exam, and laboratory tests)
● Evaluate for secondary causes
● Evaluate for familial disorders
● Consider influences of age, sex, and other CHD risk factors

Set goal LDL-cholesterol
● < 160 mg/dl or
● < 130 mg/dl – if (+) CHD or (+) two risk factors*

Go to Fig. 9-2

Figure 9-1

Classification based on low density lipoprotein (LDL)–cholesterol. Asterisk indicates that one risk factor can be male sex. CHD, Coronary heart disease; HDL, high-density lipoprotein. (Reproduced from Report of the National Cholesterol Education Program Expert Panel on Detection, Evaluation, and Treatment of High Blood Cholesterol in Adults, Arch Intern Med 148:36, 1988.)

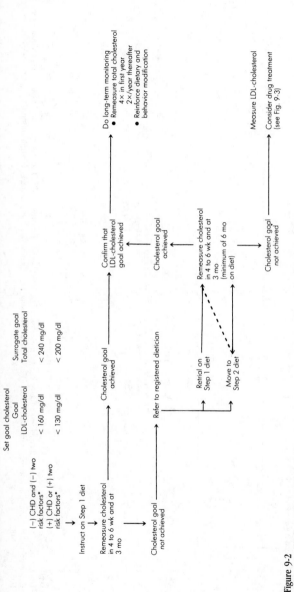

Figure 9-2

Dietary treatment. Asterisk indicates that one risk factor can be male sex. LDL, Low density lipoprotein; CHD, coronary artery disease. (Reproduced from Report of the National Cholesterol Education Program Expert Panel on Detection, Evaluation, and Treatment of High Blood Cholesterol in Adults, Arch Intern Med 148:36, 1988.)

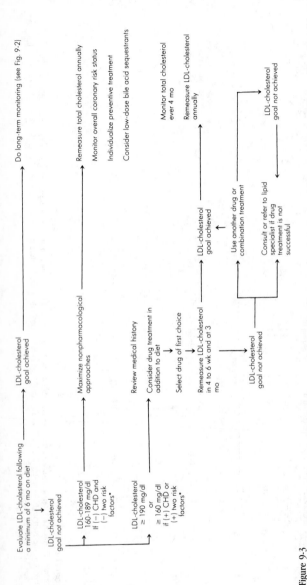

Figure 9-3
Drug treatment. Asterisk indicates that one risk factor can be male sex. LDL, Low density lipoprotein; CHD, coronary heart disease. (Reproduced from Report of the National Cholesterol Education Program Expert Panel on Detection, Evaluation, and Treatment of High Blood Cholesterol in Adults, Arch Intern Med 148:36, 1988.)

Eating Disorders

10

10.1   ANOREXIA NERVOSA

Definition

Anorexia nervosa is a prolonged illness that occurs mostly in female adolescents. It is characterized by severe self-induced weight loss, amenorrhea, and a specific psychopathology.[5]

Diagnosis[1]

1. An intense fear of becoming obese that does not diminish as weight loss progresses
2. Disturbance of body image (e.g., claiming to "feel fat" even when emaciated)
3. Weight loss of at least 25% of original body weight; if under 18 years of age, weight loss from original body weight plus weight gain expected from growth charts may be combined to make 25%
4. Refusal to maintain body weight over minimum normal weight for age and height
5. In females absence of at least three consecutive menstrual cycles when otherwise expected to occur

Clinical features

1. Amenorrhea
2. Sleep disturbances
3. Cold intolerance
4. Early satiety, abdominal pain, and constipation or diarrhea
5. Inability to interpret emotions correctly (alexithymia)

Physical exam

1. Severe malnutrition (cachexia), often masked by oversized clothes
2. Bradycardia, hypotension, hypothermia, bradypnea
3. Dry skin with excessive growth of lanugo
4. Peripheral edema may be present
5. Females represent 90% of cases

Lab results

1. Endocrine abnormalities[2]
   a. Decreased FSH, LH, T_4, T_3, estrogens, urinary 17-OH steroids, estrone, and estradiol
   b. Normal free T_4, TSH
   c. Increased cortisol, GH, rT_3, T_3RU
   d. Absence of cyclic surge of LH
2. Leukopenia, thrombocytopenia, anemia
3. Increased plasma β-carotene levels are useful to distinguish these patients from others on starvation diets

Treatment

1. Hyperalimentation of severely malnourished patients
2. Feed with assistance; patient should never eat alone and observation by the nursing staff or family is recommended
3. Psychiatric evaluation and therapy
4. Routine monitoring of patients with prolonged QT interval; sudden death in these patients is often caused by ventricular tachydysrhythmias related to QT interval prolongation[3]

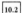 **BULIMIA**

Definition

Bulimia is characterized by episodic and uncontrollable eating binges, self-induced vomiting, repeated attempts at weight loss by severe dieting aided by vomiting and laxatives, depressed mood, and self-deprecation following binges.[2] These patients have a persistent overconcern with body shape and weight and experience at least two binge eating episodes per week for at least 3 mo.[1]

Clinical features

In a study of 275 bulimic patients, Mitchel et al.[4] noted the following features:

1. Eating binges: 100%
2. Self-induced vomiting: 88%
3. Laxative abuse: 60%
4. Diuretic abuse: 33%
5. Problems with alcohol or other drugs: 33%
6. Mean age of patients at the onset of bulimia, 17 yr

Physical exam

1. Scars on the back of the hand from rubbing against the upper incisors when inducing vomiting
2. Patient is not usually emaciated and the physical exam may be entirely normal

Lab results

1. Electrolyte abnormalities secondary to vomiting (hypokalemia and metabolic alkalosis) or to diarrhea (hypokalemia and hyperchloremic metabolic acidosis)

Therapy

1. Psychiatric evaluation and therapy
2. Management of medical complications

References

1. Diagnostic and statistical manual of mental disorders III, Washington DC, 1980, American Psychiatric Association.
2. Federman DD: Pituitary. In Rubenstein E, Federman DD (editors): Scientific American medicine, New York, 1986, Scientific American Inc.
3. Isner JM, et al: Sudden death in anorexia nervosa, Ann Intern Med 102:49, 1985.
4. Mitchell JE, et al: Characteristics of 275 patients with bulimia, Am J Psychiatry 142:482, 1985.
5. Russell GFM: Anorexia nervosa. In Wyngaarden JB, Smith LA (editors): Cecil Textbook of medicine, ed 17, Philadelphia, 1985, WB Saunders Co.

11

Adult Respiratory
Distress Syndrome

Definition

The adult respiratory distress syndrome (ARDS) is characterized by acute diffuse infiltrative lung lesions with resulting interstitial and alveolar edema, severe hypoxemia, and respiratory failure.

Etiology

1. Sepsis (bacterial, viral, fungal) >50% of cases
2. Drugs (e.g., overdose of morphine, methadone, or heroin, reaction to nitrofurantoin)
3. Aspiration (e.g., near drowning, aspiration of gastric contents)
4. Noxious inhalation (e.g., chlorine gas, high O_2 concentrations)
5. Post-resuscitation, shock, and other low-flow states
6. Trauma, burns
7. Other: Pancreatitis, head injury, blood products, miliary TB

Pathophysiology[2]

1. Early ARDS: Sequestration and degranulation of granulocytes in the pulmonary microcirculation
2. Later stages: Alveolar edema secondary to damage to the alveolar-capillary membrane is a characteristic finding; subsequently hyaline membranes can be found in the alveoli and alveolar ducts; eventually severe proliferative tissue reactions lead to progressive and diffuse fibrosis of the lungs

Clinical characteristics

1. Physical exam: tachypnea, dyspnea, tachycardia
2. Chest x-ray: initially normal, bilateral generalized interstitial infiltrates in advanced stages
3. ABGs: decreased P_{O_2}, decreased P_{CO_2}, increased alveolar-arterial O_2 difference

Management

1. Maintain $P_{O_2} \geq 60$ mm Hg with minimal FI_{O_2} (since excess O_2 per se may cause ARDS). Positive end-expiratory pressure (PEEP) is useful to

keep alveoli open. PEEP is generally started at 5 cm of H_2O and increased by increments of 2-5 cm to maintain the Po_2 ≥60 mm Hg. Insertion of a pulmonary catheter is useful to monitor cardiac output since high levels of PEEP will decrease venous return and pulmonary vascular resistance. Wedge pressure (PCWP) should be kept at 8-12 mm Hg to decrease movement of fluid in the alveoli.

2. Treat the underlying cause of ARDS (e.g., antibiotics for sepsis).
3. Nutritional support is needed to maintain adequate colloid oncotic pressure and intravascular volume.
4. High-dose methylprednisolone (30 mg/kg q6h for 24 hr) has no beneficial effect on patient survival or reversal of respiratory failure.[1]

Prognosis

The prognosis for ARDS varies with the underlying cause. Overall mortality exceeds 50%.

References

1. Bernard GR, et al: High-dose corticosteroids in patients with the adult respiratory distress syndrome, N Engl J Med 317:1565, 1987.
2. Modig J: Adult respiratory distress syndrome; pathophysiology and inflammatory mediators in bronchoalveolar lavage, Prog Clin Biol Res 308:17, 1989.

Venous Thromboembolism

Risk factors

1. Prolonged immobilization
2. Postoperative state
3. Trauma to pelvis and lower extremities
4. Birth control pill
5. Visceral cancer (lung, pancreas, alimentary tract, GU tract)
6. Age over 60 yr
7. Prior history of thromboembolic disease
8. Hematologic disorders (e.g., antithrombin III deficiency, protein C deficiency, protein S deficiency, lupus anticoagulant, dysfibrinogenemias, anticardiolipin [aCL] antibody)
9. Pregnancy and early puerperium
10. Obesity
11. Surgery, fracture, or injury involving lower leg or pelvis
12. Surgery requiring ≥30 min of anesthesia
13. Gynecological surgery (particularly gynecological cancer surgery)

Diagnosis

The clinical diagnosis of deep venous thrombosis (DVT) is inaccurate. Pain, tenderness, swelling, or color changes are not specific for DVT. Commonly used objective tests for DVT are described in Table 12-1. The suggested diagnostic approach is illustrated in Fig. 12-1.

Therapy

Guidelines for antithrombotic therapy with heparin and warfarin in venous thromboembolism are presented in Table 12-2. A 5-day course of heparin is as effective as longer courses in treating DVT and provides substantial cost savings.[1]

Prophylaxis of DVT

1. Patients undergoing hip surgery or gynecological cancer surgery: external pneumatic compression of lower extremities (intermittent pneumatic compression [IPC] boots) plus low-dose warfarin started 1-2 days prior to surgery

Table 12-1 Diagnostic tests for venous thromboembolism[2]

Diagnostic Method	Advantages	Disadvantages
Contrast venography	"Gold standard" for evaluation of DVT of lower extremity	Invasive, painful Increased risk of phlebitis, new thrombosis, renal failure, and hypersensitivity reaction to contrast media Poor visualization of deep femoral vein in thigh and internal iliac vein and its tributaries
Impedance plethysmography (IPG)	Noninvasive Can be performed repeatedly (useful to monitor suspected acute DVT) Good correlation with contrast venography for proximal DVT	Poor sensitivity in calf-vein thrombi and non-obstructive proximal thrombi False positives in patients with peripheral vascular disease, right heart failure, postoperative lower extremity swelling, excessive leg tension, and in patients receiving mechanical ventilation
Compressive duplex ultrasonography	Noninvasive Can be repeated serially (useful to monitor suspected acute DVT) Good sensitivity for proximal thrombosis and thrombosis of lower popliteal vein Fewer false positives than IPG in patients with right heart failure or on mechanical ventilation	Poor visualization of deep femoral, iliac, and pelvic veins Requires skilled operator Poor sensitivity in isolated or nonocclusive calf vein thrombi

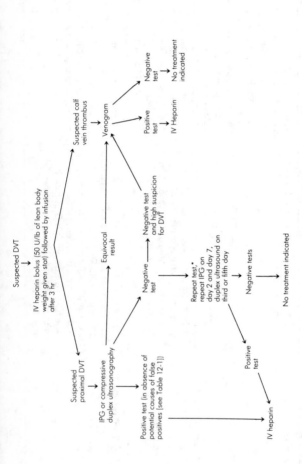

Figure 12-1
Evaluation of suspected DVT. Repeat noninvasive testing is necessary to diagnose patients with calf-vein thrombi who subsequently develop proximal thrombosis.

Table 12-2 Guidelines for Antithrombotic Therapy with Heparin and Warfarin in Venous Thromboembolism

Disease Suspected	Disease Confirmed
Obtain baseline APTT,* PT,† and platelet count and give heparin bolus (5000-10,000 U) IV; order diagnostic test, e.g., ventilation-perfusion lung scan, pulmonary angiogram, contrast venogram	Give loading dose of heparin (5000 U) and start constant IV infusion at approximately 1000 U/hr
	Monitor APTT at 6 hr and thereafter until the APTT is stabilized at 1.5-2 times control value
	Monitor platelet count every 3-4 days while administering heparin
	Start warfarin on day 1 or 2 by instituting the estimated daily maintenance dose (usually 5-10 mg)
	After at least 5 days of heparin and 4-5 days of joint therapy, stop heparin therapy and check PT 4 hr later
	Maintain PT off heparin therapy at 1.3-1.5 times control or pretreatment value
	Full-dose anticoagulation for at least 3 mo in patients without continuing risk factors, longer in other patients

*APTT, activated partial thromboplastin time.
†PT, 1-stage prothrombin time (1.3 times control performed with rabbit brain thromboplastin is roughly equal to 2 times control with human brain thromboplastin).
Reproduced from Hyers T, Hull R, Weg J: Chest 95(suppl):41S, 1989.

2. Gynecological surgery in patients over age 40 for benign conditions, urological and general abdominal surgery: low-dose heparin (5000 U SQ q8-12h) plus IPC boots or gradient elastic stockings (T.E.D. stockings)
3. Neurosurgery: gradient elastic stockings alone or in combination with IPC boots[4]; anticoagulants contraindicated
4. Patients with medical risk factors (e.g., prolonged bed rest secondary to CHF, stroke): gradient elastic stockings and/or low-dose SQ heparin

Laboratory evaluation of patients with DVT[3]

Admission laboratory evaluation (prior to anticoagulation) of young patients with venous thromboembolism, patients with recurrent thrombosis without obvious causes, and those with a family history of thrombotic disease should include protein S, protein C, fibrinogen, antithrombin III level, lupus anticoagulant, and anticardiolipin antibodies.

References

1. Hull RD, Raskob GE, et al: Heparin for 5 days as compared with 10 days in the initial treatment of proximal venous thrombosis, N Engl J Med 322:1260, 1990.
2. Moser KM: Pulmonary embolism: your challenge is prevention, J Resp Dis 10:83, 1989.
3. Rick ME: Protein C and protein S, vitamin K–dependent inhibitors of blood coagulation, JAMA 263:701, 1990.
4. Turpie AG, Hirsch J, et al: Prevention of deep vein thrombosis in potential neurosurgical patients, Arch Intern Med 149:679, 1989.

Syncope

Definition

Syncope is a temporary loss of consciousness resulting from an acute global reduction in cerebral blood flow.

Etiology[5]

1. Vasovagal (vasodepressor)
   a. Psychophysiologic (panic disorders, hysteria)
   b. Visceral reflex
   c. Carotid sinus
   d. Glossopharyngeal neuralgia
   e. Reduction of venous return due to Valsalva maneuver, cough, defecation, or micturition
2. Orthostatic hypotension
   a. Hypovolemia
   b. Hypotensive drugs
   c. Neurogenic, idiopathic
   d. Pheochromocytoma
   e. Systemic mastocytosis
3. Cardiac
   a. Reduced cardiac output
      (1) Left ventricular outflow obstruction (aortic stenosis, hypertrophic cardiomyopathy)
      (2) Obstruction to pulmonary flow (pulmonary embolism, pulmonic stenosis, primary pulmonary hypertension)
      (3) MI with pump failure
      (4) Cardiac tamponade
      (5) Mitral stenosis
   b. Dysrhythmias or asystole
      (1) Extreme tachycardia (>160-180/min)
      (2) Severe bradycardia (<30-40/min)
      (3) Sick sinus syndrome
      (4) AV block (second or third degree)
      (5) Ventricular tachycardia or fibrillation
      (6) Long QT syndrome
      (7) Pacemaker malfunction

4. Cerebrovascular
   a. Vertebrobasilar TIA, spasm
   b. Subclavian steal
   c. Basilar migraine
   d. Colloid cyst of the third ventricle
5. Other causes
   a. Mechanical reduction of venous return (atrial myxoma, ball valve thrombus)
   b. Not related to decreased blood flow: hypoxia, hypoglycemia, anemia, hyperventilation, seizure disorder, drug or alcohol abuse

Evaluation[3]

1. History
   a. Sudden loss of consciousness: consider cardiac dysrhythmias, vertebrobasilar TIA
   b. Gradual loss of consciousness: consider orthostatic hypotension, vasodepressor syncope, hypoglycemia
   c. Patient's activity at the time of syncope
      (1) Micturition, coughing, defecation: consider syncope secondary to decreased venous return
      (2) Turning his head while shaving: consider carotid sinus syndrome
      (3) Physical exertion in a patient with murmur: consider aortic stenosis
      (4) Arm exercise: consider subclavian steal syndrome
      (5) Assuming an upright position: consider orthostatic hypotension
   d. Associated events
      (1) Chest pain: consider MI, pulmonary embolism
      (2) Palpitations: consider dysrhythmias
      (3) History of aura, incontinence during episode, and transient confusion after "syncope": consider seizure disorder
   e. Current medications, particularly antihypertensive drugs
2. Physical exam
   a. Blood pressure: if low, consider orthostatic hypotension; if unequal in both arms (difference >20 mm Hg), consider subclavian steal or dissecting aneurysm; blood pressure and heart rate should be recorded in the supine, sitting, and standing positions
   b. Pulse: if patient has tachycardia, bradycardia, or irregular rhythm, consider dysrhythmia
   c. Mental status: if patient is confused after the syncopal episode consider postictal state
   d. Heart: if there are murmurs present suggestive of AS or IHSS, consider syncope secondary to left ventricular outflow obstruction; if there is JVD and distant heart sounds, consider cardiac tamponade
   e. Carotid sinus pressure can be diagnostic if it reproduces symptoms and other causes are excluded[4]; a pause ≥3 sec or a systolic BP drop >50 mm Hg without symptoms or <30 mm Hg with symptoms when sinus pressure is applied separately on each side for ≤5 sec is considered abnormal; this test should be avoided in patients with carotid bruits or cerebrovascular disease; ECG monitoring, IV access, and bedside atropine should be available when carotid sinus pressure is applied

3. Initial diagnostic tests
   a. CBC: rule out anemia, infection
   b. Electrolytes, BUN, creatinine, magnesium, and calcium: rule out electrolyte abnormalities, hypomagnesemia, and hypocalcemia; evaluate fluid status
   c. ECG: rule out dysrhythmias; may be diagnostic in 5-10% of patients
   d. Chest x-ray: evaluate cardiac size, lung fields
   e. ABG: rule out pulmonary embolus, hyperventilation
4. Additional diagnostic tests may be indicated depending on the patient's history and physical exam
   a. If dysrhythmias are suspected, a 24 hr Holter monitor and admission to a telemetry unit are appropriate; loop recorders that can be activated after a syncopal event and retrieve information about the cardiac rhythm during the preceding 4 min have added considerable diagnostic yield in patients with unexplained syncope[4]
   b. An echocardiogram is indicated in patients with a heart murmur to rule out AS, IHSS, or atrial myxoma
   c. If a seizure is suspected, a CT scan of head and an EEG are indicated
   d. If pulmonary embolism is suspected, a ventilation/perfusion scan should be done
   e. Cardiac isoenzymes should be obtained if the patient gives a history of chest pain before the syncopal episode
   f. Drug and alcohol levels when suspecting toxicity
   g. Electrophysiological studies may be indicated in patients with structural heart disease and/or recurrent syncope

Prognosis

The prognosis varies with the age of the patient and the etiology of the syncope. Various reports[1,2] indicate the following prognoses:
1. Benign prognosis (very low 1-year morbidity and mortality) in patients:
   a. Aged ≤30 and having noncardiac syncope
   b. Aged ≤70 and having vasovagal/psychogenic syncope or syncope of unknown cause
2. Poor prognosis (high morbidity and mortality) in patients with cardiac syncope

References

1. Day SC, et al: Evaluation and outcome of emergency room patients with transient loss of consciousness, Am J Med 73:15, 1982.
2. Eagle KA, et al: Evaluation and prognostic classifications for patients with syncope, Am J Med 79:455, 1985.
3. Kapoor WN: Evaluation of the patient with syncope, Cardiovasc Med, p 51, October 1985.
4. Manolis AS, Linzer M, et al: Syncope: current diagnostic evaluation and management, Ann Intern Med 112:850, 1990.
5. Plum F: Brief loss of consciousness. In Wyngaarden JB, Smith LA Jr (editors): Cecil Textbook of medicine, ed 17, Philadelphia, 1985, WB Saunders Co, vol 1.

Dementia

Marvin Garrell

Definition

The American Psychiatric Association's diagnostic criteria for delirium and dementia are described in the following lists. Delirium is mainly differentiated from the history—short onset within hours to a few weeks favors delirium, whereas chronic or gradual onset over time favors dementia. The history must be substantiated by the caregivers.

Etiology

The box on p. 111 lists the various causes of delirium and dementia.

Incidence and prevalence

The incidence and prevalence of physiologic dysfunction and psychiatric illness rise progressively with increasing age. More than a million Americans over 65 years old (and many others younger than 65) meet the criteria for dementia (see the diagnostic criteria on p. 110).

Diagnosis

Gray hair with confusion is not synonymous with dementia!

1. The elderly person whose clinical presentation suggests neuromuscular or mental derangement, whether chronic or acute, must be evaluated as if he or she has a diagnostic state of delirium
2. Physical abnormalities or dysfunctions can have an impact on cognitive and neuromuscular function and disrupt psychiatric homeostasis; systemic and metabolic abnormalities must be ruled out with thorough history, physical exam, and lab evaluation
3. The diagnostic evaluation should include the following:
   a. An attempt at the Folstein Mini–Mental State test (see box on next pages) to screen for dementia and also to document the progression of disease over time by repeating the test at 3- to 6-month intervals

DSM III Diagnostic Criteria for Delirium

A. Reduced ability to maintain attention to external stimuli (e.g., questions must be repeated because attention wanders) and to appropriately shift attention to new external stimuli (e.g., perseverates answer to a previous question)

B. Disorganized thinking, as indicated by rambling, irrelevant, or incoherent speech

C. At least two of the following:
   (1) Reduced level of consciousness (e.g., difficulty keeping awake during examination)
   (2) Perceptual disturbances: misinterpretations, illusions, or hallucinations
   (3) Disturbance of sleep-wake cycle with insomnia or daytime sleepiness
   (4) Increased or decreased psychomotor activity
   (5) Disorientation to time, place, or person
   (6) Memory impairment (e.g., inability to learn new material, such as the names of several unrelated objects after 5 min, or to remember past events, such as history of current episode of illness)

D. Clinical features develop over a short period of time (usually hours to days) and tend to fluctuate over the course of a day

E. Either (1) or (2):
   (1) Evidence from the history, physical examination, or laboratory tests of a specific organic factor (or factors) judged to be etiologically related to the disturbance.
   (2) In the absence of such evidence, an etiologic organic factor can be presumed if the disturbance cannot be accounted for by any nonorganic mental disorder (e.g., manic episode accounting for agitation and sleep disturbance)

From Diagnostic and statistical manual of mental disorders, III, Washington DC, 1987, American Psychiatric Association. Reprinted with permission.

b. One venipuncture for a profile of blood values:
   (1) Glucose
   (2) CBC
   (3) Electrolytes
   (4) AST, ALT
   (5) BUN, creatinine
   (6) VDRL
   (7) Calcium
   (8) Magnesium
   (9) HIV (selected patients)
   (10) T_4, TSH
   (11) Vitamin B_{12} level, folate

c. Depending on physical and history findings, other tests may include CT scan of head and spinal tap

DSM III Diagnostic Criteria for Dementia

A. Demonstrable evidence of impairment in short- and long-term memory. Impairment in short-term memory (inability to learn new information) may be indicated by inability to remember three objects after five minutes. Long-term memory impairment (inability to remember information that was known in the past) may be indicated by inability to remember past personal information (e.g., what happened yesterday, birthplace, occupation) or facts of common knowledge (e.g., past Presidents, well-known dates)

B. At least one of the following:
   (1) Impairment in abstract thinking, as indicated by inability to find similarities and differences between related words, difficulty in defining words and concepts, and other similar tasks
   (2) Impaired judgment, as indicated by inability to make reasonable plans to deal with interpersonal, family, and job-related problems and issues
   (3) Other disturbances of higher cortical function, such as aphasia (disorder of language), apraxia (inability to carry out motor activities despite intact comprehension and motor function), agnosia (failure to recognize or identify objects despite intact sensory function), and "constructional difficulty" (e.g., inability to copy three-dimensional figures, assemble blocks, or arrange sticks in specific designs)
   (4) Personality change, i.e., alteration or accentuation of premorbid traits

C. The disturbances in A and B significantly interfere with work or usual social activities or relationships with others

D. Not occurring exclusively during the course of Delirium

E. Either (1) or (2):
   (1) There is evidence from the history, physical examination, or laboratory tests of a specific organic factor (or factors) judged to be etiologically related to the disturbance
   (2) In the absence of such evidence, an etiologic organic factor can be presumed if the disturbance cannot be accounted for by any nonorganic mental disorder (e.g., Major Depression accounting for cognitive impairment)

Criteria for Severity of Dementia:

Mild: Although work or social activities are significantly impaired, the capacity for independent living remains, with adequate personal hygiene and relatively intact judgment

Moderate: Independent living is hazardous, and some degree of supervision is necessary

Severe: Activities of daily living are so impaired that continual supervision is required (e.g., unable to maintain minimal personal hygiene; largely incoherent or mute)

From Diagnostic and statistical manual of mental disorders, III, Washington DC, 1987, American Psychiatric Association. Reprinted with permission.

Confusion

Delirium

Drugs
Anticholinergics
Narcotics
Antidepressants
Anxiolytics
Methyldopa
β-blockers
Steroids
Non-steroidal antiinflammatory
 drugs
Phenytoin
Digoxin
Ethanol

Physical and Environmental
Stress of any type or source
Change in environment
Surgery
Anesthesia
Sleep loss
Pain
Fever or hypothermia

Fluids and Electrolytes
Hyponatremia
Hypernatremia
Hypovolemia
Hypervolemia
pH change
Hypercalcemia
Hypocalcemia
Hypomagnesemia

Systemic Changes
Infection (febrile or afebrile)
Vitamin deficiency
Fecal impaction
Urinary retention
Any abdominal disorders

Metabolic
Renal failure
Liver failure
Anemia
Thyroid dysfunction
Adrenal dysfunction
Hyperglycemia or
 hypoglycemia

CNS
Strokes
Seizure
Hematoma
Infection
Severe hypertension
Superimposed on dementia

Chest
Congestive failure
Hypercapnia
Hypoxemia
Rhythm disturbance
Acute MI

Dementia

Degenerative
Alzheimer-type disease
Parkinson's disease

Vascular
Multi-infarct
Arteritis

Infectious
HIV
Syphilis
Jakob Cruetzfeldt disease
Postencephalitic syndrome

Other
B_{12} deficiency
Vitamin deficiency
Chronic alcoholism
Subdural hematoma
Hydrocephalus
Chronic seizures
Hypothyroidism
Hearing loss
Blindness
Rule out depression

Mini–Mental State Examination

1. Orientation (maximum score 10)

   Ask, "What is today's date?" Then ask specifically for parts omitted; e.g., "Can you also tell me what season it is?"

   Ask, "Can you tell me the name of this hospital?"

   "What floor are we on?"

   "What town (or city) are we in?"

   "What county are we in?"

   "What state are we in?"

Date (e.g., January 21).	1____
Year	2____
Month.	3____
Day (e.g., Monday) . .	4____
Season	5____
Hospital	6____
Floor	7____
Town/city	8____
County	9____
State	10____

2. Registration (maximum score 3)

   Ask the subject if you may test his/her memory. Then say, "ball," "flag," "tree" clearly and slowly, about one second for each. After you have said all three words, ask subject to repeat them. This first repetition determines the score (0-3) but keep saying them (up to six trials) until the subject can repeat all three words. If (s)he does not eventually learn all three, recall cannot be meaningfully tested.

"ball"	11____
"flag"	12____
"tree"	13____

   Record number of trials:_____

3. Attention and calculation (maximum score 5)

   Ask the subject to begin at 100 and count backward by 7. Stop after five subtractions (93, 86, 79, 72, 65). Score one point for each correct number.

"93"	14____
"86"	15____
"79"	16____
"72"	17____
"65"	18____

   OR

   If the subject cannot or will not perform this task, ask him/her to spell the word "world" backwards (D, L, R, O, W). The score is one point for each correctly placed letter, e.g., DLROW = 5, DLORW = 3. Record how the subject spelled "world" backwards:

   Number of correctly placed letters . . . . . 19____

   ————
   DLROW

4. Recall (maximum score 3)
   Ask the subject to recall the three words you previously asked him/her to remember (learned in registration)

   "ball" . . . . .20___
   "flag" . . . . .21___
   "tree" . . . . .22___

5. Language (maximum score 9) Naming: show the subject a wristwatch and ask, "What is this?" Repeat for pencil. Score 1 point for each item named correctly

   Watch . . . . .23___
   Pencil . . . . .24___

   Repetition: ask the subject to repeat, "No ifs, ands, or buts." Score 1 point for correct repetition.

   Repetition . . . . . .25___

   Three-stage command: give the subject a piece of blank paper and say, "Take the paper in your right hand, fold it in half, and put it on the floor." Score 1 point for each action performed correctly

   Takes in right hand . .26___
   Folds in half . . . . .27___
   Puts on floor . . . . .28___

   Reading: on a blank piece of paper, print the sentence "Close your eyes." in letters large enough for the subject to see clearly. Ask subject to read it and do what it says. Score correct only if (s)he actually closes his/her eyes.

   Closes eyes . . . . .29___

   Writing: give the subject a blank piece of paper and ask him/her to write a sentence. It is to be written spontaneously. It must contain a subject and verb and make sense. Correct grammar and punctuation are not necessary.

   Writes sentence . . . .30___

   Copying: on a clean piece of paper, draw intersecting pentagons, each side about 1 inch, and ask subject to copy it exactly as it is. All 10 angles must be present and two must intersect to score 1 point. Tremor and rotation are ignored.

   Draws pentagons . . . .31___

Mini–Mental State Examination—cont'd

Score: Add number of correct responses. In section 3 include
items 14-18 or item 19, not both (maximum total score 30)

Total score_____

Rate subject's level of consciousness:_____(a) coma, (b)
stupor, (c) drowsy, (d) alert

Reprinted with permission from Folstein MF, et al: J Psychiatr Rev 12:189, 1975.

d. Of great importance is the identification of treatable causes of dementia (see the following list):

(1) Drug induced	(10) Stroke
(2) Depression	(11) CNS infections
(3) Hypothyroidism	(12) Generalized infections
(4) Hyperthyroidism	(13) Cerebral neoplasms
(5) Hypoglycemia	(14) Renal failure
(6) Vitamin B_{12} or folate deficiency	(15) Ethanol abuse
(7) Subdural hematoma	(16) Hypoxia
(8) Liver failure	(17) Hypercalcemia
(9) Normal-pressure hydrocephalus	(18) Vasculitis
	(19) Cardiopulmonary disorders
	(20) Anemia

Management

1. Pursue the diagnosis
2. Avoid restraints, but use them for safety
3. Control hyperactivity of delirium with haloperidol in adequate doses (i.e., 2 mg qh, IM or PO, until calm) and lorazepam 1 mg IM qh if needed

Reference

1. Folstein MF, et al: Mini–Mental State: a practical method of grading the cognitive state of the patient for the physician, J Psychiatr Rev 12:189, 1975.

Rhabdomyolysis

Definition

Rhabdomyolysis is an acute or subacute event resulting in damage or necrosis of striated muscle.

Etiology[1,2,3]

1. Trauma (e.g., crush syndrome, burns, electrical shock)
2. Muscle ischemia (e.g., thrombosis, embolism, vasculitis, sickle cell disease, pressure necrosis, tourniquet shock)
3. Drugs: drug-induced rhabdomyolysis can occur via several mechanisms
   a. Primary, toxin-induced (e.g., ethanol, methadone)
   b. Secondary to chronic intake of drugs associated with hypokalemia (e.g., thiazides)
   c. Secondary to overdose of certain drugs (e.g., barbiturates, heroin, cocaine)
   d. Malignant hyperthermia (usually seen in genetically predisposed individuals, following exposure to halothane, succinylcholine, or pancuronium)
   e. Neuroleptic malignant syndrome (associated with use of phenothiazines, butyrophenones, antipsychotics, cocaine, or diphenhydramine, usually in patients with dehydration and electrolyte imbalance)
   f. Use of certain lipid lowering agents (e.g., combination of lovastatin and gemfibrozil, use of lovastatin after cardiac transplantation, combination of lovastatin and erythromycin [rare])
4. Infections
   a. Bacterial (e.g., clostridia, *Legionella,* staphylococci, *Leptospira, Shigella*)
   b. Viral (e.g., echo, coxsackie, influenza, CMV, herpes)
   c. Parasites (trichinosis)
5. Excessive muscular stress (e.g., marathon runners, status epilepticus, DTs)
6. Genetic defects (carnitine deficiency, phosphorylase deficiency)
7. Miscellaneous: brown recluse spider bite, snake bite, hornets, polymyositis, dermatomyositis, heat stroke

Contributing factors

1. Hypokalemia
2. Hyperosmolar state[8]

Diagnostic evaluation[1,2,3]

1. History
   a. Inquire about ingestion of alcohol, caffeine, drugs
   b. Document type, intensity, and duration of exercise, recent trauma
   c. Recent or present infections
   d. Rhabdomyolysis postoperatively: halothane anesthesia
   e. Onset of reddish-brown discoloration of urine (myoglobinuria)
2. Physical exam
   a. Body temperature (elevated in malignant hyperthermia, neuroleptic malignant syndrome, infections)
   b. Hydration status (dehydration contributes to the development of rhabdomyolysis and renal failure)
   c. Muscular weakness, hypertonicity, hyperthermia, swelling
   d. Evidence of trauma (areas of ecchymoses, tenderness)
3. Laboratory evaluation
   a. Creatine kinase: elevations may exceed 1,000,000 U/L in fulminant rhabdomyolysis; the development of renal failure is not directly related to the threshold level of CK; isoenzyme fractionation is useful: if CK-MB exceeds 5% of the total CK, involvement of the myocardium is likely[4]
   b. Serum creatinine: usually elevated; the etiology of the renal failure is uncertain and probably multifactorial[6,7] (renal tubular obstruction by precipitated myoglobin, direct myoglobin toxicity, hypotension, dehydration, decreased glomerular filtration rate, intravascular coagulation)
   c. Serum potassium: preexisting hypokalemia is a contributing factor to rhabdomyolysis; fulminant rhabdomyolysis can result in life-threatening hyperkalemia secondary to increased K^+ release from damaged muscle and impaired renal excretion
   d. Calcium and phosphate: initially there is hyperphosphatemia, from muscle necrosis, and secondary hypocalcemia, from Ca^{2+} deposition in the injured muscle and decreased 1,25-dihydroxycholecalciferol; later (in the diuretic phase of renal failure), hypercalcemia is present due to remobilization of the deposited Ca^{2+} and secondary hyperparathyroidism
   e. Myoglobin: present in the serum and urine; the urine is of a brownish color, has granular casts, and is orthotoluidine-positive; a quick visual method to separate myoglobinuria from hemoglobinuria is to examine the urine and serum simultaneously: reddish brown urine and pink serum indicate hemoglobinuria whereas brown urine and clear serum suggest myoglobinuria[7]; a rise in serum myoglobin precedes the rise in CK level and is useful to estimate the risk of renal failure (serum myoglobin levels >2000 µg/L may be associated with renal insufficiency[5])

f. Other abnormalities: hyperuricemia, elevated AST, ALT, hypoalbuminemia

Therapy[1,2,3]

1. General measures
   a. Vigorous fluid replacement to maintain a good urinary output, at
      least until myoglobin disappears from the urine
   b. Administration of a single dose of mannitol (100 ml of a 25% solu-
      tion, IV over 15 min) and alkalinization of the urine with addition of
      44 mEq/L of sodium bicarbonate may improve renal perfusion and
      reduce renal toxicity in patients with oliguric myoglobinuria
   c. Hyperkalemia secondary to rhabdomyolysis is most severe 10-40 hr
      after injury; initial treatment with sodium polystyrene sulfonate is in-
      dicated (refer to Section 26.3); hyperkalemia secondary to rhabdo-
      myolysis responds poorly to treatment with glucose and insulin; at-
      tempts to correct hyperkalemia and initial hypocalcemia with cal-
      cium infusion may result in metastatic calcifications and severe hy-
      percalcemia in the recovery period; hemodialysis may be necessary
      in patients with severe hyperkalemia, volume overload, uremic peri-
      carditis, or uremic encephalopathy
2. Specific measures
   a. Immediate removal of any offending drugs
   b. Dantrolene sodium infusion in patients with malignant hyperthermia
      or neuroleptic malignant syndrome
   c. Treatment of local injury (e.g., fasciotomy for relief of compartment
      syndrome)

References

1. Better OS, Stein JH: Early management of shock and prophylaxis of acute renal
   failure in traumatic rhabdomyolysis, N Engl J Med 322:825, 1990.
2. Koppel C: Clinical features, pathogenesis, and management of drug induced rhabdomyolysis, Mod Tox Adverse Drug Exp 4:108, 1989.
3. Milne CJ: Rhabdomyolysis, myoglobinuria, and exercise, Sports Med 6:93, 1988.
4. Moss DW, et al: In Tietz NW (editor): Textbook of clinical chemistry, Philadelphia, 1986, WB Saunders Co, pp 698-700.
5. Penn AS: Myoglobinuria. In Engel AG, Banker BQ (editors): Myology, vol 2,
   New York, 1986, McGraw-Hill Book Co.
6. Roth D, et al: Acute rhabdomyolysis associated with cocaine intoxication, N Engl
   J Med 319:145, 1988.
7. Schulze VE: Rhabdomyolysis as a cause of acute renal failure, Postgrad Med
   72:145, 1990.
8. Singhal PC, et al: Rhabdomyolysis in the hyperosmolal state, Am J Med 88:9,
   1990.

Evaluation of the Patient in Shock

Definition

Shock is characterized by ineffective tissue perfusion by oxygenated blood with subsequent acidosis, alterations in cellular metabolism, and potential end-organ damage and death.

Etiology[1]

Shock can be secondary to derangement of blood volume, cardiac output, or peripheral vasomotor tone and can be subdivided into central or peripheral, based on its underlying mechanism.

1. Peripheral shock
   a. Hypovolemic: inadequate blood volume (e.g., GI bleeding, hemorrhage, burns)
   b. Distributive: maldistribution of blood volume (e.g., sepsis, anaphylaxis), neurogenic shock, endocrine shock
2. Central shock
   a. Cardiogenic: "pump" failure (e.g., MI, dysrhythmias, AS, dilated cardiomyopathy)
   b. Obstructive: impairment of blood flow (e.g., cardiac tamponade, pulmonary embolism, tension pneumothorax)

Diagnostic evaluation

1. Physical exam: generally reveals hypotension, signs of hypoperfusion (e.g., altered mental status), tachycardia, cool and clammy skin, decreased urine output; other clinical manifestations vary with the etiology of the shock (e.g., fever and chills in septic shock, chest pain and pulmonary edema in cardiogenic shock, urticaria and bronchospasm in anaphylactic shock)
2. Chest x-ray: may reveal pulmonary edema, pneumothorax, pneumonia
3. ECG: useful to identify acute MI, dysrhythmias, pulmonary embolus
4. Initial lab: CBC with differential, BUN, creatinine, electrolytes, Ca^{2+}, PO_4^{-3}, glucose, magnesium, LFTs, lactic acid, ABGs
5. Hemodynamic monitoring
   a. Arterial line to measure intraarterial pressure directly; obtain frequent labs, ABGs

    b. Foley catheter to measure urinary output

    c. Pulmonary artery (Swan-Ganz) catheter to help differentiate the cause of shock and guide therapy (See Section 5.6 for use and interpretation of pulmonary artery catheter data)

Therapeutic approach

1. General measures
   a. Insert two large-bore intravenous catheters and optimize fluid volume to maintain PCWP at 18-20 mm Hg; crystalloid solutions (saline, lactated Ringer's) plus colloid solutions (albumin, Hetastarch, dextrans) may be necessary
   b. Assess airway patency and ventilation; correct acidosis and hypoxemia; intubation may be necessary
   c. Use of beta-receptor stimulants (e.g., dopamine, dobutamine) is indicated only when volume repletion is inadequate to maintain sufficient blood pressure. Fig. 20-3 compares the hemodynamic responses to dobutamine and dopamine
   d. If military antishock trousers (the MAST suit) are used (e.g., hypovolemic shock), the lowest inflation pressure that will maintain adequate blood pressure should be used
   e. An intraaortic balloon pump (IABP) or surgery may be necessary in refractory cardiogenic shock
2. Specific measures
   a. Septic shock: see Section 25.6
   b. Cardiogenic shock: see Section 20.6
   c. Cardiac tamponade: see Section 20.7
   d. Pulmonary embolism: see Section 28.9
   e. GI bleeding: see Section 23.1

Reference

1. Peters JI, Utset O: Shock in the ICU: when to suspect, how to determine its cause, J Critical Ill 4:77, 1989.

17

Management of Alcohol Withdrawal

Alcohol withdrawal syndrome occurs when a person stops ingesting alcohol after prolonged consumption. It can result in four possible clinical patterns, depending on the severity of the patient's alcohol abuse and the time interval from the patient's previous alcohol ingestion. Although discussed separately, these alcohol withdrawal states blend together in real life.

1. Tremulous state (early alcohol withdrawal, "impending DTs," "shakes," "jitters")
   a. Time interval: usually occurs 12-48 hr after reduction of alcohol intake
   b. Manifestation: tremors, mild agitation, insomnia, tachycardia; symptoms are relieved by alcohol
   c. Treatment
      (1) Admit to medical floor (private room); monitor vital signs q4h; institute seizure precautions; maintain adequate sedation
      (2) Administer chlordiazepoxide as follows:
          Day 1: 50 mg PO q4h while awake and not lethargic
          Day 2: 25 mg PO q4h while awake and not lethargic
          Day 3: 10 mg PO q4h while awake and not lethargic
      (3) In the presence of jaundice or known liver disease, lorazepam may be substituted as follows:
          Day 1: 2 mg PO q4h while awake and not lethargic
          Day 2: 1 mg PO q4h while awake and not lethargic
          Day 3: 0.5 mg PO q4h while awake and not lethargic
          NOTE: Hold sedation for lethargy or abnormal vital or neurologic signs. The above doses are only guidelines; it is best to titrate the dose case by case.
      (4) β-Adrenergic blockers: atenolol 50-100 mg PO qd reportedly normalizes vital signs rapidly and significantly reduces the mean length of hospital stay[3] and outpatient treatment failures[2] in patients with alcohol withdrawal. However, further studies are needed to clarify the role (if any) of β-adrenergic blockers in the treatment of alcohol withdrawal. β-Blockers should be avoided in patients with contraindications to their use (e.g., bronchospasm, bradycardia, or CHF).

    (5) Hydration PO or IV (high-caloric solution); if IV: glucose with Na^+, K^+, Mg^{2+}, and PO_4^{-3} replacement prn

    (6) Vitamin replacement: thiamine 100 mg IM or PO qd; plus multivitamins

    (7) Laboratory studies

        (a) CBC and differential, platelet count, PT, PTT

        (b) Electrolytes, glucose, BUN, creatinine

        (c) Amylase, liver profile

        (d) Phosphorus and magnesium

        (e) Routine urinalysis

        (f) Serum B_{12} and folic acid (if megaloblastic features in blood smear)

    (8) X-ray studies; if subdural hematoma is suspected (evidence of trauma, persistent lethargy), a CT scan should be ordered

    (9) Social rehabilitation: group therapy such as Alcoholics Anonymous; identification and treatment of social and family problems should be initiated during the patient's hospital stay

2. Hallucinosis

  a. Manifestations: usually hallucinations are auditory, but occasionally hallucinations are visual, tactile, or olfactory; usually there is no clouding of sensorium as in delirium (clinical presentation may be mistaken for an acute schizophrenic episode)

  b. Treatment: same as for delirium tremens (see below)

3. Withdrawal seizures (rum fits)

  a. Time interval: usually occur 7-30 hr after cessation of drinking, with a peak incidence between 13-24 hr

  b. Manifestations: generalized convulsions with loss of consciousness; focal signs are usually absent; consider further investigation with CT scan of head and EEG if indicated (e.g., presence of focal neurologic deficits, prolonged postictal confusion state)

  c. Treatment

    (1) Diazepam 2.5 mg/min IV until seizure is controlled (check for respiratory depression or hypotension) may be beneficial for prolonged seizure activity; generally, withdrawal seizures are self-limited and treatment is not required; the use of phenytoin for short-term treatment of alcohol withdrawal seizures is not recommended[1]; a single loading dose of phenytoin (1000 mg at 50 mg/min IV) can be given to prevent immediate recurrence of seizure, but its need and efficacy have been questioned; chronic anticonvulsant therapy is not indicated

    (2) Thiamine 100 mg IM, followed by IV dextrose, should also be administered

    (3) Correct electrolyte imbalances ($\downarrow Mg^{2+}$, $\downarrow K^+$, $\uparrow/\downarrow Na^+$, $\downarrow PO_4^{-3}$) that may exacerbate seizures

4. Delirium tremens (DTs)

  a. Time interval: variable; usually occurs within 1 wk after reduction or cessation of heavy alcohol intake and persists for 1-3 days

  b. Manifestations: confusion, tremors, vivid visual and tactile hallucinations, autonomic hyperactivity; this is the most serious clinical presentation of alcohol withdrawal (mortality is approximately 15% in untreated patients)

c. Treatment
   (1) Admit to ICU or to unit where patient can be observed closely
   (2) Vital signs q30min (neurologic signs, if necessary)
   (3) Restrain in lateral decubitus or prone position if restraints are necessary
   (4) NPO: NG tube for abdominal distention may be necessary but should not be routinely used
   (5) Lab studies: same as for early alcohol withdrawal
   (6) Hydration: IV with glucose (Na^+, K^+, PO_4^{-3}, and Mg^{2+} replacement)
   (7) Vitamins: thiamine, 100 mg IM qd; multivitamins (may be added to the hydrating solution)
   (8) Sedation
       (a) Initially: lorazepam 2-5 mg IM/IV repeated prn
       (b) Maintenance (individualize dosage): chlordiazepoxide, 50-100 mg PO q4-6h, lorazepam 2 mg PO q4h, or diazepam 5-10 mg PO tid; withhold doses or decrease subsequent doses if signs of oversedation are apparent
   (9) Treatment of seizures (as previously described)
   (10) Diagnosis and treatment of concomitant medical, surgical, or psychiatric conditions

References

1. Alldredge BK, et al: Placebo-controlled trial of intravenous diphenyl-hydantoin for short-term treatment of alcohol withdrawal seizures, Am J Med 87:645, 1989.
2. Horwitz RL, Gottlieb LD, Kraus ML: The efficacy of atenolol in the outpatient management of alcohol withdrawal syndrome, Arch Intern Med 149:1089, 1989.
3. Kraus ML, Gottlieb LD, et al: Randomized clinical trial of atenolol in patients with alcohol withdrawal, N Engl J Med 313:905, 1985.

Disorders of Thermoregulation

18.1 ACCIDENTAL HYPOTHERMIA

Definitions

Hypothermia: rectal temperature <35° C (95.8° F)

Accidental hypothermia: unintentionally induced decrease in core temperature in absence of preoptic anterior hypothalamic conditions[9]

Clinical presentation

1. Varies with the severity of hypothermia; shivering may be absent if body temperature is <33.3° C (92° F) or in patients taking phenothiazines
2. Always measure rectal temperature with a low-reading rectal thermometer
3. Hypothermia may masquerade as CVA (ataxia, slurred speech) or the patient may appear comatose or clinically dead; there are reports in the medical literature[6] of cyanotic rigid patients with fixed pupils and no audible heart sounds who have been successfully resuscitated; therefore "no one is dead until warm and dead"[7]

Physiologic stages of hypothermia[3]

1. Mild hypothermia: 33° to 35° C (91.4° to 95° F)
   a. Dysarthria, ataxia
2. Moderate hypothermia: 27° to 32° C (80.6° to 89.6° F)
   a. Progressive decrease in level of consciousness, pulse, CO, and respiration
   b. Atrial fibrillation and other dysrhythmias (increased susceptibility to ventricular tachycardia)
   c. Elimination of shivering mechanism for thermogenesis
3. Severe hypothermia: ≤26° C (78.8° F)
   a. Absence of reflexes or response to pain
   b. ↓ Cerebral blood flow, ↓ ↓ CO
   c. ↑ Risk of ventricular fibrillation or asystole

Lab evaluation

1. Metabolic and respiratory acidosis are usually present
   a. ABGs must be corrected for temperature; correction factors as follows[17,18]:
      (1) pH ↑ 0.008 unit/° F (or 0.015 unit/° C) ↓ in temperature
      (2) Pao_2 ↑ 3.3%/° F ↓ in temperature
      (3) $Paco_2$ ↓ 2.4%/° F ↓ in temperature
2. ↓ K^+ initially, then ↑ K^+ with increasing hypothermia; extreme hyperkalemia indicates a poor prognosis
3. ↑ Hct (secondary to hemoconcentration), ↓ leukocytes, ↓ platelets (secondary to splenic sequestration)
4. ↑ Blood viscosity, ↑ clotting time

ECG[11]

1. Prolonged PR, QT, and QRS segments
2. Depressed ST segment
3. Inverted T waves
4. A V block
5. Hypothermic J waves (Osborn waves) may appear at 25° to 30° C; these waves are characterized by a notching at the junction of the QRS complex and ST segment (Fig. 18-1)

Therapy[10]

1. Treatment of hypothermia varies with the following:
   a. Degree of hypothermia
   b. Existence of concomitant diseases (e.g., cardiovascular insufficiency)
   c. Patient's age and medical condition (e.g., elderly debilitated patient vs young healthy patient)
2. General measures
   a. Secure an airway before rewarming in all unconscious patients; precede endotracheal intubation with oxygenation (if possible) to minimize the risk of dysrhythmias during the procedure
   b. Correct severe acidosis and electrolyte abnormalities; interpretation of blood gases is controversial in hypothermic patients because pH varies with temperature and it is difficult to determine the "true" core temperature; "uncorrected" pH values are generally used to assess acid-base disturbances; it is desirable to maintain the hypothermic individual at an "uncorrected" rather than a corrected pH of 7.4[17]
   c. Monitor patient, treat dysrhythmias
3. Specific treatment
   a. Mild hypothermia (rectal temperature <32.2° C [90° F])
      (1) Passive external rewarming is indicated: Place the patient in a warm room >21° C (69.8° F) and cover with insulating material after gently removing wet clothing. Recommended rewarming rates vary between 0.5° and 2.0° C/hr, but should not exceed 0.55° C/hr in elderly persons[3]
   b. Moderate to severe hypothermia
      (1) Active core rewarming

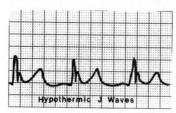

Figure 18-1
Hypothermic J waves.

    (a) Delivery of heat via fluids, such as the following:
- Warm GI irrigation (with saline enemas and via NG tube)
- Warm IV fluids[3] (usually D_5NS without potassium)
- Peritoneal dialysis with dialysate heated to 40.5° to 42.5° C[8,15]
- Hemodialysis, extracorporeal blood rewarming
    (b) Inhalation of heated humidified oxygen[4]
(2) Active external rewarming
    (a) Immersion in a bath of warm water (40° to 41° C). Active external rewarming may produce shock because of excessive peripheral vasodilation. Ideal candidates are previously healthy young patients with acute immersion hypothermia.[5]

18.2 HEAT STROKE

Clinical presentation

1. Exposure to heat load (environmental or internally generated)
2. Elevated body temperature (usually >40° C [104° F])
3. Major form of CNS dysfunction (confusion, delirium, seizures, coma)
4. Marked elevation of AST, ALT, LDH

Predisposing factors[16]

1. Exogenous heat gain (↑ ambient temperature)
2. ↑ Heat production (exercise, infection, hyperthyroidism, drugs)
3. Impaired heat dissipation (high humidity, heavy clothing, neonates or elderly patients, drugs: phenothiazines, anticholinergics, diuretics, antihistamines, butyrophenones, cocaine, amphetamines, alcohol, beta blockers)

Differential diagnosis

1. CNS pathology
   a. Infections (meningitis, encephalitis)
   b. Head trauma
   c. Epilepsy
2. Thyroid storm

3. Heat exhaustion
   a. Generalized malaise, weakness, headache, muscle cramps, nausea, vomiting, hypotension, and tachycardia
   b. Rectal temperature is usually normal
   c. Sweating is usually present
   d. Differentiated from heat stroke by the following:
      (1) Essentially intact mental functions and lack of significant fever
      (2) Mild or absent increases in CPK, AST, LDH, ALT
   e. Treatment consists of the following[1]:
      (1) Rest in a well-ventilated, cool environment
      (2) Fluid replacement. If young athlete, give NS IV (3 to 4 L over 6-8 hr); if elderly patient, consider $D_5\frac{1}{2}$ NS IV with rate titrated to cardiovascular status
4. Heat cramps[12]
   a. Severe muscle cramps, often involving the lower extremities
   b. Rectal temperature is usually normal
   c. Sweating is usually present
   d. History often reveals profuse sweating and fluid replacement with hypotonic solutions (e.g., water)
   e. Lack of acclimatization and recent use of ethanol are often contributory factors
   f. Treatment consists of the following[1]:
      (1) Rest in a cool environment
      (2) Salt replacement
         (a) PO: $\frac{1}{4}$ tsp of salt or two 10 gr salt tablets dissolved in 1 L of H_2O
         (b) IV: NS, 1 L infused over 1-4 hr depending on the patient's cardiovascular status

Clinical presentation of heat stroke

1. Neurologic manifestations (seizures, tremor, hemiplegia, coma, psychosis, and other bizarre behavior)
2. Evidence of dehydration (poor skin turgor, sunken eyeballs)
3. Tachycardia, hyperventilation
4. Skin is hot, red, and flushed
5. Sweating is often (not always) absent, particularly in elderly patients[13]
6. Lab studies reveal:
   a. ↑ BUN, ↑ creatinine, ↑ Hct, ↑/↓ Na^+, ↑/↓ K
   b. ↑ LDH, ↑ AST, ↑ ALT, ↑ CPK, ↑ bilirubin, ↓ calcium
   c. Lactic acidosis, respiratory alkalosis (secondary to hyperventilation)
   d. Myoglobinuria, hypofibrinogenemia, fibrinolysis

Treatment of heat stroke[1,14]

1. Immediate cooling: remove clothes, place the patient in a cool and well-ventilated room
2. Spray the patient with a cool mist and use fans to enhance airflow over the body (rapid evaporation method); immersion of the patient in ice water, stomach lavage with iced saline solution, intravenous administra-

tion of cooled fluids, and inhalation of cold air are advisable only when the means for rapid evaporation are not available; ice packs should not be used, because they increase peripheral vasoconstriction and may induce shivering; antipyretics are ineffective because the hypothalamic set point during heatstroke is normal despite the increased body temperature

3. Intubate a comatose patient, insert a Foley catheter, start nasal O_2, and continue ECG monitoring

4. Begin IV hydration with NS or Ringer's lactate

5. Draw initial lab studies: electrolytes, CBC, BUN, creatinine, AST, ALT, CPK, LDH, glucose, PT, PTT, platelet count, FDP, Ca^{2+}, uric acid, lactic acid, ABGs

6. Treat complications
   a. Hypotension: vigorous hydration with normal saline or Ringer's lactate
   b. Convulsions: diazepam 5-10 mg IV (slowly)
   c. Shivering: chlorpromazine 25-50 mg IV
   d. Acidosis; if pH <7.2, give sodium bicarbonate

7. Observe for evidence of hepatic, renal, or cardiac failure and treat accordingly

References

1. Callaham M: Heat illness. In Rosen P, et al (editors): Emergency medicine: concepts and clinical practice, St Louis, 1983, The CV Mosby Co.
2. Chinard FP: Accidental hypothermia: a brief review, J Med Soc NJ 75:610, 1978.
3. Danzl DF: Accidental hypothermia. In Rosen P, et al (editors): Emergency medicine: concepts and clinical practice, St Louis, 1983, The CV Mosby Co.
4. Danzl DF, Pozoj RS: Multicenter hypothermia survey, Ann Emerg Med 16:1042, 1987.
5. Golden F: Recognition and treatment of immersion hypothermia, Proc R Soc Med 66:1058, 1973.
6. Gregory RT, Doolittle WH: Accidental hypothermia. II, Clinical implications of experimental studies, Alaska Med 15:48, 1973.
7. Gregory RT, Patton JF: Treatment after exposure to cold, Lancet 1:377, 1972.
8. Klarskov P, Amter F: Hypothermia after submersion: correction with peritoneal dialysis, Ugeskr Laegr 138:1937, 1976.
9. Lloyd EL: Accidental hypothermia treated by central rewarming through the airway, Br J Anaesth 45:41, 1973.
10. MacLean D, Emslie-Smith D: Accidental hypothermia, Philadelphia, 1977, JB Lippincott Co.
11. Popvic V, Popvic P: Hypothermia in biology and in medicine, New York, 1974, Grune & Stratton Inc.
12. Proulx RP: Heat stress disease. In Schwartz GR, et al (editors): Principles and practice of emergency medicine, Philadelphia, 1978, WB Saunders Co.
13. Schoenfield Y, Udassin R: Age and sex difference in response to short exposure to extreme heat, J Appl Physiol 44:1, 1978.
14. Scott J: Heat related illness, Postgrad Med 85:154, 1989.
15. Soung LS, et al: Treatment of accidental hypothermia with peritoneal dialysis, JACEP 6:556, 1977.
16. Stine R: Heat illness, JACEP 8:154, 1978.
17. Swain JA: Hypothermia and blood pH, Arch Intern Med 148:1643, 1988.
18. Wears RL: Blood gases in hypothermia, JACEP 8:247, 1979.

Acid-Base
Disturbances

Definitions

The suffix -osis does not correspond to blood acidity but is used only to refer to the primary process generating OH^- or H^+.

Acidosis: process that generates H^+

Alkalosis: process that generates OH^-

The suffix -emia refers to blood acidity.

Acidemia: pH <7.36

Alkalemia: pH >7.44

19.1 APPROACH TO THE PATIENT WITH ACID-BASE DISTURBANCES

1. Draw ABG and electrolyte samples concomitantly; evaluate the following[3]:
   a. Plasma HCO_3^-
      (1) Increased in metabolic alkalosis or respiratory acidosis (compensated)
      (2) Decreased in metabolic acidosis or respiratory alkalosis (compensated)
   b. Serum K^+ ($\triangle pH\ 0.1 = \triangle K^+\ 0.6$)
      (1) Increased in acidemia
      (2) Decreased in alkalemia
   c. Serum Cl^-: compare with plasma sodium concentration; they should be proportionately increased or decreased if the change in Cl^- concentration is the result of a change in the hydration of the patient.
      (1) If the Cl^- is disproportionately increased, think of metabolic acidosis or respiratory alkalosis.
      (2) If the Cl^- is disproportionately decreased think of metabolic alkalosis or respiratory acidosis
2. Calculate the anion gap (AG)

$$AG = Na^+ - (Cl^- + HCO_3^-)$$
$$normal = 8\text{-}16\ mEq/L$$

The anion gap represents unmeasured anions in the plasma (negative charges on plasma proteins and negative charges contributed by organic

Table 19-1 Primary abnormality and compensatory responses in simple acid-base disorders[3]

Disorder	Primary Abnormality	Secondary Response	pH	$Paco_2$	HCO_3^-
Metabolic acidosis	Gain of H^+ or loss of HCO_3^-	↑ Ventilation (and chemical buffering)	↓	↓	↓
Respiratory acidosis	Hypoventilation	HCO_3^- generation	↓	↑	↑
Metabolic alkalosis	Gain of HCO_3^- or loss of H^+	↓ Ventilation (and chemical buffering)	↑	↑	↑
Respiratory alkalosis	Hyperventilation	HCO_3^- consumption	↑	↓	↓

and inorganic anions normally present in the plasma but not routinely measured). This measurement is important because it enables one to divide the causes of metabolic acidosis into two main categories:

1. Normal anion gap acidosis (hyperchloremic acidosis)
2. Elevated anion gap acidosis (AG acidosis)

An elevated anion gap is the result of the presence of acid ions (e.g., lactic acid) in the extracellular fluid.

3. Evaluate ABGs to determine the type of disturbance present by examining pH, $Paco_2$, and HCO_3^- (see Table 19-1)
4. Calculate if the degree of compensation is adequate:
   a. Metabolic acidosis
      (1) If adequate compensation, $Paco_2 = (1.5 \times HCO_3^-) + 8.4$[1]; usually $Paco_2$ = last 2 digits of the pH
      (2) If actual $Paco_2$ greater than calculated, then both metabolic and respiratory acidosis are present
      (3) If actual $Paco_2$ less than calculated, then metabolic acidosis and respiratory alkalosis are present
   b. Respiratory acidosis
      (1) Acute: an increase in $Paco_2$ by 10 will decrease pH by 0.08 and increase HCO_3^- by 1.0 mEq/L; usual upper limit of compensation is $HCO_3^- = 30$ mEq/L
      (2) Chronic: an increase in $Paco_2$ by 10 will decrease pH by 0.03 and will increase HCO_3^- by 3.5 mEq/L; usual upper limit of compensation is $HCO_3^- = 55$ mEq/L
   c. Metabolic alkalosis
      (1) An increase in HCO_3^- by 1.0 will increase pH by 0.015 and increase $Paco_2$ by 0.7
      (2) Limitations: the compensatory response (↑ $Paco_2$) is usually limited to a maximum $Paco_2$ of 55
      (3) There is an impaired compensatory response in patients with COPD, heart failure, and hepatic coma
   d. Respiratory alkalosis
      (1) Acute: A decrease in $Paco_2$ by 10 will increase pH by 0.08 and decrease HCO_3^- by 2.5

(2) Chronic: A decrease in $Paco_2$ by 10 will increase pH by 0.03 and decrease HCO_3^- by 5

If the degree of compensation is inadequate, consider the simultaneous presence of two or more primary abnormalities (mixed acid-base disturbances). Fig. 19-1 demonstrates the acid-base nomogram constructed from arterial pH, $Paco_2$, and HCO_3^-. The normal values are labeled N. The specific acid-base disturbance present can be determined by plotting the pH, $Paco_2$, and HCO_3^-.

The box on p. 134 presents common causes of mixed acid-base disturbances.

19.2   COMMON CAUSES OF ACID-BASE DISTURBANCES

Metabolic acidosis (Table 19-1)
1. Metabolic acidosis with increased anion gap (AG acidosis)
   a. Lactic acidosis (see box on p. 135 for causes)

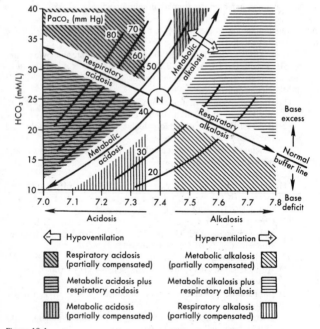

Figure 19-1
Graphic representation of the Henderson-Hasselbach equation of acid-base relationships. (From Rosen P, et al [editors]: Emergency medicine: concepts and clinical practice, St Louis, 1983, The CV Mosby Co.)

b. Ketoacidosis (diabetes mellitus, ethanol intoxication, starvation)
c. Uremia (chronic renal failure)
d. Ingestion of toxins (paraldehyde, methanol, salicylate, ethylene glycol)
e. High-fat diet (mild acidosis)
f. Refer to Fig. 19-2 and Section 22.2 for the approach to and diagnosis of anion gap acidosis

2. Metabolic acidosis with normal anion gap (hyperchloremic acidosis)
   a. Renal tubular acidosis (including acidosis of aldosterone deficiency)
   b. Intestinal loss of bicarbonate (diarrhea, pancreatic fistula)
   c. Carbonic anhydrase inhibitors (e.g., acetazolamide)
   d. Dilutional acidosis (as a result of rapid infusion of bicarbonate-free isotonic saline)
   e. Ingestion of exogenous acids (ammonium chloride, methionine, cystine, calcium chloride)
   f. Ileostomy
   g. Ureterosigmoidostomy
   h. Drugs: amiloride, triamterine, spironolactone, beta blockers

Measurement of urinary anion gap ($U_{Na^+} + U_{K^+} - U_{Cl^-}$) and urinary pH is useful in the differential diagnosis of hyperchloremic metabolic acidosis[2]:

1. Negative urinary anion gap suggests GI loss of bicarbonate
2. Positive urinary anion gap suggests altered distal urinary acidification
3. Low urinary pH and elevated plasma K^+ in patients with positive urinary anion gap suggest selective aldosterone deficiency
4. Urinary pH >5.5 and elevated plasma K^+ suggest hyperkalemic distal renal tubular acidosis
5. Urinary pH >5.5 and normal or decreased plasma K^+ indicate classic renal tubular acidosis

Therapy of metabolic acidosis

1. Correction of underlying cause (e.g., DKA, diarrhea, uremia)
2. $NaHCO_3$ therapy is the mainstay for most cases of life-threatening metabolic acidosis (pH 7.20)
3. Overaggressive $NaHCO_3$ therapy can lead to "overshoot alkalosis"; therefore the bicarbonate level should be corrected only to approximately 15 mEq/L and only half the bicarbonate deficit should be corrected over a 12 hr period
4. Hypernatremia and fluid overload following $NaHCO_3$ therapy is of concern, particularly in patients with renal failure or CHF

Respiratory acidosis

1. Pulmonary disease (COPD, severe pneumonia, pulmonary edema, interstitial fibrosis)
2. Airway obstruction (foreign body, severe bronchospasm, laryngospasm)
3. Thoracic cage disorders (pneumothorax, flail chest, kyphoscoliosis)
4. Defects in muscles of respiration (myasthenia gravis, hypokalemia, muscular dystrophy)

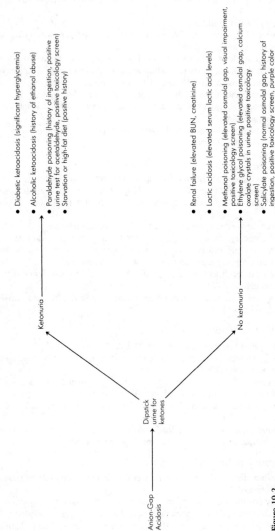

Figure 19-2
Differential diagnosis of anion gap acidosis.

5. Defects in peripheral nervous system (amyotrophic lateral sclerosis, poliomyelitis, Guillain-Barré syndrome, botulism, tetanus, organophosphate poisoning, spinal cord injury)
6. Depression of respiratory center (anesthesia, narcotics, sedatives, vertebral artery embolism or thrombosis, increased intracranial pressure)
7. Failure of mechanical ventilator

Metabolic alkalosis

It is divided into chloride-responsive (urinary chloride < 15 mEq/L) and chloride-unresponsive forms (urinary chloride level >15 mEq/L).

1. Chloride-responsive
   a. Vomiting
   b. Nasogastric suction
   c. Diuretics
   d. Post-hypercapnic alkalosis
   e. Stool losses (laxative abuse, cystic fibrosis, villous adenoma)
   f. Massive blood transfusion
   g. Exogenous alkali administration
2. Chloride-resistant
   a. Hyperadrenocorticoid states (Cushing's syndrome, primary hyperaldosteronism, secondary mineralocorticoidism [licorice, chewing tobacco])
   b. Hypomagnesemia
   c. Hypokalemia
   d. Bartter's syndrome
3. Treatment of metabolic alkalosis varies with its cause:
   a. Chloride-responsive forms are treated with saline administration and correction of accompanying hypokalemia
   b. Chloride-resistant forms require correction of underlying cause and associated potassium depletion

Respiratory alkalosis

1. Hypoxemia (pneumonia, pulmonary embolism, atelectasis, high-altitude living)
2. Drugs (salicylates, xanthines, progesterone, epinephrine, thyroxine, nicotine)
3. CNS disorders (tumor, CVA, trauma, infections)
4. Psychogenic hyperventilation (anxiety, hysteria)
5. Hepatic encephalopathy
6. Gram-negative sepsis
7. Hyponatremia
8. Sudden recovery from metabolic acidosis
9. Assisted ventilation

Therapy of respiratory alkalosis is aimed at its underlying cause: symptomatic patients with psychogenic hyperventilation often require some form of rebreathing apparatus (e.g., paper bag, breathing 5% CO_2 via mask)

Common Causes of Mixed Disturbances Associated With Metabolic Acidosis

Mixed Anion Gap Acidosis

Ketoacidosis and lactic acidosis
Methanol or ethylene glycol intoxication and lactic acidosis
Uremic acidosis and ketoacidosis

Mixed Anion Gap and Hyperchloremic Acidosis

Diarrhea and lactic acidosis or ketoacidosis
Progressive renal failure
Type IV renal tubular acidosis and diabetic ketoacidosis
Diabetic ketoacidosis during treatment

Mixed Hyperchloremic Acidosis

Diarrhea and renal tubular acidosis
Diarrhea and hyperalimentation
Diarrhea and acetazolamide or mafenide (Sulfamylon)

Anion Gap Acidosis or Hyperchloremic Acidosis and Metabolic Alkalosis

Ketoacidosis and protracted vomiting or nasogastric suction
Chronic renal failure and vomiting or nasogastric suction
Diarrhea and vomiting or nasogastric suction
Renal tubular acidosis and vomiting
Lactic or ketoacidosis plus $NaHCO_3$ therapy

Anion Gap Acidosis or Hyperchloremic Acidosis and Respiratory Alkalosis

Respiratory alkalosis
Lactic acidosis
Salicylate poisoning
Hepatic disease
Gram-negative sepsis
Pulmonary edema

Anion Gap Acidosis or Hyperchloremic Acidosis and Respiratory Acidosis

Cardiopulmonary arrest
Pulmonary edema
Respiratory failure in chronic lung disease
Phosphate depletion
Drug overdose and poisoning

From DuBose TD Jr: Med Clin North Am 67:799, 1983.

Etiology of Lactic Acidosis[4,6]

Tissue Hypoxia

Shock (hypovolemic, cardiogenic, endotoxic)
Respiratory failure (asphyxia)
Severe CHF
Severe anemia
Carbon monoxide or cyanide poisoning

Associated with Systemic Disorders

Neoplastic diseases (e.g., leukemia, lymphoma)
Liver or renal failure
Sepsis
Diabetes mellitus
Seizure activity
Abnormal intestinal flora (D-lactic acidosis)
Alkalosis

Secondary to Drugs or Toxins

Salicylates
Ethanol, methanol, ethylene glycol
Fructose and sorbitol
Biguanides (e.g., phenformin)
Isoniazid
Streptozocin

Hereditary Disorders

G_6PD deficiency and others

References

1. Albert MD, Dell RB, Winters RW: Quantitative displacement of acid-base equilibrium in metabolic acidosis, Ann Intern Med 66:312, 1964.
2. Battle DC, Hizon NM, et al: The use of urinary anion gap in the diagnosis of hyperchloremic metabolic acidosis, N Engl J Med 318:594, 1988.
3. Bia M, Thier S: Mixed acid base disturbances: a clinical approach, Med Clin North Am 65:347, 1981.
4. Cohen RD, Woods HF: Clinical and biochemical aspects of lactic acidosis, London, 1976, Blackwell Scientific Publications.
5. Dubose TD Jr: Clinical approach to patients with acid-base disorders, Med Clin North Am 67:799, 1983.
6. Narins RG, Jones ER, et al: Metabolic acid-base disorders: pathophysiology, classification, and treatment. In Arieff AI, DeFronzo RA, et al: Fluid electrolyte and acid base disorders, New York, 1985, Churchill Livingstone Inc, vol 1.

20 Cardiovascular Diseases

20.1 **ANGINA PECTORIS**

Definition

Angina pectoris is characterized by discomfort that occurs when the myocardial oxygen demand exceeds the supply. Myocardial ischemia can be asymptomatic (silent ischemia), particularly in diabetics. Angina is classified as follows:

1. Chronic (stable)
   a. Usually follows a precipitating event (e.g., climbing stairs, sexual intercourse, a heavy meal, cold weather)
   b. Generally same severity as previous attacks; relieved by the customary dose of nitroglycerin
   c. Caused by a fixed coronary artery obstruction secondary to atherosclerosis
2. Unstable (rest or crescendo)
   a. Recent onset
   b. Increasing severity, duration, or frequency of chronic angina
   c. Occurs at rest or with minimal exertion
3. Prinzmetal's variant
   a. Occurs when patient is at rest
   b. Manifests electrocardiographically as episodic ST segment elevations
   c. Caused by coronary artery spasms with or without superimposed coronary artery disease
   d. Patients also more likely to develop ventricular dysrhythmias

Risk[10,40]

1. Uncontrollable factors
   a. Age
   b. Male sex
   c. Genetic predisposition
2. Modifiable factors
   a. Smoking (risk is almost doubled)
   b. Hypertension (risk is doubled if systolic BP is > 180 mm Hg)

    c. Hyperlipidemia (see Chapter 9)
    d. Glucose intolerance or diabetes mellitus
    e. Obesity (weight > 30% over ideal)
    f. Hypothyroidism
    g. LVH
    h. Sedentary life-style
    i. Oral contraceptive use

Clinical presentation

Although there is significant individual variation, the patient usually has substernal pain (pressure, tightness, heaviness, sharp pain, sensation similar to intestinal gas or dysphagia). The pain is of short duration (30 sec to 30 min) and is often accompanied by shortness of breath, nausea, diaphoresis, and numbness or pain in the left arm or shoulder.

Differential diagnosis

Noncardiac pain mimicking angina may be caused by

1. Pulmonary diseases (pulmonary hypertension, pulmonary embolism, pleurisy, pneumothorax, pneumonia)
2. GI disorders (peptic ulcer disease, pancreatitis, esophageal spasm, esophageal reflux, cholecystitis, cholelithiasis)
3. Musculoskeletal conditions (costochondritis, chest wall trauma, cervical arthritis with radiculopathy, muscle strain, myositis)
4. Acute aortic dissection
5. Herpes zoster

Diagnostic studies

1. The most important diagnostic factor is the history
2. The physical exam is of little diagnostic help and may be totally normal in many patients
   a. Listen for the presence of heart murmurs to exclude a valvular cause for the chest pain (i.e., MVP, AS, IHSS, MS)
   b. Look for evidence of hyperlipidemia, hypertension, or cardiac decompensation
3. An ECG taken during the acute episode may show transient T wave inversion or ST segment depression/elevation, but some patients may have a normal tracing
4. Chest x-ray may show cardiomegaly or pulmonary vascular congestion
5. Echocardiography is indicated only in patients with suspected valvular abnormalities
6. Multiple gated acquisition (MUGA) scan to determine left ventricular ejection fraction (in selected patients only)
7. Exercise tolerance test
   a. Indications
      (1) Evaluation of chest pain syndromes
         (a) Typical angina or effort-induced angina
         (b) Atypical chest pain
      (2) Evaluation of exercise tolerance
         (a) Post MI (modified exercise tolerance test)

       (b) Post-CABG, postangioplasty

       (c) Evaluate effectiveness of medical therapy

    (3) Evaluation of dysrhythmias

       (a) Sick sinus syndrome

       (b) PVCs (benign PVCs usually disappear with exercise)

  b. Contraindications

    (1) Aortic stenosis

    (2) Idiopathic hypertrophic subaortic stenosis (IHSS)

    (3) Unstable angina

    (4) Poorly controlled dysrhythmias, malignant PVCs

    (5) ECG suggestive of ischemia

    (6) Severe COPD

    (7) Clinically manifested CHF

  c. Choice of protocols[11]

    (1) Bruce protocol is preferred for patients with minimum symptomatic limitation; it entails a higher initial workload and greater work increments

    (2) Naughton protocol is preferred for post-MI, post-CABG, and more debilitated patients; it entails a lower initial workload and smaller increments than the Bruce protocol

  d. Interpretation: both protocols aim at eliciting a diagnostic response within 6 to 15 min; a stress test is generally considered positive for ischemia if:

    (1) ST segment depression

       (a) ≥ 1 mm flat or downsloping ST segment depression at 0.08 sec after the J point[11]

       (b) Early onset (within 3 min of exercise)

       (c) Persists beyond 6 min of recovery phase

    (2) Patient develops chest pain

    (3) Patient develops hypotension (normally in exercise there is an increase in systolic BP because of an increase in stroke volume)

    (4) Patient develops significant dysrhythmias

    (5) ST segment elevation during exercise, although uncommon, provides reliable information about the location of the underlying coronary lesion (e.g., anterior ST segment elevation generally indicates left anterior descending coronary disease, whereas inferior ST segment elevation is suggestive of a lesion in or proximal to the posterior descending artery)[33]

8. Thallium stress test: viable myocardial cells extract thallium 201 from the blood

  a. An absent thallium uptake (cold spot on thallium scan) is an indicator of an absence of blood flow to an area of the myocardium

  b. A fixed defect on thallium scanning indicates MI at that site, whereas a defect that reperfuses suggests myocardial ischemia

  c. Increased uptake of thallium by the lungs during exercise predicts a high risk of subsequent cardiac events[22]

  d. The following are indications for thallium 201 scintigraphy:

    (1) Evaluation of patients whose resting ECG may cause false positive results on conventional stress test:

      (a) Patients with left bundle branch block (LBBB)
      (b) Patients with left ventricular hypertrophy (LVH)
      (c) Patients with sloping of ST segment secondary to digitalis administration
    (2) Evaluation of chest pain in patients with Wolff-Parkinson-White (WPW) syndrome
    (3) Evaluation of young female patients with chest pain (high rates of false positives with conventional stress test)

9. Ambulatory (Holter) electrocardiographic monitoring can detect silent ischemia (ischemic ECG changes without accompanying symptoms), which occurs in more than 50% of patients with unstable angina, despite intensive medical therapy, and identifies a subset of patients at risk for early unfavorable outcomes[24]

10. Coronary angiography is performed to define the location and extent of coronary disease; it is indicated in selected patients (Fig. 20-1) who are candidates for coronary graft bypass surgery or angioplasty

Medical therapy

1. Aggressive modification of preventable risk factors (weight reduction in obese patients, regular aerobic exercise program, diet low in cholesterol and sodium, cessation of cigarette smoking)

2. Correction of possible aggravating factors (e.g., anemia, thyrotoxicosis, hypertension, hypercholesterolemia)

3. Pharmacotherapy: the major classes of antiischemic agents are nitrates, beta adrenergic blockers, calcium channel antagonists, aspirin, and heparin; these can be used alone or in combination

   a. Nitrates cause venodilation and relaxation of vascular smooth muscle; the decreased venous return from venodilation decreases diastolic ventricular wall tension (preload) and thereby reduces the mechanical activity (and myocardial O_2 consumption) during systole. Relaxation of vascular smooth muscle increases coronary blood flow and reduces systemic pressure. Tolerance to nitrates can be minimized by avoiding sustained blood levels with a daily nitrate-free period (e.g., omission of bedtime dose of oral disosorbide dinitrate or 12 hr on/12 hr off transdermal nitroglycerin therapy). Table 33-29 describes commonly used nitrate preparations.

   b. Beta adrenergic blocking agents achieve their major antianginal effect by reducing heart rate and systolic blood pressure. Table 33-18 describes commonly used beta adrenergic blockers.

   c. Calcium channel antagonists play a major role in preventing and terminating myocardial ischemia induced by coronary artery spasm. They are particularly effective in microvascular angina[8] (cardiac pain with normal epicardial coronary arteries and dynamic vasoconstriction of prearterial intramyocardial vessels, usually seen in hypertensive patients). All calcium channel antagonists reduce the influx of calcium into the myocardial and vascular smooth muscle cells through slow channels, but they differ in their mode of action. Nifedipine exerts its antianginal effect through arterial vasodilation (both coronary and peripheral), thereby lowering left ventricular sys-

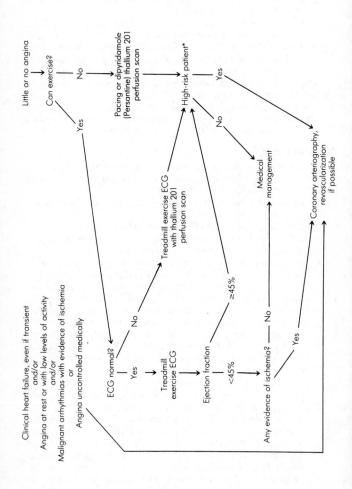

Figure 20-1
Risk stratification of patients with coronary artery disease. Included are cases of stable angina, progressive angina, prolonged myocardial ischemia, and past myocardial infarction. Asterisk (*) denotes the high-risk patient, defined as a person with at least one of the following: (1) inability to exercise 3 min on the Bruce protocol, (2) ST segment depressions of 2 mm or more with exercise, (3) decreased systolic pressure of 10 mm Hg or more with exercise, (4) failure to increase systolic pressure 10 mm Hg or more with exercise, (5) signs of congestive failure with exercise (S_3 gallop, rales), (6) large areas of decreased perfusion with exercise, especially multiple areas or with left ventricular wall or septal involvement, that fill in with rest. (From Cheitlin MD: JAMA 259:2771, 1988. Reproduced with permission.)

tolic wall tension and increasing coronary blood flow. Nicardipine produces relaxation of coronary vascular smooth muscle. Both diltiazem and verapamil produce coronary vasodilation and decrease heart rate. However, verapamil has more pronounced vasodilatory and AV nodal activity than diltiazem. Table 33-19 compares the various calcium channel antagonists.

d. Aspirin has been proved effective for prevention of myocardial infarction and coronary death in males over age 50.[49] Dosage varies from 160 to 325 mg qd or 325 mg qod. The risks of chronic salicylate use (e.g., GI bleeding, bronchospasm in susceptible patients) must be considered before starting any patient on daily aspirin.

e. Intravenous heparin is useful in unstable angina and has been shown to reduce the frequency of myocardial infarction and refractory angina.[51]

Surgical therapy

The Framingham study[10] showed that overall mortality for angina in medically treated patients is 4%. Mortality drops to 1.5% if angina is based on one- or two-vessel disease and rises to 9% if the patient has three-vessel disease and poor exercise tolerance.

Coronary artery bypass graft (CABG) surgery is recommended for patients with left main coronary disease or symptomatic three-vessel disease since the survival rate is significantly improved in these patients.[16] When CABG is done for relief of severe angina, it brings complete relief of angina in about 70% of patients and partial relief in another 20%.[28]

Percutaneous transluminal coronary angioplasty (PTCA) should be considered for patients with one- or two-vessel disease. Patients selected for PTCA must also be candidates for CABG. The types of lesions best suited for angioplasty are proximal lesions, noncalcified, concentric, and preferably shorter than 5 mm in length (should not exceed 10 mm).[27] Approximately 80% of patients will show immediate benefit after PTCA. Restenosis with recurrence of angina occurs in approximately 20% of patients, usually within the first 3 mo after PTCA. In these patients PTCA can be repeated.[23]

20.2   MYOCARDIAL INFARCTION

Definition

Myocardial infarction (MI) is characterized by necrosis resulting from an insufficient supply of oxygenated blood to an area of the heart.

1. Subendocardial (non–Q wave): area of ischemic necrosis limited to the inner third to half of myocardial wall
2. Transmural (Q wave): area of ischemic necrosis penetrates the entire thickness of the ventricular wall

Etiology

1. Coronary atherosclerosis
2. Coronary artery spasm

3. Coronary embolism (caused by infective endocarditis, rheumatic heart disease, intracavity thrombus)
4. Periarteritis and other coronary artery inflammatory diseases
5. Dissection into coronary arteries (aneurysmal or iatrogenic)
6. Congenital abnormalities of coronary circulation

Contributing factors

1. Tachycardia (increased O_2 consumption, decreased diastolic filling time)
2. Left ventricular hypertrophy (increased O_2 demand)
3. Anemia (decreased O_2-carrying capacity)
4. Increased platelet aggregation (increased risk of thrombosis, coronary artery spasm via production of thromboxane A_2)

Clinical presentation

1. Crushing substernal chest pain, usually lasting longer than 30 min
2. Pain unrelieved by rest or sublingual nitroglycerin, or it rapidly recurs
3. Pain may radiate to the left or right arm, neck, jaw, back, shoulders, or abdomen and is not pleuritic in character
4. Pain may be associated with dyspnea, diaphoresis, nausea, or vomiting
5. Approximately 20% of infarctions are painless (usually in diabetic or elderly patients)

Physical findings

1. Skin may be diaphoretic, cool, with pallor (because of decreased O_2)
2. Lungs may reveal rales at the bases (indicative of CHF)
3. Heart may have an apical systolic murmur caused by mitral regurgitation secondary to papillary muscle dysfunction; an S_3 or S_4 may also be present
4. The physical exam may be completely normal

Diagnostic studies

1. ECG
   a. In Q wave infarction there is the development of
      (1) Inverted T waves, which indicate an area of ischemia
      (2) Elevated ST segments, which indicate an area of injury
      (3) Q waves, which indicate the area of infarction; they usually develop over 12-36 hr (Table 20-1 describes location of transmural infarction based on ECG abnormalities)
   b. In non–Q wave infarction, Q waves are absent but
      (1) History and myocardial enzyme elevations are compatible with MI
      (2) ECG shows ST segment elevation, depression, or no change followed by T wave inversion
2. Serum enzyme studies: damaged necrotic heart muscle releases cardiac enzymes (CK, LDH) into the bloodstream in amounts that correlate with the size of the infarct (Fig. 20-2 and Table 20-2). Other parts of the body also have these enzymes (CK in skeletal muscle and brain; LDH in RBC, liver, skeletal muscle, kidneys, and lungs) so their presence could

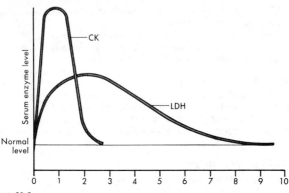

Figure 20-2
Time course of serum enzyme activity following an acute myocardial infarction.
CK, Creatine kinase; LDH, lactic dehydrogenase.

Table 20-1   ECG location of Q wave infarct

Area of Infarction	ECG Abnormality
Anterior wall	Q waves in V_1-V_4
Anteroseptal	Q waves in V_1-V_2
Anteroapical	Q waves in V_2-V_3
Anterolateral	Q waves in V_4-V_6, I, aVL
Lateral wall	Q waves in I, aVL
Inferior wall	Q waves in II, III, aVF
Posterior wall	R > S in V_1
	Q wave in V_6

Table 20-2   Serum enzyme concentration changes following acute MI

Enzyme	Rise	Peak	Return to Normal
CK	2-8 hr	12-36 hr	3-4 days
LDH	12-48 hr	3-6 days	8-14 days

KEY: CK, Creatine kinase; LDH, lactate dehydrogenase

indicate damage to extracardiac tissue. However, electrophoretic fractionation of the enzymes can pinpoint certain isoenzymes (CK-MB and
LDH_1) that are more sensitive indicators of MI than total CK or LDH.

Therapy

The goals of management during acute MI are to minimize the amount of infarcted myocardium and to prevent complications. Thrombolytic agents and early IV administration of beta-adrenergic blockers significantly reduce the incidence of recurrent infarction and ischemia.

1. Thrombolytic therapy[3]

    If the duration of pain has been short (ideally <4-6 hr), recanalization of the occluded arteries should be attempted with one of the following agents:

    a. Tissue plasminogen activator (tPA): 10 mg IV bolus followed by 50 mg over the first hour and 20 mg/hr for the next 2 hr

    b. Streptokinase: 1.5 milion units IV over 1 hr

    c. Anisoylated plasminogen/streptokinase activator complex (APSAC, Anistreplase): 30 units over 5 min

    All three of these agents are effective; however, tPA is much more expensive; adjunctive antiplatelet and anticoagulant therapy to minimize the chance of coronary reocclusion is started with

    a. Aspirin: 160-325 mg/day

    b. Heparin: 5000 U IV bolus at the time of tPA therapy followed by a continuous infusion of 1000 U/hr (adjusted to keep the APTT at 1.5-2 times control; in patients receiving streptokinase or APSAC, start the heparin when the APTT < 50 sec)

    Contraindications to thrombolytic therapy are a history of CVA, abnormal coagulation parameters, prolonged CPR, surgery, an invasive procedure within the preceding 2 wk, a systolic > 180 or diastolic > 110 mm Hg, recent head trauma or known intracranial neoplasm, pregnancy, diabetic hemorrhagic retinopathy or other hemorrhagic ophthalmic condition, suspected aortic dissection, history of bleeding disorders.

2. Use of beta-adrenergic blocking agents (Table 20-3)

    Beta blockers are useful to reduce myocardial oxygen consumption and possibly prevent tachydysrhythmias. Early intravenous beta blockade, followed by institution of an oral maintenance regimen, is also effective in reducing recurrent infarction and ischemia when used in addition to thrombolytic therapy. The timing of initiation of beta blocker therapy varies with the particular beta blocker chosen.

    Before use of beta blockers, the contraindications and side effects (i.e., exacerbation of CHF, exacerbation of asthma, CNS effects, hypotension, bradycardia) must be carefully considered.

    Patients with acute MI can also be classically subdivided into four subsets based on their clinical presentation and hemodynamic measurements[18] (Table 20-4). The therapeutic approach to each patient varies with the subset.

1. Subset I: uncomplicated MI

    a. IV nitroglycerin may be useful for pain control and can modify infarct size and early and late mortality[30]; mix 100 mg of IV NTG/500 ml of D_5W and, after a 15 μg bolus injection, begin a 6 μg/min infesion (2 ml/hr), increasing the dose by 6 μg/min q5min until

    (1) The patient is free of chest pain

    (2) Maximum dose of 200 μg/min is reached

Table 20-3 Use of beta blockers during and post-MI

Drug	Initiation of Therapy	Dosage
Metoprolol (Lopressor)	Within 24 hr in stabilized patients with acute MI	5 mg IV q2min up to 15 mg (if tolerated), followed by 50 mg PO q6h for 48 hours, followed by 100 mg PO bid
Atenolol (Tenormin)	Within 24 hr in stabilized patients with acute MI	Initial dose is 5 mg IV, followed 10 min later by repeat 5 mg IV dose (given over 5 min); 50 mg tablet then given 10 min after second IV dose, followed by another 50 mg tablet 12 hr later; daily oral dose of 100 mg started on day 2
Esmolol (Brevibloc)	Within 24 hr in stabilized patients with acute MI	Loading dose (500 μg/kg/min) infused over 1 min, followed by a 4 min infusion (usually starting with 50 μg/kg/min in saline or glucose)

Table 20-4   Clinical and hemodynamic subsets after acute MI

Subset	CI	PCWP
I: no pulmonary congestion or peripheral hypoperfusion	2.7 ± 0.5	12 ± 7
II: isolated pulmonary congestion	2.3 ± 0.4	23 ± 5
III: isolated peripheral hypoperfusion	1.9 ± 0.4	12 ± 5
IV: both pulmonary congestion and hypoperfusion	1.6 ± 0.6	27 ± 8

From Forrester JS, Diamond GA, Swan HCJ: Am J Cardiol 39:137, 1977.
KEY: CI, Cardiac index; PCWP, pulmonary capillary wedge pressure

    (3) Blood pressure decreases, below 100 mm Hg systolic
Nitroglycerin should be used with great caution in patients with inferior wall MI; nitrate usage can result in hypotension because these patients are very sensitive to change in preload[17]

  b. Nasal O_2: administer at 2-4 L/min

  c. Morphine sulfate: 2 mg IV q5min prn for severe pain unrelieved by IV nitroglycerin

    (1) Hypotension secondary to morphine can be treated with careful IV hydration

    (2) Respiratory depression caused by morphine can be reversed with naloxone (Narcan) 0.8 mg IV

  d. Lidocaine: 1 mg/kg IV bolus followed by infusion at 1-4 mg/min is indicated only if frequent (>6/min), closely coupled (R on T phenomenon), multifocal, or symptomatic PVCs are noted; prophylactic lidocaine in the initial 24 hr of MI is not recommended, particularly in patients over age 70 and those with heart failure

  e. Beta blockers: as noted previously

  f. Diet: NPO until stable; then no added salt low-cholesterol diet

  g. Stool softener: dioctyl sulfosuccinate (Colace) 100 mg PO qd; for constipation, may use milk of magnesia 30 ml PO qhs prn (do not use in patients with renal failure)

  h. Anticoagulants in patients who are not candidates for thrombolytic therapy: minidose heparin (5000 U SQ q8-12h) is indicated (barring specific contraindications) to prevent left ventricular mural thrombosis in patients with extensive acute myocardial infarction (very high peak creatine kinase levels); in patients with anterior wall MI (30% risk for developing mural thrombosis) full IV heparinization or high dose SQ heparin (12,500 U q12h) are more effective than minidose heparin in preventing left ventricular mural thrombosis; high-dose SQ heparin is generally not associated with a high frequency of hemorrhagic complications[58]; aspirin has been shown to reduce the risk of reinfarction after MI[49] and should be used barring any specific contraindications

  i. Strict bed rest: for initial 24 hr; then if patient remains stable, gradually increase the activity

  j. Sedation: use short-acting benzodiazepine (see Table 33-17)

  k. Patient education to decrease the risk of subsequent cardiac events (proper diet, cessation of smoking, regular exercise) is initiated when the patient is medically stable

2. Subset II: these patients have left ventricular dysfunction (manifested by pulmonary congestion), but can still maintain an adequate cardiac index; therapy consists of IV nitroglycerin, diuretics (to decrease PCWP), and morphine

3. Subset III: these patients often have right ventricular and inferior wall infarcts

  a. Therapy consists of careful IV hydration with normal saline until the PCWP increases to approximately 18 mm Hg

  b. The increased PCWP should increase the cardiac output unless the patient has an extremely poor ventricular function

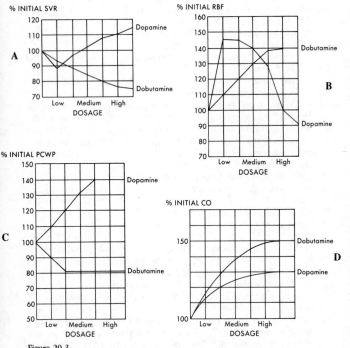

Figure 20-3

Comparison of hemodynamic responses to dobutamine and dopamine. **A,** Systemic vascular resistance. **B,** Renal blood flow. **C,** Pulmonary capillary wedge pressure. **D,** Cardiac output. (Reproduced with permission from Eli Lilly & Co.)

4. Subset IV: these patients have severe left ventricular dysfunction; therapy consists of the combined use of dobutamine and dopamine to provide inotropic stimulation
   a. Dopamine also stimulates renal vasodilatation when used at low doses (Fig. 20-3)
   b. An intraaortic balloon pump may be necessary to maintain cardiac output and coronary perfusion (see Section 5.7)

Complications

1. Dysrhythmias: see Section 20.8 for recognition and therapy
2. Mitral regurgitation: characterized by the sudden appearance of an apical systolic murmur with radiation to the axilla; a loud first heart sound is often associated with the murmur
   a. Etiology: papillary muscle dysfunction or left ventricular aneurysm (it occurs primarily in inferior, lateral, and subendocardial infarcts)
   b. Diagnostic studies: at cardiac catheterization, the pulmonary wedge tracing shows giant V waves (Fig. 20-4)
   c. Therapy[5]
      (1) IV nitroprusside to decrease PCWP
      (2) If hypotensive, will need dopamine or dobutamine combined with nitroprusside (combined use of inotropic and vasodilator agents)
      (3) Intraaortic balloon counterpulsation (IABC) provides lifesaving physiologic support by facilitating ventricular emptying during systole and increasing retrograde coronary perfusion during diastole

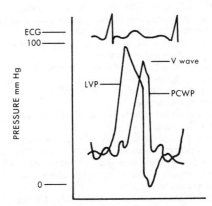

Figure 20-4
Mitral regurgitation. Note the V wave caused by regurgitation of blood in the left atrium. LVP, Left ventricular pressure; PCWP, pulmonary capillary wedge pressure.

(4) Surgical repair after stabilization of the patient

NOTE: Despite the above measures, the mortality for these patients remains extremely high.

3. Right ventricular infarct: characterized by jugular venous distention, Kussmaul's sign, and hypotension without pulmonary congestion
   a. Diagnostic studies: hemodynamic monitoring shows right atrial pressure/PCWP ≥ 0.8
   b. Right precordial ECG leads reveal ST segment elevation in V_{4R}
   c. Therapy: vigorous IV hydration

4. Ventricular septal defect (VSD): characterized by a systolic murmur at the lower left sternal border; VSD usually occurs within 2 wk after acute MI
   a. Diagnostic studies: there is an increase in oxygen content in blood samples from the pulmonary artery when compared with blood from the right atrium
   b. Therapy: same as for acute mitral regurgitation (see above)

5. Myocardial rupture: usually seen in elderly patients 2-4 days after MI; it is characterized by sudden hypotension and loss of consciousness, followed by electromechanical dissociation, and finally ending in death

6. Systemic embolism: characterized by sudden onset of neurologic deficit or pain in the involved area (e.g., flank tenderness in renal artery embolism)
   a. Etiology: mural thrombi; occur most frequently with anterior wall MI
   b. Diagnostic studies:
      (1) Echocardiography may reveal the presence of mural thrombi
      (2) Perform arteriography if peripheral embolism suspected
      (3) Perform renal scintigraphy if renal embolism suspected
   c. Therapy: IV heparinization; embolectomy if the clot is accessible

7. Pericarditis: see Section 20.7

8. Dressler's syndrome: characterized by fever, pleurisy, pericarditis, friction rub, pericardial and pleural effusions, and joint pains; usually occurs between 1 wk and 6 mo after MI
   a. Etiology: autoimmune disorder secondary to previous damage to the myocardium and pericardium
   b. Therapy: indomethacin 50 mg PO q6h or other nonsteroidal antiinflammatory agents; if no improvement, consider prednisone 30 mg PO bid initially, tapered off over several weeks

9. Left ventricular aneurysm
   a. Diagnostic studies: echocardiography; ECG shows persistent ST elevations 3-4 wk after MI
   b. Therapy: surgical excision if the aneurysm is associated with recurrent ventricular tachycardia, intractable CHF, recurrent embolization, or persistent angina despite intensive medical treatment[23]

10. Pulmonary embolism: characterized by sudden onset of tachypnea, tachycardia, and chest pain
    a. Prevention: minidose heparin (5000 U SQ q12h) and early ambulation after MI

   b. Diagnostic studies: ventilation/perfusion scan; if inconclusive, follow with arteriogram
   c. Therapy: IV heparinization

Hospital mortality during acute MI

Various attempts have been made to identify patients with an increased risk of mortality during an acute MI. The classification developed by Killip and Kimball[31] categorizes patients into four major groups (Table 20-5).

Evaluation of post-MI patients

1. Submaximal (low-level) treadmill test (done 1-3 wk after MI) in stable patients without any clinical evidence of significant left ventricular dysfunction or postmyocardial infarction angina (Fig. 20-1)
   a. Useful to assess the patient's functional capacity and formulate an at-home exercise program
   b. Helpful to determine the patient's prognosis
2. Radionuclide angiography or two-dimensional echocardiography
   a. To evaluate the patient's left ventricular ejection fraction
   b. To evaluate ventricular size and segmental wall motion
   c. Echocardiography also indicated in patients with anterior wall infarction to rule out the presence of mural thrombi
3. A 24 hr Holter monitor study to evaluate patients who have demonstrated significant dysrhythmias during their hospital stay; selected patients with complex ventricular ectopy may be candidates for programmed electrical stimulation

Prognosis after MI

The prognosis following MI depends on multiple factors:
   1. Use of beta blockers: the mortality of patients on a regular regimen of beta blockers shows a significant decrease when compared with that of control groups[29,39]
   2. Presence of dysrhythmias: frequent ventricular ectopic beats ($\geq$10/hr) or repetitive forms of ventricular ectopic beats (couplets, triplets) indicate an increased risk (two to three times greater) of sudden cardiac death[41]; however, ventricular tachycardia/fibrillation (VT/VF) occur-

Table 20-5   Killip classification during acute MI

Clinical Class	Description	Hospital Mortality
I	No heart failure (absent rales, absent S_3 gallop)	<10%
II	Heart failure (rales in $\leq$50% of lung fields or S_3 gallop and venous hypertension)	10-20%
III	Severe heart failure (rales in >50% of lung fields, pulmonary edema)	35-50%
IV	Cardiogenic shock	>80%

Adapted from Killip PT, Kimball JT: Am J Cardiol 20:457, 1967.

ring within 72 hr of MI and not associated with heart failure or hypotension does not influence prognosis; "late" VT/VF (occurring >72 hr post-MI) increases in-hospital mortality threefold though does not affect long-term mortality[55]

3. Size of infarct: the larger it is, the higher the post-MI mortality rate; there is a close correlation between the peak plasma CK values and survival over a 4 yr period[52]

4. Site of infarct: inferior wall MI carries a better prognosis than anterior wall MI, because in anterior wall MI the damage is confined exclusively to the left ventricle (resulting in severe left ventricular dysfunction), whereas in inferior wall MI the damage is shared by both ventricles and thus the hemodynamic impact on either ventricle is lessened[43]

5. Type of infarct: although the in-hospital mortality is higher for patients with Q wave infarcts, the long-term prognosis for non–Q wave MI may be worse because these patients have a higher incidence of sudden cardiac death after hospital discharge[9]; cardiac catheterization should be considered in patients with non–Q wave infarction; ST segment depressions at baseline and/or discharge identify patients at higher risk for adverse outcome who should have additional studies; diltiazem may prevent early reinfarction and severe angina after non–Q wave infarction; its use, however, should be avoided in patients with EF <40% or pulmonary congestion; calcium antagonists in general have not shown any significant benefit as an acute intervention or secondary prevention and may increase mortality in treated patients

6. Ejection fraction after MI: the lower the left ventricular ejection fraction (EF), the higher the mortality after MI; in one series[45] the probability of survival was highest in patients with an EF ≥50% and lowest in patients with EF ≤20% (a low EF associated with VPCs signifies a particularly poor prognosis)[46]

7. Presence of post-MI angina: indicates a higher mortality, particularly when angina is accompanied by new ECG changes distant from the acute infarct[47]

8. Performance on low-level exercise test: the presence of ST segment changes during the test is a predictor of higher mortality during the first year; patients with a positive test after MI should undergo coronary artery catheterization to determine if angioplasty or coronary artery bypass is indicated

9. Presence of pericarditis during the acute phase of MI: increases mortality at 1 yr (18% vs 12%)[56]

10. Type A behavior (competitive drive, ambitiousness, hostility): is associated with a lower mortality following symptomatic MI[42]

11. Thrombolytic therapy decreases mortality and increases myocardial perfusion and salvage

12. Coronary angioplasty for a patent infarct-related artery is generally not appropriate in the immediate phase after thrombolysis because of increased morbidity and mortality without improved ventricular function, sustained patency, or reduced reinfarction[54,57]

13. Additional poor prognostic factors are the following: cigarette smoking, a history of hypertension or of prior MI, increasing age, DM, and female sex

20.3 VALVULAR HEART DISEASE

Mitral stenosis

Etiology
1. Progressive fibrosis, scarring, and calcification of the valve
2. Rheumatic fever (still a common cause in underdeveloped countries)
3. Congenital defect (parachute valve)
4. Rare causes: endomyocardial fibroelastosis, malignant carcinoid syndrome, SLE

Pathophysiology
The cross-section of a normal orifice measures 4-6 cm^2. Narrowing of the valve orifice causes a pressure gradient across the valve (Fig. 20-5). A murmur becomes audible when the valve orifice becomes smaller than 2 cm^2. When the orifice approaches 1 cm^2, the condition becomes critical and symptoms appear.

Symptoms
1. Exertional dyspnea initially, followed by orthopnea and paroxysmal nocturnal dyspnea (PND)
2. Acute pulmonary edema may develop following exertion
3. Systemic emboli (caused by stagnation of blood in the left atrium) may be seen in patients with associated atrial fibrillation
4. Hemoptysis may be present due to persistent pulmonary hypertension

Physical findings
1. Prominent jugular A waves (in patients with normal sinus rhythm [NSR])

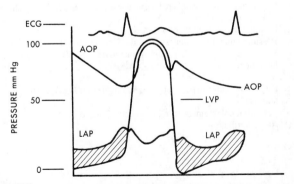

Figure 20-5
Mitral stenosis. Note the gradient between (LAP) left atrial pressure and (LVP) left ventricular pressure during diastole. AOP is aortic pressure.

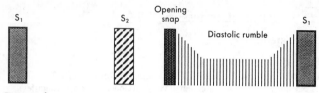

Figure 20-6
Graphic representation of a mitral stenosis murmur.

2. Opening snap occurring in early diastole; a short (<0.07 sec) A_2 to opening snap interval indicates severe mitral stenosis
3. Apical middiastolic or presystolic rumble that does not radiate (Fig. 20-6)
4. Accentuated S_1 (because of delayed and forceful closure of the valve)
5. If pulmonary hypertension is present, there may be a soft, early-diastolic, decrescendo murmur (Graham-Steell murmur) caused by pulmonic regurgitation (it is best heard along the left sternal border and may be confused with aortic regurgitation)

Diagnostic studies

1. Echocardiography: the characteristic finding on an echocardiogram is a markedly diminished E to F slope of the anterior mitral valve leaflet during diastole; there is also fusion of the commissures resulting in anterior movement of the posterior mitral valve leaflet during diastole (calcification in the valve may also be noted)
2. Chest x-ray
   a. Straightening of the left cardiac border caused by dilated left atrial appendage
   b. Left atrial enlargement on lateral chest x-ray (appearing as double density on a PA chest x-ray)
   c. Prominence of pulmonary arteries
   d. Possible pulmonary congestion and edema (Kerley-B lines)
   e. Possible elevation of left main bronchus as a result of left atrial enlargement
3. ECG
   a. Right ventricular hypertrophy, right axis deviation caused by pulmonary HTN
   b. Left atrial enlargement (broad, notched P waves)
   c. Atrial fibrillation

Therapy

1. Medical
   a. Decrease level of activity
   b. If the patient is in atrial fibrillation, control the rate response with digitalis

c. If patient has persistent atrial fibrillation (because of large left atrium), permanent anticoagulation is indicated to decrease the risk of serious thromboembolism

d. Treat CHF with diuretics and sodium restriction

e. Antibiotic prophylaxis for dental and surgical procedures

2. Surgical: valve replacement is indicated when the valve orifice < 0.7-0.8 cm^2 or if symptoms persist despite optimum medical therapy; commissurotomy may be possible if the mitral valve is not calcified and if there is pure mitral stenosis without significant subvalvular disease

3. Balloon valvuloplasty is emerging as a potential alternative, particularly in patients who are poor surgical candidates

Mitral regurgitation

Etiology

1. Papillary muscle dysfunction (as a result of ischemic heart disease)
2. Ruptured chordae tendineae
3. Infective endocarditis
4. Calcified mitral valve annulus
5. Left ventricular dilation
6. Rheumatic heart disease
7. Primary or secondary mitral valve prolapse
8. Hypertrophic cardiomyopathy
9. Idiopathic myxomatous degeneration of the mitral valve
10. Myxoma
11. SLE

Pathophysiology

A large portion of the left ventricular stroke volume is ejected in the left atrium (low-pressure chamber). Eventually there is an increase in left atrial and pulmonary pressures, with subsequent right ventricular failure.

Symptoms

1. Fatigue, dyspnea, orthopnea, frank CHF
2. Hemoptysis (caused by pulmonary hypertension)
3. Systemic emboli may occur in patients with left atrial mural thrombi associated with atrial fibrillation

Physical findings

1. Hyperdynamic apex often with palpable left ventricular lift and apical thrill
2. Holosystolic murmur at apex with radiation to base or to left axilla (Fig. 20-7); there is poor correlation between the intensity of the systolic murmur and the degree of regurgitation
3. Apical early-to-middiastolic rumble (rare)

Diagnostic studies

1. Echocardiography: enlarged left atrium, hyperdynamic left ventricle (erratic motion of the leaflet is seen in patients with ruptured chordae

Figure 20-7
Graphic representation of a mitral regurgitation murmur.

tendineae)[6]; Doppler electrocardiography will show evidence of mitral regurgitation
2. Chest x-ray
   a. Left atrial enlargement (usually more pronounced than mitral stenosis)
   b. Left ventricular enlargement
   c. Possible pulmonary congestion
3. ECG
   a. Left atrial enlargement
   b. Left ventricular hypertrophy
   c. Atrial fibrillation

Therapy

1. Medical
   a. Salt restriction, diuretics
   b. Digitalis (for inotropic effect and to control ventricular response if atrial fibrillation with fast ventricular response is present)
   c. Afterload reduction (to decrease the regurgitant fraction and to increase cardiac output) may be accomplished with nifedipine, hydralazine, or ACE inhibitors
   d. Anticoagulants, if persistent atrial fibrillation
   e. Antibiotic prophylaxis before dental and surgical procedures
2. Surgical: generally not recommended unless the patient is severely limited by the disease despite optimum medical therapy; surgery should be considered earlier in patients with moderate to severe mitral regurgitation and minimal symptoms if there is echocardiographic evidence of rapidly progressive increase in left ventricular end-diastolic dimension

Mitral valve prolapse

Incidence

1. Can be found by two-dimensional echo in 4% of the general population
2. Increased incidence is seen with autoimmune thyroid disorders, Ehlers-Danlos syndrome, Marfan's syndrome, pseudoxanthoma elasticum, pectus excavatum, anorexia nervosa, and bulimia

Symptoms (if present)

1. Chest pain
2. Palpitations
3. TIA or stroke (rare)

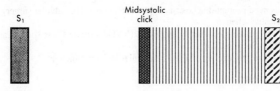

Figure 20-8
Graphic representation of a mitral valve prolapse murmur.

Physical findings

1. Usually young female patient with narrow AP chest diameter
2. Mid-to-late click, heard best at the apex (Fig. 20-8)
3. Crescendo mid-to-late systolic murmur

Echocardiography

The echocardiogram shows the anterior and posterior leaflets bulging posteriorly in systole.

Complications

1. Bacterial endocarditis
2. TIA or stroke secondary to embolic phenomena (from fibrin and platelet thrombi)
3. Cardiac dysrhythmias (usually supraventricular)
4. Sudden death
5. Mitral regurgitation

The incidence of complications in MVP is very low (less than 1% per year) and generally associated with an increase in mitral leaflet thickness to ≥ 5 mm[38]; young patients (age <45) with absence of mitral systolic murmur or mitral regurgitation on Doppler echocardiography are at low risk for any complications

Therapy[13]

1. The empirical use of antidysrhythmic drugs to prevent sudden death in patients with uncomplicated MVP is not advisable; beta blockers may be tried in symptomatic patients (e.g., palpitations, chest pain); they decrease the heart rate, thus decreasing the stretch on the prolapsing valve leaflets
2. Antibiotic prophylaxis for infective endocarditis when undergoing dental, GI, or GU procedures is indicated only in patients with MVP, systolic murmur, and echocardiographic evidence of mitral regurgitation
3. Patients should be reassured that the prognosis of this condition is generally excellent and activity should not be limited; those at high risk of complications are defined as having hemodynamically significant mitral regurgitation (2-4% of adults with MVP); they should be aggressively followed with annual Doppler echocardiography; exercise testing and 24 hr Holter monitoring should also be implemented; complex dysrhyth-

mias need prompt diagnosis and treatment; corrective valvular surgery is advisable when

a. The patient becomes symptomatic (NYHA criteria Class II or greater [see Section 20.4])
b. There is a decrease in left ventricular systolic function

Aortic stenosis

Etiology

1. Rheumatic inflammation of aortic valve
2. Progressive stenosis of congenital bicuspid valve
3. Idiopathic calcification of aortic valve
4. Congenital

Pathophysiology

The obstruction to the left ventricular outflow leads to increased left ventricular pressure (Fig. 20-9). This results in concentric hypertrophy and the subsequent decrease in contractile performance and in ejection fraction. Symptoms appear when the valve orifice decreases to less than 1 cm^2 (normal orifice is 3 cm^2). The stenosis is considered severe when the orifice is less than 0.5 cm^2/m^2 or the pressure gradient is 50 mm Hg or higher.[27]

Symptoms

1. Angina: caused by increased O_2 demand secondary to hypertrophy and decreased O_2 supply secondary to decreased coronary artery filling
2. Syncope (particularly with exertion) occurs when vasodilation in muscles during exercise causes insufficient cerebral blood flow as a result of fixed cardiac output

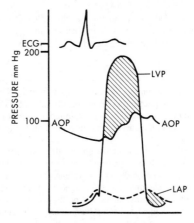

Figure 20-9
Valvular aortic stenosis. Note the gradient between (LVP) left ventricular pressure and (AOP) aortic pressure. LAP is left atrial pressure.

3. CHF: caused by left ventricular failure

   NOTE: The average duration of symptoms before death is: angina, 36 mo; syncope, 36 mo; CHF, 18 mo.

Physical findings

1. Loud, rough systolic diamond-shaped murmur, best heard at base of heart and transmitted into neck vessels (Fig. 20-10); it is often associated with a thrill or ejection click
2. Absence or diminished intensity of the sound of aortic valve closure (in severe aortic stenosis)
3. Late slow-rising carotid upstroke with decreased amplitude
4. Strong apical impulse
5. Narrowing of pulse pressure in later stages of aortic stenosis

Diagnostic studies

1. Chest x-ray
   a. Poststenotic dilation of ascending aorta
   b. Calcification of aortic cusps
   c. Pulmonary congestion (in advanced stages of aortic stenosis)
2. ECG
   a. Left ventricular hypertrophy
   b. ST-T wave changes
3. Echocardiography: thickening of the left ventricular wall; if the patient has valvular calcifications, multiple echoes may be seen from within the aortic root and there is poor separation of the aortic cusps during systole[6]
4. Cardiac catheterization: indicated in symptomatic patients; it confirms the diagnosis and estimates the severity of the disease by measuring the gradient across the valve, allowing calculation of the valve area

Therapy

1. Medical
   a. Strenuous activity should be avoided
   b. Diuretics and sodium restriction if CHF is present
   c. Antibiotic prophylaxis for surgical and dental procedures
2. Surgical: valve replacement is the treatment of choice in symptomatic patients because the 5 yr mortality after onset of symptoms is extremely

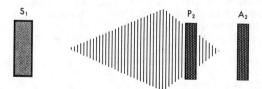

Figure 20-10
Graphic representation of an aortic stenosis murmur.

high even with optimum medical therapy; valve replacement is indicated if cardiac catheterization establishes a pressure gradient >50 mm Hg and a valve area <1.0 cm^2

3. Balloon valvuloplasty is effective in decreasing the degree of stenosis, with resulting clinical and hemodynamic improvement; restenosis after 9 mo is common, so balloon valvuloplasty should be reserved as palliative therapy for symptomatic patients who are poor surgical candidates

Aortic regurgitation

Etiology
1. Infective endocarditis
2. Rheumatic fibrosis
3. Trauma with valvular rupture
4. Congenital bicuspid aortic valve
5. Myxomatous degeneration
6. Syphilitic aortitis
7. Rheumatoid spondylitis
8. SLE

Pathophysiology
The regurgitation of blood in the left ventricle increases the left ventricular filling pressure, thereby causing left ventricular diastolic volume overload. This results in dilation and hypertrophy of the left ventricle with subsequent decompensation.

Manifestations
Aortic regurgitation (except when secondary to infective endocarditis) is generally well tolerated and patients remain asymptomatic for years; following are the common manifestations after significant deterioration of left ventricular function:
1. Dyspnea on exertion
2. Syncope
3. Chest pain
4. CHF

Physical findings
1. Widened pulse pressure (markedly increased systolic blood pressure, decreased diastolic blood pressure)
2. Bounding pulses, head "bobbing" with each systole; "water hammer" or collapsing pulse (Corrigan's pulse) can be palpated at the wrist and is caused by rapid rise and sudden collapse of the arterial pressure during late systole; capillary pulsations (Quincke's pulse) may be seen at the base of the nail beds
3. A to-and-fro "double Duroziez" murmur may be heard over femoral arteries
4. Cardiac auscultation reveals
   a. Displacement of cardiac impulse downward and to the patient's left

b. S_3 heard over the apex
c. Decrescendo, blowing diastolic murmur heard along left sternal border
d. Low-pitched, apical diastolic rumble (Austin-Flint murmur) caused by aortic regurgitation impinging on the anterior mitral leaflet
e. Early systolic apical ejection murmur

Diagnostic studies

1. Chest x-ray
   a. Left ventricular hypertrophy
   b. Aortic dilation
2. ECG: left ventricular hypertrophy
3. Echocardiography: coarse diastolic fluttering of the anterior mitral leaflet

Therapy

1. Medical
   a. Digitalis, diuretics, and sodium restriction
   b. Bacterial endocarditis prophylaxis for surgical and dental procedures
2. Surgical: reserved for
   a. Symptomatic patients with chronic aortic regurgitation despite optimum medical therapy
   b. Patients with acute aortic regurgitation (i.e., infective endocarditis) producing left ventricular failure
   c. Patients with increased cardiac enlargement, decreased fractional shortening on echocardiogram, decreasing ejection fraction

20.4 CONGESTIVE HEART FAILURE

Definition

Congestive heart failure (CHF) is a pathophysiologic state characterized by congestion in the pulmonary or systemic circulation. It is caused by the heart's inability to pump sufficient oxygenated blood to meet the metabolic needs of the tissues.

Etiology

Left ventricular failure	Right ventricular failure
Systemic hypertension	Valvular heart disease (mitral
Valvular heart disease (AS, AR, MR)	stenosis)
	Pulmonary hypertension
Cardiomyopathy, myocarditis	Bacterial endocarditis (right sided)
Bacterial endocarditis	Right ventricular infarction
MI	
IHSS	

Biventricular failure
Left ventricular failure
Cardiomyopathy
Myocarditis
Dysrhythmias
Anemia
Thyrotoxicosis
AV fistula
Paget's disease
Beri-beri

Left ventricular failure can also be differentiated according to systolic dysfunction (low EF) and diastolic dysfunction (normal or high EF, "stiff ventricle")

Systolic dysfunction	Diastolic dysfunction
Post-MI	Hypertensive cardiovascular disease
Cardiomyopathy	Valvular heart disease (AS, AR,
Myocarditis	MR, IHSS)
	Restrictive cardiomyopathy

Clinical manifestations

1. Dyspnea: initially on exertion, then with progressively less strenuous activity, and eventually manifesting when patient is at rest; it is caused by increasing pulmonary congestion; the Valsalva maneuver performed with the blood pressure cuff inflated to 15 mm Hg over systolic pressure (with ascultation in the antecubital fossa) is useful in acute dyspnea to differentiate between cardiac and pulmonary disease; a normal response is characterized by disappearance of the Korotkoff sounds during the sustained maneuver with reappearance after release; in patients with chronic heart disease an abnormal response (lack of reappearance of the Korotkoff sounds after release of the maneuver or maintenance of beats throughout the maneuver) is sensitive (80-85%) and specific (86-91%) for detection of left ventricular systolic dysfunction[64]
2. Orthopnea: caused by increased venous return in the recumbent position
3. Paroxysmal nocturnal dyspnea (PND): results from multiple factors (increased venous return in the recumbent position, decreased Pa_{O_2}, decreased adrenergic stimulation of myocardial function)
4. Nocturnal angina: results from increased cardiac work (secondary to increased venous return)
5. Cheyne-Stokes respiration: alternating phases of apnea and hyperventilation caused by prolonged circulation time from lungs to brain
6. Fatigue, lethargy: results from low cardiac output

Physical exam

Left heart failure	Right heart failure
Pulmonary rales	Jugular venous distention
Tachypnea	Peripheral edema
S_3 gallop	Perioral and peripheral cyanosis
Cardiac murmurs (AS, AR, MR)	Congestive hepatomegaly
Paradoxical splitting of S_2	Ascites
	Hepatojugular reflux

Chest x-ray

1. Pulmonary venous congestion
2. Cardiomegaly with dilation of the involved heart chamber
3. Pleural effusions

Functional classification (criteria committee, New York Heart Association)

Class I: symptomatic only with greater than ordinary activity
Class II: symptomatic during ordinary activity
Class III: symptomatic with minimal activity but asymptomatic at rest
Class IV: symptomatic at rest

Therapy

1. Determine if CHF is secondary to systolic or diastolic dysfunction and identify and correct precipitating factors (i.e., anemia, thyrotoxicosis, hypertension, infections, beta blockers or other cardiac depressants, increased sodium load, medical noncompliance)
2. Decrease cardiac workload: restrict patient to bed rest; the risk of thromboembolism during this period can be minimized by using elastic antiembolic stockings and/or heparin 5000 U SQ q12h; fluid restriction may be indicated in selected patients
3. Sodium restriction: 2-6 g/day, no added salt diet at home
4. Diuretics
   a. Furosemide: 20-80 mg/day produces prompt venodilation and diuresis; when changing from an IV to oral furosemide, a doubling of the dose is usually necessary to achieve an equal effect
   b. Thiazides are not as powerful as furosemide, but are well tolerated and useful in mild to moderate CHF
   c. The addition of metolazone to furosemide usually produces an effective diuresis; frequent monitoring of electrolytes and renal function is recommended
5. ACE inhibitors
   a. They cause dilation of the arteriolar resistance vessels and the venous capacitance vessels, thereby reducing both preload and afterload
   b. They are associated with decreased mortality and improved clinical status when used in patients with CHF due to systolic dysfunction

   c. They can be added to diuretics in patients with CHF poorly con-
      trolled with only diuretic therapy
6. Digitalis is useful because of its positive inotropic and vagotonic effect
  in patients with CHF secondary to systolic dysfunction; it is of limited
  value in patients with mild CHF and normal sinus rhythm, though more
  beneficial in patients with rapid atrial fibrillation, severe CHF, or EF
  <20%; it can be added to diuretics and ACE inhibitors in patients with
  severe CHF
    a. When digoxin is used, the loading dose is 0.5 mg IV/PO, followed
       by 0.25 mg q4-6h for 4 doses, then 0.125-0.25 mg PO qd; the dos-
       age should be reduced in elderly patients and in patients with renal
       insufficiency
    b. The serum digoxin level should be checked periodically (therapeutic
       level is 0.9-2.0 ng/ml)
    c. Major factors predisposing to digitalis toxicity are quinidine and ver-
       apamil (can cause doubling of the digitalis level), hypokalemia, and
       hypomagnesemia
7. Inotropic agents (e.g., dobutamine, nitroprusside, amrinone) are useful
  in severe heart failure; their use is reserved for patients responding
  poorly to oral therapeutic regimens

Cardiogenic pulmonary edema

Definition
Cardiogenic pulmonary edema is a life-threatening condition caused by severe left ventricular decompensation.

Physical exam
1. Dyspnea with rapid, shallow breathing
2. Diaphoresis, perioral and peripheral cyanosis
3. Pink frothy sputum
4. Moist bilateral pulmonary rales
5. Increased pulmonary second sound, S_3 gallop (in association with
  tachycardia)
6. Bulging neck veins

Diagnostic studies
1. Chest x-ray
    a. Pulmonary congestion with Kerley-B lines; fluffy perihilar infiltrates
      may be seen in the early stages
    b. Pleural effusions
2. Arterial blood gases
    a. Respiratory and metabolic acidosis: decreased Pa_{O_2}, increased P_{CO_2},
      lowered pH
    NOTE: The patient may initially show respiratory alkalosis secondary to
    hyperventilation.
3. Cardiac pressures: increased PADP and PCWP

Therapy[6,22]

All the following steps can be performed concomitantly:

1. 100% O_2 by face mask: check ABGs; if marked hypoxemia or severe respiratory acidosis, then intubate patient and place on ventilator
2. Furosemide: 40-100 mg IV bolus to rapidly establish a diuresis and decrease venous return through its venodilator action; may double the dose in 30 min if no effect
3. Vasodilator therapy
   a. Nitrates: particularly useful if the patient has concomitant chest pain
      (1) Nitroglycerin: 150-600 μg SL prn may be given immediately on arrival
      (2) 2% Nitroglycerin ointment: 1-3 inches out of the tube, applied cutaneously; absorption may be erratic
      (3) IV nitroglycerin: 100 mg/500 ml of D_5W, start at 6 μg/min (2 ml/hr)
   b. Nitroprusside: useful in hypertensive patients with decreased cardiac index (CI)
      (1) It increases the CI and decreases left ventricular filling pressure
      (2) The use of nitroprusside in patients with acute MI is controversial because it may intensify ischemia by decreasing the blood flow to the ischemic left ventricular myocardium[5]
4. Morphine: 3-10 mg IV/SQ/IM, may repeat q15min prn; it decreases venous return, anxiety, and systemic vascular resistance (naloxone should be available at bedside to reverse the effects of morphine if respiratory depression occurs)
5. Place patient in a sitting position to decrease venous return
6. Dobutamine: parenteral inotropic agent of choice in severe cases of cardiogenic pulmonary edema
7. Rotating tourniquets to the extremities helps decrease venous return
   a. Compress only three extremities at one time and every 15 min release one of the tourniquets and apply it to the free extremity
   b. The inflating pressure should exceed venous pressure (to decrease venous return), but should be lower than the arteriolar pressure
8. Aminophylline: useful *only if* patient has concomitant severe bronchospasm
9. Digitalis: limited value in acute pulmonary edema caused by MI; but is useful in pulmonary edema resulting from atrial fibrillation or flutter with a fast ventricular response
10. Identify and treat any precipitating factors, such as MI or dysrhythmias
11. Phlebotomy is indicated only when all other measures have failed

20.5 CARDIOMYOPATHIES

Cardiomyopathies are a group of diseases (three major types) primarily involving the myocardium and characterized by myocardial dysfunction that is not the result of hypertension, coronary atherosclerosis, valvular dysfunction, or pericardial abnormalities.

Dilated (congestive) cardiomyopathy

Definition

In dilated cardiomyopathy, the heart is enlarged and both ventricles are dilated.

Etiology

1. Idiopathic
2. Alcoholism
3. Collagen-vascular disease (SLE, rheumatoid arthritis, polyarteritis)
4. Postmyocarditis
5. Peripartum (last trimester of pregnancy or 6 mo postpartum)
6. Heredofamilial neuromuscular
7. Toxins (cobalt, lead, phosphorus, doxorubicin)
8. Nutritional (beri-beri, selenium deficiency, carnitine deficiency)
9. Cocaine, heroin, organic solvents ("glue sniffer's heart")
10. Irradiation
11. Acromegaly, osteogenesis imperfecta
12. Hypocalcemia

Symptoms

1. Dyspnea on exertion, orthopnea, PND
2. Palpitations
3. Systemic and pulmonary embolism

Physical findings

1. Increased jugular venous pressure
2. Small pulse pressure
3. Pulmonary rales, hepatomegaly, peripheral edema
4. S_3, S_4
5. Mitral regurgitation, tricuspid regurgitation (less common)

Diagnostic studies

1. Chest x-ray
   a. Massive cardiac enlargement
   b. Interstitial pulmonary edema
2. ECG
   a. Left ventricular hypertrophy with ST-T wave changes
   b. RBBB or LBBB
   c. Dysrhythmias (atrial fibrillation, PVC, PAC)
3. MUGA: low ejection fraction with global akinesia

Therapy

1. Treat underlying disease (SLE, alcoholism)
2. Treat CHF (cause of death in 70% of patients) with sodium restriction, diuretics, ACE inhibitors, and digitalis
3. Bed rest when CHF is present
4. Vasodilators (combined with nitrates and ACE inhibitors are effective)
5. Prevent thromboembolism with oral anticoagulants

6. Low-dose beta blockade with metoprolol (5 mg bid initially, titrated to 25-50 mg bid over several weeks) may improve ventricular function by interrupting the cycle of reflux sympathetic activity and controlling tachycardia[2]
7. Consider heart transplant for young patients who are no longer responsive to medical therapy

Restrictive cardiomyopathy

Definition

Restrictive cardiomyopathy is characterized by decreased ventricular compliance, usually secondary to infiltration of the myocardium.

Etiology

1. Infiltrative disorders (glycogen storage disease, amyloidosis, sarcoidosis, hemochromatosis)
2. Scleroderma
3. Radiation
4. Endocardial fibroelastosis
5. Endomyocardial fibrosis

Symptoms and physical findings

1. Edema, ascites, hepatomegaly, distended neck veins
2. Fatigue, weakness (secondary to low output)

Diagnostic studies

1. Chest x-ray
   a. Moderate cardiomegaly
   b. Possible evidence of CHF (pulmonary vascular congestion, pleural effusions)
2. ECG
   a. Low voltage with ST-T wave changes
   b. Frequent dysrhythmias
3. Cardiac catheterization: to distinguish restrictive cardiomyopathy from constrictive pericarditis
   a. Constrictive pericarditis: usually involves both ventricles and produces a plateau of elevated filling pressures
      (1) PCWP is equal to right atrial pressure (RAP)
      (2) Pulmonary artery systolic pressure (PASP) <50 mm Hg
      (3) Right ventricular end-diastolic pressure is greater than one third the right ventricular systolic pressure
   b. Restrictive cardiomyopathy: impairs the left ventricle more than the right
      (1) PCWP > RAP
      (2) PASP >50 mm Hg
4. MRI may be useful to distinguish restrictive cardiomyopathy from constrictive pericarditis (thickness of the pericardium is ≥5 mm in the latter)

Therapy

Cardiomyopathy caused by hemochromatosis may respond to repeated phlebotomies. There is no effective therapy for other causes of restrictive cardiomyopathy. Death usually results from CHF or dysrhythmias, and therefore therapy should be aimed at controlling CHF by restricting salt, administering diuretics, and treating potentially lethal dysrhythmias.

Hypertrophic cardiomyopathy

Pathophysiology

1. There is marked hypertrophy of the myocardium and disproportionately greater thickening of the interventricular septum than that of the free wall of the left ventricle—asymmetric septal hypertrophy (ASH)
2. During midsystole, the apposition of the anterior mitral valve leaflet against the hypertrophied septum can cause a narrowing of the subaortic area and result in left ventricular outflow obstruction; because of this, the disease has been termed idiopathic hypertrophic subaortic stenosis (IHSS) or hypertrophic obstructive cardiomyopathy (HOCM)

Epidemiology

The disease occurs in two major forms:
1. A familial form, usually diagnosed in young patients and gene-mapped to chromosome 14q[1]
2. A sporadic form, usually found in elderly patients

Factors influencing obstruction[1][2]

Increase obstruction	Decrease obstruction
Drugs: digitalis, beta adrenergic stimulators (isoproterenol, dopamine, epinephrine), nitroglycerin, vasodilators, and diuretics	Drugs: beta adrenergic blockers, calcium channel blockers, α-adrenergic stimulators (phenylephrine)
Hypovolemia	Volume expansion
Tachycardia	Bradycardia
Valsalva maneuver	Handgrip exercise
Standing position	Squatting position

Symptoms

1. Dyspnea
2. Syncope (usually seen with exercise)
3. Angina (decreased angina in recumbent position)
4. Palpitations
5. Sudden death may be the only manifestation (usually seen in young adults during physical exercise)

Physical findings

1. Harsh, systolic, diamond-shaped murmur at the left sternal border or

apex that increases with Valsalva maneuver and decreases with squatting
2. Paradoxic splitting of S_2 (if left ventricular obstruction is present)
3. S_4
4. Double or triple apical impulse

Diagnostic studies

1. Chest x-ray: normal or cardiomegaly
2. ECG
   a. Left ventricular hypertrophy
   b. Abnormal Q waves may be seen in anterolateral and inferior leads
3. Echocardiography
   a. Ventricular hypertrophy
   b. Ratio of septum thickness to left ventricular wall thickness greater than 1.3 : 1
4. MUGA: increased ejection fraction

Treatment[12]

1. Propranolol 160-240 mg/day decreases outflow tract obstruction by lowering the force of contraction
2. Verapamil also decreases left ventricular outflow obstruction
3. IV saline infusion in addition to propranolol and verapamil is indicated in patients with CHF
4. 24 hr Holter monitoring to screen for potentially lethal dysrhythmias (the principal cause of syncope or sudden death in obstructive cardiomyopathy)
   a. Electrophysiological studies may be used to select prophylactic therapy[32]
   b. Disopyramide is a useful antidysrhythmic
5. Surgical myectomy is used only when optimum medical therapy fails to relieve symptoms; the risk of sudden death from dysrhythmias is not altered by surgery
6. Antibiotic prophylaxis for surgical procedures
7. Screening of family members with echocardiography is indicated
8. Avoid use of digitalis, diuretics, nitrates, and vasodilators

20.6 MYOCARDITIS

Definition

Myocarditis is an inflammatory condition of the myocardium that can result from a variety of etiological factors:
1. Infection
   a. Viral (coxsackie B virus, echovirus, poliovirus, adenovirus, mumps)
   b. Bacterial (*Staphylococcus aureus, Clostridium perfringens*)
   c. *Mycoplasma*
   d. Mycotic (*Candida, Mucor, Aspergillus*)
   e. Parasitic (*Trypanosoma cruzi, Trichinella, Echinococcus,* amebic)
   f. Rickettsial (*Rickettsia rickettsii*)
   g. Spirochetal (*Borrelia burgdorferi*–Lyme carditis)

2. Rheumatic fever
3. Secondary to drugs (emetine, doxorubicin)
4. Toxins (carbon monoxide, diphtheria toxin)
5. Collagen-vascular disease (SLE, scleroderma)
6. Sarcoidosis

Symptoms

1. Fatigue, palpitations, dyspnea
2. Precordial discomfort
3. Myalgias

Physical exam

1. Persistent tachycardia, out of proportion to fever
2. Faint S_1
3. Murmur of mitral regurgitation
4. Pericardial friction rub if associated with pericarditis
5. Signs of biventricular failure (hypotension, hepatomegaly, peripheral edema, distention of neck veins)

Diagnostic studies

1. Chest x-ray: enlargement of cardiac silhouette
2. ECG: sinus tachycardia with nonspecific ST-T wave changes
3. Lab results
   a. Increased CK (with elevated MB fraction), LDH, and AST secondary to myocardial necrosis may be seen
   b. Increased erythrocyte sedimentation rate (nonspecific, but may be of value in following the progress of the disease and the response to therapy)
   c. Increased WBC, increased eosinophils if parasitic infection
   d. Viral titers (acute and convalescent)
   e. Cold-agglutinin titer, ASLO titer, blood cultures
   f. Lyme disease antibody titer
4. Cardiac catheterization and angiography
   a. To rule out coronary artery and valvular disease
   b. A right ventricular endomyocardial biopsy can confirm the diagnosis, although a negative biopsy does not exclude myocarditis

Therapy

1. Treat underlying cause (e.g., specific IV antibiotics for bacterial infection)
2. Supportive care
3. Restrict physical activity (to decrease cardiac work)
4. Treat CHF with digitalis, diuretics, ACE inhibitors, and salt restriction
5. If dysrhythmias are present, treat with quinidine or procainamide
6. Anticoagulation to prevent thromboembolism
7. Preload and afterload reducing agents for treating cardiac decompensation
8. Corticosteroids are contraindicated in early infectious myocarditis; their

use is justified only in selected patients with intractable CHF, severe systemic toxicity, and severe life-threatening dysrhythmias

9. Corticosteroids and azathioprine (immunosuppressive therapy) may be beneficial in selected patients with inflammatory infiltrates on myocardial biopsy[61]

 PERICARDITIS

Definition

Pericarditis is inflammation (or infiltration) of the pericardium associated with a wide variety of etiological factors:

1. Idiopathic (possibly postviral)
2. Infectious (viral, bacterial, tuberculous, fungal, amebic, toxoplasmosis)
3. Collagen-vascular disease (SLE, rheumatoid arthritis, scleroderma)
4. Drug-induced lupus syndrome (procainamide, hydralazine)
5. Acute MI
6. Trauma
7. After MI (Dressler's syndrome)
8. After pericardiotomy
9. After mediastinal radiation (e.g., patients with Hodgkin's disease)
10. Uremia
11. Sarcoidosis
12. Neoplasm (primary or metastatic)
13. Leakage of aortic aneurysm in pericardial sac
14. Familial Mediterranean fever
15. Rheumatic fever

Symptoms and signs

1. Severe constant pain that localizes over the anterior chest and may radiate to arms and back; it can easily be mistaken for myocardial ischemia; characteristically, however, the pain intensifies with inspiration and is relieved by sitting up and leaning forward
2. Pericardial friction rub is best heard with the patient upright and leaning forward and by pressing the stethoscope firmly against the chest; it classically consists of three short, scratchy sounds:
   a. Systolic component
   b. Diastolic component
   c. Late diastolic component (associated with atrial contraction)
3. Cardiac tamponade is occurring if the following are observed:
   a. Tachycardia
   b. Low blood pressure and pulse pressure
   c. Distended neck veins
   d. Paradoxical pulse

Diagnostic studies

1. ECG: varies with the evolutionary stage of pericarditis (see Fig. 5-4, *C*)
   a. Acute phase: there are diffuse ST segment elevations (particularly

evident in the precordial leads); this can be distinguished from acute MI by:
   (1) Absence of reciprocal ST segment depression in oppositely oriented leads (reciprocal ST segment depression may be seen in aVR and V_1)
   (2) The elevated ST segments are concave upward
   (3) Absence of Q waves
   b. Intermediate phase: the ST segment returns to baseline and T wave inversion is seen in leads previously showing ST segment elevation
   c. Latent phase: there is resolution of the T wave changes
2. Lab tests (in the absence of an obvious cause):
   a. CBC with differential
   b. Viral titers (acute and convalescent)
   c. Erythrocyte sedimentation rate (nonspecific, but may be of value in following the course of the disease and the response to therapy)
   d. ANA, rheumatoid factor (RF)
   e. Purified protein derivative (PPD), ASLO titers
   f. BUN, creatinine
   g. Blood cultures
   h. Cardiac isoenzymes are usually normal, but mild elevations of CK-MB may occur
3. Echocardiogram is indicated if pericardial effusion is suspected

Treatment

1. Antiinflammatory therapy (salicylates 3-5 g/day or indomethacin 25-50 mg tid)
2. Prednisone 30 mg bid for severe forms of acute pericarditis (before using prednisone, tuberculous pericarditis must be excluded)
3. Codeine 15-60 mg PO qid for pain refractory to salicylates or indomethacin
4. Observe patient closely for signs of cardiac tamponade
5. Avoid anticoagulants (↑ risk of hemopericardium)
6. Treat underlying cause
   a. Bacterial pericarditis
      (1) Commonly caused by streptococci, meningococci, staphylococci, *Haemophilus*, gram-negative bacteria, anaerobic bacteria
      (2) Therapy: systemic antibiotics and surgical drainage of pericardium
   b. Fungal pericarditis
      (1) Caused by histoplasmosis, coccidioidomycosis, candidiasis, blastomycosis, or aspergillosis
      (2) Therapy: IV amphotericin B and drainage of pericardial space (if indicated)
   c. Tuberculous pericarditis
      (1) Therapy: antituberculous drugs for a minimum of 9 mo
      (2) Pericardiectomy may be necessary 2-4 wk after antituberculous drugs have been started

Complications

1. Pericardial effusion: the time required for a pericardial effusion (fluid

within the pericardial space) to develop is of critical importance; if the rate of fluid accumulation is slow, the pericardium can gradually stretch and accommodate a large effusion (up to 1000 ml), whereas a rapid accumulation (e.g., traumatic hemopericardium) can cause tamponade even with 200 ml of fluid

2. Chronic constrictive pericarditis
    a. Pathophysiology: fibrous scarring and adhesions of the two pericardial layers obliterate the pericardial cavity and cause the pericardium to become rigid and thickened; this prevents the ventricles from adequately filling during diastole and causes increased venous pressures and decreased stroke volume
    b. Etiology
        (1) Idiopathic
        (2) After pericardiotomy
        (3) After radiation therapy
        (4) Uremia
        (5) Tuberculous pericarditis
        (6) After idiopathic pericarditis
    c. Physical exam
        (1) Jugular venous distention, Kussmaul's sign (increase in jugular venous distention during inspiration due to increased venous pulse)
        (2) Pericardial knock (early diastolic filling sound heard 0.06-0.1 sec after S_2)
        (3) Clear lungs
        (4) Tender hepatomegaly
        (5) Pedal edema, ascites
        (6) ±Pulsus paradoxus
    d. Diagnostic studies
        (1) Chest x-ray: clear lung fields, normal or slightly enlarged heart; pericardial calcification may be seen
        (2) ECG: low-voltage QRS complexes
        (3) Echocardiography: may show pericardial thickening or may be normal
        (4) Cardiac catheterization: there is an M or W contour of the central venous pattern (Fig. 20-11) caused by both systolic *(x)* and diastolic *(y)* dips (this differs from cardiac tamponade, which does not display a prominent diastolic *[y]* descent); in chronic constrictive pericarditis there are also increased right ventricular and pulmonary arterial pressures (for differentiation of constrictive pericarditis from restrictive cardiomyopathy refer to Section 20.5)
        (5) In addition to lab evaluation of pericarditis (see above), obtain a TSH level (myxedema) and serum albumin and urine protein measurement (nephrotic syndrome)
    e. Therapy: surgical stripping and removal of both layers of the constricting pericardium

3. Cardiac tamponade
    a. Definition: pericardial effusion that significantly impairs diastolic filling of the heart

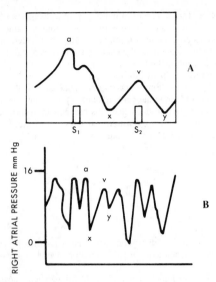

Figure 20-11

Atrial pressure curves in normal patients, **A**, and in patients with constrictive pericarditis, **B**. Letter designations are as follows: a, increased pressure with atrial contraction; x, fall in right atrial pressure seen at the beginning of ventricular systole; v, increased pressure in the right atrium due to continuous venous return; y, fall in right atrial pressure seen with the beginning of diastole.

 b. Symptoms
   (1) Dyspnea, orthopnea
   (2) Interscapular pain
 c. Physical exam
   (1) Distended neck veins
   (2) Distant heart sounds, decreased apical impulse
   (3) Diaphoresis, tachypnea
   (4) Tachycardia (compensatory to maintain cardiac output)
   (5) Ewart's sign: an area of dullness at the angle of the left scapula; it is caused by compression of the lung by the pericardial effusion
   (6) Pulsus paradoxus (decrease in systolic blood pressure >10 mm Hg during inspiration)
   (7) Hypotension
   (8) Narrowed pulse pressure
 d. Diagnostic studies
   (1) Chest x-ray: cardiomegaly (water bottle configuration of the cardiac silhouette) with *clear* lung fields; the chest x-ray film may be normal when acute tamponade occurs rapidly in absence of prior pericardial effusion

(2) ECG
  (a) Decreased amplitude of the QRS complex
  (b) Variation of the R wave amplitude from beat to beat (electrical alternans); this results from the heart oscillating in the pericardial sac from beat to beat and is frequently seen with neoplastic effusions
(3) Echocardiography: detects effusions as small as 30 ml (they are seen as an echo-free space), paradoxical wall motion can also be seen
  (a) Two-dimensional echocardiography may reveal prolonged diastolic collapse or inversion of right atrial free wall
  (b) Early diastolic collapse of right ventricular wall is also suggestive of cardiac tamponade
  (c) Echocardiography may miss localized effusions laterally adjacent to right atrium
(4) Cardiac catheterization
  (a) Equalization of pressures within chambers of the heart
  (b) Elevation of right atrial pressure with a prominent x but no significant y descent
(5) MRI can also be used to diagnose pericardial effusions
e. Therapy
  (1) Immediate pericardiocentesis; in patients with recurrent effusions (e.g., neoplasms), placement of a percutaneous drainage catheter or pericardial window draining into the pleural cavity may be necessary
  (2) Send aspirated fluid for analysis and cultures (protein, LDH, cytology, cell count, Gram stain, AFB stain, cultures, and sensitivity)

20.8 DYSRHYTHMIAS

Supraventricular dysrhythmias

Paroxysmal supraventricular tachycardia (SVT)

1. Definition: group of dysrhythmias that generally originate as reentrant rhythm from the AV node and are characterized by sudden onset and abrupt termination
2. Etiology
  a. Young patients without evidence of cardiac disease
  b. Preexcitation syndromes (e.g., Wolff-Parkinson-White syndrome [WPW])
  c. Atrial septal defect
  d. Acute MI
3. ECG
  a. Absolutely regular rhythm at a rate between 150-220 bpm (Fig. 20-12)
  b. P waves may or may not be seen (the presence of P waves depends on the relationship of atrial to ventricular depolarization)

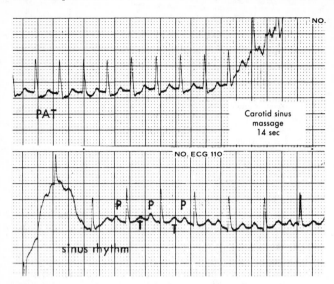

Figure 20-12
Supraventricular tachycardia (PAT). The upper and lower rows are part of one continuous strip. In the upper row no definite P waves are visible. The diagnosis of this ECG is therefore merely "supraventricular tachydysrhythmia." The ventricular rate is approximately 185/min. In the lower strip, taken at the end of the carotid sinus massage, sinus rhythm has appeared. However, the heart rate is still rapid (approximately 135/min). (From Goldberger E: Treatment of cardiac emergencies, ed 5, St Louis, 1990, The CV Mosby Co.)

c. Wide QRS complex (>0.12 sec) with initial slurring (delta wave) during sinus rhythm and short PR interval (≤0.12 sec) is characteristic of WPW syndrome (Fig. 20-13); the syndrome is due to an accessory AV pathway (bundle of Kent), which preexcites the ventricular muscle earlier than would be expected if the impulse reached the ventricles by way of the normal conduction system; dysrhythmias associated with WPW are narrow-complex SVT, atrial fibrillation, and ventricular fibrillation; digoxin and verapamil should be avoided because they can lead to dysrhythmia acceleration

d. See Table 20-6 for differentiation of PAT from sinus tachycardia
4. Symptoms
   a. Usually asymptomatic; the patient may be aware of "fast heart beat"
   b. May precipitate CHF or hypotension during acute MI
5. Therapy
   a. Valsalva maneuver in the supine position is the most effective way to terminate SVT; carotid sinus massage (after excluding occlusive

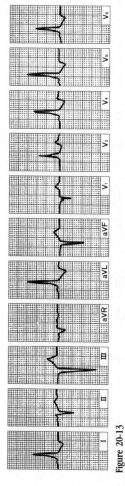

Figure 20-13
Wolff-Parkinson-White syndrome (accelerated conduction). Short PR (<0.12 sec); initial segment of the QRS slurred (delta wave); may simulate an inferior MI, with Q waves in II, III, and aVF; the QRS is prolonged, with secondary ST segment and T wave changes. (Courtesy Merck, Sharp & Dohme.)

Table 20-6 Differentiation of PAT from sinus tachycardia[22]

Rhythm	Ventricular Rate	Effect of Deep Inspiration	Onset and Disappearance	Comparison of P Waves Before and After Tachycardia
Sinus tachycardia	Usually <140/min	Momentary slowing of heart rate	Gradual	P waves remain unchanged
PAT	Usually >160/min	No response	Abrupt	Usually there is aberration of P wave and PR interval

carotid disease) is also commonly used to elicit vagal efferent impulses

b. Synchronized DC shock if patient shows signs of cardiogenic shock, angina, or CHF

c. Verapamil 5-10 mg IV over 5 min; if no effect, may repeat in 30 min
   (1) Verapamil should be used cautiously in patients with SVT associated with hypotension
   (2) Slow injection of calcium chloride (10 ml of a 10% solution given over 5-8 min) before verapamil administration decreases the hypotensive effect without compromising its antidysrhythmic effect[26]

d. Repeat carotid massage after IV verapamil if SVT persists

e. Adenosine (Adenocard), an endogenous nucleoside, is useful for treatment of paroxysmal SVT, particularly that associated with WPW; it is considered by many to be first choice therapy for treatment of almost all episodes of SVT that are unresponsive to vagal maneuvers; the dose is 6 mg given as a rapid IV bolus; tachycardia is usually terminated within few seconds; if necessary, may repeat with 12 mg IV bolus; contraindications are second- or third-degree AV block, sick sinus syndrome (SSS), atrial fibrillation, and ventricular tachycardia; adenosine may cause bronchospasm in asthmatics; patients receiving theophylline (a competitive antagonist of adenosine receptors) are usually refractory to treatment; dipyridamole enhances the effect of adenosine; therefore patients receiving dipyridamole should be started on lower doses

f. IV digitalization (0.75-1 mg slow IV loading)
   (1) Repeat carotid sinus massage 30 min later; if not successful, give additional 0.25 mg IV digoxin and repeat carotid sinus massage 1 hr later
   (2) Digoxin should be avoided in patients with WPW syndrome and narrow QRS tachycardia (increased risk of atrial fibrillation during AV reentrant tachycardia)

Multifocal atrial tachycardia (MAT)

1. Definition: chaotic, irregular atrial activity at rates between 100-180 bpm
2. Etiology
   a. Chronic obstructive pulmonary disease
   b. Metabolic disturbances (hypoxemia, hypokalemia, hypomagnesemia)
   c. Sepsis
   d. Theophylline toxicity
3. ECG
   a. Variable P-P intervals
   b. Morphology of the P wave varies from beat to beat (Fig. 20-14), with a minimum of three different forms of P wave besides those from the sinus node
   c. Each QRS complex is preceded by a P wave

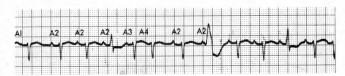

Figure 20-14

Multifocal atrial tachycardia (MAT). Letter designations A1, A2, A3, and A4 show premature atrial contractions from varying foci. Notice that the fourth, eighth, and eleventh QRS complexes are aberrant. (From Goldberger E: Treatment of cardiac emergencies, ed 5, St Louis, 1990, The CV Mosby Co.)

4. Therapy
   a. Treat the underlying cause (e.g., improve oxygenation, correct electrolyte abnormalities)
   b. Verapamil 5 mg IV at a rate of up to 1 mg/min (may repeat after 20 min); calcium gluconate 1 g IV, given 5 min before treatment with verapamil, may reduce drug-induced hypotension without preventing the antidysrhythmic effect[44]
   c. Metoprolol or esmolol has also been used in absence of COPD, CHF, or bronchospasm[30a]

Atrial fibrillation

1. Definition: totally chaotic atrial activity caused by simultaneous discharge of multiple atrial foci
2. Etiology
   a. CAD
   b. MS, MR, AS, AR
   c. Thyrotoxicosis
   d. Pulmonary embolism, COPD
   e. Pericarditis
   f. Myocarditis, cardiomyopathy
   g. Tachycardia-bradycardia syndrome
   h. Alcohol abuse
   i. MI
   j. Wolff-Parkinson-White syndrome
   k. Other causes: left atrial myxoma, atrial septal defect, carbon monoxide poisoning, pheochromocytoma, idiopathic
3. Diagnostic studies of new-onset atrial fibrillation should include echocardiography, to evaluate left atrial size and detect valvular disorders, and thyroid function studies, to rule out thyrotoxicosis
   a. ECG
      (1) Irregular, nonperiodic wave forms (best seen in V_1) reflecting continuous atrial reentry
      (2) Absence of P waves
      (3) Conducted QRS complexes show no periodicity (Fig. 20-15)

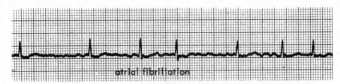

Figure 20-15
Atrial fibrillation with slow ventricular response (From Goldberger E: Treatment of cardiac emergencies, ed 5, St Louis, 1990, The CV Mosby Co.)

4. Therapy (of new-onset atrial fibrillation)
   a. Digoxin 0.5 mg IV loading dose (slow), then 0.25 mg IV q2h until the ventricular rate is controlled; daily dosage varies from 0.125-0.25 mg (decrease dosage in patients with renal insufficiency and elderly patients); digoxin should be avoided in WPW with atrial fibrillation; these patients are better treated with IV procainamide or cardioversion; electrophysiologic testing and transcatheter or surgical ablation of the accessory pathway are curative measures
   b. Conversion to normal sinus rhythm (NSR) with initial digitalization is successful in only 15-20% of patients; in the remainder quinidine sulfate 300 mg q6h should be added to help convert the patient to normal sinus rhythm
   c. In acute atrial fibrillation when the rate is not controlled by digoxin, propranolol 0.5 mg IV (slowly) may be given followed by IV boluses of 1 mg q5min to a total of 5 mg
   d. Cardioversion is indicated if the ventricular rate is >140 bpm and the patient is symptomatic (particularly in acute MI, chest pain, dyspnea, CHF), or when there is no conversion to NSR after 3 days of therapy with digoxin and quinidine
      (1) Cardioversion will restore sinus rhythm in 90% of patients
      (2) Points to remember when preparing the patient for cardioversion:
         (a) Start quinidine at least 24 hr before cardioversion to help maintain NSR once it is achieved
         (b) If left atrial size ≥4.5 cm, there is little chance of achieving or maintaining NSR
         (c) Hold digoxin and check serum digoxin level on morning of cardioversion
         (d) The patient should be NPO for 8 hr before cardioversion
         (e) Anticoagulation is advisable for 3 wk before and 3 wk after cardioversion, particularly in patients with mitral valve disease or a history of thromboembolism
   e. Complications of cardioversion
      (1) Ventricular fibrillation (if shock applied on T waves)
      (2) Thromboembolism (seen mainly in nonanticoagulated patients with long-standing atrial fibrillation)
      (3) Myocardial damage secondary to the current (rare)

    (4) Erythema on the chest wall

    (5) Recurrence of prior dysrhythmia; factors associated with maintenance of sinus rhythm are left atrium diameter <60 mm, absence of mitral valve disease, short duration of atrial fibrillation, and conversion to NSR with drug therapy alone[7]

5. Long-term anticoagulation is indicated in patients with atrial fibrillation and the following associated conditions[63]:

  a. Rheumatic valvular disease

  b. Mitral stenosis (MS)

  c. Prosthetic mitral valve (any type)

  d. History of previous embolism

  e. Known cardiac thrombus

  f. CHF

  g. Cardiomyopathy with poor left ventricular function

  h. Nonrheumatic heart disease (e.g., hypertensive cardiovascular disease, coronary artery disease)

6. Anticoagulation is not recommended in younger patients with lone atrial fibrillation (defined as occurring with no evidence of associated cardiovascular disease except hypertension)[63]

Atrial flutter

1. Definition: rapid atrial rate of 280-340 bpm with varying degrees of atrioventricular block

2. Etiology

  a. Atherosclerotic heart disease

  b. MI

  c. Thyrotoxicosis

  d. Pulmonary embolism

  e. Mitral valve disease

  f. Cardiac surgery

  g. COPD

3. ECG

  a. Regular "sawtooth" or "F wave" pattern best seen in II, III, and aVF and secondary to atrial depolarization (Fig. 20-16)

  b. AV conduction block (2:1, 3:1, or varying)

  c. Valsalva maneuver or carotid sinus massage usually slows the ventricular rate (increases grade of AV block) and may make flutter waves more evident

4. Therapy

  a. Electrical cardioversion at low energy levels (20-25 J)

  b. In the absence of cardioversion, IV digitalization may be tried to slow the ventricular rate and convert flutter to fibrillation

  c. Atrial pacing may also terminate atrial flutter

AV conduction defects

First-degree AV block

1. Definition: prolongation of the PR interval >0.20 sec (at a rate of 70 bpm), which remains constant from beat to beat (Fig. 20-17)

Cardioversion Procedure

1. Use short-acting barbiturate or IV diazepam to induce amnesia and have anesthesiologist in attendance at the procedure.
2. Have adequate IV line in place and continuous ECG monitoring
3. Select energy levels:

Dysrhythmia	Initial energy level	Subsequent shocks (if necessary)
Atrial fibrillation	100 joules (J)	200 J, 300 J, 360 J
Atrial flutter	20-25 J	50 J, 100 J, 200 J

4. Synchronize the defibrillator to prevent the electrical shock from being applied during repolarization of the ventricles (T wave) and causing ventricular fibrillation.

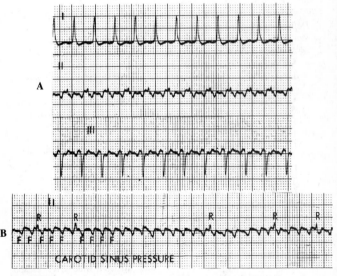

Figure 20-16
Atrial flutter waves (F). **A,** The flutter waves are not apparent in lead I but are obvious in leads II and III. **B,** Carotid sinus pressure slowed the ventricular rate but did not change the atrial flutter rate. (From Goldberger E: Treatment of cardiac emergencies, ed 5, St Louis, 1990, The CV Mosby Co.)

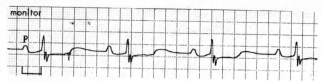

Figure 20-17
First-degree AV block. The PR interval is 0.32 sec. (From Goldberger E: Treatment of cardiac emergencies, ed 5, St Louis, 1990, The CV Mosby Co.)

2. Etiology
   a. Vagal stimulation
   b. Degenerative changes in the AV conduction system
   c. Ischemia at the AV nodes (seen particularly in inferior wall MI)
   d. Drugs (digitalis, quinidine, procainamide)
   e. Cardiomyopathies
   f. Aortic regurgitation
   g. Lyme carditis
3. Therapy: none

Second-degree AV block

1. Definition: blockage of some (but not all) impulses from the atria to the ventricles
2. Mobitz type I (Wenckebach)
   a. Definition
      (1) Progressive prolongation of the PR interval before an impulse is completely blocked; the cycle repeats periodically
      (2) Cycle with dropped beat is less than 2 times the previous cycle
   b. Site of block: usually AV nodal (proximal to the bundle of His)
   c. Etiology: same as for first-degree AV block
   d. ECG
      (1) Gradual prolongation of PR interval leading to a blocked beat (Fig. 20-18)
      (2) Shortened PR interval after the dropped beat
   e. Therapy
      (1) Usually transient, no treatment necessary
      (2) If symptomatic (e.g., dizziness), atropine 1 mg (may repeat once after 5 min) may be tried to increase AV conduction; if no response, insert temporary pacemaker
      (3) If block is secondary to drugs (e.g., digitalis), discontinue the drug
      (4) If associated with anterior wall MI and wide QRS escape rhythm, consider insertion of a temporary pacemaker
3. Mobitz type II
   a. Definition: sudden interruption of AV conduction without prior prolongation of the PR interval
   b. Site of block: infranodal

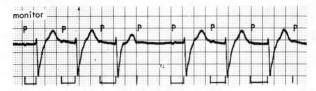

Figure 20-18
Mobitz I second-degree AV block (Wenckebach). (From Goldberger E: Treatment of cardiac emergencies, ed 5, St Louis, 1990, The CV Mosby Co.)

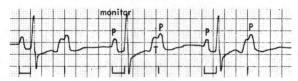

Figure 20-19
Mobitz II second-degree AV block. Notice that every alternate P wave is blocked. (From Goldberger E: Treatment of cardiac emergencies, ed 5, St Louis, 1990, The CV Mosby Co.)

   c. Etiology
     (1) Degenerative changes in His-Purkinje system
     (2) Acute anterior wall MI
     (3) Calcific aortic stenosis
   d. ECG
     (1) Fixed duration of PR interval
     (2) Sudden appearance of blocked beats (Fig. 20-19)
   e. Therapy: pacemaker insertion, since this type of block is usually permanent and often progresses to complete AV block

Third-degree AV block (complete AV block)

1. Definition: all AV conduction is completely blocked, and the atria and ventricles have separate independent rhythms
2. Etiology
   a. Same as for Mobitz II
   b. Cardiomyopathy
   c. Trauma
   d. Cardiovascular surgery
   e. Congenital
3. ECG
   a. P waves constantly change their relationship to the QRS complexes (Fig. 20-20)

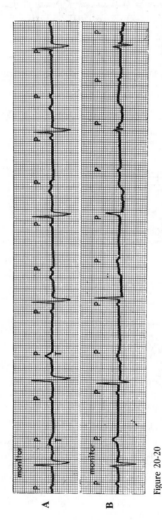

Figure 20-20

Third-degree block. **A** and **B** taken several hours apart. **A**, Atrial rate of 75 bpm. The ventricles are beating independently at a slow rate of approximately 40 bpm. **B**, A few hours later, same patient; variations in the shape of QRS complex from beat to beat. (From Goldberger E: Treatment of cardiac emergencies, ed 5, St Louis, 1990, The CV Mosby Co.)

b. Ventricular rate usually <50 bpm (may be higher in congenital forms)
c. Ventricular rate generally lower than the atrial rate
d. QRS wide
4. Symptoms
   a. Dizziness, palpitations
   b. Stokes-Adams syncopal attacks
   c. CHF
   d. Angina
5. Therapy: immediate pacemaker insertion unless the patient has congenital third-degree AV block and is completely asymptomatic

Ventricular dysrhythmias

Ventricular tachycardia

1. Definition: three or more consecutive beats of ventricular origin (wide QRS) at a rate between 100-200 bpm (Fig. 20-21)
2. Differentiation between ventricular beats and supraventricular tachycardia with aberrant ventricular conduction may be very difficult; wide-QRS tachycardia in the conscious adult should be considered ventricular tachycardia until proved otherwise
   a. Factors favoring ventricular tachycardia[1]
      (1) Similar morphology to premature ventricular contraction (PVC)
      (2) Initiating event is a PVC
      (3) Usually no response to vagal maneuvers

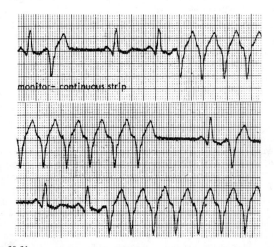

Figure 20-21
Ventricular tachycardia. (From Goldberger E: Treatment of cardiac emergencies, ed 5, St Louis, 1990, The CV Mosby Co.)

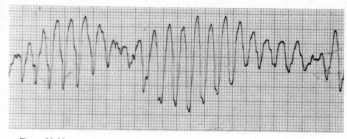

Figure 20-22
Torsade de pointes. (From Cerra FB: Manual of critical care, St Louis, 1987, The CV Mosby Co.)

    (4) Presence of AV dissociation
    (5) QRS duration >140 millisec with an RBBB and >160 millisec with an LBBB pattern
    (6) Extreme left axis deviation (less than −90 to ±180 degrees)
    (7) Combination of LBBB and right axis deviation
    (8) Different QRS pattern during tachycardia compared to a baseline ECG in patients with preexisting BBB
    (9) QRS concordance (the QRS waves are in same direction in all precordial leads)
  b. Factors favoring supraventricular rhythm
    (1) Similar morphology to baseline rhythm
    (2) Initiating event is a premature atrial contraction (PAC)
    (3) The rhythm can slow or break with vagal stimuli
    (4) Physical exam demonstrating ventriculoatrial dissociation (e.g., variation in loudness of S_1 and systolic blood pressure on successive beats)
    (5) ECG may reveal biphasic or monophasic QRS in V_1 with a right bundle branch block (RBBB), QRS >0.14 sec, left axis deviation

3. Torsade de pointes (Fig. 20-22) is a form of ventricular tachycardia manifested by episodes of alternating electrical polarity with the amplitude of the QRS complex twisting around an isoelectric baseline; rhythm usually starts with a PVC and is preceded by widening of the QT interval
  a. It may be caused by electrolyte disturbances, antidysrhythmic drugs that prolong the QT interval (procainamide, quinidine, disopyramide), phenothiazines, and tricyclic antidepressants
  b. Treatment includes the following:
    (1) Electrical termination of the tachycardia
    (2) IV infusion of isoproterenol to decrease the QT interval and prevent recurrences

(3) Elimination of contributing factors (correction of electrolyte abnormalities, discontinuation of suspected drugs)

(4) IV magnesium sulfate may be helpful

4. Therapy: guidelines for treatment of ventricular tachycardia are outlined in Appendix X; Table 20-7 lists the major IV agents useful in ventricular dysrhythmias; Table 33-36 lists the commonly used oral agents; and Table 20-8 describes the major electrophysiological effects of commonly used antidysrhythmic agents

NOTE: The erroneous administration of verapamil in ventricular tachycardia often results in a poor outcome; when in doubt, IV procainamide is preferred because it is effective in slowing and terminating ventricular tachycardia and also tachycardia originating in the atrium, AV node, or tachycardia via an accessory pathway.[60]

Ventricular fibrillation

Ventricular fibrillation (VF) is characterized by a chaotic ventricular rhythm with disorganized spread of impulses throughout the ventricles (Fig. 20-23). Therapy is outlined in Appendix X.

Accelerated isochronic (isorhythmic) ventricular rhythm

1. Ventricular rate 60-100 bpm, at times interspersed with brief runs of sinus rhythm (Fig. 20-24)
2. Usually seen in acute MI
3. Generally benign and transient, not requiring any therapy
4. Atrioventricular sequential pacing may be necessary if the dissociation between atria and ventricles impairs ventricular filling and decreases cardiac output

20.9   CARDIAC PACEMAKERS

The indications for temporary pacemaker in an acute MI setting are as follows:

1. Complete heart block with anterior wall MI
2. Alternating bundle branch block
3. Bifascicular block (new RBBB with LAHB or LPHB)
4. Mobitz II
5. Mobitz I with anterior wall MI or inferior wall MI with wide QRS escape rhythm
6. Symptomatic sinus bradycardia unresponsive to atropine or isoproterenol
7. New RBBB with anterior wall MI
8. New LBBB with anterior wall MI

Indications for permanent pacemaker

1. Sick sinus syndrome
2. Third-degree heart block
3. Mobitz II heart block
4. Symptomatic block at any site of the conduction system
5. Bifascicular block and recurrent syncope

Table 20-7 IV agents used in ventricular dysrhythmias

Drug	Indications	Dosage	Onset of Action	Therapeutic Plasma Level
Lidocaine (Xylocaine)	Ventricular tachydysrhythmias	Loading 1 mg/kg bolus followed by infusion at 1-4 mg/min	Immediate	2-5 µg/ml
Bretylium (Bretylol)	Life-threatening refractory ventricular fibrillation or tachycardia	5 mg/kg slow bolus followed by infusion at 2 mg/min	5 minutes for significant antifibrillatory effect; may be delayed up to 2 hr for prevention of ventricular dysrhythmias	1.33 µg/ml
Procainamide (Pronestyl)	Ventricular tachydysrhythmias	100 mg slow IV bolus followed by infusion at 1-4 mg/min	Immediate	3-10 µg/ml
Phenytoin (Dilantin)	Digitalis-induced ventricular dysrhythmias	125-250 mg slow bolus q15min prn to maximum of 750 mg/hr	Immediate	5-20 µg/ml

Table 20-8 Electrophysiologic effects of common antidysrhythmic agents

Drug	Interval			Sinus Rate	Class
	PR	QRS	QT		
Lidocaine	N	N	N	N	Ib
Procainamide	N/↑	↑	↑	N	Ia
Bretylium	N	N	N	N	III
Quinidine	N/↑	↑	↑	N/↓	Ia
Disopyramide	N/↑	↑	↑	N/↑	Ia
Digitalis	N/↑	N	N/↓	N/↓	—
Propranolol	N/↑	N	N/↓	↓	II
Verapamil	↑	N	N	↓	IV

KEY: ↑, Increase; ↓, decrease; N, no change.

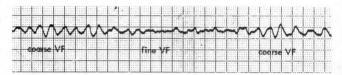

Figure 20-23
Ventricular fibrillation. Coarse and fine fibrillatory waves are shown. (From
Goldberger E: Treatment of cardiac emergencies, ed 5, St Louis, 1990, The CV
Mosby Co.)

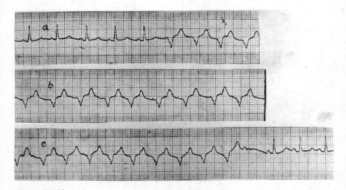

Figure 20-24
Accelerated isochronic (isorhythmic) ventricular rhythm. (From Cerra FB: Manual of
critical care, St Louis, 1987, The CV Mosby Co.)

Table 20-9 Classification of pacemakers (Intersociety Commission for Heart Disease)[48]

Chamber(s) Paced	Chamber(s) Sensed	Modes of Response	Programmable Function
V (ventricle)	V	+ (triggered)	P (limited rate, or output, or both)
A (atrium)	A	I (inhibited)	M (multiprogrammable)
D (double)	D	D*; 0 (none)	R (rate modulated)
S (single)	0 (none)	R (reverse)	0 (none)

*Double, triggered, and inhibited.

Classifications

Pacemakers are best classified using a three-letter code. The first letter indicates the chamber(s) paced, the second letter the chamber(s) sensed, and the third letter the mode of response. A fourth letter may be used to indicate the programmable function (Table 20-9).

Common types of pacemakers

1. VVI (ventricular inhibited): it paces the ventricle at a set rate, senses the ventricle, and is inhibited by the patient's own QRS complex; indicated in complete AV block, slow ventricular rate associated with atrial fibrillation or flutter, sick sinus syndrome, and sinus arrest
2. DDD (universal pacemaker): most technologically advanced pacemaker; paces both chambers, senses both chambers, and may trigger or inhibit output depending on the chamber sensed and paced; contraindicated in the presence of atrial fibrillation

References

1. Akhtar M, Shenasa M, et al: Wide QRS tachycardia; re-appraisal of a common clinical problem, Ann Intern Med 109:905, 1988.
2. Anderson JL, Lutz JR, et al: A randomized trial of low-dose beta-blockade therapy for idiopathic dilated cardiomyopathy, Am J Cardiol 55:471, 1985.
3. Antem EM, Braunwald E: Acute MI management in the 1990s, Hosp Pract 7:65, 1990.
4. Baker FJ II, Strauss R, Walter JJ: Cardiac arrest. In Rosen P, et al (editors): Emergency medicine, St Louis, 1983, The CV Mosby Co.
5. Boden WE, Capone RJ: Coronary care, Philadelphia, 1984, WB Saunders Co.
6. Braunwauld E: In Petersdorf RG, et al (editors): Harrison's Principles of internal medicine, ed 10, New York, 1983 McGraw-Hill Book Co.
7. Brodsky MA, et al: Maintenance of sinus rhythm after conversion of chronic atrial fibrillation, Am J Cardiol 63:1065, 1989.
8. Brush JE Jr, Cannon RO, Schenke WH, et al: Angina due to coronary microvascular disease in hypertensive patients without left ventricular hypertrophy, N Engl J Med 319:1302, 1988.
9. Cannom DS, Levy W, Cohen LS: The short- and long-term prognosis of patients with transmural and non-transmural myocardial infarction, Am J Med 61:452, 1976.
10. Dawber TR: The Framingham study: The epidemiology of atherosclerotic disease, Cambridge Mass, 1980, Harvard University Press.
11. DeBusk RF: Techniques of exercise testing. In Hurst JW, et al (editors): The heart, ed 6, New York, 1985, McGraw-Hill Book Co, vol 2.
12. DeSanctis RW: Cardiomyopathies. In Rubenstein E, Federman DD (editors): Scientific American medicine, New York, 1985, Scientific American Inc.
13. Devereux R, et al: Mitral valve prolapse: causes, clinical implications, and management, Ann Intern Med 111:305, 1989.
14. Deleted in proofs.
15. Deleted in proofs.
16. European Coronary Surgery Group: Prospective randomized study of coronary artery bypass in stable angina pectoris; second interim report, Lancet 2:491, 1980.
17. Ferguson JJ, et al: Significance of nitroglycerin-induced hypotension with inferior wall acute myocardial infarction, Am J Cardiol 64:311, 1989.
18. Forrester JS, et al: Medical therapy of acute myocardial infarction by application of hemodynamic subsets, N Engl J Med 295:1404, 1976.

19. Deleted in proofs.
20. Deleted in proofs.
21. Deleted in proofs.
22. Gill JB, Ruddy TD, et al: Prognostic importance of thallium uptake by the lungs during exercise in coronary artery disease, N Engl J Med 317:1485, 1987.
23. Goldberger E: Treatment of cardiac emergencies, ed 5, St Louis, 1991, The CV Mosby Co.
24. Gottlieb SO, et al: Silent ischemia as a marker for early unfavorable outcomes in patients with unstable angina, N Engl J Med 314:1214, 1986.
25. Haft JI, Habbab MA: Treatment of atrial arrhythmias: effectiveness of verapamil when preceded by calcium infusion, Arch Intern Med 146:1085, 1986.
26. Deleted in proofs.
27. Hancock EW: Valvular heart disease. In Rubenstein E, Federman DD (editors): Scientific American medicine, New York, 1985, Scientific American Inc.
28. Hutter AM Jr: Angina pectoris. In Rubenstein E, Federman DD (editors): Scientific American medicine, New York, 1985, Scientific American Inc.
29. Hjalmarson A, et al: Effect on mortality of metoprolol in acute myocardial infarction: a double-blind randomized trial, Lancet 2:823, 1981.
30. Jugdutt BI, Warnica JW: Intravenous nitroglycerin therapy to limit myocardial infarct size, expansion, and complications: effect of timing, dosage, and infarct location, Circulation 78:906, 1988.
30a. Kastor JA: Multifocal atrial tachycardia, N Engl J Med 322:1713, 1990.
31. Killip T, Kimball JT: Treatment of myocardial infarction in a coronary care unit, Am J Cardiol 20:457, 1967.
32. Kowey PR, Eisenberg R, Engel TR: Sustained arrhythmias in hypertropic obstructive cardiomyopathy, N Engl J Med 310:1566, 1984.
33. Mark DB, et al: Localizing coronary obstruction with the exercise treadmill test, Ann Intern Med 106:53, 1987.
34. Deleted in proofs.
35. Deleted in proofs.
36. Deleted in proofs.
37. Deleted in proofs.
38. Nishimura RA, et al: Echocardiographically documented mitral valve prolapse: long-term follow-up of 237 patients, N Engl J Med 313:1305, 1985.
39. Norwegian Multicenter Study Group: Timolol-induced reduction in mortality and re-infarction in patients surviving acute myocardial infarction. I, Mortality results, JAMA 247:1701, 1982.
40. Pooling Project Research Group: Relationship of blood pressure, serum cholesterol, smoking habits, relative weight, and ECG abnormalities to incidence of major coronary events: final report of the pooling project, J Chron Dis 31:201, 1978.
41. Pratt CM, Seals AA, Luck JC: The clinical significance of ventricular arrhythmias after myocardial infarction: symposium on prognosis after MI, Cardiol Clin 2:3, 1984.
42. Ragland DR, Brand RJ: Type A behavior and mortality from coronary heart disease, N Engl J Med 318:65, 1988.
43. Roberts R, Pratt CM: The influence of the site and locus of myocardial damage on prognosis: symposium on prognosis after MI, Cardiol Clin 2:21, 1984.
44. Salerno DM, Anderson B, et al: Intravenous verapamil for treatment of multifocal atrial tachycardia with and without calcium pre-treatment, Ann Intern Med 107:623, 1987.
45. Sanz G, et al: Determinants of prognosis in survivors of myocardial infarction: a prospective clinical angiographic study, N Engl J Med 306:1065, 1982.

46. Schulze RA, Schulze RA Jr, Strauss HW, Pitt B: Sudden death in the year following myocardial infarction: relation to ventricular premature contractions in the late hospital phase and left ventricular ejection fraction, Am J Med 62:182, 1977.
47. Schuster EH, Buckley BH: Early post-infarction angina: ischemia at a distance and ischemia in the infarct zone, N Engl J Med 305:1101, 1981.
48. Shively B, Goldsch N: Progress in cardiac pacing. II, Arch Intern Med 145:2238, 1985.
49. Steering Committee of the Physicians' Health Study Research Group: Final report on the aspirin component of the ongoing physicians' health study, N Engl J Med 321:129, 1989.
50. Deleted in proofs.
51. Theroux P, Ouimet H, et al: Aspirin, heparin, or both to treat acute unstable angina, N Engl J Med 319:1105, 1988.
52. Thompson PL, Fletcher EE, Katavatis V: Enzymatic indices of myocardial necrosis: influence on short- and long-term prognosis after myocardial infarction, Circulation 59:113, 1979.
53. Deleted in proofs.
54. The TIMI Study Group: Comparison of invasive and conservative strategies after treatment with intravenous tissue plasminogen activator in acute myocardial infarction, N Engl J Med 320:618, 1989.
55. Tofler GH: Prognosis after cardiac arrest due to ventricular tachycardia or ventricular fibrillation associated with acute myocardial infarction (The MILIS study), Am J Cardiol 60:755, 1987.
56. Tofler GH, et al: Clinical significance of pericardial friction rubs after MI, Am Heart J 117:86, 1989.
57. Topol EJ: Coronary angioplasty for acute myocardial infarction, Ann Intern Med 109:970, 1988.
58. Turpie AG, Robinson·JG, et al: Comparison of high dose with low dose subcutaneous heparin to prevent left ventricular mural thrombosis in patients with acute transmural anterior myocardial infarction, N Engl J Med 320:352, 1989.
59. Deleted in proofs.
60. Wellens HJ: The wide QRS tachycardia, Ann Intern Med 104:879, 1986.
61. Wenger NK, Abelmann WH, Roberts WWC: Myocarditis. In Hurst JW, Longe RB, et al (editors): The heart, New York, 1985, McGraw-Hill Book Co.
62. Deleted in proofs.
63. Wipf JE, Lipsky BA: Atrial fibrillation: thromboembolic risk and indications for anticoagulation, Arch Intern Med 150:1598, 1990.
64. Zema MJ: Heart failure and bedside Valsalva maneuver, Chest 97:772, 1990.

Dermatology

Cutaneous diseases vary in appearance with their stage and the effect of various environmental factors. It is useful to divide skin lesions into three categories:

1. Primary—initial basic lesions
2. Secondary—may result from evolution of the primary lesions or may be created by scratching or infection
3. Special—unique skin lesions that cannot be classified as primary or secondary

These lesions have been summarized in Tables 21-1, 21-2, and 21-3. Table 21-4 provides a classification of urticaria, a frequently encountered problem in medical patients. Cutaneous lesions associated with internal malignancy are noted in Table 21-5. The detailed description and therapeutic approach to these various skin disorders is beyond the scope of this book. The reader is referred to the many excellent dermatology texts, in particular, to *Clinical Dermatology, A Color Guide to Diagnosis and Therapy,* by T.P. Habif (1990, Mosby).

Table 21-1 Primary skin lesions

Description	Differential Diagnosis
Macule A circumscribed flat discoloration, which may be brown, blue, red, or hypopigmented 	**Brown** Becker's nevus Café-au-lait spot Erythrasma Fixed drug eruption Freckle Junction nevus Lentigo Lentigo maligna Melasma Photoallergic drug eruption Phototoxic drug eruption Stasis dermatitis Tinea nigra palmaris **Blue** Ink (tattoo) Maculae caeruleae (lice) Mongolian spot Ochronosis **Red** Drug eruptions Juvenile rheumatoid arthritis (Still's disease) Rheumatic fever Secondary syphilis Viral exanthems **Hypopigmented** Idiopathic guttate hypomelanosis Piebaldism Postinflammatory (psoriasis) Radiation dermatitis Nevus anemicus Tinea versicolor Tuberous sclerosis Vitiligo

Continued.

From Habif PF: Clinical dermatology, a color guide to diagnosis and therapy, ed 2, St Louis, 1990, The CV Mosby Co.

Table 21-1 Primary skin lesions—cont'd

Description	Differential Diagnosis
Pustule	
A circumscribed collection of leukocytes and free fluid that varies in size	Acne Candidiasis Dermatophyte infection Dyshidrosis Folliculitis Gonococcemia Hidradenitis suppurativa Herpes simplex Herpes zoster Impetigo Psoriasis Pyoderma gangrenosum Rosacea Varicella

Vesicle

A circumscribed collection of free
fluid up to 0.5 cm diameter

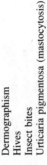

Bulla

A circumscribed collection of free
fluid more than 0.5 cm diameter

Wheal

A firm edematous plaque resulting
from infiltration of the dermis
with fluid; it is transient and may
last only a few hours

Angioedema
Dermographism
Hives
Insect bites
Urticaria pigmentosa (mastocytosis)

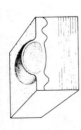

Table 21-1 Primary skin lesions—cont'd

Description	Differential Diagnosis
Papule	
An elevated solid lesion up to 0.5 cm in diameter; color varies; papules may become confluent and form plaques	Flesh colored, yellow, or white
	Adenoma sebaceum
	Basal cell epithelioma
	Closed comedone (acne)
	Flat warts
	Granuloma annulare
	Lichen nitidus
	Lichen sclerosis et atrophicus
	Molluscum contagiosum
	Milium
	Nevi (dermal)
	Neurofibroma
	Pearly penile papules
	Pseudoxanthoma elasticum
	Sebaceous hyperplasia
	Skin tags
	Syringoma
	Red
	Acne
	Atopic dermatitis
	Cholinergic urticaria
	Chondrodermatitis nodularis chronica helicis
	Eczema
	Folliculitis
	Insect bites
	Keratosis pilaris
	Leukocytoclastic vasculitis
	Miliaria
	Polymorphic light eruption
	Psoriasis
	Pyogenic granuloma
	Scabies
	Urticaria
	Blue or violaceous
	Angiokeratoma
	Blue nevus
	Lichen planus
	Lymphoma
	Kaposi's sarcoma
	Melanoma
	Mycosis fungoides
	Venous lake
Brown	
Dermatofibroma	Seborrheic keratosis
Keratosis follicularis	Urticaria pigmentosa
Melanoma	Warts
Nevi	

Plaque

A circumscribed, elevated, superficial, solid lesion more than 0.5 cm in diameter, often formed by the confluence of papules

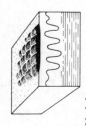

Eczema
Mycosis fungoides
Papulosquamous (papular and scaling)
Discoid lupus erythematosus
Lichen planus
Pityriasis rosea
Psoriasis
Seborrheic dermatitis
Syphilis (secondary)
Tinea corporis
Tinea versicolor

Nodule

A circumscribed, elevated, solid lesion more than 0.5 cm in diameter; a large nodule is referred to as a tumor

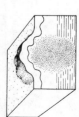

Basal cell epithelioma
Erythema nodosum
Furuncle
Hemangioma
Kaposi's sarcoma
Keratoacanthoma
Lipoma
Lymphoma
Melanoma
Metastatic carcinoma
Mycosis fungoides
Neurofibromatosis
Prurigo nodularis
Sporotrichosis
Squamous cell carcinoma
Warts
Xanthoma

Table 21-2   Secondary skin lesions

Description	Differential Diagnosis
Scale	
Excess dead epidermal cells that are produced by abnormal keratinization and shedding	Fine to stratified
	Eczema craquele
	Ichthyosis (quadrangular)
	Lupus erythematosus (carpet tack)
	Pityriasis rosea (collarette)
	Psoriasis (silvery)
	Scarlet fever (fine on trunk)
	Seborrheic dermatitis (greasy)
	Syphilis (secondary)
	Tinea (dermatophytes)
	Tinea versicolor
	Xerosis (dry skin)
	Scaling in sheets
	Scarlet fever (hands and feet)
	Staphylococcal scalded skin syndrome

Crust

A collection of dried serum and cellular debris; a scab

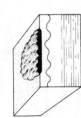

Acute eczematous inflammation
Atopic (face)
Impetigo (honey colored)
Pemphigus foliaceus
Tinea capitis

Erosion

A focal loss of epidermis; it does not penetrate below dermal-epidermal junction and therefore heals without scarring

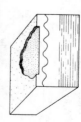

Candidiasis
Dermatophyte infection
Eczematous diseases
Intertrigo
Perlèche
Senile skin
Toxic epidermal necrolysis
Vesiculobullous diseases

From Habif PF: Clinical dermatology, a color guide to diagnosis and therapy, ed 2, St Louis, 1990, The CV Mosby Co.

Continued.

Table 21-2 Secondary skin lesions—cont'd

Description		Differential Diagnosis
Ulcer A focal loss of epidermis and dermis; it heals with scarring		Aphthae Chancroid Decubitus Factitial Ischemic Necrobiosis lipoidica diabeticorum Neoplasms Pyoderma gangrenosum Radiodermatitis Syphilis (chancre) Stasis ulcers
Fissure A linear loss of epidermis and dermis with sharply defined nearly vertical walls		Chapping (hands, feet) Eczema (fingertip) Intertrigo Perlèche

Atrophy

A depression in skin resulting from thinning of epidermis or dermis

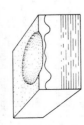

Aging
Dermatomyositis
Discoid lupus erythematosus
Lichen sclerosis et atrophicus
Morphea
Necrobiosis lipoidica diabeticorum
Radiodermatitis
Striae
Topical and intralesional steroids

Scar

An abnormal formation of connective tissue implying dermal damage; when following injury or surgery it is initially thick and pink but with time becomes white and atrophic

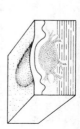

Acne
Burns
Herpes zoster
Hidradenitis suppurativa
Porphyria
Varicella

Table 21-3 Special skin lesions

Description	Differential Diagnosis
Excoriation	
An erosion caused by scratching; are often linear	—
Comedone	
A plug of sebaceous and keratinous material lodged in the opening of a hair follicle; the follicular orifice may be dilated (blackhead) or narrowed (whitehead) or closed (comedone)	—
Milia	
Small superficial keratin cysts with no visible openings	—
Cyst	
A circumscribed lesion having a wall and a lumen; the lumen may contain fluid or solid matter	—
Burrow	
A narrow, elevated, tortuous channel produced by a parasite	—
Lichenification	
An area of thickened epidermis induced by scratching; the skin lines are accentuated so the surface looks like a washboard	—

Telangiectasia

Dilated superficial blood vessels

Actinically damaged skin
Adenoma sebaceum
Ataxia-telangiectasia
Basal cell carcinoma
Bloom's syndrome
CRST syndrome
Hereditary hemorrhagic telangiectasia
Keloid
Lupus erythematosus
Necrobiosis lipoidica diabeticorum
Of the proximal nail fold
   Dermatomyositis
   Lupus erythematosus
   Scleroderma
Poikiloderma
Radiodermatitis
Rosacea
Scleroderma
Vascular spiders
   Pregnancy
   Cirrhosis
Xeroderma pigmentosum

Continued.

From Habif PF: Clinical dermatology, a color guide to diagnosis and therapy, ed 2, St Louis, 1990, The CV Mosby Co.

Table 21-3 Special skin lesions—cont'd

Description	Differential Diagnosis
Petechiae Circumscribed deposits of blood less than 0.5 cm diameter	Gonococcemia Leukocytoclastic vasculitis Meningococcemia Platelet abnormalities Progressive pigmentary purpura Rocky Mountain spotted fever Scurvy Senile (traumatic)
Purpura A circumscribed deposit of blood greater than 0.5 cm diameter	

Table 21-4 Etiologic Classification of Urticaria

Foods
  Fish, shellfish, nuts, eggs, chocolate, strawberries, tomatoes,
    pork, cow's milk, cheese, wheat, yeast
Food additives
  Salicylates, benzoates, penicillin, dyes such as tartrazine
Drugs
  Penicillin, aspirin, sulfonamides; also drugs that cause
    nonimmunologic release of histamine (e.g., morphine, codeine,
    polymyxin, dextran, curare, quinine)
Infections
  Chronic bacterial infections (e.g., sinus, dental, chest,
    gallbladder, urinary tract), fungal infections (dermatophytosis,
    candidiasis), viral infections (viral hepatitis, infectious
    mononucleosis, coxsackie), protozoal and helminth infections
    (intestinal worms, malaria)
Inhalants
  Pollens, mold spores, animal danders, house dust, aerosols,
    volatile chemicals
Internal disease
  Serum sickness, systemic lupus erythematosus, hyperthyroidism,
    carcinomas, lymphomas, juvenile rheumatoid arthritis (Still's
    disease), leukocytoclastic vasculitis, polycythemia vera (acne
    urticata—urticarial papule surmounted by a vesicle), rheumatic
    fever
Physical stimuli (the physical urticarias)
  Dermographism, pressure urticaria, cholinergic urticaria, solar
    urticaria, cold urticaria, urticarias induced by heat, vibration,
    water (aquagenic)
Nonimmunologic contact urticaria
  Plants (nettles), animals (caterpillars, jellyfish), medications
    (cinnamic aldehyde, compound 48/80, dimethyl sulfoxide)
Immunologic or uncertain mechanism contact urticaria
  Ammonium persulfate used in hair bleaches, chemicals, foods,
    textiles, wood, saliva, cosmetics, perfumes
Skin diseases
  Urticaria pigmentosa (mastocytosis), dermatitis herpetiformis,
    pemphigoid, amyloidosis
Pregnancy
Genetic, autosomal dominant (all rare)
  Hereditary angioedema, cholinergic urticaria with progressive
    nerve deafness and amyloidosis of the kidney, familial cold
    urticaria, vibratory urticaria

From Habif PF: Clinical dermatology, a color guide to diagnosis and therapy, ed 2, St Louis, 1990, The CV Mosby Co.

Table 21-5 Cutaneous lesions and internal malignancy

Syndrome	Clinical Presentation	Malignancy
Ataxia telangiectasia	Cerebellar ataxia, telangiectasia (pinna, bulbar conjunctiva, etc.)	Reticulum cell sarcoma, Hodgkin's, gastric
Alopecia mucinosa	Patch of follicular papules and boggy infiltrate, face, trunk, scalp	Mycosis fungoides
Amyloidosis	Macroglossia; smooth tongue; shiny, translucent, waxy papules on eyelids, nasolabial folds, lips, and intertriginous areas; "pinch purpura"—skin bleeds with trauma	Multiple myeloma
Acanthosis nigricans	Adult onset in absence of obesity, endocrinopathy, and family history; hyperkeratotic, hyperpigmented skin folds in flexural areas (neck, axillae, antecubital fossa, breast, groin)	Abdominal cancer, other adenocarcinomas
Bazex's syndrome (acrokeratosis para neoplastica)	Three stages: 1. psoriasiform lesions, tips of fingers and toes; 2. keratoderma, hands and feet; 3. lesions extend locally and new lesions appear on knees, legs, thighs, arms	Carcinoma of esophagus, tongue, lower lip, upper lobes of the lungs
Bloom's syndrome	Erythema face ("butterfly area"), stunted growth	Acute leukemia

Carcinoid syndrome	Episodes of flushing (face, neck, chest), dyspnea, asthma, diarrhea, murmur of pulmonary stenosis and insufficiency	Serotonin-containing tumor of appendix, small intestine, bronchus, etc.
Cowden's syndrome (multiple hamartoma syndrome)	Warty papules on face, hands, mouth	Breast, thyroid
Dermatomyositis (adult)	Heliotrope erythema eyelids, bluish-red plaques on knuckles	Breast, gastrointestinal, genitourinary, lung, ovary
Erythema gyratum repens	Rapidly moving waxy bands of erythema with a serpiginous outline and "wood grain" pattern	Breast, lung, stomach, bladder, prostate
Gardner's syndrome	Epidermal cysts, cutaneous osteomas and fibromas, polyps in small and large intestine	Adenocarcinoma of colon
Glucagonoma syndrome	Migratory necrolytic erythema in intertriginous and dependent areas, elevated serum glucagon levels	Glucagon secreting alpha cell tumor of the pancreas
Hypertrichosis lanuginosa (acquired)	Long hair on face and trunk	Bronchus, gallbladder, rectum
Ichthyosis (acquired)	Generalized scaling, prominent on extremities, spares the flexural area	Hodgkin's disease; other lymphoproliferative malignancies; cancer of lung, breast, cervix
Kaposi's sarcoma	Red papular and nodular neoplasms most common on lower legs	Internal organ Kaposi's sarcoma, high incidence of other cancers
Leser-Trélat sign	Sudden appearance (3-6 mo) and rapid increase in size and number of seborrheic keratoses	Colon, breast

Continued.

Table 21-5   Cutaneous lesions and internal malignancy—cont'd

Syndrome	Clinical Presentation	Malignancy
Melanosis (generalized)	Generalized cutaneous melanosis	Metastatic melanoma
Metastasis to the skin	Metastasis to any cutaneous site	Variety of tumors
Paget's disease (breast)	Eczematous crusted lesion of nipple, areola	Breast
Paget's disease (extramammary)	Eroded scaling plaques of vulva, scrotum, axilla, perianal, groin	Cervical cancer and adenocarcinoma of anus and rectum
Palmoplantar keratoderma (tylosis)	Skin thickening of palms and soles	Gastrointestinal carcinomas
Peutz-Jeghers syndrome	Pigmented macules on lips and oral mucosa; polyposis of small intestine	Adenocarcinoma of stomach, duodenum, colon
Sipple's syndrome	Multiple mucosal neuromas	Medullary carcinoma of thyroid, C cell neoplasia, pheochromocytoma
Torre's syndrome	Multiple sebaceous adenomas	Visceral carcinomas
Urticaria pigmentosa (disseminated maculopapular form)	Brown-red macules and papules that contain mast cells and urticate when traumatized	Hematologic malignancies
von Hippel–Lindau	Angiomas of skin, angiomatosis of cerebellum or medulla	Hypernephroma, pheochromocytoma
von Recklinghausen's neurofibromatosis	Café-au-lait spots, white macules, multiple cutaneous neuromas, internal neuromas	Malignant neurilemoma, astrocytoma, pheochromocytoma
Wiskott-Aldrich syndrome	Eczematous lesions in atopic dermatitis distribution	Reticuloendothelial malignancy

From Habif PF: Clinical dermatology, a color guide to diagnosis and therapy, ed 2, St Louis, 1990, The CV Mosby Co.

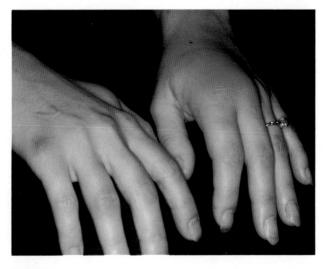

Plate 1

Gonococcal septicemia. Note the erythema and joint swelling on the left hand. A single vesicle is present on the right hand. (From Habif TP: Clinical dermatology. A color guide to diagnosis and therapy, ed 2, St Louis, 1990, The CV Mosby Co.)

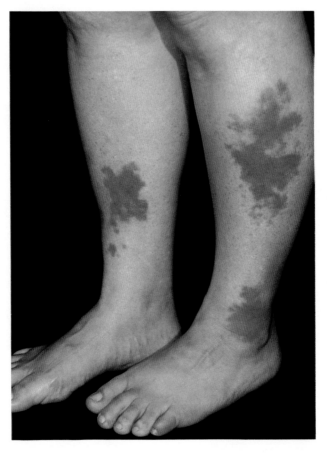

Plate 2

Necrobiosis lipoidica diabeticorum. Erythematous violaceous plaques on the anterior surfaces of the lower legs. (From Habif TP: Clinical dermatology. A color guide to diagnosis and therapy, ed 2, St Louis, 1990, The CV Mosby Co.)

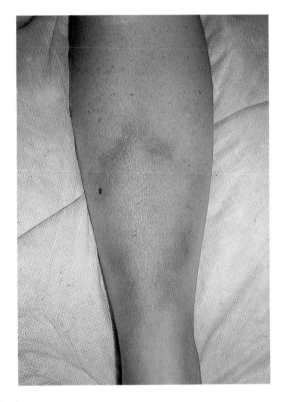

Plate 3

Erythema chronicum migrans. Broad oval area of erythema has slowly migrated from the central area. (From Habif TP: Clinical dermatology. A color guide to diagnosis and therapy, ed 2, St Louis, 1990, The CV Mosby Co.)

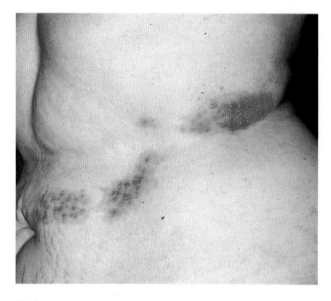

Plate 4
Herpes zoster. A common presentation with involvement of a single thoracic dermatome. (From Habif TP: Clinical dermatology. A color guide to diagnosis and therapy, ed 2, St Louis, 1990, The CV Mosby Co.)

Endocrinology

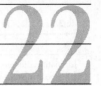

22

DIABETES MELLITUS
H. Christina Hanley

Diabetes mellitus (DM) affects approximately 5% of the American population. It is characterized by an imbalance between the factors that elevate and the counterregulatory factors that lower the blood glucose level:

Increased glucose	Decreased glucose
Food intake	Insulin
Glucagon	Exercise
Cortisol	Cellular glucose uptake
Growth hormone	
Catecholamines	
Hepatic gluconeogenesis	

Classification

Table 22-1 gives a recent classification of DM based on newer insights into the causes and conditions associated with diabetes.

Diagnosis

Table 22-2 gives the criteria used by the National Diabetes Data Group and the WHO for blood glucose limits on an oral glucose tolerance test.[23,48] Because of the disagreement on criteria, the nonstandardization of the test (many patients have not eaten 300 g carbohydrate/day diet for 3 days preceding the test), and the day-to-day blood glucose level variation within the same individual, many physicians measure the *glycosylated hemoglobin* (HbA_{1c}) to determine glucose intolerance and to diagnose DM.[26] However, the use of HbA_{1c} to screen for DM has been questioned by many endocrinologists.

Treatment of the patient with nonacute DM

The goal of treatment is to normalize the serum glucose level. This can be achieved with the following modalities:
1. Diet

213

Table 22-1 Classification of diabetes mellitus

Type	Associated Factors
Idiopathic diabetes	
Type I: insulin-dependent diabetes mellitus (IDDM)	Hereditary factors: Islet cell antibodies (found in 90% of patients within the first year of diagnosis) Higher incidence of HLA types DR3, DR4 50% concordance in identical twins Environmental factors: Viral infection (possibly coxsackievirus, mumps virus)
Type II: non–insulin-dependent diabetes mellitus (NIDDM)	Hereditary factor: 90% concordance in identical twins Environmental factor: obesity
Diabetes secondary to	
Hormonal excess	Cushing's syndrome, acromegaly, glucagonoma, pheochromocytoma
Drugs	Glucocorticoids, diuretics, oral contraceptives
Insulin receptor unavailability	With or without circulating antibodies
Pancreatic disease	Pancreatitis, pancreatectomy, hemochromatosis
Genetic syndromes	Hyperlipidemias, myotonic dystrophy, lipoatrophy
Gestational diabetes	

Table 22-2 Diagnostic criteria for diabetes mellitus

Lab Test	National Diabetes Data Group	WHO
Fasting blood sugar (FBS)	$\geq$140 mg/dl	$\geq$140 mg/dl
Glucose level 30 or 60 minutes after a 75 g glucose load (Glucola)	$\geq$200 mg/dl	
Glucose level 2 hours after 75 g glucose load (Glucola)	$\geq$200 mg/dl	$\geq$200 mg/dl

a. Calories
   (1) The diabetic patient can be started on 15 calories/lb of ideal body weight; this number can be increased to 20 calories/lb for an active person and 25 calories/lb if the patient does heavy physical labor
   (2) The calories should be distributed as 55-60% carbohydrates, 25-35% fat, and 15-20% protein
   (3) The emphasis should be on complex carbohydrates rather than simple and refined starches, and on polyunsaturated instead of saturated fats in a ratio of $2:1$
b. Seven food groups
   (1) The exchange diet of the American Diabetes Association includes: protein, bread, fruit, milk, fat, and low and intermediate carbohydrate vegetables
   (2) The diet should be well balanced and may include one or more foods from each of these groups, unless otherwise contraindicated (e.g., milk in a patient with lactose intolerance)
   (3) The name of each exchange is meant to be all inclusive (e.g., cereal, muffins, spaghetti, potatoes, rice are in the bread group; meats, fish, eggs, cheese, peanut butter are in the protein group)
c. The *glycemic index*[20] compares the rise in blood sugar after the ingestion of simple sugars and complex carbohydrates with the rise that occurs after the absorption of glucose; equal amounts of starches do not give the same rise in plasma glucose (pasta equal in calories to a baked potato causes less of a rise than the potato); thus it is helpful to know the glycemic index of a particular food product
d. Fiber: insoluble fiber (bran, celery) and soluble globular fiber (pectin in fruit) delay glucose absorption and attenuate the postprandial serum glucose peak; they also appear to lower the elevated triglyceride level often present in uncontrolled diabetics
2. Exercise increases the cellular glucose uptake by increasing the number of cell receptors[77]; the following points must be considered:
   a. Exercise programs must be individualized and built up slowly
   b. Insulin is more rapidly absorbed when injected into a limb that is then exercised, and this can result in hypoglycemia (patients who have experienced hypoglycemia during exercise should eat a snack before the activity and, if necessary, reduce the insulin dose that peaks at that time of day)
3. Weight loss: to ideal weight if the patient is overweight
4. Oral hypoglycemic agents
   a. When the above measures fail to normalize the serum glucose, a sulfonylurea should be added to the regimen (Table 33-33 lists the commonly used sulfonylureas)
   b. Oral hypoglycemic agents work best when given before meals (e.g., 15 min before breakfast) because they increase the postprandial output of insulin from the pancreas
   c. All sulfonylureas are contraindicated in patients allergic to sulfa
   d. Second-generation sulfonylureas are generally safer than previous agents because of their alternative excretion routes (e.g., their excretion in bile permits a safer use in patients with renal disease)

5. Insulin is indicated for the treatment of all DM type I (insulin dependent) and DM type II patients who cannot be adequately controlled with diet and sulfonylureas
    a. Insulin treatment progresses from the administration of once-a-day intermediate-acting insulin (NPH, lente) to twice-a-day insulin, then bid doses of NPH or lente plus regular insulin, to basal insulin with multiple doses of regular[62]
    b. Table 33-26 describes the various types of insulin preparations; human insulin (Humulin) is recommended for first-time diabetic patients to avoid inducing antiinsulin antibodies, and it is now available at prices comparable with pork or beef insulin
    c. Insulin therapy should start with the simplest regimen and advance to the next step only when adequate glucose control cannot be otherwise achieved
    d. Patients receiving insulin should initially monitor their glucose in the morning (before breakfast), before lunch, before dinner, and before bedtime; insulin dosage should be adjusted accordingly
    e. Rotating insulin injections from site to site increases variability in the blood glucose concentration; the abdomen is the preferred site for insulin injections since it produces less variability in absorption[5]

Determination of NPH insulin dosage

1. Measure the blood glucose qid (before meals and before bed); urine glucose measurements should not be used because of their inherent inaccuracies (variable renal glucose threshold, glycosuria reflects blood glucose of several hours not glucose level at time of insulin administration)
2. Cover blood glucose qid with regular insulin based on a sliding-scale coverage:

Blood glucose level (mg/dl)	Regular insulin dose (U)
351-400	12
301-350	10
251-300	7
200-250	5

3. Determine the total amount of regular insulin given and give 2/3 of this dosage as NPH insulin qAM before breakfast
4. An alternate method is to arbitrarily give 20 U NPH qAM (0.3 U/kg body weight) before breakfast and adjust this amount by 2, 5, or 10 U every 3 days depending on the serum glucose levels (a change in insulin dosage takes about 3 days to stabilize; therefore the dosage should not be changed before then)

Example:

Time	AM	Before Lunch	Before Dinner	Before Bedtime	Insulin Adjustment
Glucose level	Normal	↑	Normal	Normal	Add 4 U of regular insulin to AM NPH dose
	↑	Normal	Normal	Normal	Change to bid NPH insulin (prebreakfast and either predinner or at bedtime)

As noted in the above example, bid insulin is necessary when the plasma glucose is inadequately controlled with only one NPH insulin injection; regular insulin may be added to the NPH doses as needed

5. One of the complications of bid NPH insulin is the *Somogyi effect*, which is characterized by early morning (3 AM) hypoglycemia followed by rebound hyperglycemia in the AM. The hypoglycemia is caused by an excessive evening NPH insulin dose (peak effect seen at approximately 3 AM). The rebound hyperglycemia is secondary to the effects of counterregulatory hormones. If the Somogyi effect is suspected (sweating, tremors, tachycardia during the night and increased FBS or awakening in AM with headache and wet clothing), the diagnosis can be confirmed by checking a 3 AM plasma glucose level (markedly decreased). The treatment is to reduce the evening NPH insulin dose. The "dawn phenomenon" is characterized by hyperglycemia between 4:00 AM and 7:00 AM *in absence* of the Somogyi effect. It is believed to be secondary to nocturnal release of growth hormone. Treatment (after excluding Somogyi effect) consists of increasing the pre-bedtime NPH (or lente insulin) dose or giving the second insulin injection at bedtime if it was being given before supper. If a patient requires three insulin injections/day (and the patient is compliant), best control of the hyperglycemia can be achieved by dividing the total insulin dosage in the following manner:
   a. ⅔ of the total daily dosage before breakfast, subdivided in:
      (1) ⅔ intermediate-acting insulin
      (2) ⅓ short-acting insulin
   b. ⅙ of the dosage before dinner (regular insulin)
   c. ⅙ of the dosage at bedtime (intermediate-acting insulin)
For example, if the total daily insulin dosage is 36 U:
a. 24 U given before breakfast
   (1) 16 U NPH insulin
   (2) 8 U regular insulin
b. 6 U regular insulin given before dinner
c. 6 U NPH insulin given at bedtime
   Table 22-3 lists insulin dosage corrections based on the time of the abnormal glucose levels

Table 22-3 Correction of insulin dosage

Time	Plasma Glucose	Insulin Adjustment
AM	↑	↓ Evening NPH insulin initially, ↑ NPH insulin when the Somogyi effect has been ruled out
	↓	↓ Evening NPH insulin
Lunch	↑	↑ AM regular insulin
	↓	↓ AM regular insulin
Dinner	↑	↑ AM NPH insulin
	↓	↓ AM NPH insulin
Bedtime	↑	↑ Predinner regular insulin
	↓	↓ Predinner regular insulin

Monitoring adequacy of glucose control

Since normalization of serum glucose is the ultimate goal, the patient should have a mechanism to measure the degree of control (this will act as a motivator).

1. Urine testing can be done on a qid basis (before meals and at bedtime) on double-voided specimens until the urine is consistently negative, indicating a serum glucose level below 180-200 mg/dl; urine testing is a mediocre assay of blood glucose since it cannot differentiate among mild hyperglycemia, euglycemia, and hypoglycemia. It should be used only in stable NIDDM when compliance with blood glucose testing is a problem. It should also be supplemented by periodic HbA$_{1c}$ and fasting plasma glucose determinations[60]

2. Blood glucose monitoring is the optimal test for glycemia. Glucose oxidase strips can be compared with the color chart on the container, or they can be used in conjunction with a meter to give a digital reading. The testing can be done once a day, but vary the time each day so that over a period of time the serum glucose level before meals and at bedtime can frequently be assessed without pricking the patient's fingers qid

3. Glycosylated hemoglobin (HbA$_{1c}$): nondiabetic patients normally have 3-8% of their hemoglobin glycosylated (sugar attached to the hemoglobin molecule); this depends on the ambient sugar concentration over the preceding 4-8 wk, and therefore the higher the average serum glucose the higher the glycohemoglobin level. HbA$_{1c}$ levels greater than 9-10% indicate poor glycemic control over the previous 4-8 wk. This test can be obtained at any time of the day and requires no fasting. Factors (other than serum glucose) that can alter HbA$_{1c}$ are

Decreased HbA$_{1c}$	Increased HbA$_{1c}$
Chronic blood loss	Increased HbF
Anemia (hemolytic)	Chronic renal failure
Presence of abnormal Hb (S,C,D)	Splenectomy
	Dialysis
	Thalassemia
	Increased triglycerides

Complications

Retinopathy is found in approximately 15% of type I diabetics and in 6% of type II diabetics after 15 years.

1. Nonproliferative retinopathy (background diabetic retinopathy)
   a. Initially: microaneurysms, capillary dilation, waxy or hard exudates, dot and flame hemorrhages, AV shunts
   b. Advanced stage: microinfarcts with macular edema, cotton wool exudates
   c. Most common form (80% of all diabetic retinopathy) results in legal blindness in 5-20% of patients within 5 yr
2. Proliferative retinopathy: formation of new vessels; if untreated, it will result in legal blindness in 50% of patients within 5 yr
3. Complications of retinopathy: vitreal hemorrhages, fibrous scarring, retinal detachment
4. Diagnosis: diabetic patients should have a yearly examination by an ophthalmologist
5. Therapy: photocoagulation treatment (laser beam therapy) can greatly improve the prognosis in diabetic retinopathy; vitrectomy may be necessary when hemorrhage or retinal detachment occurs in proliferative retinopathy
6. Cataracts and glaucoma occur with increased frequency in diabetics

Neuropathy is common in diabetics, its frequency in type II approaching 70-80%.

1. Peripheral neuropathy
   a. Manifestations
      (1) Paresthesias of extremities (feet more than hands); the symptoms are symmetric, bilateral, and associated with intense burning pain (particularly during the night)
      (2) Mononeuropathies involving cranial nerves III, IV, VI, intercostal nerves, and femoral nerve are also common
   b. Physical exam
      (1) Decreased pinprick sensation, sensation to light touch, and pain sensation
      (2) Decreased vibration sense
      (3) Loss of proprioception (leading to ataxia)
      (4) Motor disturbances (decreased DTR, weakness and atrophy of interossei muscles); when the hands are affected, the patient has trouble picking up small objects, with dressing, and with turning pages in a book
      (5) Diplopia, abnormalities of visual fields

   c. Therapy
- (1) Use mild analgesics (avoid narcotics); capsaicin 0.075% cream (Axsain) applied tid-qid may provide some relief of painful diabetic neuropathy
- (2) Additional modalities include amitriptyline (25-75 mg hs), or carbamazepine 100 mg PO bid initially
- (3) Mononeuropathies usually resolve spontaneously within 3 months and require no treatment (an eye patch may be helpful in patients with diplopia)

2. Autonomic neuropathy
   a. GI disturbances
     (1) Manifestations
- (a) Disturbances of esophageal motility
- (b) Gastroparesis with delayed gastric emptying
- (c) Diarrhea (usually nocturnal)

     (2) Treatment
- (a) Metoclopramide (Reglan) 10 g qid or bethanechol 5-10 mg tid-qid to treat impaired esophageal and gastric motility
- (b) H_2 blockers (cimetidine, ranitidine) to decrease gastric acidity
- (c) Clonidine (α-2 adrenergic agonist) to control diarrhea resulting from autonomic neuropathy; initial dosage is 0.1 mg q12h and may be increased to 0.5 mg q12h over 3 days

   b. GU disturbances
     (1) Neurogenic bladder is characterized by hesitancy, weak stream, and dribbling
- (a) Treatment consists of frequent voidings (q4h), manual pressure suprapubically to facilitate voiding, and bethanechol 10-50 mg PO tid or qid to increase the tone of the detrusor urinae muscle
- (b) Prompt antibiotic therapy in suspected UTI

     (2) Impotence occurs frequently in diabetic men
- (a) Sexual desire is normal and ejaculation is preserved, but erection is affected; other causes of impotence should also be ruled out
- (b) Treatment is disappointing, but many patients have been helped by a penile prosthesis implant or penile injection of papaverine[80]

   c. Orthostatic hypotension
     (1) Manifestations: postural syncope, dizziness, lightheadedness
     (2) Treatment
- (a) Ensure adequate hydration, liberalize salt intake if indicated
- (b) Fludrocortisone 0.05-0.1 mg qd or bid is helpful in some patients
- (c) Antiembolic stockings to prevent pooling of blood in the lower extremities
- (d) Have patient avoid sudden movement from recumbent to erect position

Nephropathy occurs in 10-15% of diabetics (higher prevalence in Type I diabetics)

1. Manifestations: proteinuria occurs approximately 3 yr before a marked reduction in creatinine clearance is evident and approximately 5 yr before renal failure
2. Treatment
   a. Rigidly controlling the plasma glucose level from the onset of diabetes may prevent or delay the onset of nephropathy
   b. Dietary restriction in protein and phosphates and maintenance of fluid balance is also essential in patients with renal insufficiency
   c. Hypertension, if present, should be treated aggressively; ACE inhibitors have been shown to decrease the degree of albuminuria and may delay the development of diabetic nephropathy
   d. Contrast material (IVP, CT scan dye) should be avoided (particularly if the serum creatinine is >2.0 mg/dl); prior hydration is mandatory
   e. Urinary tract infections should be treated aggressively
   f. When renal failure has occurred, chronic dialysis or kidney transplant may be possible, depending on whether other complications are present

• • •

Infections are generally more common in diabetics because of multiple factors, such as impaired leukocyte function, decreased tissue perfusion secondary to vascular disease, repeated trauma because of loss of sensation, and urinary retention secondary to neuropathy; Table 22-4 lists infections that have an increased incidence in diabetics.

Following are other complications seen in diabetic patients:

1. Foot ulcers occur frequently and are usually secondary to peripheral vascular insufficiency, repeated trauma (unrecognized because of the sensory loss), and superimposed infection; treatment includes
   a. Have the patient eliminate weight bearing on the area of the ulcer; bed rest and use of heel protectors may be necessary to prevent repeated microtrauma
   b. Have the patient avoid tight-fitting shoes and keep feet clean; whirlpool therapy may be helpful
   c. Apply povidone-iodine (Betadine) solution to the area and cover with a sterile dressing (change dressing two or three times per day)
   d. If the ulcer is significant, surgical debridement will be necessary; IV antibiotics are indicated if there is evidence of infection
   e. The infection is usually polymicrobial (staphylococci, gram-negative bacilli, streptococci, anaerobes)
   f. Broad spectrum antibiotic therapy with imipenem/cilastin or combination of penicillinase-resistant penicillin and aminoglycoside or ciprofloxacin is indicated
   g. Evaluate the adequacy of the vasculature; noninvasive studies with differential Doppler analysis[32] and consult with a vascular surgeon are suggested; arterial reconstruction may be necessary for ulcer healing

Table 22-4   Infections with increased prevalence in diabetics

Site of Infection	Organism
Skin and connective tissue	*Candida albicans* and other dermatophytes
	Staphylococcus sp, streptococci, and gram-negative bacilli
	Anaerobes (e.g., *B. fragilis*)
Nasal mucosa	Fungi of genera *Mucor, Rhizopus,* and *Absidia* (rhinocerebral mucormycosis)
Ears	*Pseudomonas aeruginosa* (malignant external otitis)
Lungs	*Staphylococcus* sp
	Klebsiella sp
	Mycobacterium tuberculosis
Gallbladder	*Clostridium* sp and other anaerobic and aerobic organisms (emphysematous cholecystitis)
Urinary tract	*Escherichia coli,* staphylococci, *Torulopsis glabrata*
Vagina	*Candida albicans* (vaginal moniliasis)

   h. In patients with vascular compromise, bone biopsy to exclude osteo-myelitis may result in bone necrosis

2. Neuropathic arthropathy (Charcot joints): bone or joint deformities from repeated trauma (secondary to peripheral neuropathy); limitation of weight bearing is indicated; short leg cast immobilization or ankle-foot orthosis may be necessary
3. Osteoporosis has an increased incidence in diabetics
4. Necrobiosis lipoidica-diabeticorum: plaquelike reddened areas with a central area that fades to white-yellow found on the anterior surfaces of the legs; in these areas, the skin becomes very thin and can ulcerate readily; the patient should avoid any trauma to the affected area (see Fig. 21-2)

22.2   DIABETIC KETOACIDOSIS

Definition

Diabetic ketoacidosis (DKA) results from severe insulin deficiency. It is manifested clinically by severe dehydration and alterations in the sensorium. The various pathophysiologic events leading to DKA are described in Fig. 22-1.

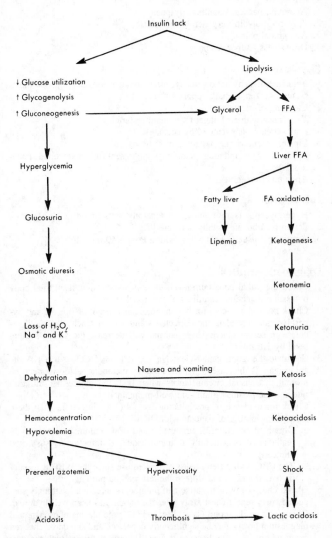

Figure 22-1
Pathophysiological events leading to diabetic ketoacidosis. (From Felts PW: Med Clin North Am 67:831, 1983.)

Symptoms

1. Anorexia, nausea, vomiting, dyspnea
2. Polyuria, polydipsia, generalized malaise
3. Abdominal pain
4. Drowsiness, stupor, coma

Physical exam

1. Evidence of dehydration (tachycardia, hypotension, dry mucous membranes, sunken eyeballs, poor skin turgor)
2. Clouding of mental status
3. Tachypnea with air hunger (Kussmaul respiration)
4. Fruity breath odor (caused by acetone)
5. Lipemia retinalis may be noted in some patients
6. Evidence of precipitating factors may be present (infected wound, pneumonia)
7. Abdominal tenderness

Lab results

1. Hyperglycemia (serum glucose is generally >300 mg/dl)
2. Serum bicarbonate usually <15 mEq/L
3. Arterial pH usually below 7.3, with a P_{CO_2} <40 mm Hg
4. Ketosis

Diagnostic studies

1. Check the initial potassium level; there is always significant total body potassium depletion regardless of the initial level
2. Check the sodium level for hyponatremia as a result of lipemia and hyperglycemia; calculate the corrected sodium level (each 100 mg/dl increase in serum glucose over normal will decrease the serum sodium level by 1.6 mEq/L)
3. Calculate the anion gap: $AG = Na^+ - (Cl^- + HCO_3^-)$; in DKA the anion gap is increased; hyperchloremic metabolic acidosis may be present in unusual circumstances when both the glomerular filtration rate and the plasma volume are well-maintained
4. Check for evidence of precipitating factors (e.g., infection, MI); these are present in 50% of patients with DKA
   a. Obtain blood cultures, urinalysis, and urine culture and sensitivity (catheterize patient only if unconscious) if infection is suspected clinically
   b. The CBC with differential is of limited use since the WBC is usually increased and a mild shift to the left may be present
5. Obtain chest x-ray; if negative and pulmonary infection is strongly suspected, may repeat chest x-ray after the patient has been well hydrated
6. Obtain admission serum Ca^{2+}, Mg^{2+}, PO^{-3}; the plasma phosphate and magnesium levels may be significantly depressed and should be checked again within 24 hours because they will decrease further with the correction of DKA
7. Obtain admission BUN (↑), creatinine (↑)

8. The admission ECG is extremely valuable for the immediate diagnosis of electrolyte abnormalities and can serve as a useful guide to the rate of potassium administration; the following ECG changes may be noted[15]:
   a. Hypokalemia: ST segment depression, decreased amplitude of the T wave (or inverted T waves), increased amplitude of the U wave, apparent prolongation of the QT and PR interval
   b. Hyperkalemia: tall, narrow or tent-shaped T waves, decreased or absent P waves, short QT intervals, widening of the QRS complex
   c. Hypocalcemia: QT interval prolongation, flat or inverted T waves
   d. Hypercalcemia: short or absent ST segment, decreased QT_c interval
   e. Magnesium deficiency: ventricular and supraventricular dysrhythmias

Differential diagnosis

1. Alcoholic ketoacidosis: usually seen in poorly nourished alcoholics with vomiting, abdominal pain, and only minimal food intake over several days
   a. Lab values
      (1) Increased AG metabolic acidosis (due to increased hydroxybutyric acid > acetoacetic acid)
      (2) Low or absent serum ethanol level
      (3) Positive nitroprusside test
      (4) Normal to low serum glucose
   b. Therapy mainly consists of glucose infusion
2. Uremic acidosis: absent ketosis, markedly elevated BUN
3. Metabolic acidosis secondary to methyl alcohol, ethylene glycol
   a. Lab shows an increased osmolar gap (measured serum osmolality − calculated osmolality)

$$\text{Calculated osmolality} = 2(Na^+ + K^+) + \left(\frac{\text{Glucose}}{18}\right) + \left(\frac{\text{BUN}}{2.8}\right)$$

   b. In methyl alcohol poisoning, the patient complains of blindness or decreased visual acuity
   c. In ethylene glycol poisoning, the urine contains Ca oxalate crystals
   d. Ketosis is absent
4. Salicylate poisoning: history of aspirin ingestion; combined respiratory alkalosis and metabolic acidosis are present

Therapy

1. Fluid replacement: the usual fluid deficit is 6-8 L
   a. Do not delay fluid replacement until lab results have been received
   b. Use 0.45% saline infusion in elderly patients or patients with a history of CHF; may use 0.9% saline in young or hypotensive patients
   c. The rate of fluid replacement varies with the age of the patient and the presence of severe heart or renal disease
      (1) The usual rate of infusion is 500 ml–1L over the first hour, 300-500 ml/hr for the next 12 hr
      (2) Continue the infusion at a rate of 200-300 ml/hr until the serum glucose level is below 250-300 ml/hr, and then change the hydrating solution to D_5W to prevent hypoglycemia, replenish free

water, and introduce additional glucose substrate (necessary to suppress lipolysis and ketogenesis)

2. Insulin administration
   a. The patient should be given an initial loading IV bolus of 0.15-0.2 U/kg of regular insulin followed by a constant infusion at a rate of 0.1 U/kg/hr (e.g., 25 U of regular insulin in 250 ml of 0.9% saline at 70 ml/hr = 7 U/hr for 70 kg patient)
   b. Monitor serum glucose hourly for the first 2 hours then q2-4h
   c. The goal is to decrease serum glucose level by 50 mg/dl/hr (following an initial drop because of rehydration); if the serum glucose level is not decreasing at the expected rate, increase the rate of insulin infusion
   d. When the serum glucose level approaches 250-300 mg/dl, decrease the rate of insulin infusion to 2-3 U/hr and continue this rate until the patient has received adequate fluid replacement
   e. Approximately 30 min before stopping the IV insulin infusion, administer an IM dose of regular insulin (dose varies with patient's demonstrated insulin sensitivity); this IM dose of regular insulin is necessary because of the extremely short life of the insulin in the IV infusion[73]

3. Potassium replacement:
   a. Total body potassium loss in DKA is approximately 300-500 mEq; the rate of replacement varies with the patient's serum potassium level, degree of acidosis ($\downarrow$ pH = $\uparrow$ K level), and renal function (potassium replacement should be used with caution in patients with renal failure)
   b. Table 22-5 lists some guidelines for potassium replacement therapy in patients with normal renal function (as a rule of thumb, potassium administration may be started when there is no ECG evidence of hyperkalemia)
   c. Monitor serum potassium level hourly for the initial 2 hr, then q2-4h
   d. Monitor urine output hourly

Table 22-5   Initial potassium replacement in patients with DKA and normal renal function

Initial Serum Potassium Level (mEq/L)	Suggested Potassium Replacement* (mEq KCl/L)
>5.3	No KCl added to first liter of IV hydrating solution
5.0-5.3	10
4.5-5.0	20
4.0-4.5	30
3.5-4.0	40
<3.5	>40

*Per liter of hydrating solution.

4. Correct metabolic acidosis
   a. Vigorous hydration and correction of hyperglycemia usually restores normal pH
   b. Use bicarbonate judiciously (bicarbonate therapy in patients with severe DKA [arterial blood pH 6.9 to 7.15] may not shorten clinical recovery time or significantly improve biochemical variables[46]); restrict bicarbonate use only to severe metabolic acidosis (e.g., arterial pH ≤7.1)
5. Obtain a serum phosphorus level on admission and after 24 hr of therapy; correct significant hypophosphatemia; Neutra-Phos capsules or powder contain 250 mg of phosphorus and 7.1 mEq of potassium; dosage is bid-qid
6. Use lab data flow sheet to closely monitor the patient (Table 22-6)

Complications

1. Cerebral edema should be suspected when the patient's sensorium remains impaired despite improvement of metabolic parameters
   a. Etiology is controversial; it may be secondary to an extremely rapid decrease in the serum glucose level and to osmotic disequilibrium caused by rapid and early use of hypotonic fluids
   b. Diagnosis: a CT scan of the brain will demonstrate narrowing of the ventricular system compatible with cerebral edema
   c. Therapy
      (1) Mannitol and low–molecular weight dextran
      (2) Large doses of corticosteroids (controversial)
2. Cardiac dysrhythmias
   a. Caused by electrolyte abnormalities and acidosis
   b. Closely monitor potassium, magnesium, and calcium levels and correct any abnormalities
3. Shock: caused by severe hypovolemia, infection, or cardiac dysfunction; monitor with a pulmonary artery catheter if not readily corrected with fluid replacement

Table 22-6 DKA flow sheet

Time (hr)	0	1	2	4	6	8	10	12	16	20	24
Serum glucose											
Serum potassium											
pH or HCO_3^-											
Insulin infusion (U/hr)											
IV fluids (ml/hr)											
Type of IV solution											
Urine output (ml/hr)											
Mental status											
Pulse											
Respiration											
Blood pressure											

4. Hypoglycemia
5. MI
6. Acute pancreatitis (caution must be used in interpreting serum amylase, as its elevation may be secondary to salivary amylase and not pancreatitis)

22.3   HYPEROSMOLAR COMA

Definition

Hyperosmolar coma is a state of extreme hyperglycemia, marked dehydration, serum hyperosmolarity, altered mental status, and absence of severe ketoacidosis. It occurs in non–insulin dependent diabetics.

Etiology

1. Infections (20-25%), e.g., pneumonia, urinary tract infection, sepsis
2. New or previously unrecognized diabetes (30-50%)
3. Reduction or omission of diabetic medication
4. Stress (MI, CVA)
5. Drugs
   a. Phenytoin, diazoxide may lead to impaired insulin secretion
   b. Diuretics may result in excessive dehydration
   c. Hypertonic alimentation may cause dehydration secondary to osmotic diuresis

• • •

The patient is usually an elderly or bed-confined diabetic with impaired or no ability to communicate thirst presenting after an interval of 1-2 wk of prolonged osmotic diuresis. Fig. 22-2 illustrates the pathophysiology of hyperosmolar coma.

Symptoms

1. Mental obtundation, seizures
2. Polyuria
3. Nausea and vomiting (not as severe as in patients with DKA)

Physical exam

1. Evidence of extreme dehydration (poor skin turgor, sunken eyeballs, dry mucous membranes)
2. Neurologic defects (reversible hemiplegia, focal seizures)
3. Orthostatic hypotension, tachycardia
4. Evidence of precipitating factors (pneumonia, infected skin ulcer)

Lab results[74]

1. Hyperglycemia: serum glucose usually >600 mg/dl
2. Hyperosmolarity: serum osmolarity usually >340 mOsm/L
3. Serum sodium: may be low, normal, or high; if normal or high the patient is severely dehydrated since normally an elevated blood sugar will draw fluid from intracellular space decreasing the serum sodium; the corrected serum sodium adjusts for the dilutional effect of hyperglycemia; it is obtained by increasing the serum sodium concentration

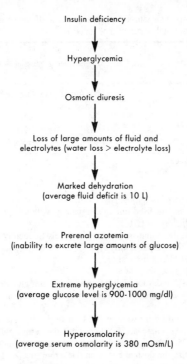

Figure 22-2
Pathophysiology of the hyperosmolar state.

by 1.6 mEq/dl for every 100 mg/dl increase in the serum glucose level
4. Serum potassium: may be low, normal, or high; regardless of the initial serum level, the total body loss is approximately 5-15 mEq/kg
5. Serum bicarbonate: usually >12 mEq/L (average is 17 mEq/L)
6. Arterial pH: usually >7.2 (average 7.26); both serum bicarbonate and arterial pH may be lower if lactic acidosis is present
7. BUN: azotemia (prerenal) is usually present (BUN = 60-90 mg/dl)
8. Phosphorus: hypophosphatemia (average loss is 70-140 mM)
9. Calcium: hypocalcemia (average loss is 50-100 mEq)
10. Magnesium: hypomagnesemia (average loss is 50-100 mEq)

Therapy

1. Vigorous fluid replacement: infuse 1000-1500 ml/hr for the initial 1-2 L, then decrease the rate of infusion to 500 ml/hr and monitor urine output, blood chemistries, and blood pressure; use normal saline (0.9% sa-

Table 22-7 Suggested potassium replacement in diabetics with hyperosmolar state and normal renal function

Initial Serum Potassium Level (mEq/L)	Suggested Initial Potassium Replacement (mEq KCl/hr)*
>5.2	No initial potassium replacement necessary
4-5.2	10
3.2-4.0	20
<3.2	≥30

*If urine output is adequate.

line) if the patient is hypotensive, otherwise use 0.45% saline (slower infusion rate may be used initially in patients with compromised cardiac status and a history of CHF)[72]

2. Replace electrolytes and monitor serum levels frequently (Table 22-7)
   a. Monitor urine output hourly
   b. Monitor ECG continuously
3. Correct hyperglycemia
   a. Vigorous IV hydration will decrease the serum glucose level in most patients by 20 mg/dl/hr; a regular insulin IV bolus is often not necessary
   b. Low dose insulin infusion at 1-2 U/hr (e.g., 25 U regular insulin in 250 ml 0.9% saline at 20 ml/hr) until the serum glucose level approaches 250-300 mg/dl, then the patient is started on regular insulin SQ q6h with the dosage based on the serum glucose level:
      <200 mg/dl: no insulin coverage
        201-250 mg/dl: 2 U
        251-300 mg/dl: 4 U
        301-350 mg/dl: 6 U
        351-400 mg/dl: 8 U
      >400 mg/dl: notify physician for insulin orders
   c. There is no need to give an IM dose of regular insulin when the infusion is stopped (unlike in DKA) since the majority of patients will not need any further insulin therapy for at least 6 hr
4. Rule out precipitating factors: obtain blood and urine cultures and chest x-ray
5. Monitor all critical parameters (see Table 22-6)

22.4 HYPOGLYCEMIA
Iradj Nejad

Definition

Hypoglycemia can be arbitrarily defined as a plasma glucose level <50 mg/dl. To establish the diagnosis, the following three criteria are necessary:
1. Presence of symptoms
   a. Adrenergic: sweating, anxiety, tremors, tachycardia, palpitations

b. Neuroglycopenic: seizures, fatigue, syncope, headache, behavior changes, visual disturbances
2. Low plasma glucose level in symptomatic patient
3. Relief of symptoms following ingestion of carbohydrates

Classification

1. Reactive hypoglycemia
   a. Hypoglycemia usually occurs 2-4 hr after a meal rich in carbohydrates
   b. These patients never have symptoms in the fasting state and rarely experience loss of consciousness secondary to their hypoglycemia
   c. Patients who have had subtotal gastrectomy will rapidly absorb carbohydrates causing an early and very high plasma glucose level followed by a late insulin surge that reaches its peak when most of the glucose has been absorbed and results in hypoglycemia
   d. Congenital deficiencies of enzymes necessary for carbohydrate metabolism and functional (idiopathic) hypoglycemia are additional causes of reactive hypoglycemia
2. Fasting hypoglycemia
   a. Symptoms usually appear in the absence of food intake (at night or during early morning)
   b. Etiology: factitious hypoglycemia, insulinoma, non–islet cell neoplasms, hormonal deficiency, liver disease, renal disease, and ethanol-induced hypoglycemia

Diagnosis

In a normal person, when the plasma glucose level is low (e.g., fasting state) the plasma insulin level is also low. Any patient presenting with fasting hypoglycemia of unexplained cause should have the following tests drawn during the hypoglycemic episode (see Table 22-8 for interpretation of results).

1. Plasma insulin level
2. Insulin antibodies
3. Plasma and urine sulfonylurea levels
4. C-peptide

Factitious hypoglycemia should be considered, especially if the patient has ready access to insulin or sulfonylureas (e.g., medical/paramedical per-

Table 22-8 Lab differentiation of factitious hypoglycemia and insulinoma

Lab Test	Insulinoma	Exogenous Insulin	Sulfonylurea
Plasma insulin level	↑	↑ ↑	↑
Insulin antibodies	None*	Present	None*
Plasma/urine sulfonylurea levels	Absent	Absent	Present
C-peptide	↑	N/↓	↑

*May be present if the patient has had prior insulin injections.
KEY: ↑, Increased; ↓, decreased; N, normal.

sonnel, family members who are diabetic or who are in the medical profession).

1. To diagnose factitious hypoglycemia secondary to sulfonylureas, screen serum and urine to determine the presence of sulfonylureas.
2. To diagnose factitious hypoglycemia secondary to insulin, measure:
   a. Plasma free insulin level, which is markedly increased following exogenous insulin injection.
   b. Insulin antibodies, which are usually present after an exogenous insulin injection, but may be absent if a more purified insulin preparation or if human insulin has been used (this test is not useful if the patient has a history of previous insulin use).
   c. C-peptide (connecting peptide): insulin is synthesized by the pancreas as a single chain polypeptide formed of A and B chains joined by the C-peptide. This single chain polypeptide (proinsulin) is broken down and secreted into the bloodstream as insulin and C-peptide in a 1:1 ratio. Exogenous insulin does not contain C-peptide, thus C-peptide levels are elevated in patients with insulinoma, but not following exogenous insulin injection.

Pancreatic islet cell neoplasms (insulinoma) are usually small (<3 cm in size), single, insulin-producing adenomas. Measurement of inappropriately elevated serum insulin levels despite an extremely low plasma glucose level after prolonged fasting (24-72 hr) is pathognomonic for these neoplasms.

The insulinoma can be located by CT scanning of pancreas and abdomen; if inconclusive, angiography or percutaneous transportal venous sampling (to measure a step up in insulin levels) can be attempted.

Other causes of hypoglycemia are as follows:

1. Non-islet cell neoplasms: tumors of mesodermal origin located in the peritoneal or retroperitoneal cavity. It is believed that they cause hypoglycemia or inhibit hepatic glucose production via a nonsuppressible insulin-like activity (NSILA).
2. Deficiency of counterregulatory hormones (e.g., glucagon, catecholamines, cortisol, growth hormone) can also cause hypoglycemia.
3. Liver disease can deplete hepatic glycogen storage.
4. Chronic renal disease can result in increased insulin level and poor nutritional status.

22.5 ANTERIOR PITUITARY DISORDERS

Hypopituitarism

Etiology and classification

1. Primary hypopituitarism
   a. Postpartum vascular insufficiency of anterior pituitary (Sheehan's syndrome)
      (1) Seen in postpartum patients with a history of hemorrhagic crisis at delivery or in the immediate postpartum period
      (2) Suspect in any postpartum patient who fails to resume menses or does not lactate

b. Ischemic necrosis of pituitary secondary to sickle cell anemia, vasculitis, diabetes mellitus

c. Neoplasms (primary or metastatic)

d. Granulomatous diseases (sarcoidosis, Wegener's granulomatosis)

e. Cavernous sinus thrombosis

f. Infections (TB, mycoses, syphilis, meningitis)

g. "Empty sella syndrome"

    (1) Primary "empty sella syndrome": protrusion of the third ventricle (subarachnoid cistern) in the sella turcica; it is difficult to diagnose by conventional CT scan because the CSF fluid in the empty sella has the same density as fluid from a cystic pituitary tumor, but it can be readily diagnosed by magnetic resonance imaging (MRI)[33] or by injecting metrizamide (a water-soluble, iodine contrast agent) into the subarachnoid space via LP and outlining the parasellar contents

    (2) Secondary "empty sella syndrome": decrease in size of the pituitary caused by various etiologies (irradiation, surgery)

h. Aneurysmal dilation of internal carotid artery

i. Radiation therapy for neck and head tumors

j. Other: surgical destruction, lymphocytic hypophysitis, hemochromatosis, chronic renal failure, familial

2. Secondary hypopituitarism

a. Hypothalamic abnormalities: tumors, inflammation (sarcoidosis, TB), trauma, radiation, subarachnoid hemorrhage, infections (encephalitis, meningitis), lipid storage diseases

b. Lesions of pituitary stalk: trauma, surgery, aneurysms, or tumor compression

Clinical presentation

1. Symptoms secondary to mass effect

a. Visual disturbances

    (1) Bitemporal hemianopsia: most common defect; it is caused by compression of the optic chiasm

    (2) Superior bitemporal defect: earliest defect

    (3) Loss of central vision: caused by pressure on the posterior part of the chiasm (location of the papulomacular bundle of fibers)

b. Headaches

c. Seizures (rare)

2. Hormonal effects

a. Growth hormone deficiency: initial hormonal deficiency; there are no clinical manifestations in adults

b. Gonadal dysfunction: amenorrhea in menstruating women, impotence in men; hypogonadotropic hypogonadism is the earliest and most frequent presentation

c. Hypothyroidism: often mistaken for depression

d. ACTH deficiency: develops in later stages of hypopituitarism; can manifest with an addisonian crisis during a period of stress, such as surgery or infection

Diagnosis

1. Endocrine tests

   a. Demonstration of target gland deficiency (e.g., measurement of testosterone levels in an impotent man)

   b. Measurement of pituitary hormones (e.g., decreased plasma FSH and LH levels in an impotent man with low testosterone levels indicate hypogonadism caused by central defect [secondary hypogonadism])

   c. Tests of pituitary reserve: cortisol and GH levels fluctuate widely in response to stress or diurnal variation, but their deficiency can be demonstrated by using the following provocative testing methods:

      (1) Metyrapone test (Fig. 22-3)

         (a) Metyrapone competitively inhibits the adrenal enzyme 11-β hydroxylase necessary for the conversion of 11-deoxycortisol to cortisol; the resulting low cortisol level stimulates the normal pituitary (via feedback mechanism) to release ACTH, and thereby increases adrenal production of 11-deoxycortisol until the 11-deoxycortisol levels are sufficiently elevated to compete with all the metyrapone available (thus eliminating the block to cortisol formation)

         (b) An elevated plasma 11-deoxycortisol level following 3 g PO dose of metyrapone overnight is proof of adequate ACTH reserve

         (c) Caution: the metyrapone test produces adrenal insufficiency and can result in an addisonian crisis in patients with known primary or secondary insufficiency

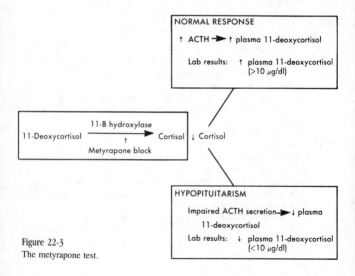

Figure 22-3
The metyrapone test.

    (2) Insulin tolerance test (ITT)
       (a) Obtain fasting plasma glucose, cortisol level, and GH level
       (b) Start the patient on an insulin infusion at 0.1 U/kg/hr
       (c) Measure plasma glucose, cortisol, and GH at 30, 45, 60, and 90 min
       (d) Stop the insulin infusion when the blood sugar falls to half the control value or if the patient becomes symptomatic
       (e) Interpretation: the induced hypoglycemia should result in a rise in cortisol (>7 μg/dl) and growth hormone (>9 ng/dl) in a patient with an intact hypothalamic-pituitary-adrenal axis
       (f) Caution: this test must be performed only under close medical supervision; it is contraindicated in patients suspected of having adrenal insufficiency, seizure disorders, or cardiovascular disease
    (3) The ACTH (cosyntropin) stimulation test is useful to distinguish pituitary from adrenal causes of adrenal insufficiency (see p. 270).

2. Additional tests
   a. A lateral skull x-ray may be useful in screening for large pituitary tumors; it can identify erosions or abnormalities in the shape of the sella and may also show lytic lesions in the skull, directing the diagnosis toward a primary breast or lung neoplasm, but its value is limited by many false-positive and false-negative results
   b. CT of head (with coronal views and contrast enhancement) or MRI; the latter has greater sensitivity for detecting pituitary adenomas

Therapy

Therapy is aimed at treating the cause of the pituitary failure and providing adequate hormone replacement.

Anterior pituitary hyperfunction secondary to pituitary neoplasms

The diagnosis and therapy of hormone-secreting pituitary adenomas varies with the type of hormone secreted. This section will discuss hypersecretion of growth hormone, ACTH, and prolactin.

Growth hormone

Excessive growth hormone (GH) secretion will result in *gigantism* (extreme height, wide hands and feet, prognathism) if it occurs before closure of the epiphyses or *acromegaly* if it occurs after epiphyseal closure.

1. History: obtain old photos for comparison and inquire about family history (acromegaly can present as a manifestation of multiple endocrine neoplasia [MEN]) (see Section 22.12)
2. Physical exam
   a. Excessive size of hands and feet with "spade-like" digits (because of increased width of distal bone tufts), sausage-shaped fingers
   b. Characteristic facies (broad jaw, protrusion of supraorbital ridges, gap teeth, prominent forehead)

   c. Oily skin, acanthosis nigricans, excessive sweating

   d. Enlargement of skeletal muscles, increase in size of visceral organs

   e. Deep voice, weakness

   f. Diastolic hypertension, decreased libido, galactorrhea

   g. Abnormalities secondary to pituitary enlargement (headaches, visual disturbances)

   h. Carpal tunnel syndrome secondary to increase in soft tissue

3. X-ray findings: degenerative arthritis

   a. Thickening of outer skull table, enlarged sella turcica

   b. Tufting of phalanges, narrowed carpal tunnels

4. Lab results

   a. Elevated fasting serum GH level (>10 ng/ml)

   b. Nonsuppression of GH secretion (failure to decrease GH concentration below 2 ng/ml) after an oral glucose tolerance test; if the glucose tolerance test is equivocal, thyrotropin-releasing hormone (TRH) injection will paradoxically stimulate GH secretion in acromegalic patients

   c. Glucose intolerance and hypercalciuria may also be present

   d. Increased plasma somatomedin C level can be used as a screening test for acromegaly in adult patients

5. Therapy

   a. Surgery

     (1) Transfrontal surgery if there is suprasellar extension of the tumor

     (2) Transsphenoidal surgery if the tumor is confined to the sella turcica[68]

   b. Pituitary irradiation results in a higher incidence of hypopituitarism than surgery, therefore in patients in whom fertility is an important consideration (e.g., young patients) it should be regarded as a second choice

   c. Bromocriptine (dopamine agonist) will paradoxically reduce GH levels in some patients with acromegaly; however, shrinkage of tumor size is uncommon in these patients

   d. Combination of above treatments

ACTH

Glucocorticoid excess secondary to an ACTH-secreting pituitary adenoma will result in Cushing's disease. This is one of the many causes of Cushing's syndrome described in Section 22.9. Therapy of ACTH-secreting pituitary adenomas:

1. Transsphenoidal microsurgery can result in selective removal of the adenoma, preservation of pituitary function, and minimal morbidity if performed by an experienced neurosurgeon[14]

2. Pituitary irradiation

   a. Heavy-particle irradiation produces high cure rates but also a greater incidence of hypopituitarism than conventional irradiation; its availability is also limited

   b. Conventional radiation therapy may be preferred to heavy-particle irradiation in children[30]

3. Neuropharmacotherapeutic drugs
    a. Cyproheptadine (serotonin antagonist) controls ACTH secretion in some patients with Cushing's disease
    b. Metyrapone inhibits adrenal cortisol biosynthesis and may be useful in debilitated patients who cannot tolerate surgery

Prolactin

Prolactin secretion, unlike other pituitary hormones, is regulated by tonic inhibition. Dopamine is the major prolactin inhibiting factor.

1. Etiology of hyperprolactinemia
    a. Pituitary tumors: microadenomas (<10 mm diameter) or macroadenomas (>10 mm diameter)
    b. Drugs: phenothiazines, methyldopa, reserpine, MAO inhibitors, androgens, progesterone, cimetidine, tricyclic antidepressants, haloperidol, meprobamate, chlordiazepoxide, estrogens, narcotics, metoclopramide, verapamil, amoxapine, cocaine
    c. Hepatic cirrhosis, renal failure, primary hypothyroidism
    d. Ectopic prolactin-secreting tumors (hypernephroma, bronchogenic carcinoma)
    e. Infiltrating diseases of the pituitary (sarcoidosis, histiocytosis)
    f. Head trauma, chest wall injury, spinal cord injury
    g. Pregnancy, nipple stimulation
    h. Idiopathic hyperprolactinemia, stress
2. Clinical manifestations
    a. Men: decreased libido, impotence, decreased facial and body hair, small testicles, delayed puberty (due to decreased testosterone secondary to inhibition of gonadotropin secretion)
    b. Women: amenorrhea and galactorrhea, oligomenorrhea, anovulation
    c. Both sexes: headache, visual field defects (caused by tumor expansion)
3. Diagnosis
    a. Lab results
        (1) Elevated serum prolactin level
            (a) Normal mean levels are 8 ng/ml (women) and 5 ng/ml (men)
            (b) Levels >300 ng/ml are virtually diagnostic of prolactinomas
        (2) TRH stimulation test: the normal response is an increase in serum prolactin levels by 100% within 1 hr of TRH infusion; failure to demonstrate an increase in prolactin level is suggestive of pituitary lesion
    b. Magnetic resonance imaging (MRI) is the procedure of choice in the radiographic evaluation of pituitary disease[33]; in absence of MRI, a radiographic diagnosis is best accomplished with a high-resolution CT scanner and special coronal cuts through the pituitary region; angiography should be considered to rule out aneurysm in patients with a large soft tissue mass in the sellar region and prolactin levels <100 ng/ml
4. Therapy
    a. Transsphenoidal resection: the success rate is dependent on the location of the tumor (entirely intrasellar), experience of the neurosur-

geon, and size of the tumor (<10 mm in diameter); the recurrence
rate may reach 80% within 5 yr
b. Medical therapy is preferred when fertility is an important consideration
(1) Bromocriptine (dopamine agonist): dosage is 2.5-10 mg/day; it
decreases the size of the tumor and lowers the prolactin level
into the normal range when the initial serum prolactin is <200
ng/ml, but initial values greater than 1000 ng/ml may be difficult
to reduce[51]
(2) Pergolide mesylate is also effective and may be better tolerated
than bromocriptine
c. Pituitary irradiation is useful as adjunctive therapy of macroade-
nomas (≥10 mm diameter)

22.6 | FLUID HEMOSTASIS DISORDERS

Diabetes insipidus

Definition

Diabetes insipidus (DI) is a polyuric disorder resulting from insufficient
production of antidiuretic hormone (ADH) (pituitary [neurogenic] diabetes
insipidus) or unresponsiveness of the renal tubules to ADH (nephrogenic
diabetes insipidus).

Etiology

1. Neurogenic diabetes insipidus
   a. Idiopathic
   b. Neoplasms of brain or pituitary fossa (craniopharyngiomas, meta-
      static neoplasms from breast or lung)
   c. Posttherapeutic neurosurgical procedures (e.g., hypophysectomy)
   d. Head trauma (e.g., basal skull fracture)
   e. Granulomatous disorders (sarcoidosis or tuberculosis)
   f. Histiocytosis (Hand-Schüller-Christian disease, eosinophilic granu-
      loma)
   g. Familial (autosomal dominant)
   h. Other: interventricular hemorrhage, aneurysms, meningitis, posten-
      cephalitis, multiple sclerosis
2. Nephrogenic diabetes insipidus
   a. Drugs: lithium, amphotericin B, demeclocycline, methoxyflurane an-
      esthesia
   b. Familial (X-linked recessive)
   c. Metabolic: hypercalcemia or hypokalemia
   d. Other: sarcoidosis, amyloidosis, pyelonephritis, polycystic disease,
      sickle cell disease, postobstructive

Clinical manifestations (usually seen when vasopressin secretory capacity is reduced <20% of normal)

1. Polyuria: urine volumes usually range 2.5-6 L/day
2. Polydipsia (predilection for cold or iced drinks)
3. Neurologic manifestations (seizures, headaches, visual field defects)
4. Evidence of volume contraction

Lab results

1. Decreased urine specific gravity (≤1.005)
2. Decreased urine osmolarity (usually <200 mOsm/kg)
3. Hypernatremia, increased plasma osmolarity, hypercalcemia, hypokalemia

Differential diagnosis

1. Diabetes insipidus
2. Primary polydipsia
3. Osmotic diuresis (glucose, mannitol, urea)

Diagnosis

Fig. 22-4 illustrates the diagnostic approach to a patient with suspected diabetes insipidus.

Therapy

1. Partial neurogenic diabetes insipidus
   a. Chlorpropamide (Diabinese) 250-375 mg PO qd; it potentiates the ADH effect on the kidney
   b. If chlorpropamide is inadequate to control the polyuria, the patient will require ADH replacement (see below)
2. Severe neurogenic diabetes insipidus: various ADH preparations are available
   a. Vasopressin tannate in oil: 2.5-5 U IM q24-72h; useful for long-term management because of its long life (the ampule must be shaken well before injection)
   b. DDAVP desmopressin: 2.5-20 μg administered intranasally q12-24h is useful for long-term treatment of ambulatory patients
   c. Aqueous vasopressin: 5-10 U SQ/IM q4-6h; short acting, useful only for short-term therapy
3. Nephrogenic diabetes insipidus
   a. Adequate hydration
   b. Low-sodium diet and chlorothiazide to induce mild sodium depletion
   c. Polyuria of DI secondary to lithium can be ameliorated by using amiloride (5 mg PO bid initially, increased to 10 mg PO bid after 2 wk)

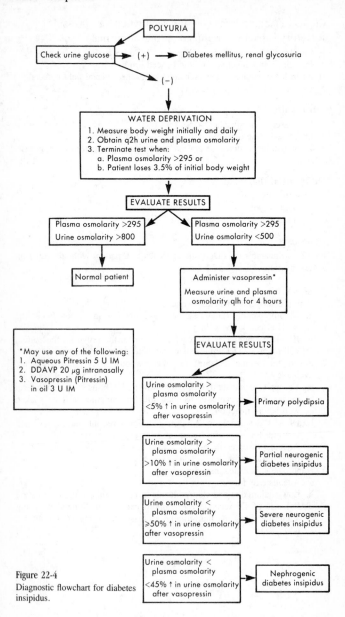

Figure 22-4
Diagnostic flowchart for diabetes insipidus.

Syndrome of inappropriate antidiuretic hormone secretion

Definition

The syndrome of inappropriate antidiuretic hormone secretion (SIADH) is characterized by excessive secretion of ADH in absence of normal osmotic or physiologic stimuli (increased serum osmolarity, decreased plasma volume, hypotension).

Etiology

1. Neoplasms: lung, duodenum, pancreas, brain, thymus, bladder, prostate mesothelioma, lymphoma, Ewing's sarcoma
2. Pulmonary disorders: pneumonia, TB, bronchiectasis, emphysema, status asthmaticus
3. Intracranial pathology: trauma, neoplasm, infections (meningitis, encephalitis, brain abscess), hemorrhage, hydrocephalus
4. Postoperative period: surgical stress, ventilators with positive pressure, anesthetic agents
5. Drugs: chlorpropamide, thiazide diuretics, vasopressin, oxytocin, chemotherapeutic agents (vincristine, vinblastine, cyclophosphamide), carbamazepine, phenothiazines, MAO inhibitors, tricyclic antidepressants, narcotics, nicotine, clofibrate, haloperidol
6. Other: acute intermittent porphyria, Guillain-Barré syndrome, myxedema, psychosis, delirium tremens, ACTH deficiency (hypopituitarism)

Clinical manifestations

1. The patient is generally normovolemic or slightly hypervolemic; edema is absent
2. Confusion, lethargy, and seizures may be present if the hyponatremia is severe or of rapid onset
3. Manifestations of the underlying disease may be evident (e.g., fever from an infectious process, or headaches and visual field defects from an intracranial mass)

Lab results

1. Hyponatremia
2. Urine osmolarity greater than serum osmolarity
3. Urinary sodium usually >30 mEq/L
4. Normal BUN, creatinine (indicate normal renal function and absence of dehydration), decreased uric acid
5. Other criteria: normal thyroid, adrenal, and cardiac function; no recent or concurrent use of diuretics

Therapy

1. Fluid restriction to 500-750 ml/day
2. Demeclocycline (Declomycin) 300-600 mg PO bid may be useful in patients with chronic SIADH (e.g., secondary to a neoplasm), but use with caution in patients with hepatic disease; its side effects include nephrogenic DI and photosensitivity

3. In emergency situations (seizures, coma), SIADH can be treated with a combination of hypertonic saline and furosemide; this increases the serum sodium by causing diuresis of urine that is more dilute than plasma[29]; the rapidity of correction varies depending on the degree of hyponatremia and if the hyponatremia is acute or chronic; generally the serum sodium should be corrected only halfway to normal in the initial 24 hr

22.7 | THYROID DISORDERS

Interpretation of thyroid function studies (Fig. 22-5)

1. Serum thyroxine (T_4)
   a. Thyroid function screening test; if results are within 75-80% of the lab reference value, any further testing of asymptomatic patients is not likely to be productive[52]
   b. Test measures both circulating thyroxine bound to protein (represents >99% of circulating T_4) and unbound (free) thyroxine
   c. Values vary with protein binding; changes in the concentration of T_4, secondary to changes in thyroxine binding globulin (TBG), can be caused by the following:

Increased TBG ($\uparrow T_4$)	Decreased TBG ($\downarrow T_4$)
Pregnancy	Androgens, glucocorticoids
Estrogens	Nephrotic syndrome, cirrhosis
Acute infectious hepatitis	Acromegaly
Oral contraceptives	Hypoproteinemia
Familial	Phenytoin, ASA, high-dose
Fluorouracil, clofibrate, heroin,	penicillin, asparaginase
methadone	Chronic debilitating illness
	Familial

   d. To eliminate the suspected influence of protein binding on thyroxine values, two additional tests are available: T_3 resin uptake, free thyroxine
2. T_3 resin uptake (T_3RU) measures the percentage of free T_4 (not bound to protein); it does not measure serum T_3 concentration; T_3RU and other tests reflecting thyroid hormone binding to plasma protein are also known as thyroid hormone–binding ratio (THBR)
3. Serum free T_4 directly measures unbound thyroxine; the free thyroxine index (FTI) can also be easily calculated by multiplying $T_4 \times T_3RU$ and dividing the result by 100; the FTI corrects for any abnormal T_4 values secondary to protein binding:

$$FTI = \frac{T_4 \times T_3RU}{100}$$

Normal values = 2-5

4. Thyroid stimulating hormone (TSH) is used primarily to diagnose primary hypothyroidism (the increased TSH level is the earliest thyroid ab-

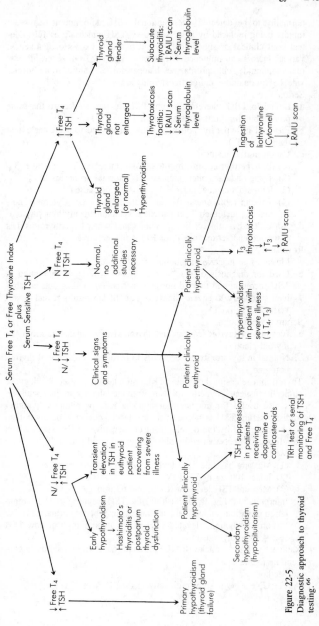

Figure 22-5
Diagnostic approach to thyroid testing. [66]

normality to be detected); conventional TSH radioimmunoassays are rapidly being replaced by new "sensitive" TSH which are useful to detect both clinical or subclinical thyroid hormone excess or deficiency; various factors can influence TSH levels: recovery from severe illness, metoclopramide, chlorpromazine, haloperidol, and amiodarone all elevate TSH; dopamine and corticosteroids lower it[66]

5. Serum T_3
   a. Bound to TBG, therefore serum T_3 levels are subject to the same protein binding limitations as serum T_4
   b. Elevated in hyperthyroidism (usually earlier and to a greater extent than serum T_4)
   c. Useful in diagnosing:
      (1) T_3 hyperthyroidism (thyrotoxicosis): increased T_3, normal FTI
      (2) Toxic nodular goiter: increased T_3, normal or increased T_4
      (3) Iodine deficiency: normal T_3, possibly decreased T_4
      (4) Thyroid replacement therapy with liothyronine (Cytomel): normal T_4, increased T_3 if patient is symptomatically hyperthyroid
   d. Not ordered routinely, but it is indicated when hyperthyroidism is suspected and serum free T_4 or FTI is inconclusive

6. Reverse T_3
   a. Measures an inactive metabolite of T_4
   b. Used for diagnosis of the "sick euthyroid syndrome" (alteration in TSH secretion and thyroid hormone peripheral binding and metabolism secondary to severe illness or stress); lab results reveal ↑ reverse T_3, ↓ T_3RIA

7. Serum thyroglobulin
   a. Elevated in thyroid cancer and thyrotoxicosis emanating from the thyroid gland
   b. Normal in thyrotoxicosis secondary to iatrogenic ingestion of thyroid hormone

8. Thyrotropin releasing hormone (TRH) stimulation is used to diagnose clinically suspected hyperthyroidism when the lab tests are inconclusive; it is also useful for diagnosis of hypothalamic or pituitary hypothyroidism (serum TSH is normal); its use in diagnosing hyperthyroidism has been limited by the development of "sensitive" TSH assays which can distinguish between euthyroid and hyperthyroid patients[66]
   a. Method
      (1) Measure baseline TSH level
      (2) Inject 400 μg of TRH IV
      (3) Measure TSH levels at 0, 30, and 60 min
   b. Interpretation: Fig. 22-6 illustrates the TSH response to TRH stimulation in various endocrine disturbances; in general: normal TSH rise = normal function; elevated TSH rise = hypothyroidism; low TSH rise = hyperthyroidism

9. Radioactive iodine uptake (RAIU) measures the thyroid's ability to concentrate iodine
   a. Method
      (1) Give a PO dose of radioactive iodine (^{123}I or ^{131}I)

(2) Measure the amount of iodine taken up by the thyroid 24 hr later
b. Interpretation
  (1) Normal 24 hr RAI uptake is 10-30%
  (2) An overactive thyroid shows an increased uptake whereas an underactive thyroid (hypothyroidism, subacute thyroiditis) shows a decreased uptake
    (a) Increased homogeneous uptake: Graves' disease, iodine deficiency
    (b) Increased heterogeneous uptake: multinodular goiter
    (c) Single focus of increased uptake: hot nodule (p. 255)
c. Indications
  (1) Iatrogenic ingestion of thyroid hormone by a clinically hyperthyroid patient ("thyrotoxicosis factitia") will result in increased serum T_4 and serum T_3RU, but the RAIU is decreased instead of increased, as it would be in other causes of hyperthyroidism; serum thyroglobulin levels will also be decreased in thyrotoxicosis factitia and elevated in thyrotoxicosis emanating from the thyroid gland
  (2) Subacute thyroiditis: the patient will have increased serum free T_4 or FTI, but decreased RAIU because of the follicular cells' inability to concentrate iodine
  (3) Pre-^{131}I-therapy for hyperthyroidism to calculate the ^{131}I dose to be administered

Hyperthyroidism

Etiology

1. Graves' disease
2. Toxic multinodular goiter
3. Toxic adenoma
4. Iatrogenic and factitious
5. Transient hyperthyroidism
  a. Subacute thyroiditis
  b. Hashimoto's thyroiditis
6. Rare causes: hypersecretion of TSH (e.g., pituitary neoplasms), struma ovarii, ingestion of large amounts of iodine in a patient with preexisting thyroid hyperplasia or adenoma (Jod-Basedow phenomenon), hydatidiform mole, carcinoma of thyroid, amiodarone

Graves' disease

1. Definition: hypermetabolic state characterized by thyrotoxicosis, diffuse goiter, and infiltrative ophthalmopathy; infiltrative dermopathy is occasionally present
2. Pathogenesis: abnormalities are caused by thyroid-stimulating antibodies (TS Ab), which activate thyroid adenylate cyclase and compete with TSH for receptors on thyroid cell membranes; there is an increased prevalence of HLA-B8 and HLA-DR3 in caucasians with Graves' disease

3. Symptoms
   a. Tachycardia (resting rate >90 beats/minute), palpitations, atrial fibrillation
   b. Tremor, anxiety, irritability, emotional lability, panic attacks
   c. Proximal muscle weakness
   d. Heat intolerance, sweating
   e. Increased appetite, diarrhea
   f. Weight loss, weight gain from increased appetite (rare)
   g. Insomnia
   h. Menstrual dysfunction (oligomenorrhea, amenorrhea)
4. Physical exam
   a. General features
      (1) Tachycardia, tremor, hyperreflexia
      (2) Fine, smooth, or velvety skin, warm and moist hands
      (3) Onycholysis (brittle nails)
      (4) Diffuse goiter, bruit over thyroid
   b. Features unique to Graves' disease
      (1) Infiltrative ophthalmopathy: exophthalmos, lid retraction, lid lag
      (2) Infiltrative dermopathy: pretibal myxedema (raised, hyperpigmented areas involving the pretibial region and the feet)
      (3) Thyroid acropathy: clubbing of fingers associated with periosteal new bone formation in other skeletal areas
   NOTE: Elderly hyperthyroid patients may have only subtle signs (weight loss, tachycardia, fine skin, brittle nails) this form is known as *apathetic hyperthyroidism.* An enlarged thyroid gland may be absent. Coexisting medical disorders (most commonly cardiac disease), may also mask the symptoms. These patients often have unexplained CHF, worsening of angina or new onset atrial fibrillation that is resistant to treatment.
5. Lab results
   a. Increased Free T_4 (or FTI), decreased "sensitive" TSH
   b. Increased T_3
   c. TRH stimulation test diagnostic of hyperthyroidism: use this test only when the serum Free T_4 (or FTI) and "sensitive" TSH are inconclusive
6. Medical therapy
   a. Antithyroid drugs (thionamides): propylthiouracil (PTU) and methimazole (Tapazole) inhibit thyroid hormone synthesis by blocking production of thyroid peroxidase (PTU and methimazole) or inhibit peripheral conversion of T_4 to T_3 (PTU)
      (1) Dosage
         (a) PTU: 100-200 mg PO q8h
         (b) Methimazole: 10-20 mg PO q8h or 30-60 mg/day given as a single dose
      (2) Side effects
         (a) Granulocytopenia occurs in 0.5% of patients (obtain baseline WBC before starting therapy); monitoring of WBC is generally not helpful because granulocytopenia is an idiosyncratic reaction of sudden onset
         (b) Aplastic anemia

       (c) Skin rash (3-5% of patients), arthralgias, myalgias

       (d) Patients should be instructed to stop the medication immediately and notify the physician if they develop mouth ulcers or symptoms of infections (pharyngitis, fever)

    (3) Comments

       (a) Both drugs cross the placenta and inhibit the fetal thyroid gland, therefore patient should be advised against pregnancy while taking thionamides; if patient is pregnant, use the smallest effective dose

       (b) PTU is preferred over methimazole during pregnancy because it crosses the placenta to a lesser degree[45]

       (c) Clinical response may be delayed up to 2 wk after onset of therapy because of the stored supply of thyroid hormone

       (d) Euthyroid state is usually achieved in 2-4 mo; prolonged therapy may cause hypothyroidism

    (4) Duration of therapy

       (a) Continue treatment for 6 mo to 1 yr after the patient becomes clinically euthyroid and the T_4 level returns to normal

       (b) After discontinuation, measure the T_4 level periodically to confirm the euthyroid state

       (c) If the T_4 level begins to rise (indicating early hyperthyroidism), restart the patient on antithyroid therapy or give radioactive iodine

       (d) If the patient becomes hypothyroid, start L-thyroxine (see therapy for hypothyroidism)

  b. Propranolol: alleviates the β-adrenergic symptoms of hyperthyroidism (tachycardia, tremor)

    (1) Initial dosage: 20-40 mg PO q6h; dosage is gradually increased until symptoms are controlled

    (2) Contraindications: bronchospasm, CHF

  c. Radioactive iodine (^{131}I)

    (1) Treatment of choice for men and for women over the age of 30 and in younger patients who have not achieved remission after 1 yr of thionamide therapy

    (2) High incidence of postradiotherapy hypothyroidism[64]; therefore these patients should be frequently evaluated for the onset of hypothyroidism

    (3) Radioactive iodine therapy is contraindicated during pregnancy (can cause fetal hypothyroidism)

7. Surgical therapy: subtotal thyroidectomy

  a. Indications

    (1) Pregnant patient who cannot be adequately managed with low doses of PTU, or who develops side effects with antithyroid medication

    (2) Any patient who refuses radioactive iodine and cannot be adequately managed with thionamides

    (3) Obstructing goiters

  b. Complications: hypothyroidism (28-43% after 10 yr), hypoparathyroidism, and damage to recurrent laryngeal nerve

8. Graves' ophthalmopathy
   a. High-dose corticosteroids, external radiation, or orbital decompression are used for severe exophthalmos
   b. Methylcellulose eye drops (e.g., Tears Naturale) are useful to protect against excessive eye dryness

Toxic multinodular goiter

1. Incidence: usually seen in women over the age of 55 with a history of multinodular goiter for many years, whereas Graves' disease is typically seen in young women
2. Clinical presentation: onset is usually insidious and clinical phenomena (tachycardia, tremor, heat intolerance) may be masked by manifestations of coexisting diseases (e.g., a patient with ASHD may have CHF secondary to atrial fibrillation with a fast ventricular response)
3. Therapy: Radioactive iodine (^{131}I) after the initiation of beta blockers

Toxic adenoma

1. Diagnosis: thyroid scan demonstrates increased uptake (hot nodule)
2. Therapy
   a. Surgical removal of the adenoma is preferred in young hyperthyroid patients and patients with very large adenoma
   b. Medical: radioactive iodine (^{131}I) therapy is used in all other patients

Thyroid storm

Definition

Thyroid storm is characterized by an abrupt, severe exacerbation of thyrotoxicosis.

Etiology

1. Major stress (e.g., infection, MI, surgery, DKA) in an undiagnosed hyperthyroid patient
2. Inadequate therapy in a hyperthyroid patient

Symptoms

1. Fever (>100° F)
2. Marked anxiety and agitation, psychosis
3. Hyperhidrosis, heat intolerance
4. Marked weakness and muscle wasting
5. Tachydysrhythmias, palpitations
6. Diarrhea, nausea, vomiting
7. Elderly patients may have a combination of tachycardia, CHF, and mental status changes

Physical exam

1. Goiter
2. Tremor, tachycardia, fever

3. Warm moist skin
4. Lid lag, lid retraction, proptosis
5. Altered mental status (psychosis, coma, seizures)
6. Other: evidence of precipitating factors (infection or trauma)

Lab results

1. Increased serum free T_4 or FTI, decreased "sensitive" TSH
2. Blood and urine cultures should be obtained to rule out sepsis

Therapy[38]

If the diagnosis is strongly suspected, start immediate therapy without waiting for lab confirmation.
1. Specific therapy
   a. To inhibit hormonal synthesis
      (1) Propylthiouracil (PTU) 400 mg initially (PO or via NG tube) then 400 mg PO q6h
      (2) If the patient has gastric or intestinal obstruction or vomiting, methimazole (Tapazole) 80-100 mg can be administered PR followed by 30 mg PR q8h
   b. To inhibit release of stored thyroid hormone
      (1) Iodide (sodium iodide) 250 mg IV q6h, potassium iodide (SSKI) 5 gtt PO q8h, or Lugol's solution 10 gtt q8h; administer a thionamide (PTU or methimazole) 1 hr *before* the iodide to prevent the oxidation of iodide to iodine and its incorporation in the synthesis of additional thyroid hormone
      (2) Corticosteroids: dexamethasone 2 mg IV q6h or hydrocortisone 100 mg IV q6h for approximately 48 hr
         (a) Inhibit thyroid hormone release
         (b) Impair peripheral generation of T_3 from T_4
         (c) Provide additional adrenal cortical hormone to correct deficiency (if present)
   c. To suppress peripheral effects of thyroid hormone
      (1) Beta adrenergic blockers: propranolol 10-40 mg PO q4-6h; in acute situations propranolol may also be given IV 1 mg/min for 2-10 min under continuous ECG and blood pressure monitoring
      (2) Beta adrenergic blockers must be used with caution in patients with CHF or bronchospasm
      (3) Cardioselective beta blockers (e.g., atenolol 100 mg PO qd) may be more appropriate for patients with bronchospasm, but these patients must be closely monitored for exacerbation of bronchospasm since these agents lose their cardioselectivity at high doses
2. Supportive therapy
   a. Control fever: use acetaminophen 300-600 mg q4h or cooling blanket if necessary, but do not use aspirin because it displaces thyroid hormone from its binding protein
   b. Digitalize patients with CHF: these patients may require higher than usual digitalis dosages, particularly to control atrial fibrillation

    c. Nutritional care: replace fluid deficit aggressively; use solutions containing glucose and add multivitamins to the hydrating solution

    d. Rule out and treat any precipitating factors: obtain blood and urine cultures; use IV antibiotics if infection is strongly suspected

Hypothyroidism

Etiology

1. Primary hypothyroidism (thyroid gland dysfunction) is the cause of >90% of the cases of hypothyroidism
   a. Hashimoto thyroiditis (chronic lymphocytic thyroiditis); this is the commonest cause of hypothyroidism after 8 yr of age
   b. Idiopathic myxedema (possibly a nongoitrous form of Hashimoto's thyroiditis)
   c. Previous treatment of hyperthyroidism (^{131}I therapy, subtotal thyroidectomy)
   d. Subacute thyroiditis
   e. Radiation therapy of the neck (usually for malignant disease)
   f. Iodine deficiency or excess
   g. Drugs (lithium, PAS, sulfonamides, phenylbutazone, amiodarone, thiourea)
   h. Congenital (approximately 1:4000 live births)
   i. Prolonged treatment with iodides
2. Secondary hypothyroidism: pituitary dysfunction, postpartum necrosis, neoplasm, infiltrative disease causing deficiency of TSH
3. Tertiary hypothyroidism: hypothalamic disease (granuloma, neoplasm, or irradiation causing deficiency of TRH)
4. Tissue resistance to thyroid hormone (rare)

Symptoms

1. Fatigue, lethargy, weakness
2. Constipation, weight gain (usually <15 lb)
3. Muscle weakness, muscle cramps, arthralgias
4. Cold intolerance
5. Slow speech with hoarse voice (caused by myxedematous changes in the vocal cords)
6. Slow cerebration with poor memory

Physical exam

1. Skin is dry, coarse, thick, cool, sallow (yellow color caused by carotenemia); nonpitting edema in the skin of the eyelids and hands (myxedema) secondary to infiltration of the subcutaneous tissues by a hydrophilic mucopolysaccharide substance
2. Hair is brittle and coarse; loss of outer one third of eyebrows
3. Facies: dulled expression, thickened tongue, and thick slow-moving lips
4. Thyroid gland may or may not be palpable (depending on the cause of the hypothyroidism)
5. Heart sounds are distant; pericardial effusion may be present

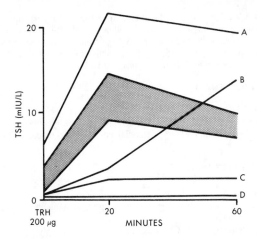

Figure 22-6
TSH response to TRH. The shaded area indicates normal response; the letter A, primary hypothyroidism; B, hypothalamic (tertiary) hypothyroidism; C, pituitary (secondary) hypothyroidism; D, hyperthyroidism with suppressed TSH. (From Rock RC: Geriatrics 40:61, 1985.)

6. Pulse: bradycardia
7. Neurologic
   a. Delayed relaxation phase (return phase) of deep tendon reflexes
   b. Cerebellar ataxia
   c. Hearing impairment, poor memory
   d. Peripheral neuropathies with paresthesias, carpal tunnel syndrome

Lab results

1. Decreased free T_4 or FTI
2. Increased TSH (TSH level may be normal if patient has secondary or tertiary hypothyroidism or is receiving dopamine or corticosteroids, or following severe illness)
3. Increased serum cholesterol, triglycerides, LDH, ALT, AST, and MM band of CPK
4. Decreased Hb/Hct, hyponatremia
5. Elevated antimicrosomal and antithyroglobulin antibody titers are characteristic of hypothyroidism associated with Hashimoto's thyroiditis
6. TRH stimulation test is useful to distinguish secondary from tertiary hypothyroidism (see Fig. 22-6)

Therapy

Start replacement therapy with L-thyroxine (Synthroid) 25-100 μg/day depending on the patient's age and the severity of the disease. May increase dose q4-6 wk depending on the clinical response. Elderly patients and patients with coronary artery disease should be started with 25 µg/day (higher doses may precipitate angina). The average maintenance dose of L-thyroxine is 1.6 µg/kg/day (100-150 µg/day in adults, 50-75 µg/day in the elderly). Monitor sensitive TSH for adequacy of replacement.

Myxedema coma

Definition
Myxedema coma is a life-threatening complication of hypothyroidism characterized by profound lethargy or coma and usually accompanied by hypothermia.

Contributing factors
1. Sepsis
2. Exposure to cold weather
3. CNS depressants (sedatives, narcotics, antidepressants)
4. Trauma, surgery
5. CVA, hypoglycemia, CO_2 narcosis

Symptoms
1. Elderly patients, profoundly lethargic or comatose
2. Hypothermia (rectal temperature <35° C [95° F]); hypothermia is often missed by using ordinary thermometers graduated only to 34.5° C or if the mercury is not shaken below 36° C
3. Bradycardia, hypotension (secondary to circulatory collapse)
4. Delayed relaxation phase of DTR, areflexia

Lab results
1. Markedly increased TSH (if primary hypothyroidism)
2. Decreased serum free T_4
3. Other: CO_2 retention, hypoxia, acidosis, hyponatremia, macrocytic anemia, hypoglycemia
4. Draw cortisol level and blood cultures on admission to rule out adrenal insufficiency and sepsis

Therapy
If diagnosis is strongly suspected, initiate immediate treatment without waiting for confirmatory lab results (mortality in myxedema coma is 20-50%).
1. L-Thyroxine: 2 µg/kg IV infused over 5-15 min, then 100 µg IV q24h
2. Hydrocortisone hemisuccinate: 100 mg IV bolus, then 50 mg IV q12h or 25 mg q6h IV until plasma cortisol level is normal; glucocorticoids are given to treat possible associated adrenocortical insufficiency, but avoid large doses because they may impair conversion of T_4 to T_3
3. IV hydration: usually with D_5NS to correct hypotension and hypoglycemia (if present); avoid overhydration and possible water intoxication because clearance of free water is impaired in these patients
4. Prevent further heat loss, cover the patient but avoid external rewarming because it may produce vascular collapse

5. Support respiratory function: intubation and mechanical ventilation may be required
6. Rule out and treat precipitating factors, such as sepsis
7. Monitor patient in an intensive care unit

Thyroiditis[27]

Thyroiditis is an inflammatory disease of the thyroid. It is clinically categorized as acute, subacute, and chronic thyroiditis.

Acute suppurative thyroiditis

1. Etiology: bacterial thyroid infection (usually seen in immunocompromised host) or following a penetrating injury to neck
2. Symptoms: fever, malaise, tenderness over thyroid
3. Lab results: increased WBC with "shift to left," normal thyroid function studies, normal 24 hr RAI uptake
4. Therapy: IV antibiotics, drainage of abscess (if present)

Subacute thyroiditis

Subacute granulomatous thyroiditis
1. Etiology: possibly postviral; usually follows a respiratory illness
2. Symptoms: exquisitely tender, enlarged thyroid, fever, and generalized malaise
3. Lab results: markedly increased sedimentation rate, increased WBC with "shift to left," low RAI uptake, increased serum thyroglobulin levels, and increased or normal T_4 level
4. Treatment
   a. The disease is self-limited, hyperthyroidism is transient and resolves spontaneously over a few weeks in >90% of patients; relapses may occur
   b. Serial measurements of serum thyroglobulin (Tg) levels are useful in monitoring the course of subacute thyroiditis[42]
   c. Pain can be treated with aspirin 650 mg qid; prednisone 20-40 mg qd may be used if aspirin is insufficient, but it should be gradually tapered off over several weeks
   d. Symptoms of hyperthyroidism can be controlled with beta adrenergic blockers
   e. Thionamides are not indicated in subacute thyroiditis
   f. Some patients will develop transient hypothyroidism requiring thyroxine therapy for 3-6 mo

Subacute lymphocytic thyroiditis (painless thyroiditis)
1. Etiology unknown, but probably autoimmune; usually seen postpartum
2. Symptoms
   a. Normal or slightly enlarged nontender thyroid gland
   b. Tachycardia, tremor, heat intolerance, insomnia, anxiety, and other signs of hyperthyroidism
3. Lab results
   a. Increased free T_4 or FTI
   b. Decreased 24 hr RAI uptake

   c. Increased serum thyroglobulin (acute phase)

   d. Low or absent antimicrosomal antibody

4. Therapy: self-limited disease; symptoms of initial hyperthyroid phase can be controlled with beta adrenergic blockers; hypothyroid phase should be treated with thyroid hormone replacement therapy; recovery is generally seen in about 75% of patients

Chronic thyroiditis

Hashimoto's thyroiditis

1. Pathophysiology
   a. Autoimmune disease involving a defect in suppressor T lymphocytes (patient may also have pernicious anemia or other autoimmune disorders)
   b. There is progressive destruction of thyroid gland by an inflammatory process
   c. Histologically there is marked lymphocytic infiltration of thyroid
   d. Antimicrosomal antibodies are detected in over 90% of patients
   e. Goitrous Hashimoto's thyroiditis is associated with increase in HLA-DR5 whereas atrophic Hashimoto's thyroiditis has increased prevalence of HLA-B8 and HLA-DR3

2. Symptoms
   a. Diffuse, firm enlargement of the thyroid gland; thyroid gland may also be of normal size (atrophic form with clinically manifested hypothyroidism)
   b. Patient may have signs of hyper- or hypothyroidism, depending on the stage of the disease

3. Therapy: if patient is hypothyroid, L-thyroxine therapy will correct hypothyroidism and suppress goiter

Riedel's thyroiditis

1. A rare condition characterized by fibrous infiltration of the thyroid, with subsequent hypothroidism

2. May be mistaken for carcinoma of the thyroid

Evaluation of patient with thyroid nodule

History and physical exam

1. History of prior head and neck irradiation (increased risk of thyroid cancer)
2. Family history of pheochromocytoma, carcinoma of the thyroid, and hyperparathyroidism (medullary carcinoma of the thyroid is a component of multiple endocrine neoplasia II)
3. Dysphagia/hoarseness (may indicate infiltrative malignant neoplasm)
4. Increased likelihood that nodule is malignant
   a. Nodule increasing in size or larger than 2 cm
   b. Regional lymphadenopathy
   c. Fixation to adjacent tissues
   d. Age less than 40, male sex

Diagnostic tests

1. Fine-needle aspiration (FNA) biopsy is the best initial diagnostic study; the accuracy can be as high as 97%,[53,71] but it is directly related to the level of experience of the physician and the cytopathologist interpreting the aspirate

   Evaluation of results

   a. Normal cells: may repeat biopsy during present evaluation or reevaluate patient after 3-6 mo of suppressive therapy (L-thyroxine, 100-200 μg PO qd)
      (1) Failure to regress indicates increased likelihood of malignancy
      (2) Reliance on repeat needle biopsy is preferable to routine surgery for nodules not responding to thyroxine[28]
   b. Malignant cells: surgery
   c. Hypercellularity: thyroid scan
      (1) Hot nodule: [131]I therapy if the patient is hyperthyroid
      (2) Warm or cold nodule: surgery (follicular adenoma vs carcinoma)
   d. FNA biopsy is less reliable with thyroid cystic lesions; surgical excision should be considered for most thyroid cysts not abolished by aspiration
2. Thyroid ultrasound to evaluate the size of the thyroid, and the number, composition (solid vs cystic), and dimensions of the thyroid nodule(s); solid thyroid nodules have a higher incidence of malignancy, but cystic nodules can also be malignant
3. Thyroid scan with ([99mTc]) pertechnetate
   a. Classifies nodules as hyperfunctioning (hot), normally functioning (warm), or nonfunctioning (cold); cold nodules have a higher incidence of malignancy
   b. Scan has difficulty evaluating nodules near the thyroid isthmus or at the periphery of the gland
   c. Normal tissue over a nonfunctioning nodule may mask the nodule as "warm" or normally functioning
4. Serum thyroglobulin level should be obtained prior to thyroidectomy
   a. A return to normal following thyroidectomy suggests absence of functional metastatic thyroid tissue
   b. Persistent or new elevation following thyroidectomy indicates functional metastases
5. Serum calcitonin at random or after pentagastrin stimulation is useful when suspecting medullary carcinoma of the thyroid
6. Total body scan using sodium iodide 131 is useful for the evaluation of residual or recurrent disease following initial therapy of well-differentiated thyroid cancer[44]

Both thyroid scan and ultrasound provide information regarding the risk of malignant neoplasia based on the characteristics of the thyroid nodule, but their value in the initial evaluation of a thyroid nodule is limited because neither one provides a definite tissue diagnosis.

Thyroid carcinoma

There are four major types of thyroid carcinomas: papillary, follicular, anaplastic, and medullary.

Papillary carcinoma

1. Characteristics
   a. Most common type (50-60%)
   b. Most frequent in women during second or third decade
   c. Histologically "psammoma bodies" (calcific bodies present in the papillary projections) are pathognomonic; they are found in 35-45% of papillary thyroid carcinomas
   d. Majority are not pure papillary lesions, but are mixed papillary follicular carcinomas
   e. Spread is via lymphatics and by local invasion
2. Therapy
   a. Total thyroidectomy is indicated if the patient has:
      (1) Extrapyramidal extension of carcinoma
      (2) Papillary carcinoma limited to thyroid, but a positive history of irradiation to the head and neck
      (3) Lesion larger than 2 cm
   b. Lobectomy with isthmectomy (associated with careful exploration of the other lobe) may be considered in patients with intrathyroidal papillary carcinoma smaller than 2 cm and no history of neck and head irradiation; must follow surgery with suppressive therapy of thyroid hormone because these tumors are TSH responsive
   c. Radiotherapy with ^{131}I (after total thyroidectomy), followed by thyroid suppression therapy with triiodothyronine can be used in metastatic papillary carcinoma

Follicular carcinoma

1. Characteristics
   a. More aggressive than papillary carcinoma
   b. Incidence increases with age
   c. Tends to metastasize hematogenously to bone, producing pathologic fractures
   d. Tends to concentrate iodine (useful for radiation therapy)
2. Therapy
   a. Total thyroidectomy
   b. Radiotherapy with ^{131}I followed by thyroid suppression therapy with triiodothyronine is useful in patients with metastases

Anaplastic carcinoma

1. Characteristics
   a. Very aggressive neoplasm
   b. Two major histologic types
      (1) Small cell: less aggressive (5 yr survival approximately 20%)
      (2) Giant cell: death usually within 6 mo of diagnosis
2. Therapy
   a. At diagnosis, this neoplasm is rarely operable; palliative surgery is indicated for extremely large tumor compressing the trachea
   b. Management is usually restricted to radiation therapy or chemother-

apy with combination of doxorubicin, cisplatin, and other antineoplastic agents; these measures rarely provide significant palliation

Medullary carcinoma

1. Characteristics
   a. Unifocal lesion: found sporadically in elderly patients
   b. Bilateral lesions: associated with pheochromocytoma and hyperpara-
      thyroidism; this combination is known as multiple endocrine neopla-
      sia II (MEN II) and is inherited as an autosomal dominant disorder
      (see Section 22.12)
2. Diagnosis
   a. Increased plasma calcitonin assay (these tumors produce thyrocalci-
      tonin)
   b. Screen family members; normal family members who are at risk can
      be identified by using provocative testing with IV pentagastrin or
      calcium infusion to stimulate thyrocalcitonin release from neoplastic
      cells; a genetic marker on chromosome 10 has also been identified
3. Treatment
   a. Thyroidectomy
   b. Patients and their families should be screened for pheochromocy-
      toma and hyperparathyroidism

| 22.8 | CALCIUM HOMEOSTASIS DISORDERS |

Physiology

1. Serum calcium levels are controlled mainly by parathyroid hormone
   (PTH) and vitamin D (1,25 dihydroxy vitamin D), and to a lesser extent
   by calcitonin
   a. The three organs involved in calcium metabolism are bone, kidneys,
      and intestine
   b. The effects of calcium-regulating hormones on each are summarized
      in Table 22-9
2. Calcium is found in plasma in three major forms:
   a. Bound to plasma proteins, particularly albumin (35-40%)
   b. Free (ionized) calcium (45-50%)
   c. Bound to complexing ions: phosphate, citrate, carbonate (10-15%)
3. The standard serum calcium level measures the total serum calcium
   level, but the only physiologically active form is the free (ionized) calcium; any factor that decreases the free (ionized) calcium (e.g., alkalosis) can produce hypocalcemic crises, whereas factors that affect only
   the protein-bound calcium will not provoke symptoms of hypocalcemia
   (Table 22-10)

Hypercalcemia

Etiology

1. Malignancy: increased bone resorption via osteoclast-activating factors,
   secretion of PTH-like substances, prostaglandin E_2, direct erosion by tumor cells, transforming growth factors, colony-stimulating activity[47];
   hypercalcemia is common in the following neoplasms:

Table 22-9 Hormonal action in calcium homeostasis

Hormone	Action			Result	
	Bone	Kidneys	Intestine	Serum Ca	Serum PO₄
PTH	↑ Ca²⁺ resorption ↑ PO₄⁻³ resorption	↑ Ca²⁺ resorption ↑ Phosphate excretion ↑ Conversion of vitamin D to active form	↑ Ca²⁺ absorption (via vitamin D)	↑	↓
1,25 dihydroxyvitamin D	↑ Ca²⁺ resorption	↑ Ca²⁺ reabsorption	↑ Ca²⁺ absorption ↑ Po₄⁻³ absorption	↑	↑
Calcitonin	↑ Ca²⁺ resorption	↑ Excretion of Ca²⁺ ↑ PO₄⁻³ reabsorption	—	↓	↑

KEY: Ca²⁺, calcium; PO₄⁻³, phosphorus; ↑, increase; ↓, decrease

Table 22-10   Effects of hypoalbuminemia and alkalosis on serum calcium

Condition	Effect	Result	Symptoms of Hypocalcemia
Decreased albumin	Decreased protein-bound Ca^{2+}	Decreased total serum, but normal free (ionized) Ca^{2+}	Absent
Alkalosis	Increased protein-bound Ca^{2+}	Normal total serum Ca^{2+}, but decreased free (ionized) Ca^{2+}	May be present

    a. Solid tumors: breast, lung, pancreas, kidneys, ovary
    b. Hematologic cancers: myeloma, lymphosarcoma, adult T-cell lymphoma, Burkitt's lymphoma
2. Hyperparathyroidism: increased bone resorption, GI absorption, and renal absorption; etiology:
    a. Parathyroid hyperplasia, adenoma
    b. Hyperparathyroidism of renal failure
3. Granulomatous disorders: increased GI absorption (e.g., sarcoidosis)
4. Paget's disease: increased bone resorption, seen only during periods of immobilization
5. Vitamin D intoxication, milk-alkali syndrome: increased GI absorption
6. Thiazides: increased renal absorption
7. Other causes: familial hypocalciuric hypercalcemia, thyrotoxicosis, adrenal insufficiency, prolonged immobilization, vitamin A intoxication, recovery from acute renal failure, lithium administration, pheochromocytoma, disseminated SLE

Symptoms (vary with rapidity of development and degree of hypercalcemia)

1. GI: constipation, anorexia, nausea, vomiting, pancreatitis, ulcers
2. CNS: confusion, obtundation, psychosis, lassitude, depression, coma
3. Genitourinary: nephrolithiasis, renal insufficiency, polyuria, decreased urine-concentrating ability, nocturia, nephrocalcinosis
4. Musculoskeletal: myopathy, weakness, osteoporosis, pseudogout, bone pain
5. Other: hypertension, metastatic calcifications, band keratopathy, pruritus
6. Most patients are asymptomatic at time of diagnosis

Diagnostic studies

1. History
    a. Family history of hypercalcemia, such as MEN syndromes or *familial hypocalciuric hypercalcemia* (latter is a benign autosomal dominant condition of increased serum Ca^{2+}, low urinary calcium, de-

creased fractional excretion of Ca^{2+}, and a normal PTH level; parathyroidectomy is not indicated)

b. Inquire about intake of milk and antacids (milk-alkali syndrome), intake of thiazides, lithium, large doses of vitamin A or D

c. Inquire whether patient has any bone pain (multiple myeloma, metastatic disease), or abdominal pain (pancreatitis, PUD)

2. Physical exam
   a. Look for evidence of primary neoplasm (e.g., breast, lung)
   b. Check eyes for evidence of band keratopathy (found in medial and lateral margins of the cornea)

3. Lab results
   a. Initial lab studies should include: serum calcium, albumin, PO_4^{-3}, magnesium, alkaline phosphatase, electrolytes, BUN, creatinine, and 24 hr urine calcium (see Table 22-11 for interpretation of results)
   b. If the history is suggestive of excessive intake of vitamin D (e.g., food faddists with intake of megadoses of fat-soluble vitamins), a serum vitamin D level (1,25 dihydroxyvitamin D) is indicated
   c. The iPTH distinguishes primary hyperparathyroidism from hypercalcemia caused by malignancy when the serum calcium level is >12 mg/dl; below this value there is considerable overlap and the differentiation between these two major causes of hypercalcemia is extremely difficult[31]
   d. A very high level of urinary cyclic AMP is strongly suggestive of primary hyperparathyroidism, although certain nonparathyroid malignancies have also been shown to produce elevated levels of urinary cyclic AMP[65]; parathyroid hormone–like protein (PLP) is increased in hypercalcemia associated with solid malignancies (e.g., squamous, breast, renal tumors)
   e. Table 22-12 describes the use of PTH, cyclic AMP, and iPLP in the differential diagnosis of hypercalcemia

4. Radiologic evaluation
   a. Bone survey may show evidence of subperiosteal bone resorption (suggesting PTH excess)
   b. Bone scan may show hot spots in association with lytic lesions

5. ECG: shortening of the QT interval

Table 22-11   Interpretation of initial lab studies

Lab Test	Hyperparathyroidism	Familial Hypocalciuric Hypercalcemia	Sarcoidosis	Metastatic Carcinoma
Serum Ca^{2+}	↑	↑	↑	↑
Serum PO_4^{-3}	↓	↓	N/↑	N
24 hr urine Ca^{2+}	N/↑	↓ *	N/↑	↑
Alkaline phosphatase	N/↑	N	N/↑	N/↑

KEY: ↑, Increased; ↓, decreased; N, normal; Ca^{2+}, calcium; PO_4^{-3}, phosphate
*The ratio of calcium clearance/creatinine clearance is <0.01.

Table 22-12 Use of iPTH and urinary cyclic AMP in the differential diagnosis of hypercalcemia

iPTH	Urinary Cyclic AMP	iPLP	Diagnosis
↑ ↑	↑ ↑	N	Primary hyperparathyroidism
N/↓	N/↓	↑	Probable occult malignancy

KEY: ↑, Increased; ↓, decreased; N, normal; iPTH, parathyroid hormone by radioimmunoassay; iPLP, parathyroid hormone–like protein by radioimmunoassay.

Therapy

1. Acute severe hypercalcemia (serum calcium >13 mg/dl or symptomatic patient)
   a. Vigorous IV hydration with normal saline followed by IV furosemide q4-6h
      (1) Normal saline infusion will increase urinary calcium excretion by inhibiting proximal tubular sodium and calcium reabsorption; the addition of a loop diuretic further inhibits calcium and sodium transport downstream from the proximal tubule
      (2) Use normal saline with caution in patients with cardiac or renal insufficiency to avoid fluid overload
      (3) Monitor serum electrolytes and magnesium and calcium levels frequently; complications of the above regimen include decreased potassium, magnesium, and sodium
   b. Calcitonin: 4 U/kg q12h
      (1) The initial dose is given IV following initial skin testing for allergy; subsequent doses may be given SQ
      (2) Particularly useful in hypercalcemia associated with hyperphosphatemia because it also increases urinary phosphate excretion; however, it is indicated only when saline hydration and furosemide are ineffective
   c. Mithramycin: 25 μg/kg by slow IV infusion (over 6 hr); this is the most potent of all antihypercalcemic agents
      (1) It lowers serum calcium within 12-24 hr by inhibiting bone resorption
      (2) Its use should be restricted to emergency treatment of severe hypercalcemia
      (3) May cause hepatotoxicity, nephrotoxocity, and thrombocytopenia (usually seen following repeated IV doses)
   d. Etidronate disodium (Didronel): 7.5 mg/kg/day in 250 ml of saline, infused over 2 hr on 1 to 4 consecutive days
      (1) Etidronate and other diphosphonates inhibit bone resorption by osteoclasts and are effective in lowering hypercalcemia in patients with malignant disease
      (2) The serum calcium level will be lowered to normal range within 2-5 days in approximately 75% of patients

2. Chronic hypercalcemia
   a. Identify and treat underlying disease (e.g., vitamin D intoxication, sarcoidosis)
   b. Discontinue potential hypercalcemic agents (e.g., thiazide diuretics)
   c. If the hypercalcemia is caused by a parathyroid adenoma, parathyroidectomy is the treatment of choice; medical follow-up is preferred in elderly patients with mild asymptomatic hyperparathyroidism
   d. Unless contraindicated, these patients should maintain a high daily intake of fluids (3-5 L/day) and of sodium chloride (>400 mEq/day) to increase renal calcium excretion
   e. Medications
      (1) Glucocorticoids: hydrocortisone 3-5 mg/kg/day IV initially, then prednisone 30 mg PO bid
          (a) The calcium-lowering action of corticosteroids occurs via decreased intestinal calcium absorption; they are very effective in hypercalcemia secondary to breast carcinoma, myeloma, sarcoidosis, and vitamin D intoxication
          (b) Their use in acute hypercalcemia is limited because it takes 48-72 hr before the serum calcium shows a significant decline
      (2) Oral phosphates: 1-3 g/day in divided doses (e.g., Neutra-Phos 250-500 mg PO q6h)
          (a) Phosphates lower serum calcium by decreasing GI calcium absorption and bone resorption
          (b) Not useful in acute hypercalcemia because their calcium-lowering effect will not be apparent for 2-3 days
          (c) Oral phosphates are contraindicated in renal insufficiency or any other medical conditions with elevated serum phosphate levels
      (3) Indomethacin: 75-150 mg/day
          (a) Prostaglandin synthetase inhibitor
          (b) It is only effective in prostaglandin-mediated hypercalcemia

Hypocalcemia

Etiology

1. Renal insufficiency: hypocalcemia caused by
   a. Increased calcium deposits in bone and soft tissue secondary to increased serum PO_4^{-3} level
   b. Decreased production of 1,25 dihydroxyvitamin D
   c. Excessive loss of 25-OHD (nephrotic syndrome)
2. Hypoalbuminemia: each decrease in serum albumin (g/L) will decrease serum calcium by 0.8 mg/dl but will not change free (ionized) calcium
3. Vitamin D deficiency
   a. Malabsorption (most common cause)
   b. Inadequate intake
   c. Decreased production of 1,25 dihydroxyvitamin D (vitamin D–dependent rickets, renal failure)
   d. Decreased production of 25-OHD (parenchymal liver disease)

    e. Accelerated 25-OHD catabolism (phenytoin, phenobarbital)

    f. End-organ resistance to 1,25 dihydroxyvitamin D

4. Hypomagnesemia: hypocalcemia caused by
    a. Decreased PTH secretion
    b. Inhibition of PTH effect on bone

5. Pancreatitis, hyperphosphatemia, osteoblastic metastases: hypocalcemia is secondary to increased calcium deposits (bone, abdomen)

6. Pseudohypoparathyroidism (PHP): autosomal recessive disorder characterized by short stature, shortening of metacarpal bones, obesity, and mental retardation; the hypocalcemia is secondary to congenital end-organ resistance to PTH

7. Idiopathic hypoparathyroidism, surgical removal of parathyroids (e.g., neck surgery)

8. "Hungry bones syndrome": rapid transfer of calcium from plasma into bones following removal of a parathyroid tumor

9. Sepsis

Symptoms

1. Neuromuscular irritability
    a. Chvostek's sign: facial twitch following gentle tapping over the facial nerve
    b. Trousseau's sign: carpedal spasm following inflation of blood pressure cuff above the patient's systolic blood pressure for a 2-3 min duration
    c. Tetany, paresthesias, myopathy, seizures, muscle spasm or weakness

2. Psychiatric disturbances: psychosis, depression, impaired cognitive function

3. Soft-tissue calcifications, ocular cataracts

4. Cardiovascular manifestations: dysrhythmias, CHF (caused by decreased myocardial contractility), increased QT interval, hypotension

Diagnostic tests

1. Serum albumin: to rule out hypoalbuminemia

2. BUN, creatinine: to rule out renal failure

3. Serum magnesium: to rule out severe hypomagnesemia

4. Serum PO_4^{-3}, alkaline phosphatase: to differentiate hypoparathyroidism from vitamin D deficiency (see Table 22-13)

5. Serum PTH level by radioimmunoassay should be ordered only when above tests are inconclusive

Table 22-13 Differentiation of hypoparathyroidism from vitamin D deficiency

Disorder	Serum Ca^{2+}	Serum PO_4^{-3}	Alkaline Phosphatase
Hypoparathyroidism	↓	↑	N
Vitamin D deficiency	↓	↓	↑

KEY: ↑, Increase; ↓, decrease; N, normal

    a. Markedly increased PTH: pseudohypoparathyroidism
    b. Increased PTH: vitamin D deficiency
    c. Decreased PTH: hypoparathyroidism

Therapy

1. Hypoalbuminemia
   a. Improve nutritional status
   b. Calcium replacement is not indicated since the free (ionized) calcium is normal
2. Hypomagnesemia: correct the magnesium deficiency
   a. Severe hypomagnesemia (serum magnesium level <0.8 mEq/L): give 1 g (8 mEq) of a 10% magnesium sulfate solution IV slowly (over 15 min)
   b. Moderate-to-severe hypomagnesemia (serum magnesium level 0.8-1.3 mEq/L): give one 2 ml ampule of a 50% magnesium solution IM; may repeat q4-6h
3. Acute, severe symptomatic hypocalcemia caused by hypoparathyroidism or vitamin D deficiency: give a slow IV bolus (over 15 min) of 10-30 ml of a 10% calcium gluconate solution
4. Chronic hypocalcemia caused by hypoparathyroidism or vitamin D deficiency
   a. Calcium supplementation: 1-4 g/day of elemental calcium (e.g., calcium carbonate 650 mg PO qid will provide 1 g of elemental calcium/day)
   b. Vitamin D replacement (e.g., calcitriol 0.25 μg/day)
5. Chronic hypocalcemia caused by renal failure
   a. Reduction of hyperphosphatemia with phosphate binding antacids (Amphojel, Basojel, Alternajel)
   b. Vitamin D and oral calcium supplementation (as noted above)

22.9 | ADRENAL GLAND DISORDERS

Cushing's syndrome

Definition

Cushing's syndrome is characterized by glucocorticoid excess secondary to exaggerated adrenal cortisol production or chronic glucocorticoid therapy.

Etiology

1. Chronic glucocorticoid therapy
2. Pituitary ACTH excess (Cushing's disease)
3. Adrenal neoplasms
4. Ectopic ACTH production (neoplasm of lung, pancreas, kidney, thyroid, thymus)

Symptoms

1. Hypertension
2. Obesity
3. Hirsutism, menstrual irregularities, hypogonadism, infertility
4. Diabetes mellitus, osteoporosis (bone pain and fractures)
5. Psychosis, emotional lability
6. Skin fragility, hemorrhagic diathesis, poor wound healing

Physical exam

1. Ecchymoses, red-purple abdominal striae, acne, facial plethora, hyperpigmentation (when there is ACTH excess)
2. Central obesity with rounding of the facies (moon facies), thin extremities
3. Fat accumulation in dorsocervical spine (buffalo hump) and supraclavicular areas
4. Muscle wasting with proximal myopathy

NOTE: The above characteristics are not commonly present in Cushing's syndrome secondary to ectopic ACTH production. Many of these tumors secrete a biologically inactive ACTH that does not activate adrenal steroid synthesis.[28] The patients may have only weight loss and weakness.

Initial lab results

1. Hypokalemia, hypochloremia, metabolic alkalosis, hyperglycemia, hypercholesterolemia
2. Increased 24-hour urinary free cortisol (>100 µg/24 hr)

Diagnosis

1. The classic diagnostic approach is outlined in Fig. 22-7
2. An overnight high-dose dexamethasone suppression test has been developed by Tyrrell et al.[70] to diagnose Cushing's syndrome
   a. Measure baseline plasma cortisol level (7 AM)
   b. Give patient 8 mg of dexamethasone PO at 11 PM
   c. Measure cortisol level at 7 AM the following morning
   d. Interpretation: suppression of plasma cortisol level to $>50\%$ of baseline indicates Cushing's disease
   e. This test has a sensitivity of 92%, a specificity of 100%, and diagnostic accuracy of 93%; these values equal or exceed those of the standard 2 day test whether based on suppression of plasma cortisol or urinary 17-hydroxysteroids
   f. Continuous IV dexamethasone infusion (1 mg/hr) for 7 hr can also be used for the differential diagnosis of Cushing's syndrome; a cortisol decrease of at least 190 mmol/L defines a positive response; false test results can occur in patients with CRH-secreting tumors[9]
3. Metyrapone test (see Fig. 22-3): an increase in plasma 11-deoxycortisol level differentiates Cushing's disease from other causes of Cushing's syndrome
4. Corticotropin releasing hormone (CRH) stimulation test: useful to distinguish pituitary from adrenal causes of Cushing's syndrome

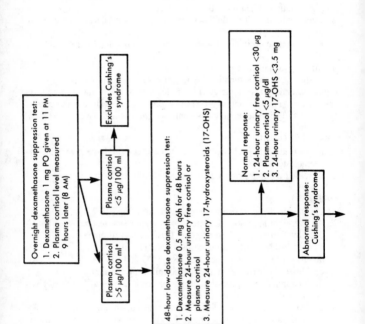

Overnight dexamethasone suppression test:
1. Dexamethasone 1 mg PO given at 11 PM
2. Plasma cortisol level measured 9 hours later (8 AM)

Plasma cortisol <5 μg/100 ml → Excludes Cushing's syndrome

Plasma cortisol >5 μg/100 ml*

48-hour low-dose dexamethasone suppression test:
1. Dexamethasone 0.5 mg q6h for 48 hours
2. Measure 24-hour urinary free cortisol or plasma cortisol
3. Measure 24-hour urinary 17-hydroxysteroids (17-OHS)

Normal response:
1. 24-hour urinary free cortisol <30 μg
2. Plasma cortisol <5 μg/dl
3. 24-hour urinary 17-OHS <3.5 mg

Abnormal response: Cushing's syndrome

Continued.

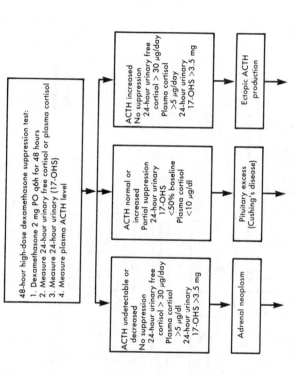

48-hour high-dose dexamethasone suppression test:
1. Dexamethasone 2 mg PO q6h for 48 hours
2. Measure 24-hour urinary free cortisol or plasma cortisol
3. Measure 24-hour urinary (17-OHS)
4. Measure plasma ACTH level

ACTH undetectable or decreased
No suppression
24-hour urinary free cortisol > 30 µg/day
Plasma cortisol >5 µg/dl
24-hour urinary 17-OHS >3.5 mg

ACTH normal or increased
Partial suppression
24-hour urinary 17-OHS <50% baseline
Plasma cortisol <10 µg/dl

ACTH increased
No suppression
24-hour urinary free cortisol > 30 µg/day
Plasma cortisol >5 µg/day
24-hour urinary 17-OHS >3.5 mg

Adrenal neoplasm

Pituitary excess (Cushing's disease)

Ectopic ACTH production

Figure 22-7
Diagnostic approach to Cushing's syndrome.

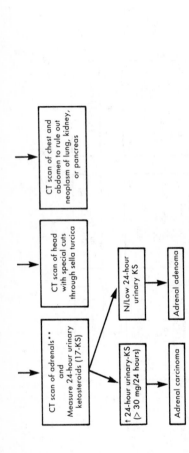

CT scan of chest and abdomen to rule out neoplasm of lung, kidney, or pancreas

CT scan of head with special cuts through sella turcica

CT scan of adrenals** and Measure 24-hour urinary ketosteroids (17-KS)

N/Low 24-hour urinary KS

Adrenal adenoma

↑ 24-hour urinary-KS (> 30 mg/24 hours)

Adrenal carcinoma

*Failure to suppress endogenous cortisol secretion can also be seen in patients with agitated depression, severe stress, alcoholism, anorexia nervosa, and in patients taking oral contraceptives. Corticotropin–releasing factor (CRF) is useful in evaluating Cushing's syndrome and in differentiating it from hypercortisolism of psychiatric origin.[59]

**A ''routine'' CT scan of the abdomen (with cuts >1 cm) is inappropriate to identify adrenal masses. The radiographer must be instructed to perform multiple small tomographic cuts through the adrenal area.[14]

Figure 22-7, cont'd
Diagnostic approach to Cushing's syndrome.

5. Inferior petrosal sinus sampling: to reveal elevated ACTH concentration in patients with pituitary adenoma. This test is indicated only when biochemical and radiographic data have not clearly defined the cause of Cushing's syndrome

Therapy

1. Pituitary adenoma: transsphenoidal resection is the therapy of choice in adults
2. Adrenal neoplasm
   a. Surgical resection of the affected adrenal
   b. Glucocorticoid replacement therapy for approximately 9-12 months after the surgery to allow time for the contralateral adrenal to recover from its prolonged suppression
   c. Mitotane 6-12 g/day in divided doses blocks glucocorticoid synthesis and can be used to control cortisol excess in patients with residual or nonresectable carcinoma[59]
   d. Metyrapone and aminoglutethimide also inhibit adrenal synthesis of steroids and can be used in patients who do not respond to or are unable to tolerate mitotane
3. Ectopic ACTH
   a. Surgical resection of the ACTH-secreting neoplasm
   b. Control of cortisol excess with metyrapone, aminoglutethimide, or ketaconazole[59]
   c. Control of the mineralocorticoid effects of cortisol and 11-deoxycorticosteroid with spironolactone[69]

Primary adrenocortical insufficiency

Definition

Primary adrenocortical insufficiency (Addison's disease) is characterized by inadequate secretion of corticosteroids resulting from partial or complete destruction of the adrenal glands.

Etiology

1. Autoimmune destruction of the adrenals
2. Tuberculosis
3. Carcinomatous destruction of the adrenals
4. Adrenal hemorrhage (anticoagulants, trauma, coagulopathies, pregnancy, sepsis)
5. Adrenal infarction (arteritis, thrombosis)
6. Other: sarcoidosis, amyloidosis, postoperative, fungal infection

Symptoms[7]

1. Weakness, anorexia, weight loss (100%)
2. Increased pigmentation (>90%)
3. Hypotension (85-90%)
4. GI disturbances (abdominal pain, diarrhea, constipation) (>50%)
5. Other: hypoglycemic manifestations, salt craving, poor response to stress

Physical exam

1. Hyperpigmentation: more prominent in palmar creases, buccal mucosa, pressure points (elbows, knees, knuckles), perianal mucosa, and around areolas of nipples
2. Hypotension
3. Generalized weakness
4. Amenorrhea and loss of axillary hair in females

Lab results

1. Increased K^+, decreased Na^+ and Cl^-
2. Decreased glucose
3. Increased BUN/creatinine ratio (prerenal azotemia)
4. Mild normocytic, normochromic anemia, neutropenia, lymphocytosis, eosinophilia (significant dehydration may mask the hyponatremia and anemia)
5. Decreased 24 hr urine cortisol, 17-OHCS, and 17-KS, and increased ACTH (if primary adrenocortical insufficiency)

Radiological evaluation

1. Chest x-ray: may reveal a small-sized heart
2. Abdominal x-ray: adrenal calcifications may be noted if the adrenocortical insufficiency is secondary to TB or fungus
3. Abdominal CT scan: small adrenal glands generally indicate either idiopathic atrophy or long-standing TB whereas enlarged glands are suggestive of early TB or potentially treatable diseases[75]

Diagnosis

1. A screening test can be performed for primary adrenal insufficiency
   a. Give 0.25 mg of cosyntropin (synthetic ACTH) IV after measuring the basal cortisol level
   b. Measure the plasma cortisol levels again after 60 min
   c. A rise <7 μg/dl is suggestive of primary adrenal insufficiency if the patient's basal cortisol level is <20 μg/dl
2. If the clinical picture is highly suggestive of adrenocortical insufficiency, the diagnosis can be made with the following test[24]
   a. On day before starting the test and on each day of the test collect 24 hr urine for 17-OHCS, and for creatinine (to evaluate adequacy of collection)
   b. Each day of the test (3 days) the patient is given dexamethasone 0.5 mg IV bid and fludrocortisone 0.1 mg PO qd; these are continued daily until the test results are known to avoid acute adrenal insufficiency
   c. ACTH 0.4 mg mixed in 500 ml of D_5NS is infused over 8 hr each day of the test
3. The interpretation of the above test is summarized in Table 22-14
4. Secondary adrenocortical insufficiency can be distinguished from primary adrenal insufficiency by
   a. Absence of hyperpigmentation
   b. Decreased plasma ACTH level

Table 22-14   Interpretation of 3-day ACTH infusion test for adrenocortical insufficiency

Interpretation	Cortisol (Baseline)	ACTH (Baseline)	17-OHCS (Baseline)	17-OHCS (Day 1)	17-OHCS (Day 2)	17-OHCS (Day 3)
Normal response	N	N	N	↑	↑↑	↑↑
Primary adrenocortical insufficiency (Addison's disease)	↓	↑	N/↓	No increase or small increase	No increase or small increase	No increase or small increase
Secondary adrenocortical insufficiency (caused by pituitary dysfunction)	↓	↓	N/↓	↑	↑↑	↑↑↑

KEY: N, Normal; ↑, increase; ↓, decrease; ACTH, adrenocorticotropin; 17-OHCS, 17-hydroxycorticosteroid

   c. No significant impairment of aldosterone secretion (since aldosterone
      secretion is under control of the renin-angiotensin system)
   d. There may be additional evidence of hypopituitarism (e.g., hypogo-
      nadism, hypothyroidism)
   e. Absence of 11-deoxycortisol response to metyrapone

Therapy

1. Chronic adrenocortical insufficiency
   a. Hydrocortisone 15-20 mg PO qAM and 5-10 mg in late afternoon, or
      prednisone 5 mg in AM and 2.5 mg at hs
   b. 9-α-fludrohydrocortisone 0.05-0.1 mg PO qAM; this mineralocorti-
      coid replacement is necessary if the patient has primary adrenocorti-
      cal insufficiency
   c. Periodic monitoring of serum electrolytes, vital signs, and body
      weight; liberal sodium intake
   d. Instruct patient to increase glucocorticoid replacement in times of
      stress and to receive parenteral glucocorticoids if diarrhea or vomit-
      ing occurs
2. Addisonian crisis: acute complication of adrenal insufficiency characterized by circulatory collapse, dehydration, nausea, vomiting, hypoglycemia, and hyperkalemia
   a. Draw plasma cortisol level; do not delay therapy until confirming lab
      results are obtained
   b. Administer hydrocortisone 100 mg IV q6h for 24 hr; if patient shows
      good clinical response, gradually taper dosage and change to oral
      maintenance dose (usually prenisone 7.5 mg/day)
   c. Provide adequate volume replacement with D_5NS until hypotension,
      dehydration, and hypoglycemia are completely corrected
   d. Identify and correct any precipitating factor (e.g., sepsis, hemor-
      rhage)

Disorders of mineralocorticoid secretion

Physiology

1. Mineralocorticoids participate in the regulation of sodium and potassium
   balance by promoting
   a. Reabsorption of sodium in the cortical collecting tubules
   b. Secretion of potassium in the cortical collecting tubules
   c. Secretion of hydrogen ion in the collecting tubules
2. The principal sodium-retaining hormone, aldosterone, is regulated by
   several mechanisms[8]: renin-angiotensin system, ACTH, and potassium
   a. The concentration of renin in the blood is the principal regulator
   b. Renin is secreted in response to several signals (renal perfusion pres-
      sure, beta adrenergic activity, fluid composition of the distal nephron
      at the macula densa)
   c. Renin stimulates aldosterone secretion by acting on angiotensinogen
      and splitting off a decapeptide, angiotensin I, which is then con-
      verted to angiotensin II by an enzyme; angiotensin II stimulates ad-
      renal production of aldosterone and also produces arterial vasocon-
      striction

Hypoaldosteronism

1. Etiology
   a. Hyporeninemic hypoaldosteronism: decreased aldosterone production secondary to decreased renin production; the typical patient has renal disease secondary to various factors (e.g., diabetes mellitus, interstitial nephritis, multiple myeloma)
   b. Aldosterone deficiency found in association with deficiency of adrenal glucocorticoid hormones (e.g., Addison's disease, bilateral adrenalectomy)
   c. Rarer causes: idiopathic hypoaldosteronism, unresponsiveness to aldosterone (pseudohypoaldosteronism)
2. Initial lab results[6]
   a. Increased potassium, normal or decreased sodium
   b. Hyperchloremic metabolic acidosis (caused by absence of hydrogen-secreting action of aldosterone)
   c. Increased BUN and creatinine (secondary to renal disease)
   d. Hyperglycemia (diabetes mellitus is common in these patients)
3. Treatment
   a. Treat primary condition
   b. Judicious use of 9-α-fluorocortisol (0.05-0.1 mg PO q$_{AM}$) in patients with aldosterone deficiency associated with deficiency of adrenal glucocorticoid hormones
   c. Furosemide is useful to correct hyperkalemia of hyporeninemic hypoaldosteronism

Hyperaldosteronism

1. Classification
   a. Primary aldosteronism (Conn's syndrome): aldosterone hypersecretion secondary to bilateral adrenal hyperplasia or aldosterone-secreting adenomas
   b. Secondary aldosteronism: excessive aldosterone secretion secondary to stimulation of the renin-angiotensin system; it is seen in association with chronic liver disease, chronic diuretic therapy, pregnancy, renal artery stenosis, renin-secreting neoplasms, Bartter's syndrome, hypovolemia, sodium depletion, and malignant hypertension
2. Diagnosis: hyperaldosteronism should be suspected in patients with hypertension and signs of hypokalemia (muscle weakness, cramping); Fig. 22-8 describes a simplification of the various tests necessary for the diagnosis for diagnostic evaluation of hypertensive patients with suspected aldosteronism
3. Therapy[6]
   a. Aldosterone secreting adenoma: unilateral adrenalectomy after correction of blood pressure and hypokalemia with:
      (1) Spironolactone (aldosterone antagonist): 200-400 mg/day or
      (2) Amiloride (potassium-sparing diuretic): 20-40 mg/day
   b. Bilateral hyperplasia
      (1) Control hypokalemia with spironolactone or amiloride
      (2) Control hypertension with antihypertensive agents

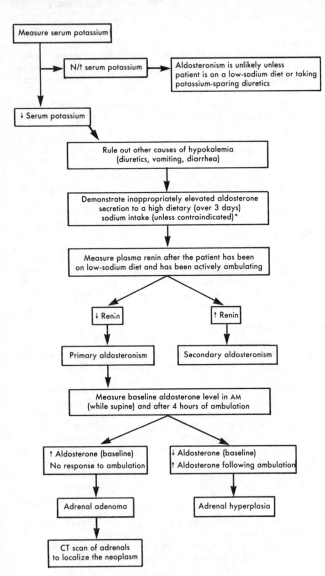

Measure serum potassium

→ N/↑ serum potassium → Aldosteronism is unlikely unless patient is on a low-sodium diet or taking potassium-sparing diuretics

↓ Serum potassium

Rule out other causes of hypokalemia (diuretics, vomiting, diarrhea)

Demonstrate inappropriately elevated aldosterone secretion to a high dietary (over 3 days) sodium intake (unless contraindicated)*

Measure plasma renin after the patient has been on low-sodium diet and has been actively ambulating

↓ Renin

↑ Renin

Primary aldosteronism

Secondary aldosteronism

Measure baseline aldosterone level in AM (while supine) and after 4 hours of ambulation

↑ Aldosterone (baseline)
No response to ambulation

↓ Aldosterone (baseline)
↑ Aldosterone following ambulation

Adrenal adenoma

Adrenal hyperplasia

CT scan of adrenals to localize the neoplasm

*For a noncompliant patient, it may be necessary to use a short-term saline infusion (2 L of normal saline over 4 hours) unless contraindicated. Measure baseline and postinfusion serum renin and aldosterone levels. A positive test for primary aldosteronism is failure of aldosterone suppression and no change in low renin level. [33]

Figure 22-8

Diagnostic evaluation of hypertensive patients with suspected aldosteronism.

22.10   PHEOCHROMOCYTOMA

Pathophysiology

Pheochromocytomas are catecholamine-producing tumors that originate from chromaffin cells of the adrenergic system. They generally secrete both norepinephrine and epinephrine, but norepinephrine is usually the predominant amine.

Characteristics[43]

1. "Rough rule of 10"

   10% are extraadrenal   10% involve both adrenals
   10% are malignant   10% are multiple (other than
   10% are familial   bilateral adrenal)
   10% occur in children

2. Clinical presentation: "Five H's"

   Headache   Hyperglycemia
   Hypertension   Hypermetabolism
   Hyperhidrosis

Symptoms

1. Hypertension can be sustained (55%) or paroxysmal (45%)
2. Headache (80%): usually paroxysmal in nature and described as "pounding" and severe
3. Palpitations (70%): can be present with or without tachycardia
4. Hyperhidrosis (60%): most evident during paroxysmal attacks of hypertension

   These symptoms may often arise in a dramatic and explosive fashion following sudden catecholamine release in response to a particular stimulus (e.g., sudden pressure in the area of the tumor, exercise, ingestion of certain foods, surgery). The paroxysms can last from less than 1 min to several hours. Their frequency varies from once every few months to multiple daily episodes.

Diagnosis

1. Obtain family history: approximately 10% of pheochromocytomas are familial (see MEN, Section 22.12)
2. Screening for pheochromocytoma should be considered in patients with any of the following[10,35]:
   a. Malignant hypertension
   b. Poor response to antihypertensive therapy
   c. Paradoxical hypertensive responses
   d. Hypertension during induction of anesthesia, parturition, surgery, or thyrotropin-releasing hormone testing

e. Hypertension associated with imipramine or desipramine
f. Neurofibromatosis (increased incidence)
g. von Hippel–Lindau disease (increased incidence)
3. Physical exam may be entirely normal if done in a symptom-free interval; during a paroxysm the patient may demonstrate marked increase in both systolic and diastolic pressure, profuse sweating, visual disturbances (caused by hypertensive retinopathy), dilated pupils (secondary to catecholamine excess), paresthesias in the lower extremities (caused by severe vasoconstriction), tremor, tachycardia
4. Lab results
   a. 24 hr urine metanephrine (↑) and vanillylmandelic acid (VMA) (↑) are usually done to screen for pheochromocytoma; measurement of 24 hr urinary levels of free norepinephrine have been reported to provide better accuracy for the diagnosis of pheochromocytoma[21]
   b. Increased plasma catecholamines: according to some investigators[10] this test has the highest sensitivity for detecting pheochromocytoma
   c. Clonidine suppression test[11]: clonidine administration will cause a decrease in plasma catecholamine levels in patients with essential hypertension but have no effect in patients with pheochromocytoma

Locating the pheochromocytoma

1. Abdominal CT scan: useful in locating pheochromocytomas >0.5 inches in diameter
2. Magnetic resonance imaging (MRI): pheochromocytomas demonstrate a distinctive MRI appearance; MRI may become the diagnostic imaging modality of choice[18]
3. Scintigraphy with ^{131}I-MIBG[61]: this norepinephrine analog localizes in adrenergic tissue; it is particularly useful in localizing extraadrenal pheochromocytomas
4. Selective vena cava sampling for norepinephrine levels: useful when CT scan and scintigraphy are unsuccessful; some investigators report a 97% success rate with this procedure[2]

Surgical therapy

1. Preoperative stabilization
   a. Volume expansion: done to prevent postoperative hypotension
   b. α Blockade to control hypertension: phenoxybenzamine (Dibenzyline) 10 mg PO bid-qid; metyrosine 250 mg PO qid or prazosin can be used when phenoxybenzamine therapy alone is not effective or is not well tolerated
   c. Beta blockade with propranolol 20-40 mg PO q6h, to be used only following α blockade
      (1) Useful to prevent catecholamine-induced dysrhythmias
      (2) Some investigators[11] do not recommend routine preoperative β blockade in absence of documented dysrhythmias; they advocate the use of IV propranolol (1-2 mg) intraoperatively if dysrhythmias develop during surgery

2. Hypertensive crises pre- and intraoperatively should be controlled with phentolamine (Regitine) 2-5 mg IV every 1-2 hr prn; second drug of choice is nitroprusside used in combination with beta adrenergic blockers
3. Combination chemotherapy with cyclophosphamide, vincristine, and dacarbazine is effective for advanced malignant pheochromocytoma[4]

22.11 CARCINOID SYNDROME

Definition

Carcinoid syndrome is characterized by paroxysmal vasomotor disturbances, diarrhea, and bronchospasm.

Pathophysiology

The symptoms are caused by the action of amines and peptides (serotonin, bradykinin, histamine) produced by tumors arising from enterochromaffin cells.

Organ distribution and characteristics

1. Carcinoids are principally found in the following organs:
   Appendix (40%)
   Small bowel (20%, 15% in ileum)
   Rectum (15%)
   Bronchi (12%)
   Esophagus, stomach, colon (10%)
   Ovary, biliary tract, pancreas (3%)
2. Carcinoid tumors do not usually produce the syndrome unless liver metastases are present or primary tumor does not involve the gastrointestinal tract
3. The appearance of the carcinoid syndrome often correlates directly with the tumor burden (increased tumor size = increased incidence of carcinoid syndrome) and with the presence of metastases
4. Carcinoids of the appendix and rectum have a low malignancy potential and rarely produce the clinical syndrome; metastases are also uncommon if the size of the primary lesion is less than 2 cm in diameter

Clinical manifestations

1. Cutaneous flushing (75-90%)
   a. The patient usually has red-purple flushes involving face, neck, and upper trunk
   b. The flushing episodes last from a few minutes to hours (longer lasting flushes are usually associated with bronchial carcinoids)
   c. Flushing may be triggered by emotion, alcohol, or foods or may occur spontaneously
   d. Dizziness, tachycardia, and hypotension may be associated with the cutaneous flushing
   e. The carcinoid syndrome must be distinguished from idiopathic flushing (IF); patients with IF are more often females, younger, and with a longer duration of symptoms; palpitations, syncope, and hypotension occur primarily in patients with IF[1]

2. Diarrhea (>70%): often associated with abdominal cramping and audible peristaltic rushes
3. Intermittent bronchospasm (25%): characterized by severe dyspnea and wheezing
4. Facial telangiectasia
5. Endocardial fibrosis: predominantly involves the endocardium, chordae, and valves of the right heart and can result in right-sided CHF

Diagnosis

1. Increased 24 hr urinary 5-hydroxyindoleacetic acid (5-HIAA): a metabolite of serotonin (5-hydroxytryptamine)
2. False elevations can be seen with ingestion of certain foods (bananas, pineapples, eggplant, avocados, walnuts) and certain medications (acetaminophen, caffeine, guaifenesin, reserpine); therefore, these patients should be on a restricted diet when the test is ordered
3. CT of abdomen or liver/spleen radionuclide scan is useful to detect liver metastases (palpable in over 50% of cases)

Therapy

1. Surgical resection of tumor
   a. Can be palliative and result in prolonged asymptomatic periods
   b. Percutaneous embolization and ligation of the hepatic artery can decrease the bulk of the tumor in the liver and provide palliative treatment of the carcinoid syndrome
   c. Surgical manipulation of the tumor can cause severe vasomotor abnormalities and bronchospasm (carcinoid crisis): somatostatin is effective in reversing some of the symptoms[67]
2. Cytotoxic chemotherapy: combination chemotherapy with 5-fluorouracil and streptozotocin can be used in patients with unresectable or recurrent carcinoid tumors[12]
3. Control of clinical manifestations
   a. Diarrhea: usually responds to Lomotil (diphenoxylate with atropine)
   b. Flushing: can be controlled by the combined use of histamine H_1 and H_2 receptor antagonists (e.g., diphenhydramine 50 mg PO q6h and cimetidine 300 mg PO q6h)[50]
   c. Somatostatin analogue (SMS 201-995) is useful for both flushing and diarrhea in most patients with carcinoid syndrome[19]
   d. Bronchospasm can be treated with aminophylline and/or albuterol
4. Nutritional support: supplemental niacin therapy is used to prevent pellagra because these patients utilize dietary tryptophan for serotonin synthesis

22.12   MULTIPLE ENDOCRINE NEOPLASIA

Definition

The syndrome of multiple endocrine neoplasia (MEN) occurs familially in an autosomal dominant pattern. The endocrine neoplasms may be expressed as hyperplasia, adenoma, or carcinoma, and may develop synchronously or metachronously.[57]

Classification

1. MEN I (Wermer's syndrome)
    a. Tumors or hyperplasia of pituitary, pancreatic islet cells (insulinoma, gastrinoma, glucagonoma), or parathyroid
    b. Possible associated conditions
        (1) Adrenocortical adenoma or hyperplasia
        (2) Thyroid adenoma or hyperplasia
        (3) Renal cortical adenoma
        (4) Carcinoid tumors
        (5) Gastrointestinal polyps
        (6) Multiple lipomas
    c. Clinical manifestations[57]
        (1) Peptic ulcer and its complications
        (2) Hypoglycemia
        (3) Hypercalcemia and/or nephrocalcinosis
        (4) Headache, visual field defects, secondary amenorrhea
        (5) Multiple subcutaneous lipomas
        (6) Other: flushing, acromegaly, Cushing's syndrome, hyperthyroidism
2. MEN II (Sipple's syndrome, MEN IIa)
    a. Associated with medullary thyroid carcinomas (MTC), pheochromocytoma, and hyperparathyroidism
    b. Clinical manifestations[15]
        (1) Neck mass (due to MTC)
        (2) Hypertension
        (3) Headache, palpitations, sweating
        (4) Hypercalcemia, nephrocalcinosis, osteitis fibrosa cystica
    c. Relatives of affected persons should be screened to detect medullary carcinoma at an early stage; screening can be accomplished with[63]
        (1) Pentagastrin test
        (2) Identification of a genetic marker on chromosome 10
3. MEN III (multiple mucosal neuroma syndrome, MEN IIb)
    a. Associated with[35] medullary thyroid carcinoma (MTC), pheochromocytoma, and multiple mucosal neuromas
    b. Possible associated conditions: intestinal ganglioneuromatosis, marfanoid habitus
    c. Clinical manifestations[39]
        (1) Neck mass (due to MTC)
        (2) Headache, palpitations, sweating, hypertension
        (3) Mucosal neuromas (initially noted as whitish, yellow-pink nodules involving lips and anterior third of tongue[13])
        (4) Marfan-like habitus (with absence of cardiovascular abnormalities and lens subluxation)
        (5) Peripheral neuropathy (caused by neuromatous plaques overlying the posterior columns of the spinal cord, cauda equina, and sciatic nerve)[22]

References

1. Aldrich LB, et al: Distinguishing features of idiopathic flushing and carcinoid syndrome, Arch Intern Med 148:2614, 1988.

2. Allison DJ, Brown MJ: Role of venous sampling in locating a pheochromocytoma, Br Med J 286:1122, 1983.

3. A.M.A. Division of Drugs and American Society for Clinical Pharmacology and Therapeutics: AMA drug evaluations, ed 5, Philadelphia, 1983, WB Saunders Co.

4. Averbuch SD, et al: Malignant pheochromocytoma: effective treatment with a combination of cyclophosphamide, vincristine, and dacarbazine, Ann Intern Med 109:267, 1988.

5. Bantle JP, Weber MS, et al: Rotation of the anatomic regions used for insulin injections and day-to-day variability of plasma glucose in type I diabetic subjects, JAMA 263:1802, 1990.

6. Baxter JD: Adrenocortical hypofunction. In Wyngaarden JB, Smith LH Jr (editors): Cecil Textbook of medicine, ed 17, Philadelphia, 1985, WB Saunders Co.

7. Baxter JD, Tyrrell JB: The adrenal cortex. In Felig P, Baxter JD, et al (editors): Endocrinology and metabolism, New York, 1981, McGraw-Hill Book Co.

8. Best CH: Best and Taylor's Physiological basis of medical practice, ed 11, Baltimore, 1985, The Williams & Wilkins Co.

9. Biemond P, DeJong FA, et al: Continuous dexamethasone infusion for seven hours in patients with the Cushing syndrome, Ann Intern Med 112:738, 1990.

10. Bravo EL, Gifford RW Jr: Pheochromocytoma: diagnosis, localization, and management, N Engl J Med 311:1298, 1984.

11. Bravo EL, et al: Clonidine-suppression test: a useful aid in the diagnosis of pheochromocytoma, N Engl J Med 305:623, 1981.

12. Brennan M, MacDonald J: Carcinoid tumors. In DeVita V Jr, Hellman S, Rosenberg S (editors): Cancer; principles and practice of oncology, Philadelphia, 1985, JB Lippincott Co.

13. Brown RS, et al: The syndrome of multiple mucosal neuromas and medullary thyroid carcinoma in childhood: importance of recognition of the phenotype for the early detection of malignancy, J Pediatr 86:77, 1975.

14. Burch WM: Cushing's disease: a review, Arch Intern Med 145:1106, 1985.

15. Cance WG, Wells SA: Multiple endocrine neoplasia. Type IIa, Curr Probl Surg 22(5):1, 1985.

16. Carpenter PC: Cushing's syndrome: update of diagnosis and management, Mayo Clin Proc 61:49, 1986.

17. Chava NR: Use of the ECG in the clinical management of diabetic ketoacidosis, Pract Cardiol 12:77, 1986.

18. Chezmar JL, et al: Adrenal masses: characterization with T1-weighted MR imaging, Radiology 166:357, 1988.

19. Comi RJ: Somatostatin and somatostatin analogue (SMS 201-995) in the treatment of hormone secreting tumors of the pituitary and GI tract and non-neoplastic disease of the gut, Ann Intern Med 110:35, 1989.

20. Crapo PO, Reuven G, Plefsky J, Alto P: Post-prandial plasma-glucose and insulin response to different complex carbohydrates, Diabetes 26:1178, 1977.

21. Duncan MW, et al: Measurement of norepinephrine and 3,4-dihydroxy-phenylglycol in urine and plasma for the diagnosis of pheochromocytoma, N Engl J Med 319:136, 1988.

22. Dyck PJ, et al: Multiple endocrine neoplasia, type 2b: phenotype recognition, neurological features, and their pathological basis, Ann Neurol 6:302, 1979.

23. Expert committee on diabetes mellitus, World Health Organization, WHO Tech Rep Ser, p 646, 1980.

24. Federman DD: The adrenal. In Rubenstein E, Federman DD (editors): Scientific American medicine, New York, 1985, Scientific American Inc.

25. Flier JS, Underhill LH: Pathogenesis and management of lipoprotein disorders, N Engl J Med 312:1300, 1985.

26. Hall PM, Cook J, et al: Proteins in the diagnosis of diabetes mellitus and impaired glucose tolerance, Diabetes Care 7:147, 1984.

27. Hamburger JI: The various presentations of thyroiditis, Ann Intern Med 104:219, 1986.

28. Hamburger J: Consistency of sequential needle biopsy findings for thyroid nodules, Arch Intern Med 147:97, 1987.

29. Hsu TH: Disorders of the pituitary gland. In Harvey AM, Johns RJ, et al (editors): The principles and practice of medicine, ed 21, New York, 1984, Appleton-Century-Crofts.

30. Jennings AS, Liddle GW, Orth DN: Results of treating childhood Cushing's disease with pituitary irradiation, N Engl J Med 297:957, 1977.

31. Kao PC: Parathyroid hormone assay, Mayo Clin Proc 57:596, 1982.

32. Karanfillian RG, et al: The value of laser Doppler velocimetry and transcutaneous oxygen tension determinations in predicting healing of ischemic forefoot ulcerations and amputations in diabetic and non-diabetic patients, J Vasc Surg 4:511, 1986.

33. Kaufman B: Magnetic resonance imaging of the pituitary gland, Radiol Clin North Am 22:795, 1984.

34. Kem D, et al: Saline suppression of plasma aldosterone in hypertension, Arch Intern Med 128:380, 1971.

35. Khairi MR, et al: Mucosal neuroma, pheochromocytoma, and medullary thyroid carcinoma: multiple endocrine neoplasia, type 3, Medicine 54:89, 1985.

36. Knoben JE, Anderson PO: Handbook of clinical drug data, ed 5, Washington DC, 1983, Drug Intelligence Publications Inc.

37. Krane RJ, et al: Impotence, N Engl J Med 321:1648, 1990.

38. Larsen PR: The thyroid. In Wyngaarden JB, Smith LH (editors): Cecil Textbook of medicine, ed 17, Philadelphia, 1985, WB Saunders Co, vol 2.

39. Leshin M: Multiple endocrine neoplasia. In Wilson JD, Foster DW (editors): Williams Textbook of endocrinology, ed 7, Philadelphia, 1985, WB Saunders Co.

40. Levy RI, Morganroth J, Rifkind BM: Treatment of hyperlipidemias, N Engl J Med 290:1295, 1974.

41. Levy RI, Rifkind BM: Lipid lowering drugs and hyperlipidemias, Drugs 6:12, 1973.

42. Maddedu G, et al: Serum thyroglobulin levels in the diagnosis and follow-up of subacute "painful" thyroiditis, Arch Intern Med 145:243, 1985.

43. Manger WM, Gifford RW Jr, Hoffman BB: Pheochromocytoma: a clinical and experimental overview, Curr Probl Cancer 9(5):1, 1985.

44. Manni A, Aiello DP: Thyroglobulin measurement vs iodine-131 total-body scan for follow-up of well-differentiated thyroid cancer, Arch Intern Med 150:437, 1990.

45. Marchant B, et al: The placental transfer of propylthiouracil, methimazole, and carbimazole, J Clin Endocrinol Metab 45:1187, 1977.

46. Morris LR, et al: Bicarbonate therapy in severe diabetic ketoacidosis, Ann Intern Med 105:836, 1986.

47. Mundy GR, et al: The hypercalcemia of cancer, N Engl J Med 310:1718, 1984.

48. National Diabetes Data Group: Classification and diagnosis of diabetes mellitus and other categories of glucose intolerance, Diabetes 28:1039, 1979.

49. Ney RL: Disorders of the adrenal gland. In Harvey AM, Johns RJ, et al (editors): Principles and practice of medicine, ed 21, New York, 1984, Appleton-Century-Crofts.

50. Pyles JD, et al: Histamine antagonists and carcinoid flush, N Engl J Med 302:234, 1980.

51. Robbins RJ: Medical management of prolactinomas. In Olefsky JM, Robbins RJ (editors): Prolactinomas, New York, 1986, Churchill Livingstone Inc.

52. Rock RC: Interpreting thyroid tests in the elderly: updated guidelines, Geriatrics 40:61, 1985.

53. Rojeski M, Gharib H: Nodular thyroid disease; evaluation and management, N Engl J Med 313:428, 1985.
54. Ryzen E, et al: Intravenous etidronate in the management of malignant hypercalcemia, Arch Intern Med 145:449, 1985.
55. Samuel P: Drug treatment of hyperlipidemia, Am Heart J 109:873, 1980.
56. Schimke RN: Disorders affecting multiple endocrine systems. In Petersdorf RG, et al (editors): Harrison's Principles of internal medicine, ed 10, New York, 1983, McGraw-Hill Book Co.
57. Schimke RN: Genetic aspects of multiple endocrine neoplasia, Annu Rev Med 35:25, 1984.
58. Schuermeter TH: Pharmacologic and pharmacokinetic properties of corticotropin-releasing factor in humans. In Chrousos GP (moderator): Clinical applications of corticotropin-releasing factor, Ann Intern Med 102:344, 1985.
59. Shepherd FA, et al: Ketoconazole; use in the treatment of ectopic adrenocorticotropic hormone production in Cushing's syndrome in small-cell lung cancer, Arch Intern Med 145:863, 1985.
60. Singer DE, et al: Tests of glycemia in diabetes mellitus; their use in establishing diagnosis and in treatment, Ann Intern Med 110:125, 1989.
61. Sisson JC, et al: Locating pheochromocytomas by scintigraphy using[131]I-metaliodobenzylguanidine, CA 34:86, 1984.
62. Skyler JS, Siegler DE, Reeves ML: A comparison of insulin regimens in insulin-dependent diabetes mellitus, Diabetes Care 5:11, 1982.
63. Sobol H, et al: Screening for multiple endocrine neoplasia Type 2 with DNA-polymorphism analysis, N Engl J Med 321:996, 1989.
64. Sridama V, et al: Long-term follow-up study of compensated low dose[131]I therapy for Graves' disease, N Engl J Med 311:426, 1984.
65. Stewart AF, et al: Biochemical evaluation of patients with malignancy-associated hypercalcemia: evidence for humoral and non-humoral groups, N Engl J Med 303:1377, 1980.
66. Surks MI, Chopra IJ, et al: American Thyroid Association guidelines for use of laboratory tests in thyroid disorders, JAMA 263:1529, 1990.
67. Thulin L, et al: Efficacy of somatostatin in a patient with carcinoid syndrome, Lancet 2:43, 1978.
68. Tucker H, et al: The treatment of acromegaly by transsphenoidal surgery, Arch Intern Med 140:795, 1980.
69. Tyrrell JB: Cushing's syndrome. In Wyngaarden JB, Smith LA Jr (editors): Cecil Textbook of medicine, ed 17, Philadelphia, 1985, WB Saunders Co.
70. Tyrrell JB, et al: An overnight high-dose dexamethasone suppression test for rapid differential diagnosis of Cushing's syndrome, Ann Intern Med 104:180, 1986.
71. Van Herle AJ, et al: The thyroid nodule, Ann Intern Med 96:221, 1982.
72. Vignati L, et al: Diabetic ketoacidosis. In Chapter 26 (Coma in diabetes) of Marble A, Krall LP, et al (editors): Joslin's Diabetes mellitus, ed 12, Philadelphia, 1985, Lea & Febiger, p 526.
73. Vignati L, et al: Hyperglycemic hyperosmolar nonketotic coma. In Chapter 26 (Coma in diabetes) of Marble A, Krall LP, et al (editors): Joslin's Diabetes mellitus, ed 12, Philadelphia, 1985, Lea & Febiger, p 543.
74. Vita JA, et al: Clinical clues to the cause of Addison's disease, Am J Med 78:461, 1985.
75. Williams GH, Dluhy RG: Diseases of the adrenal cortex. In Petersdorf RG, et al (editors): Harrison's Principles of internal medicine, ed 10, New York, 1983, McGraw-Hill Book Co, p 634.
76. Zinman B, Zuniga-Guajardo S, Kelly D: Comparison of the long-term effects of exercise in glucose control in Type I diabetes, Diabetes Care 7:515, 1984.

Gastroenterology

23.1 ACUTE GASTROINTESTINAL BLEEDING
Saul Feldman

Patients with acute GI hemorrhage must be approached in a multidisciplinary manner. The evaluating team should include the family physician/internist, a gastroenterologist, a radiologist, and a gastrointestinal surgeon. The initial assessment is directed toward:
1. Evaluating the extent (severity) of the bleeding
2. Locating the site of the bleeding:
   a. Upper GI bleeding (above ligament of Trietz)
   b. Lower GI bleeding (below ligament of Treitz)

After a brief initial assessment, the physician should immediately stabilize the patient with volume expanders (Ringer's lactate or normal saline) until blood is available (after patient's blood is typed and cross-matched).

History and physical exam

Although the history and the physical exam may be somewhat limited by the patient's condition, they should be performed to help identify the severity, duration, location, and cause of the bleeding (see Section 6.15 for the differential diagnosis of GI bleeding). The following are some salient points to note when taking the patient's history:
1. Drug history (aspirin, steroids, "blood thinners," nonsteroidal antiinflammatory drugs [NSAID])
2. Prior GI or vascular surgery
3. History of GI diagnosis or bleeding
4. History of smoking (increased risk of PUD)
5. Alcohol intake (gastritis, esophageal varices)
6. Symptoms of peptic ulcer
7. Associated diseases (ASHD, diabetes, hypertension, hematologic disorders, renal failure)
8. Protracted retching and vomiting (consider gastric or gastroesophageal tear [Mallory-Weiss])
9. Weight loss, anorexia (consider carcinoma)

283

10. Color and character of stool
11. Presence or absence of hematemesis

Physical exam

1. Vital signs
   a. Document tachycardia, hypotension, and postural changes; a pulse increase of more than 20 bpm or a postural fall in systolic blood pressure greater than 10-15 mm Hg usually indicates blood loss greater than 1 L
   b. Patients taking beta adrenergic blockers or vasodilators may not demonstrate significant variations of the vital signs
2. Cardiorespiratory exam: murmurs (increased incidence of angiodysplasia in patients with aortic stenosis), pulmonary rales, JVD (to determine rapidity of volume replacement)
3. Abdominal exam
   a. Observe for masses, tenderness, distention
   b. Auscultate for bowel sounds or abdominal bruits
   c. Look for evidence of liver disease (hepatomegaly, splenomegaly, abnormal vascular patterns, gynecomastia, spider angiomata, palmar erythema, testicular atrophy)
4. Digital rectal exam: check for masses, strictures, hemorrhoids; test stool for occult blood and inspect it for abnormalities (tarry, blood-streaked, bright red, mahogany color)
5. Skin: check for jaundice (liver disease), ecchymoses (coagulation abnormality), cutaneous telangiectasia (Rendu-Osler-Weber disease), buccal pigmentation (Peutz-Jeghers syndrome), and other mucocutaneous changes (Ehlers-Danlos syndrome)
6. Look for evidence of metastatic disease (cachexia, firm nodular liver)
7. Insert NG tube to determine if the bleeding is emanating from the upper GI tract (presence of bright red blood clots or coffee ground guaiac-positive aspirate); however, a negative aspirate does not rule out UGI bleeding since it could have subsided or the patient could be bleeding from the duodenal bulb without reflux into the stomach; make note of the presence of bile in the aspirate

Initial management

1. Stabilize patient: insert a large-bore (16 gauge) IV catheter and administer Ringer's lactate or normal saline; the rate of volume replacement is based on the estimated blood loss, clinical condition, and history of cardiovascular disease
2. Type and cross-match for 2-8 units of packed RBC (depending on estimated blood loss) and transfuse prn
3. Initial lab evaluation
   a. Hemoglobin/hematocrit
      (1) Initial value should be considered as erroneously high until blood volume is replaced
      (2) After bleeding ceases, the hemogram may continue to decrease for up to 6 hr and full equilibration may require 24 hr
      (3) The hematocrit generally falls by about 2-3 points for every 500 ml of blood lost

b. BUN: in absence of renal disease, a BUN may help determine the severity of the bleeding; a simultaneous creatinine level may also be of value, as the disparity in the BUN/creatinine ratio will reveal the extent of the bleeding more accurately; a BUN/Cr $\geq$ 36 is suggestive of UGI bleeding

c. Prothrombin time (PT), partial thromboplastin time (PTT), and platelet count should be done to exclude bleeding disorders; they should also be assessed before endoscopy or other invasive procedures

d. Other initial lab measurements to be drawn include LFTs, serum electrolytes, glucose, and WBC

e. ECG to rule out myocardial ischemia or silent MI

Investigational tools (Fig. 23-1)

Endoscopic evaluation

1. Upper endoscopy is indicated when blood or guaiac-positive material is obtained from NG tube aspirate or if lower endoscopy is negative; if an invasive procedure (e.g., bipolar heater-probe, laser cauterization, or injection sclerotherapy) is considered, endoscopy should be done emergently

2. Flexible sigmoidoscopy should be performed initially if lower GI bleeding is suspected; it helps to diagnose anal disease, colitis, and neoplasms in the lower colon

3. Colonoscopy should be performed if sigmoidoscopy is not diagnostic and bleeding appears to be colonic in origin; most useful in cases of AV malformations, colitis, neoplasms, and intussusception

Radiologic evaluation

1. Barium enema (BE)
   a. It should not be performed initially because it precludes other modes
   b. A double-contrast BE may be initiated after sigmoidoscopy, colonoscopy, arteriography, and nuclear scanning have been done
   c. The BE may be therapeutic in some cases of bleeding secondary to diverticular disease or intussusception

2. Upper GI series should be ordered only after utilizing endoscopy, arteriography, and nuclear scans; when ordering a GI series, the investigator must specify whether an esophagram and/or a small bowel series is desired

3. Radionuclide scans
   a. Technetium 99 pertechnetate scan (Meckel scan) selectively tags acid-secreting cells (gastric mucosa); it is used most often in unexplained bleeding in infants and young adults
   b. Technetium sulfur colloid scan is very sensitive in detecting lesions with low bleeding rates; its major drawbacks are:
      (1) Short half-life (difficulty in detecting intermittent bleeding)
      (2) Affinity of the colloid for liver and spleen (colonic bleeding may be missed if it originates in a region superimposed on areas of liver or spleen uptake)
   c. Technetium (^{99m}Tc)-labeled red blood cell scan: its major advantage over the sulfur colloid scan is its long duration; it is useful for inter-

Figure 23-1
Management of acute GI bleeding.

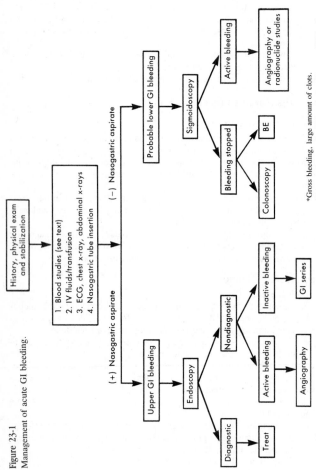

*Gross bleeding, large amount of clots.
†See text for negative NG aspirate with upper GI bleeding.

mittent bleeding because the patient can be monitored for GI bleeding for up to 24 hr

4. Selective angiography
   a. Occasionally first test ordered in actively bleeding patients
   b. May also be therapeutic since vasoconstrictors, autologous clots, or Gelfoam emboli can be administered intraarterially at the time of angiography to occlude the bleeding vessel
   c. Major drawbacks are high rate of bleeding (>0.5 ml/min) necessary for diagnosis and the risk of allergic reaction to contrast dye

Therapy

The treatment of acute GI bleeding may require multiple modalities and will be mentioned only briefly.

1. Correct bleeding abnormalities by administering fresh frozen plasma or vitamin K if the patient has a coagulopathy and platelets if patient is severely thrombocytopenic
2. H_2-receptor antagonists, sucralfate, and antacids are indicated only in cases of probable peptic ulcer or gastritis; H_2 blockers can cause liver toxicity, confusion, and many serious drug interactions, so they should be used with caution
3. Vasopressin (Pitressin) infusion is used in the management of significant variceal bleeding
   a. Mix 20 U of vasopressin in 100 ml of D_5W (0.2 U/ml)
   b. The infusion rate initially is 0.2 U/min (1 ml/min via continuous infusion pump), but it can be increased by 0.2-0.3 U q30min prn to control esophageal bleeding; maximum dosage is 0.9 U/min
   c. Relative contraindications are severe coronary artery disease and peripheral or cerebrovascular disease because of increased risk of angina, MI, tachycardia, TIA, CVA, and hypertension
   d. Concomitant administration of nitrates reverses the cardiotoxic effects of vasopressin and potentiates the reduction in portal pressure; nitroglycerin is particularly recommended in patients with ASHD and may be given IV, transdermally (e.g., 2.5 cm q4h), or SL (150 µg q30min for up to 6 hr)
   e. Vasopressin is only a temporizing measure; many patients will experience rebleeding when vasopressin is stopped
4. Endoscopy
   a. Sclerotherapy for bleeding varices
   b. Laser therapy (directed through the endoscope) may be used in proven bleeding from ulcerations, AV malformations, or neoplasms
   c. Cauterization with bipolar electrode is a useful modality to stop bleeding from ulcerations
5. Balloon tamponade by inserting a Sengstaken-Blakemore (SB) tube or Minnesota quadruple tube (modification of SB tube with a port to suction above the esophageal balloon)
   a. Balloon tamponade is indicated for severe bleeding from esophageal varices
   b. It should be inserted only by experts since it can result in esophageal

rupture, pulmonary aspiration or rupture, and upper airway obstruction if dislodged

6. Radiologic modalities: localized infusion of vasopressin, autologous clots, or foreign coagulating substances (e.g., Gelfoam) in the bleeding vessel during or following arteriography

7. Surgery is indicated at the onset of diagnosis of aortoduodenal fistula, but it is not suggested as the initial therapy in other causes of GI bleeding until a definitive diagnosis is made and other noninvasive modalities are attempted; exceptions to the conservative approach are
   a. Rebleeding in a hospitalized patient
   b. Bleeding episode requiring transfusion of more than 6 units of blood
   c. Endoscopic visualization of a "naked" vessel in a peptic ulcer

23.2   PEPTIC ULCER DISEASE (PUD)

Etiology

Peptic ulcers result from an imbalance between mucosal defense mechanisms (protective factors) and various mucosal damaging mechanisms (Table 23-1).

Table 23-1   Factors involved in the pathogenesis of peptic ulcers[42]

Protective Factors	Aggressive Factors
Mucosal barrier: pH-mucus gradient formed by a mixture of bicarbonate (secreted by gastric and duodenal epithelia) and gastric mucus	Acid secreted by parietal cells
	Pepsin secreted as pepsinogen by chief cells
	Bile acids play a significant role in the pathogenesis of gastric ulcer and esophagitis
Adequate blood supply to gastric mucosa and submucosa	Decreased blood flow to gastric mucosa
Competent sphincters (pyloric and LES) block reflux of bile salts into the stomach and esophagus	Incompetent pylorus or LES
	Medications
Medications	Aspirin
Histamine H_2-receptor antagonists	Nonsteroidal antiinflammatory drugs (NSAIDs)
Antacids	Glucocorticoids
Sucralfate	Cigarette smoking
Colloidal bismuth suspension	Gastrinoma
Anticholinergics	Stress (particularly following trauma)
Inhibitors of parietal cell secretion (misoprostol)	Alcohol
Proton pump inhibitors (omeprazole)	Impaired proximal duodenal bicarbonate secretion
Antimuscarinic agents (pirenzepine)	(?) *Helicobacter pylori*

Anatomic location

1. Duodenal ulcers: 90-95% occur in the first portion of the duodenum
2. Gastric ulcers: occur most frequently in the lesser curvature, near the incisura angularis

Clinical manifestations

1. Duodenal ulcer: patient usually has epigastric pain occurring 3-4 hr after eating; the pain is described as a burning, aching, boring, gnawing "pressure on the abdomen" that awakens the patient from sleep and is usually relieved by ingesting antacids or food (however, many patients with active duodenal ulcers may be asymptomatic)
2. Gastric ulcer: patient has epigastric pain similar to duodenal ulcer, but pain is not usually relieved by food; food may actually precipitate the symptoms

Physical exam

The physical exam is often unremarkable. The patient may have epigastric tenderness, tachycardia, pallor, hypotension (from acute or chronic blood loss), nausea and vomiting (if the pyloric channel is obstructed), boardlike abdomen and rebound tenderness (if perforated), and hematemesis or melena (if bleeding ulcer).

Diagnostic modalities

1. Endoscopy
   a. Highest accuracy (approximately 90-95%)
   b. Useful to identify superficial or very small ulcerations
   c. Essential to diagnose gastric ulcers (1-4% of gastric ulcers diagnosed as benign by UGI series are eventually diagnosed as gastric carcinoma)
   d. Additional advantages over UGI series include:
      (1) Possible biopsy of suspicious looking ulcers
      (2) Electrocautery of bleeding ulcers
      (3) Measurement of gastric pH in suspected gastrinoma (e.g., patient with multiple ulcers)
      (4) Diagnosis of esophagitis, gastritis, duodenitis
      (5) Detection of *Helicobacter pylori* (formerly *Campylobacter pylori*)*
   e. Its major disadvantage is its higher cost
2. UGI series: conventional UGI barium studies identify approximately 70-80% of PUD; accuracy can be increased to about 90% by using double contrast

Complications

1. GI bleeding (20%)
   a. Clinical manifestations: hematemesis, melena, hematochezia (if rapid transit time)
   b. Physical exam: pallor, hypotension, tachycardia, diaphoresis
   c. Diagnosis: endoscopy (after the patient has been stabilized)

*Note: *Campylobacter* is still the designation for lower gastrointestinal organisms.

    d. Therapy
       (1) IV hydration with NS, blood transfusion
       (2) Surgery if bleeding persists
2. Perforation (10%)
    a. Clinical manifestations: severe abdominal pain, epigastric pain with radiation to back or RUQ (if penetrating ulcer)
    b. Physical exam: boardlike abdomen, rebound tenderness, severe epigastric tenderness, absent bowel sounds
    c. Diagnosis: x-ray studies of abdomen may reveal free air in the peritoneal cavity
    d. Therapy: surgery
3. Gastric outlet obstruction (5%)
    a. Clinical manifestations: nausea, vomiting of undigested food, epigastric pain unrelieved by food or antacids
    b. Physical exam: large amount of air and fluid in the stomach, "succussion splash" may be heard
4. Posterior penetrations: manifested by severe back pain, pancreatitis

Medical therapy

Medical treatment is aimed at neutralizing gastric acidity (antacids), reducing acid production (H_2 blockers, misoprostol), increasing mucosal protection (sucralfate, misoprostol), and decreasing risk factors (e.g., cigarette smoking).
1. Antacids[16]
    a. They decrease the hydrogen ion concentration; the duration of their effect is directly related to their potency (Table 33-3) and to the length of time the antacid remains in the stomach (duration is prolonged if given after meals)
    b. Dosage is 30 ml of antacid given 1 and 3 hr after meals and hs
    c. Duration of therapy is 6-8 wk
2. Histamine H_2-receptor antagonists[28]
    a. They decrease gastric acid secretion by blocking histamine H_2 receptors on parietal cells
    b. For comparison of various H_2 blockers, refer to Table 33-25
    c. Duration of therapy is 8 wk
3. Sucralfate (Carafate)[33]
    a. Sucralfate is a disaccharide with negatively charged radicals that adhere to positively charged proteins on the surface of the ulcer crater and form a protective coating that shields the ulcer from acid and pepsin
    b. The action of sucralfate requires an acidic environment, therefore simultaneous ingestion of H_2-blockers or antacids should be avoided
    c. Dosage is 1 g 30-60 min before meals and at hs
    d. Duration of therapy is 6-8 wk
    e. Maintenance therapy is 1 g bid
4. Misoprostol (Cytotec)
    a. Misoprostol is a synthetic prostaglandin E_1 analog; it decreases gastric acid production and increases mucus and bicarbonate secretion
    b. It is indicated for the prevention of NSAID induced gastric ulcers in patients at high risk of complications from a gastric ulcer

c. It is contraindicated in women of childbearing age because of its abortifacient properties

d. Initial dosage is 100 μg qid with food, increased to 200 μg qid if well-tolerated; high incidence of diarrhea

e. Therapy with misoprostol is continued for the duration of NSAID therapy

5. Omeprazole (Prilosec)

a. Omeprazole suppresses gastric acid secretion by specific inhibition of the H^+/K^+-ATPase enzyme system at the secretory surface of the gastric parietal cell

b. It is indicated for the treatment of severe erosive esophagitis and poorly responsive gastroesophageal reflux disease (GERD); dosage is 20 mg daily for 4-8 wk

c. Omeprazole is also the drug of choice in Zollinger-Ellison syndrome; dosage is 60 mg daily, continued for as long as clinically indicated

6. Colloidal bismuth subcitrate (120 mg qid) or combination of bismuth and tinidazole may be useful in patients not responding to the above measures and with documented presence of *Helicobacter pylori* (via endoscopic biopsy, urea breath test, or specific antibodies); however, the significance (if any) of *H. pylori* infection in peptic ulcer disease remains to be fully defined

Ancillary therapy

1. Stop cigarette smoking[48]; cigarette smoking increases the risk of PUD, decreases the healing rate, and increases the frequency of recurrence

2. Avoid salicylates and nonsteroidal antiinflammatory drugs (NSAIDs)

3. Prophylaxis of patients at risk for PUD[45]: patients on prolonged mechanical ventilation, ICU patients receiving steroids, or persons admitted following severe trauma should receive a prophylactic regimen of antacids, H_2 blockers, or sucralfate to prevent upper GI bleeding

4. Special diets have been proved *unrelated* to ulcer development or healing; however, avoid foods that cause symptoms

Medical and ancillary therapy will result in complete healing of approximately 80-90% of peptic ulcers. Surgery should be performed when the patient has undergone an adequate course of medical therapy with an unsatisfactory response (inadequate healing, multiple recurrences).

Surgical treatment consists of highly selective vagotomy for duodenal ulcers or ulcer removal with antrectomy or hemigastrectomy without vagotomy for gastric ulcers.

Maintenance therapy in duodenal ulcer patients

Indicated in the following situations:

1. Persistent smokers

2. Recurrent ulceration

3. Chronic treatment with NSAIDs, glucocorticoids

4. Elderly or debilitated patients

5. Aggressive or complicated ulcer disease (e.g., perforation, hemorrhage).

6. Asymptomatic bleeders

Recurrence

The recurrence rate for untreated PUD is approximately 60% (>70% in smokers). Treatment will decrease the recurrence rate approximately 20-30%. Patients with recurrent ulcers should be retreated for an additional 8 wk and then placed on maintenance therapy with H_2 blockers, sucralfate, or antacids. Screening for hypersecretory disorders (e.g., Zollinger-Ellison syndrome) should be considered. In Z-E patients measurement of basal acid output is usually >15 mEq/hr and fasting serum gastrin concentration >1000 pg/ml.

Suggested follow-up

1. Duodenal ulcer: no further evaluation necessary if patient is asymptomatic after 8 wk of therapy
2. Gastric ulcer: repeat endoscopy should be done after 4-6 wk of therapy; further management will depend on the results of the endoscopy:
   a. Completely healed ulcer requires no further follow-up
   b. Partially healed ulcer
      (1) >50% healing and exfoliative cytology negative for carcinoma requires continued medical therapy for 6 more wk and then re-evaluate patient
      (2) >50% healing but exfoliative cytology positive for carcinoma requires surgery
      (3) <50% healing requires surgery

23.3 INFLAMMATORY BOWEL DISEASE

Inflammatory bowel disease (IBD) is a chronic disorder of the GI tract of undetermined etiology. The incidence is increased in young adults and Jews, but decreased in blacks. IBD is subdivided into two major groups:
1. Crohn's disease
2. Ulcerative colitis/proctitis
   Table 23-2 compares the clinical manifestations and physical exam in patients with Crohn's disease and ulcerative colitis.

Lab results

1. Decreased hemoglobin/hematocrit, potassium, magnesium, calcium, albumin
2. Vitamin B_{12} deficiency, folate deficiency (more common in Crohn's disease)

Differential diagnosis

1. Bacterial infections
   a. Acute: *Campylobacter, Yersinia, Salmonella, Shigella,* gonococcal proctitis, *Chlamydia, E. coli* (toxigenic), *C. difficile* (pseudomembranous colitis)
   b. Chronic: Whipple's disease, TB enterocolitis
2. Irritable bowel syndrome
3. Protozoal and parasitic infections (amebiasis, giardiasis)
4. Intestinal lymphoma

Table 23-2 Comparison of inflammatory bowel diseases

Crohn's Disease	Ulcerative Colitis
Clinical manifestations	
RLQ abdominal pain	Diarrhea often bloody and accompanied by tenesmus
Fever, dehydration, weight loss	Constipation may be present in some patients with significant rectal involvement
Anorexia, nausea, vomiting	
Diarrhea	Fever, dehydration, weight loss
	Abdominal pain, anorexia, nausea, vomiting
Physical Exam	
RLQ tenderness	Abdominal distention
Abdominal mass may be present (usually formed by adjacent loops of bowel)	Abdominal tenderness
	Extraintestinal manifestations may be present: liver disease, sclerosing cholangitis, iritis, uveitis, episcleritis
Anorectal disease (perirectal abscesses, fissures, fistulas)	
Extraintestinal manifestations same as in ulcerative colitis	Arthritis
	Erythema nodosum
	Pyoderma gangrenosum
	Aphthous stomatitis

5. Carcinoma of ileum or colon
6. Carcinoid tumors
7. Celiac sprue
8. Mesenteric adenitis
9. Diverticulitis
10. Appendicitis
11. Polyarteritis nodosa
12. Radiation enteritis
13. Collagenous colitis
14. Fungal infections (*Histoplasma, Actinomyces*)
15. α Chain disease
16. Endometriosis
17. "Gay bowel syndrome," gonococcal proctitis
18. Ischemic bowel disease

Complications

1. Intestinal obstruction (in Crohn's disease)
2. Intestinal perforation with peritonitis and/or abscess (in Crohn's disease)
3. Malabsorption
4. Electrolyte abnormalities (secondary to diarrhea)

5. GI hemorrhage
6. Anemia (from chronic blood loss), hypoproteinemia, vitamin B_{12} and folate deficiencies
7. Carcinoma of bile ducts, primary sclerosing cholangitis, and pericholangitis
8. Fistulas (in Crohn's disease)
9. Toxic megacolon (associated with danger of perforation)
10. Carcinoma of colon (both ulcerative colitis and Crohn's disease, but a higher percentage in ulcerative colitis)

Diagnosis

1. Sigmoidoscopy is done to establish the presence of mucosal inflammation; Table 23-3 describes the endoscopic differences between ulcerative colitis and Crohn's disease
2. Air-contrast barium enema: see Table 23-4 for interpretation of results
3. Pathologic differences: Crohn's disease can be further distinguished from ulcerative colitis by
   a. Presence of transmural involvement
   b. Frequent presence of noncaseating granulomas and lymphoid aggregates

Table 23-3   Endoscopic features of Crohn's disease and ulcerative colitis

Crohn's Disease	Ulcerative Colitis
Asymmetric and discontinuous disease	Very friable mucosa
Deep, longitudinal fissures	Diffuse, uniform erythema replacing the usual mucosal vascular pattern
Cobblestone appearance	
Aphthous ulcers	Rectal involvement invariably present if disease is active
Mucosa friability not usually present	Pseudopolyp
Strictures	

Table 23-4   Radiographic differences between Crohn's disease and ulcerative colitis

Crohn's Disease	Ulcerative Colitis
Deep ulcerations (often longitudinal and transverse)	Fine superficial ulcerations
Segmental lesions (skip lesions)	Continuous involvement (including rectum)
Strictures	Shortening of the bowel
Fistulas	Symmetric bowel contour
Cobblestone appearance of mucosa (caused by submucosal inflammation	Decreased mucosal pattern
	Pseudopolyp
"Thumbprinting" common	

4. In 5-10% of patients with IBD a clear distinction between ulcerative colitis and Crohn's disease cannot be made

Therapy

Medical therapy

1. Control of inflammatory process
    a. Avoid oral feedings during acute exacerbation to decrease colonic activity; a low-roughage diet may be helpful in *early* relapse
    b. Sulfasalazine[4] is effective in ulcerative colitis and in Crohn's disease confined to the colon; dosage is 500 mg PO bid initially, increased qd or qod by 1 g until therapeutic dosages of 4-6 g/day are achieved
    c. Steroids: methylprednisolone[28] or prednisone (e.g., prednisone 40-60 mg/day); steroid retention enemas may be useful in patients with ulcerative colitis limited to the rectum and accompanied by severe tenesmus
    d. Immunosuppressants (azathioprine, 6-mercaptopurine, cyclosporine) have been used in severe IBD refractory to above measures; however, their role has been questioned
    e. Mesalamine (5-aminosalicylic acid) enemas are as effective as corticosteroid enemas for treatment of mild to moderate distal ulcerative colitis; dosage is 4 g (60 ml) enemas at hs
2. Correction of nutritional deficiencies
    a. Correct existing electrolyte disorders, anemia, and vitamin deficiencies
    b. TPN with bowel rest may be necessary in severe cases
    c. Folate supplementation may reduce the incidence of dysplasia and cancer in chronic ulcerative colitis
3. Psychotherapy is very important because of the chronicity of the diseases and the relatively young age of the patients
4. Because of the increased risk of colon carcinoma, colonoscopic surveillance and multiple biopsies should be instituted approximately 10 yr after diagnosis in all patients with IBD
5. Treatment of complications
    a. Fulminant colitis or toxic megacolon (midtransverse colon $\geq$6 cm in diameter)
        (1) IV corticosteroids
        (2) Broad spectrum IV antibiotics (e.g., cefoxitin plus gentamicin)
        (3) Vigorous IV hydration, correction of any electrolyte abnormalities, and TPN
        (4) Nasogastric suction
        (5) Correct anemia and metabolic and nutritional abnormalities
        (6) Surgical intervention if there is no marked improvement with above measures
    b. Anal fistulas and other perineal diseases
        (1) IV metronidazole (Flagyl) 20 mg/kg/day in divided doses
        (2) Surgical repair
        (3) Extensive bowel resection if patient develops recurrent retrovaginal or rectovesicular fistulae

 c. Intestinal obstruction
  (1) Nasogastric suction
  (2) IV hydration
  (3) IV steroids and IV antibiotics
  (4) Surgical intervention if no improvement
 d. Abscess formation
  (1) IV antibiotics
  (2) IV steroids
  (3) IV hydration

Surgical therapy

Surgery is indicated in patients with ulcerative colitis who fail to respond to intensive medical therapy. Colectomy is usually curative in these patients and it also eliminates the high risk of developing adenocarcinoma of the colon (10-20% of patients develop it after 10 yr with the disease). Newer surgical techniques allow for preservation of the sphincter. In Crohn's disease, surgery is generally not curative (postoperative recurrence rate >50%); therefore it is generally reserved for treatment of severe complications (e.g., intractable recurrent rectovaginal, rectovesicular fistulae or intractable obstruction).

 DIARRHEA

Definition

Diarrhea is said to exist when the patient has frequent passage of loose or watery stools.

Diagnostic approach to new-onset diarrhea

History

1. Travel history (traveler's diarrhea)
 a. Recent travel to areas or countries with poor sanitation: consider toxigenic and invasive *E. coli*, parasites *(Giardia, Entamoeba histolytica)*
 b. See Table 23-5 for causes of acute bacterial diarrheas and Table 23-6 for clues to common parasitic diarrheas
 c. Outdoor living in wilderness areas with ingestion of water from streams: consider *Giardia* (particularly in Rocky Mountains region)
 d. *Yersinia enterocolitica* is found predominantly in cooler geographic areas (e.g., Canada)
2. Temporal characteristics
 a. Duration of diarrhea: diarrhea of short duration (1-3 days) associated with mild symptoms is usually of viral etiology (rotavirus, Norwalk agent); diarrhea lasting longer than 3 wk is unlikely to be bacterial
 b. Time of day: nocturnal diarrhea is common with diabetic neuropathy
 c. Relationship to meals
  (1) Sudden onset within hours after a particular meal: consider diarrhea secondary to toxins *(Staphylococcus aureus,* toxigenic *E.*

    coli, Clostridium perfringens, Bacillus cereus, Vibrio parahae-molyticus)

    (2) Diarrhea secondary to *Salmonella, Shigella, Campylobacter,* and *Yersinia* has a longer incubation period

  d. Related to stress: consider "functional" diarrhea

  e. Diarrhea alternating with constipation: consider irritable bowel syndrome (IBS)

3. Diet
   a. Ingestion of foods containing sorbitol or mannitol may cause osmotic diarrhea
   b. Diarrhea following ingestion of dairy food products may be caused by lactose intolerance
   c. Shellfish ingestion: Norwalk agent, *Vibrio cholerae, V. mimicus, V. parahaemolyticus, Plesiomonas shigelloides*
   d. Chinese food: *Bacillus cereus*
   e. Undercooked hamburger: *E. coli* serotype 0157:H7

4. Activities
   a. Long distance runners may experience bloody diarrhea secondary to bowel ischemia
   b. Institutionalized patients have a higher incidence of bacterial and parasitic infections

5. Medications
   a. Almost any drug can cause diarrhea; following is a list of the commonly used agents that may:
      (1) Magnesium-containing antacids
      (2) Methylxanthines (caffeine, theophylline)
      (3) Laxatives
      (4) Lactulose
      (5) Colchicine
      (6) Quinidine, digitalis, propranolol, and other antidysrhythmic agents
      (7) Nutritional supplements
      (8) Chenodiol (Chenix)
      (9) Artificial sweeteners (sorbitol, mannitol)
   b. Antibiotic—induced pseudomembranous colitis should be suspected in any patient receiving antibiotics: a positive test for *C. difficile* toxin confirms the diagnosis

6. Sexual habits: male homosexuals have a high incidence of bacterial and parasitic intestinal infections (e.g., *Giardia lamblia, Entamoeba histolytica,*[27] *Cryptosporidium, Salmonella, Neisseria gonorrhoeae, Campylobacter*)

7. Relevant medical history
   a. Surgical history (ileal resection, gastrectomy, cholecystectomy)
   b. Abdominal irradiation
   c. Diabetes mellitus
   d. Hyperthyroidism
   e. Watery diarrhea in an elderly patient with chronic constipation may be caused by fecal impaction or obstructing carcinoma
   f. AIDS: *Cryptosporidium, Salmonella,* CMV, *Mycobacterium intra-*

Table 23-5 Acute bacterial diarrheas

	S. aureus	C. perfringens	Enterotoxigenic E. coli	V. cholerae	Salmonella (nontyphoid)	Shigella	Campylobacter fetus ssp jejuni
Stool volume	Moderate to large	Moderate	Moderate to large	Large	Variable	Variable	Small to moderate
Blood	−	−	−	−	±	−	71%
Fecal WBCs	−	−	−	−	85%	51%	87%
Vomiting	++	±	±	−	−	69%-91%	29%
Fever	−	−	Low-grade	−	+	+	57%
Abdominal pain	−	+	+	−	+	+	86%
Rapid diagnosis*	−	−	−	−	−	≅	Dark-field microscopy or fuchsin stain
Incubation period	2-4 hr	12-16 hr	1-2 wk	6 hr-5 days	6-24 hr	24-48 hr	2-11 days
Duration of illness†	Few hours	Few hours	3-7 days	4-5 days	1-7 days	4 days-2 wk	4-5 days
Duration of shedding†	−	−	−	−	Variable	Variable	Few days to 7 wk

	Food	Meat, poultry	Food, water	Water	Food, animals, humans	Fecal-oral	Food, pets, humans
Mode of transmission	Food	Meat, poultry	Food, water	Water	Food, animals, humans	Fecal-oral	Food, pets, humans
Enterotoxin	+	+	+	+	±	–	Role in disease is unclear
Therapy*	Supportive	Supportive	Bismuth subsalicylate; tetracycline may be helpful	Supportive	Contraindicated except in life-threatening cases	Ampicillin or trimethoprim-sulfamethoxazole or ciprofloxacin	Erythromycin or ciprofloxacin
Comments		Generally mild illness	History of recent travel is suggestive	Very high stool volume; rare in children <1 year old	Generally mild illness	Peripheral differential WBC count may show increased band: segmented ratio	Reactive arthritis may occur, especially associated with HLA-B27 antigen

Modified from Appenheimer AT: Primary Care Emergency Decisions, p 21, September 1985.
*Within first few hours of presentation.
†In untreated cases.

Table 23-6 Clues to common parasitic diarrheas

	Organism	
	Giardia	*E. histolytica*
Stool volume	Variable	Small to moderate
Stool consistency	Bulky, foul-smelling	Watery and mild to explosive and purulent
Blood	–	39%
Fecal WBCs	–	7%
Vomiting	Nausea	–
Fever	–	Low-grade
Abdominal symptoms	Distention, cramps, flatulence	Pain
Rapid diagnosis*	Stool exam†	Stool exam†
Incubation	Unknown	Unknown
Duration	Weeks	Weeks-years
Duration of shedding (if untreated)	Prolonged	Years
Transmission	Water, humans	Fecal-oral
Enterotoxin	–	–
Therapy	In adults, quinacrine or metronidazole, in children furazolidone	Metronidazole and diiodohydroxyquin
Comments	Malabsorption is common	Proctoscopy may be necessary for diagnosis

Modified from Appenheimer AT: Primary Care Emergency Decisions, p 21, September 1985.
*Within first few hours of presentation.
†High incidence of false-negatives.

cellulare avium (MIA), Kaposi's sarcoma involving the gut, AIDS enteropathy
   g. History of laxative abuse (patient may deny)
8. Associated symptoms
   a. Tenderness, fever, weight loss (inflammatory bowel disease)
   b. Abdominal pain and significant weight loss (carcinoma of pancreas or other malignancies)
   c. Weight loss despite good appetite (malabsorption, hyperthyroidism)
   d. Diarrhea and PUD (Zollinger-Ellison syndrome, gastrinoma)
   e. Flushing and bronchospasm (carcinoid syndrome)
   f. LLQ pain, fever +/− bloody diarrhea (diverticulitis)
9. Characteristics of the stool (from patient's history)
   a. Large, foul smelling (malabsorption)
   b. Increased mucus (irritable bowel syndrome)
   c. Watery stools (psychosomal disturbances, fecal impaction, colon carcinoma, IBD, pancreatic cholera [VIP])

Physical exam

1. Rectal fistulas, RLQ abdominal mass (Crohn's disease)
2. Arthritis, iritis, uveitis, erythema nodosum (IBD)
3. Abdominal masses (neoplasms of colon, pancreas, or liver, diverticular abscess [LLQ mass], IBD)
4. Flushing, bronchospasm (carcinoid syndrome)
5. Buccal pigmentation (Peutz-Jeghers syndrome)
6. Increased pigmentation (Addison's disease)
7. Ammoniacal or urinary breath odor (renal failure)
8. Ecchymosis (vitamin K deficiency secondary to malabsorption of fat soluble vitamins)
9. Fever (IBD, infectious diarrhea)
10. Goiter, tremor, tachycardia (hyperthyroidism)
11. Lymphadenopathy (neoplasm, lymphoma, TB)
12. Macroglossia (amyloidosis)
13. Kaposi's sarcoma (AIDS)

Initial evaluation

1. Lab tests
   a. CBC: markedly increased WBC with "shift to left" may indicate infectious process; decreased hemoglobin/hematocrit may indicate anemia from blood loss, increased hematocrit, dehydration
   b. Serum electrolytes: decreased potassium from diarrhea, increased sodium from dehydration
   c. BUN, creatine: indicated if physical exam shows evidence of significant dehydration
   d. pH: hyperchloremic acidosis may be present
   e. Stool sample
      (1) Occult blood (positive in IBD, bowel ischemia, some bacterial infections)
      (2) Löffler's alkaline methylene blue stain for fecal leukocytes (positive in inflammatory diarrhea caused by *Salmonella, Campylobacter, Yersinia*)

(3) Bacterial cultures and sensitivity *(Salmonella, Shigella, Campylobacter, Yersinia);* cultures for *Neisseria gonorrhoeae* in active homosexual patients

(4) Ova and parasites, stool examination; indirect hemagglutination test for *E. histolytica* is useful when suspecting amebiasis and stool examination is inconclusive

(5) *Clostridium difficile* toxin assay to rule out pseudomembranous colitis in patients receiving antibiotics; although associated with any antibiotic, it occurs most frequently with clindamycin, ampicillin, and cephalosporins

(6) Modified Ziehl-Nielsen stain or auramine stain in immunocompromised patients with suspected *Cryptosporidium* infection

2. Procedures
   a. Sigmoidoscopy (without cleansing enema) is indicated in patients with
      (1) Bloody diarrhea (sigmoidoscopy may reveal neoplasm, inflammatory changes caused by IBD, bacterial agents, or amebiasis)
      (2) Suspected antibiotic-induced pseudomembranous colitis (sigmoidoscopy will show raised white-yellow exudative plaques adherent to the colonic mucosa)
   b. Abdominal x-rays (flat plate and upright) are indicated in patients with abdominal pain or evidence of obstruction to rule out toxic megacolon and bowel ischemia; pancreatic calcifications are suggestive of pancreatic insufficiency

Initial treatment

1. NPO; fasting usually results in cessation of osmotic diarrhea
2. IV hydration
3. Correct electrolyte abnormalities
4. Discontinue possible causative agents (e.g., antacids containing magnesium, antibiotics)
5. Antiperistaltic agents (e.g., diphenoxylate) should be used with caution in patients suspected of having IBD or infectious diarrhea; loperamide (Imodium) or bismuth subsalicylate (Pepto-Bismol) may be helpful in mild diarrhea
6. If diarrhea persists and a bacterial or parasitic organism is identified, antibiotic therapy should be started
   a. *Giardia:* metronidazole 250 mg tid for 5-10 days
   b. *E. histolytica:* metronidazole 750 mg tid for 10 days
   c. *Shigella:* trimethoprim-sulfamethoxazole 160 mg and 800 mg, respectively, bid for 5 days or ciprofloxacin 500 mg bid for 10 days
   d. *Campylobacter:* erythromycin 250 mg qid for 5 days or ciprofloxacin 500 mg bid for 7 days
   e. *Clostridium difficile:* If diarrhea persists after other antibiotics have been discontinued, treat with either
      (1) Metronidazole 250 mg PO bid for 10-14 days
      (2) Vancomycin 125 mg PO qid for 10-14 days
   Cholestyramine 4 g PO qid for 10 days or bacitracin 25,000 U PO qid has also been reported effective but is not recommended as initial therapy

7. Traveler's diarrhea is best treated with the combination of sulfamethoxazole/trimethoprim (800 mg/160 mg) bid for 3 days and loperamide, 4 mg PO loading and 2 mg after each loose bowel (max or 16 mg/day).[15] Prevention of traveler's diarrhea can be achieved by careful selection of food and beverages and by using two tablets of bismuth subsalicylate qid (ac and hs) for periods up to 3 wk. Patients should be warned to avoid concomitant use of salicylate-containing products to minimize the occurrence of salicylate toxic effects.[17]

NOTE: Antibiotics are contraindicated in *Salmonella* infections unless caused by *S. typhosa* or the patient is septic. Empirical antibiotic therapy is generally not indicated for patients with acute diarrhea; however, the use of ciprofloxacin (before the results of stool cultures are known) may be appropriate in more severely ill patients with suspected bacterial enteric pathogens.[20]

Evaluation of patient with chronic or recurrent diarrhea

Etiology of chronic diarrhea

1. Drug-induced (including laxative abuse)
2. Irritable bowel syndrome
3. Inflammatory bowel disease
4. Lactose intolerance
5. Malabsorptive diseases (e.g., mucosal disease, pancreatic insufficiency, bacterial overgrowth)
6. Parasitic infections (giardiasis, amebiasis)
7. Functional diarrhea
8. Postsurgical (partial gastrectomy, ileal resection, cholecystectomy)
9. Endocrine disturbances
   a. Diabetes mellitus (decreased sympathetic input to the gut)
   b. Hyperthyroidism
   c. Addison's disease
   d. Gastrinoma (Zollinger-Ellison syndrome)
   e. Vipoma (pancreatic cholera)
   f. Carcinoid tumors (serotonin)
   g. Medullary carcinoma of thyroid (calcitonin)
10. Pelvic irradiation
11. Colonic carcinoma (e.g., villous adenoma)

Diagnosis

1. History, physical exam, and initial lab evaluation are the same as for new onset diarrhea
2. Additional lab evaluation
   a. Examine stool for presence of fat droplets (use Sudan III stain) and meat fibers, their presence indicates malabsorption
   b. If CBC shows macrocytic anemia, then obtain vitamin B_{12} and RBC folate levels to rule out megaloblastic anemia secondary to malabsorption
   c. Sodium hydroxide test for laxative-derived phenolphthalein should be done in patients suspected of laxative abuse

Obtain 24 hr stool collection and measure the following:

1. Volume (normal <250 ml/day); if increased, make patient NPO and observe effect on diarrhea
   a. Persistence of high volume indicates *secretory* diarrhea
   b. Decreased volume indicates *osmotic* diarrhea
2. pH; if less than 5.5, indicates carbohydrate malabsorption, thus *osmotic* diarrhea
3. Osmolality (normal <290 mOsm): if greater than 290 mOsm, indicates *osmotic* diarrhea
4. Electrolytes (Na^+, K^+); there are two methods to differentiate osmotic from secretory diarrhea based on stool electrolyte values:
   a. Multiply the sum of Na^+ and K^+ by 2 and compare with stool osmolality and serum osmolality

      If $2\times (Na^+ + K^+)$ = Measured stool osmolality, indicates *secretory* diarrhea

      If $2\times (Na^+ + K^+) + 25$ mmol/L < Measured serum osmolality, indicates *secretory* diarrhea
   b. Calculate the stool osmotic gap (OG)

      If stool osmolality $- 2\times (Na^+ + K^+) > 100$, indicates *osmotic* diarrhea

When all the above lab tests indicate malabsorption, additional work-up for malabsorption should proceed as indicated in Section 23.5

---

d. If Sudan stain is suggestive of malabsorption, additional lab exams indicative of malabsorption are: decreased serum albumin, carotene, cholesterol, calcium, and phosphate, and increased prothrombin time
e. 24 hr urine collection for 5-HIAA in patients with suspected carcinoid syndrome; serum gastrin level in patients suspected of Zollinger-Ellison syndrome
f. Define mechanism of diarrhea
   (1) Secretory diarrhea results from impaired absorption or excessive intestinal secretion of electrolytes (fecal fluid contains large amounts of electrolytes); following is a list of common causes of secretory diarrhea:
       (a) Enteric infections
       (b) Neoplasms of exocrine pancreas (VIP, GIP, secretin, glucagon)
       (c) Bile salt enteropathy
       (d) Villous adenoma
       (e) Inflammatory bowel disease
       (f) Carcinoid tumor
       (g) Celiac sprue
       (h) Ingestion of cathartic agents (e.g., phenolphthalein)

(2) Osmotic diarrhea results from impaired water absorption secondary to osmotic effect of nonabsorbable intraluminal molecules; following is a list of common causes of osmotic diarrhea:
   (a) Lactose and other disaccharide deficiencies
   (b) Drug induced (lactulose, sorbitol, sodium sulfate, antacids)
   (c) Postsurgical (gastrojejunostomy, vagotomy and pyloroplasty, intestinal resection)

23.5 MALABSORPTION SYNDROME

Definition

Malabsorption syndrome is defined as impaired intestinal absorption manifested by steatorrhea and various nutritional deficiencies.

Etiology

1. Pancreatic exocrine insufficiency
   a. Chronic pancreatitis
   b. Pancreatic resection
   c. Pancreatic carcinoma
   d. Cystic fibrosis
2. Mucosal absorptive defect
   a. Gluten-induced enteropathy (celiac disease)
   b. Tropical spruce
   c. Whipple's disease
   d. Intestinal lymphangiectasia (lymphatic obstruction is also present)
   e. Lymphoma (lymphatic obstruction is also present)
   f. Amyloidosis
   g. Scleroderma
   h. Crohn's disease
   i. Intestinal resection (inadequate absorptive surface)
3. Bacterial proliferation in small bowel
   a. Afferent loop stasis (Billroth II subtotal gastrectomy)
   b. Blind loops, fistulas, strictures, multiple diverticula
   c. Diabetic neuropathy, hypothyroidism, vagotomy, and other causes of motor abnormalities
4. Other
   a. Endocrine and metabolic disorders (hyperthyroidism, carcinoid, vipoma, gastrinoma)
   b. Drugs (neomycin, cholestyramine)
   c. Liver disease, *Giardia* infection, disaccharide deficiency, abetalipoproteinemias

Signs and symptoms

1. Steatorrhea: foul-smelling, bulky, greasy stools
2. Diarrhea: often preceded by abdominal cramps
3. Malnutrition, weight loss
4. Excessive gas and bloating
5. Edema secondary to hypoalbuminemia
6. Generalized weakness, fatigue secondary to anemia (iron, folate, vitamin B_{12} deficiencies)

7. Neuropathy secondary to malabsorption of vitamin B group
8. Pathologic fractures secondary to decreased calcium and vitamin D
9. Ecchymoses secondary to vitamin K deficiency

Lab results

1. Decreased serum albumin, serum carotene, and serum cholesterol
2. Decreased serum calcium and serum phosphorus
3. Increased prothrombin time
4. Decreased hemoglobin/hematocrit, increased MCV, decreased vitamin B_{12}, RBC folate, and serum iron

Diagnostic studies

1. History of recurrent pancreatitis or evidence of pancreatic calcifications on abdominal x-ray suggests pancreatic insufficiency
2. An x-ray of the small bowel is useful in the initial evaluation of malabsorption; the classic finding in malabsorption is a nonspecific segmentation of barium in the small bowel (moulage sign); a small bowel series can also detect intestinal fistulas, multiple diverticuli, motility problems, and other contributing factors to bacterial overgrowth
3. Bentiromide (Chymex) test[52]: bentiromide is a synthetic peptide attached to PABA; chymotrypsin separates bentiromide from PABA, and a by-product of the latter is excreted in the urine as arylamine; decreased arylamine urinary excretion following ingestion of bentiromide is suggestive of pancreatic insufficiency (chymotrypsin deficiency)
4. Serum trypsin-like immunoreactivity test shows decreased immunoreactivity in pancreatic insufficiency

   The diagnosis of pancreatic insufficiency can be confirmed by adding pancreatic extract preparations (e.g., pancrease) to the patient's meals. A repeat 72 hr stool examination for fat (on an 80 g fat/day diet) will demonstrate increased fat absorption.

Treatment

The therapeutic approach varies with the etiology of the malabsorption.

1. Pancreatic insufficiency is treated by adding pancreatic extract and sodium bicarbonate to the patient's diet
2. Intestinal bacterial overgrowth is treated with broad-spectrum antibiotics (tetracycline, ampicillin) and surgical repair of strictures or other lesions causing stasis
3. In mucosal abnormalities, treat the specific disorder (e.g., antibiotic therapy for Whipple's disease; gluten-free diet [no wheat, barley, or oat grain] in patients with celiac disease)

Additional lab evaluation (Fig. 23-2)

1. Examine stool for fat droplets (use Sudan III stain) and meat fibers; their presence indicates malabsorption
2. Quantitate the degree of steatorrhea with a 72 hr fecal fat measurement on a diet of 80 g fat/day
   a. Normal excretion is ≤6 g fat/24 hr (>95% absorption)
   b. Excretion of more than 6 g fat/day indicates malabsorption

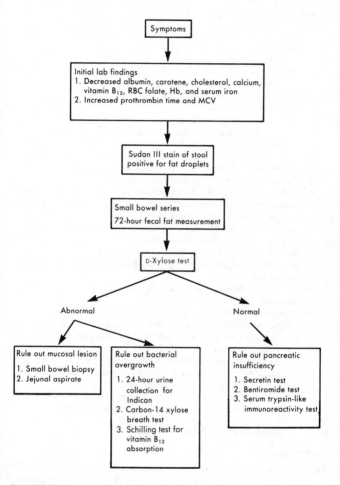

Figure 23-2
Diagnostic approach to malabsorption.

3. Perform a D-xylose absorption test to determine if the malabsorption is due to a mucosal lesion; a 5-hour urine xylose excretion less than 4.5 g following ingestion of 25 g of D-xylose indicates mucosal disease or bacterial overgrowth
4. Further define the mucosal lesion with a small bowel biopsy
   a. Following is a list of mucosal abnormalities identifiable with small bowel biopsy.
      (1) Celiac and tropical sprue
      (2) Whipple's disease
      (3) Lymphoma
      (4) Intestinal parasites
      (5) Amyloidosis
      (6) Eosinophilic gastroenteritis
      (7) Other: intestinal lymphangiectasia, abetalipoproteinemias, systemic mastocytosis, agammaglobulinemia, collagenous sprue
   b. A jejunal aspirate should be obtained at the time of biopsy and examined for the presence of intestinal parasites *(Giardia)*
5. Useful tests in suspected bacterial overgrowth are:
   a. 24-hour urine collection for Indican (by-product of the action of intestinal bacteria on tryptophan); increased 24-hour Indican excretion is suggestive of bacterial overgrowth
   b. Carbon-14 xylose or carbon-14 glycocolate breath test; elevated level is suggestive of bacterial overgrowth
   c. Schilling test (see Fig. 24-1) demonstrating vitamin B_{12} malabsorption with subsequent correction after tetracycline or ampicillin administration
6. If the D-xylose absorption test is normal, pancreatic insufficiency should be suspected
7. Secretin test is useful to document pancreatic insufficiency
   a. Under fluoroscopic guidance, a tube is placed in the second part of the duodenum and pancreatic secretions are collected
   b. The patient is then given an IV dose of secretin (pancreatic secretagogue) and pancreatic secretions are again measured
   c. Pancreatic exocrine deficiency is proven by a decreased total pancreatic fluid output and decreased bicarbonate secretion
   d. This test is very sensitive and specific for pancreatic insufficiency, but it is invasive and requires excellent patient cooperation

23.6   POLYPOSIS SYNDROMES

Definition

Polyposis is a hereditary syndrome characterized by multiple colonic adenomas and is further subdivided by the presence or absence of extracolonic signs.[32]

Clinical importance

The identification of colonic adenomatous polyps is extremely important because there is evidence that adenomatous tissue can transform into colorectal cancer. The chance of a polyp's becoming cancerous depends on

1. The histologic type: villous adenoma carries the highest malignant potential; incidence of malignant degeneration can be found in up to 60% of villous adenomas at the time of diagnosis
2. Size of the polyp: 1-2 cm polyps have a 5-10% incidence of malignancy; the malignant potential increases to 10-40% for polyps larger than 2 cm

Characteristics and classification

Table 23-7 compares the characteristics of the various types of polyps. Familial adenomatous polyposis coli is a syndrome defined as the presence of > 100 adenomatous polyps in the colon by the end of the third decade of life. Genetic analysis has localized the gene responsible for this condition to the long arm of chromosome 5.[29] Table 23-8 describes the major inherited gastrointestinal polyposis syndromes. The risk of colon cancer varies with each syndrome. It is very high in patients with Gardner's syndrome and Turcot's syndrome, and in familial polyposis it approaches nearly 100% by the age of 40.

Identification and treatment

Patients with polyposis syndromes should be regularly examined for colon carcinoma, beginning in the second decade of life. The exams should consist of biannual fecal occult blood test, an annual sigmoidoscopy, and colonoscopy every 1 to 3 years (depending on the age of the patient). Asymptomatic carriers of the familial polyposis genotype can be identified by the presence of increased levels of ornithine decarboxylase in biopsy specimens of colonic mucosa.[31] Sulindac (Clinoril) has been reported to cause both regression and suppression of colorectal polyps in patients with familial polyposis coli and Gardner's syndrome.[53] Surgical treatment varies from total colectomy and ileostomy to subtotal colectomy with regular endoscopic rectal exams. The latter is preferred by the majority of patients because it enables them to have normal bowel movements. However, the rate of carcinoma recurring in the rectal stump is extremely high and many surgeons prefer total colectomy.

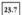 **CARCINOMA OF THE COLON**

Risk factors

1. Hereditary polyposis syndromes
   a. Familial polyposis (high risk)
   b. Gardner's syndrome (high risk)
   c. Turcot's syndrome (high risk)
   d. Peutz-Jeghers syndrome (low-moderate risk)
2. Inflammatory bowel disease, both ulcerative colitis and Crohn's disease
3. Family history of "cancer family syndrome"
4. Heredofamilial breast cancer and colon carcinoma
5. History of previous colorectal carcinoma
6. Women undergoing irradiation for gynecological cancer
7. First-degree relatives with colorectal carcinoma
8. Age over 40

Table 23-7   Comparison of polyp types

	Juvenile	Peutz-Jeghers	Hyperplastic	Hyperplastic Adenomatous	Adenomatous
Size (cm)	0.1 to 3.0	0.1 to 3.0	Range from several microscopic crypts to 0.5	0.3 to 3.0+	Unicryptal to 100+
Sessile	±	±	+	+	+
Pedunculated	+	+	±*	+	+
Gland architecture	Disorganized	Disorganized	Organized	Organized	Tubular, villous, mixed
Relation to cancer	±	±	−	?	+
Polyposis syndrome	+	+	−	?	+

Modified from Fenoglio-Preiser CM, Hutter RVP: CA 35:338, 1985.

KEY: +, Present; −, absent; ±, sometimes present.

*Predunculated lesions have been described, but the figures suggest that they are mixed hyperplastic adenomatous polyps.

Table 23-8 Multiple polyposis syndromes

Location	FP	GS	TS	JPC	CCS	GJP	PJS	CD
Esophagus	–	–	–	–	–	–	–	+
Small intestine	+	+	–	–	+	+	+++	+
Colon-rectum	+++	+++	+++	+	+++	+++	++	+
Nose	–	–	–	–	–	–	+	
Bronchi	–	–	–	–	–	–	+	
Urinary system	–	–	–	–	–	–	+	
Polyp type	A	A	A	J	J	J	H	H
Present at birth	±	±	±	+	+	+	+	+
Extraintestinal manifestations	None	Epidermoid cysts Fibromas Dental abnormalities Osteomas Lymphoid polyps Gastric manifestations Abdominal desmoids Retroperitoneal fibrosis Thyroid, adrenal carcinoma Duodenal carcinoma	Medulloblastoma Glioblastoma Ependymoma Cancer of thyroid				Gonadal stromal tumors Mucocutaneous pigmentation Endocervical lesions	Congenital anomalies Thyroid tumors Breast hypertrophy

From Fenoglio-Preiser CM, Hutter RVP: CA 35:338, 1985.

KEY: FP, Familial polyposis, GS, Gardner's syndrome; TS, Turcot's syndrome; CD, Cowden's disease; JPC, juvenile polyposis coli; CCS, Cronkhite-Canada syndrome; GJP, generalized juvenile polyposis; PJS, Peutz-Jeghers syndrome; A, adenomatous polyp; J, juvenile polyp; H, hamartomatous polyp

9. Possible dietary factors (high fat or meat diet, beer drinking, reduced vegetable consumption)

Distribution

1. 70%-75%
   a. Rectosigmoid and rectum (30-33%)
   b. Descending colon (40-42%)
2. 25%-30%
   a. Transverse colon (10-13%)
   b. Cecum and ascending colon (25-30%)
3. 50% of rectal cancers are within reach of the examiner's finger
4. 50% of colon cancers are within reach of the flexible sigmoidoscope

Clinical presentation

Initially vague and nonspecific (weight loss, anorexia, malaise). It is useful to divide colon cancer symptoms into those commonly associated with the right colon and those commonly associated with the left colon since the clinical presentation varies with the location of the carcinoma.

1. Right colon
   a. Anemia (iron deficiency secondary to chronic blood loss)
   b. Dull, vague, uncharacteristic abdominal pain may be present or patient may be completely asymptomatic
   c. Rectal bleeding is often missed because blood is admixed with feces
   d. Obstruction and constipation are unusual because of large lumen and more liquid stools
2. Left colon
   a. Change in bowel habits (constipation, diarrhea, tenesmus, pencil-thin stools)
   b. Rectal bleeding (bright red blood coating the surface of the stool)
   c. Intestinal obstruction is frequent because of small lumen

Physical exam

1. May be completely unremarkable
2. Digital rectal exam can detect approximately 50% of rectal cancers
3. Palpable abdominal masses indicate metastases or complications of colorectal carcinoma (abscess, intussusception, volvulus)
4. Abdominal distention and tenderness are suggestive of colonic obstruction
5. Hepatomegaly is indicative of hepatic metastases

Staging and prognosis (Table 23-9)

Diagnosis

Early identification of patients with surgically curable disease (Dukes' A,B) is necessary since survival is directly related to the stage of the carcinoma at the time of diagnosis (see Table 23-9). The suggested screening intervals for colorectal cancer in the general population are described in Chapter 4. An asymptomatic patient age 45 or older with a positive Hemoccult II test has a 1 in 10 chance of having colorectal carcinoma and a 1 in 3 chance of having either a colorectal carcinoma or a polyp; the same patient

Table 23-9   Staging of colon cancers: Dukes' classification (modified)

Stage	Tumor Involvement	Approximate 5 yr Survival
A	Confined to mucosa	80%
B_1	Confined to muscularis	66%
B_2	Penetrates the muscularis	50-54%
C_1	Confined to bowel wall	30-43%
C_2	Penetrates the bowel wall	15-22%
D	Distant metastases	0-14%

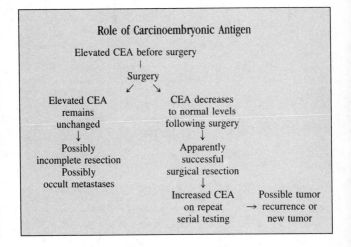

Role of Carcinoembryonic Antigen

Elevated CEA before surgery

Surgery

Elevated CEA remains unchanged
↓
Possibly incomplete resection
Possibly occult metastases

CEA decreases to normal levels following surgery
↓
Apparently successful surgical resection
↓
Increased CEA on repeat serial testing → Possible tumor recurrence or new tumor

with a negative Hemoccult test has a 0.2% chance of having a colorectal carcinoma diagnosed within 2 yr of testing and a 0.7% chance of having a polyp[1] (refer to Fig. 23-3 for evaluation of the patient with positive fecal occult blood)

Therapy

1. Surgical resection
2. Radiation therapy is a useful adjunct for rectal and anal carcinoma
3. Adjuvant chemotherapy with combination of 5-fluorouracil (5-FU) and levamisole (an antihelminthic) has been reported to improve survival in a patient with Dukes' Stage C colon cancer[34]

Follow-up

1. Fecal occult blood testing every 6 mo for 4 yr, then yearly

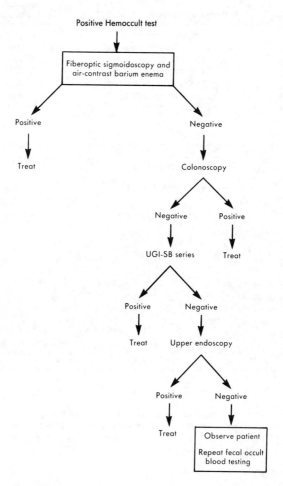

Figure 23-3
Evaluation of asymptomatic patients with positive fecal occult blood.

2. Colonoscopy yearly for initial 2 yr, then every 3 yr
3. CEA levels

Role of carcinoembryonic antigen[19]

1. CEA should not be used as a screening test for colorectal cancer since it can be elevated in many other conditions (smoking, IBD, alcoholic liver disease)
2. A normal CEA level does not exclude the diagnosis of colorectal cancer
3. A baseline CEA level is indicated in all patients with colorectal cancer since it can be used postoperatively as a measure of completeness of tumor resection or to monitor tumor recurrence; if used to monitor tumor recurrence, CEA should be obtained every 2 mo for 2 yr, then every 4 mo for 2 yr, and then yearly

23.8 DIVERTICULAR DISEASE

Definition

Colonic diverticula are herniations of mucosa and submucosa through the muscularis. They are generally found along the colon's mesenteric border at the site where the vasa recta penetrate the muscle wall (anatomic weak point).

Characteristics

1. More common in elderly patients (incidence increases with age)
2. Found most commonly in sigmoid colon (area of highest intraluminal pressure)
3. Increased incidence in western nations is believed to be secondary to low intake of dietary fiber, which results in lessened fecal bulk, narrowing of colonic lumen, increased intraluminal pressure, and evagination of colonic mucosa and submucosa through anatomically weak areas

Clinical manifestations[3]

1. Diverticulosis: asymptomatic presence of multiple colonic diverticula
   a. Physical exam is generally normal
   b. Usually discovered as an incidental finding on barium enema
   c. No specific treatment, high-fiber diet is helpful
2. Painful diverticular disease: caused by distortion of the colonic lumen secondary to muscular hypertrophy
   a. Usual complaint is LLQ pain, often relieved by defecation
   b. Constipation is common; it often alternates with diarrhea
   c. Distinguished from diverticulitis by absence of fever, leukocytosis, or other evidence of peritoneal inflammation
   d. Barium enema will demonstrate multiple diverticula and muscle spasm ("saw-tooth" appearance of the lumen)
   e. Treatment consists of high-fiber diet; bulk laxatives (e.g., psyllium preparations) are helpful in most patients
3. Diverticulitis: inflammatory process or localized perforation of diverticulum

    a. Main clinical features are fever and LLQ pain

    b. Digital rectal exam reveals muscle spasm, guarding, and rebound and significant tenderness

    c. Lab results reveal leukocytosis and left shift

    d. Diagnosis can be confirmed by barium enema (pericolonic mass, fistula, or stricture formation); barium enema can be hazardous and should not be performed in the acute stage because it may produce free perforation

    e. A CT scan can also be used to diagnose acute diverticulitis; typical findings are evidence of inflammation outside the bowel wall, fistulas, or abscess formation

    f. Treatment of diverticulitis consists of

       (1) IV antibiotics

          (a) Ampicillin (to cover *Enterococcus*) in mild diverticulitis

          (b) In moderate to severe diverticulitis, gram-negative aerobes and *Bacteroides fragilis* should be aggressively covered (possible antibiotic choices are cefotetan, cefoxitin, or an aminoglycoside plus clindamycin or metronidazole)

       (2) Liquid diet and stool softener for mild disease; bowel rest for moderate to severe disease

       (3) Surgical treatment consists of resection of involved area and reanastomosis (if feasible), otherwise a diverting colostomy is performed and reanastomosis performed when the infection has been controlled; surgery should be considered in patients with:

          (a) Repeated episodes of diverticulitis

          (b) Poor response to full medical therapy

          (c) Abscess or fistula formation

          (d) Obstruction

          (e) Peritonitis

          (f) Immunocompromised patients[40]

4. Hemorrhage: 70% of diverticular bleeding occurs in the right colon[2]

    a. Bleeding is painless and stops spontaneously in the majority of patients; it is usually caused by erosion of a blood vessel by a fecalith present within the diverticular sac

    b. Medical therapy consists of blood replacement and correction of volume and any clotting abnormalities

    c. The bleeding site can be identified by:

       (1) Arteriography if the bleeding is faster than 1 ml/minute; advantages of arteriography are the possible infusion of vasopressin directly into the artery supplying the bleeding vessel[5] or selective arterial embolization

       (2) Technetium-99m sulfur colloid

       (3) Technetium-99m labeled RBC

       (4) Emergent colonoscopy after rapid cleansing of the colon with a nonabsorbable solution ingested by the patient or instilled into the stomach via nasogastric tube

    d. Surgical resection is necessary if bleeding does not stop spontaneously after administration of four to five units of packed RBC or recurs with severity within few days[25]

    e. BE may be therapeutic (stoppage of bleeding)

23.9 ACUTE PANCREATITIS

Etiology

1. In more than 90% of all cases:
   a. Biliary tract disease
   b. Alcohol
2. Drugs (thiazides, azathioprine, furosemide, sulfonamides, corticosteroids, tetracycline, estrogens, valproic acid, metronidazole, L-asparaginase, methyldopa, pentamidine, ethacrynic acid, procainamide)
3. Abdominal trauma
4. Surgery
5. ERCP
6. Infections (predominantly viral infections)
7. Peptic ulcer (penetrating duodenal ulcer)
8. Pancreas divisum (congenital failure to fuse of dorsal and ventral pancreas)
9. Idiopathic
10. Pregnancy
11. Vascular (vasculitis, ischemia)
12. Hyperlipoproteinemias (Types I, IV, V)
13. Hypercalcemia
14. Pancreatic carcinoma (primary or metastatic)
15. Renal failure
16. Hereditary pancreatitis
17. Occupational exposure to chemicals: methanol, cobalt, zinc, mercuric chloride, chlorinated naphthalenes, cadmium, cresol, lead
18. Other: scorpion bite, obstruction at ampullar region (neoplasm, duodenal diverticula, Crohn's disease), hypotensive shock

Diagnosis

History

1. History of alcohol abuse or recent abdominal trauma
2. Patient taking drugs that may cause pancreatitis
3. Any associated illnesses
   a. Cholelithiasis: possible impacted stone or passage of stone
   b. PUD: possible posterior penetrating ulcer
   c. Hyperlipoproteinemias, renal failure, and hypercalcemia all have an increased incidence of pancreatitis
4. History of recurrent abdominal pains
   a. Pancreatitis usually manifests with boring abdominal pain located in the epigastrium
      (1) The pain may be localized or radiate to back and RUQ
      (2) Partial relief is at times obtained by sitting forward
      (3) Nausea and vomiting are prominent symptoms
   b. Patients with pancreas divisum often have recurrent abdominal pain following ingestion of small amounts of alcohol

Differential diagnosis

1. PUD
2. Acute cholecystitis, biliary colic
3. High intestinal obstruction
4. Early acute appendicitis
5. Mesenteric vascular obstruction
6. DKA
7. Pneumonia (basilar)
8. MI (inferior wall)
9. Renal colic
10. Ruptured or dissecting aortic aneurysm

Physical exam

1. Epigastric tenderness and guarding
2. Hypoactive bowel sounds (secondary to ileus)
3. Tachycardia, shock (secondary to decreased intravascular volume)
4. Confusion (secondary to metabolic disturbances)
5. Fever
6. Tachycardia, decreased breath sounds (atelectasis, pleural effusions, ARDS)
7. Jaundice (secondary to obstruction or compression of biliary tract)
8. Ascites (secondary to tear in pancreatic duct, leaking pseudocyst)
9. Palpable abdominal mass (pseudocyst, phlegmon, abscess, carcinoma)
10. Evidence of hypocalcemia (Chvostek's sign, Trousseau's sign)
11. Evidence of intraabdominal bleeding (hemorrhagic pancreatitis)
    a. Bluish discoloration around the umbilicus (Cullen's sign)
    b. Bluish discoloration involving the flanks (Grey-Turner sign)
12. Tender subcutaneous nodules (caused by subcutaneous fat necrosis)

Lab results

1. Pancreatic enzymes
   a. Amylase
      (1) Increased serum amylase: usually elevated in the initial 3-5 days of acute pancreatitis; normal serum amylase levels may be found in acute pancreatitis in:
         (a) Patients presenting 3-5 days after onset of symptoms
         (b) Hyperlipemia (will mask elevated amylase)
         (c) Up to 31% of cases of acute alcoholic pancreatitis[49]
         NOTE: Serum amylase is not specific for pancreatitis and may be elevated in other illnesses (salivary gland dysfunction, mesenteric infarction, diabetic ketoacidosis)
      (2) Isoamylase determination[27]: separation of pancreatic and salivary isoenzyme components of amylase is helpful in excluding occasional cases of salivary hyperamylasemia
      (3) Urinary amylase determinations
         (a) To diagnose acute pancreatitis in patients with lipemic serum
         (b) To rule out elevated serum amylase secondary to macroamylasemia
   b. Serum lipase levels are elevated in acute pancreatitis and the elevation is less transient than serum amylase; concomitant evaluation of serum amylase and lipase increases the diagnostic accuracy of acute pancreatitis[39]

   c. Elevated serum trypsin levels are diagnostic of pancreatitis (in absence of renal failure); measurement is made by radioimmunoassay (this test is not readily available in most labs)
1. Additional lab tests
   a. CBC
     (1) WBC: an increase may indicate sepsis or abscess
     (2) Hematocrit: initially increased secondary to hemoconcentration; decreased hematocrit may indicate hemorrhage or hemolysis (DIC)
   b. BUN: usually increased secondary to dehydration or renal impairment caused by pancreatitis
   c. Serum glucose: elevation in a previously normal patient correlates with the degree of pancreatic malfunction
   d. Liver profile
     (1) AST and LDH: increased secondary to tissue necrosis
     (2) Bilirubin and alkaline phosphatase: increased secondary to common bile duct obstruction
   e. Serum calcium: decreased secondary to saponification, precipitation, and decreased PTH response
   f. ABG
     (1) Pao_2: decreased secondary to ARDS, atelectasis, or pleural effusion
     (2) pH: decreased secondary to lactic acidosis, respiratory acidosis, and renal insufficiency
   g. Serum electrolytes
     (1) Potassium is increased secondary to acidosis or renal insufficiency
     (2) Sodium is increased because of dehydration

Radiographic evaluation of suspected acute pancreatitis

1. Abdominal plain film may reveal
   a. Localized ileus (sentinel loop)
   b. Pancreatic calcifications
   c. Blurring of left psoas shadow
   d. Dilation of transverse colon
   e. Calcified gallstones
2. Chest x-ray may reveal
   a. Elevation of one or both diaphragms
   b. Pleural effusion(s)
   c. Basilar infiltrates
   d. Plate-like atelectasis
3. Abdominal ultrasonography is useful in detecting gallstones and pancreatic pseudocysts; its major limitation is the presence of distended bowel loops overlying the pancreas
4. Computed tomography (CT) is superior to ultrasonography in identifying pancreatitis and defining its extent,[36] and it also plays a role in diagnosing pseudocysts (they appear as well-defined areas surrounded by a high-density capsule[37]); GI fistulation or infection of a pseudocyst can also be identified by the presence of gas within the pseudocyst[35]

Endoscopic retrograde cholangiopancreatography (ERCP)

The generally accepted indications for ERCP in pancreatitis are as follows:
1. Recurrent pancreatitis of unknown etiology
2. Preoperative planning in patients with chronic pancreatitis
3. Suspicion of pseudocyst not detected by sonography or CT scanning

NOTE: ERCP should not be performed during the acute stage of disease unless necessary to remove an impacted stone.

Determination of prognosis

When the illness is mild and self-limited with edema as the predominant inflammatory response, mortality is usually less than 5%.[8] Ranson[41] has listed the "early objective criteria" (see box, facing page) that permit early identification of the risk of major complications or death from acute pancreatitis. The mortality varies with the numbers of risk factors present:
1. Less than three risk factors: mortality is approximately 1%
2. Three to four risk factors: 15% mortality
3. Five to six risk factors: 40% mortality
4. More than seven risk factors: mortality approaches 100%

Treatment

General measures
1. Maintain adequate intravascular volume with vigorous IV hydration
2. NPO until the patient is clinically improved, stable, and hungry
3. Nasogastric suction is useful in severe pancreatitis to decompress the abdomen in patients with vomiting or ileus
4. Control pain: all analgesics may effect the sphincter of Oddi; meperidine (Demerol) is preferred because it produces less constriction of the sphincter
5. Correct metabolic abnormalities (e.g., replace calcium and magnesium if necessary)
6. TPN may be necessary in severe prolonged pancreatitis

Specific measures
1. IV antibiotics should not be used prophylactically; their use is justified if the patient has evidence of septicemia, pancreatic abscess, or pancreatitis secondary to biliary calculi
Appropriate antibiotic therapy should cover:
   a. *Bacteroides fragilis* and other anaerobes (cefotetan, cefoxitin, metronidazole, or clindamycin, plus aminoglycoside)
   b. *Enterococcus* (ampicillin)
2. Surgical therapy has a limited role in acute pancreatitis
   a. Gallstone-induced pancreatitis: cholecystectomy is indicated when the acute pancreatitis subsides
   b. Perforated peptic ulcer
   c. Excision or drainage of necrotic or infected foci
3. Identification and treatment of complications
   a. Pseudocyst[9]

Prognostic Signs in Acute Pancreatitis

At Admission or Diagnosis

Age >55 yr (70 for gallstones)
WBC >16,000/mm^3
Blood glucose >200 mg/dl
Serum LDH >350 IU/L
Aspartate aminotransferase (AST) >250 IU

During Initial 48 hr

Hematocrit fall >10%
BUN rise >5 mg/dl
Serum calcium level <8 mg/dl
Arterial oxygen pressure <60 mm Hg
Base deficit >4 mEq/L
Estimated fluid sequestration >6000 ml

From Ranson JHC: Am J Gastroenterol 77:633, 1982.

    (1) Definition: round or spheroid collection of fluid, tissue, pancreatic enzymes, and blood; it is distinct from adjacent structures
    (2) Diagnosis: CT scan or sonography
    (3) Therapy: CT scan or ultrasound-guided percutaneous drainage (with a pigtail catheter left in place for continuous drainage) has been used by some,[26] but the recurrence rate is high; the conservative approach is to reevaluate the pseudocyst (with CT scan or sonography) after 6-7 wk and surgically drain it if the pseudocyst has not decreased in size (pseudocysts ≥5 cm diameter have an increased incidence of perforation, hemorrhage, or infection)
  b. Phlegmon
    (1) It represents pancreatic edema
    (2) Diagnosis: CT scan or sonography
    (3) Treatment: general supportive measures; it usually resolves spontaneously
  c. Pancreatic abscess
    (1) Diagnosis: CT scan demonstrates presence of air bubbles in the retroperitoneum[18]; cultures of fluid obtained from percutaneous aspiration usually identify the bacterial organism
    (2) Therapy: surgical (or catheter) drainage and IV antibiotics
  d. Pancreatic ascites
    (1) Etiology: usually caused by leaking pseudocyst or tear in pancreatic duct; increased incidence is seen in pancreatitis secondary to trauma or alcohol
    (2) Diagnosis: paracentesis reveals very high amylase and lipase lev-

els in the pancreatic fluid; ERCP may demonstrate the lesion (e.g., ductal rupture)
    (3) Treatment: surgical correction may be necessary; exudative ascites from severe pancreatitis usually resolves spontaneously
  e. GI bleeding: caused by alcoholic gastritis, bleeding varices (secondary to cirrhosis or portal vein thrombosis following inflammation of tail of the pancreas), stress ulceration, or disseminated intravascular coagulation (DIC)
  f. Renal failure: caused by hypovolemia resulting in oliguria or anuria, cortical or tubular necrosis (shock, DIC), or thrombosis of renal artery or vein
  g. Hypoxemia: caused by ARDS, pleural effusion(s), or atelectasis

| 23.10 | **ACUTE VIRAL HEPATITIS** |

Etiology
Acute viral hepatitis may be caused by any of the following (Table 23-10):
1. Hepatitis A virus (HAV)
2. Hepatitis B virus (HBV)
3. Hepatitis non-A, non-B viruses (hepatitis C virus [HCV] and others)
4. Delta agent (needs HBV for replication)

Diagnostic criteria
1. History
  a. Blood transfusions: HCV hepatitis; hepatitis B (now rare since testing of blood for HBV)
  b. IV drug abuse: hepatitis B; HCV, HDV hepatitides
  c. Travel history to underdeveloped countries: hepatitis A
  d. Ingestion of raw shellfish: hepatitis A
  e. Contact with children attending a day care center: hepatitis A
  f. Exposure to others with hepatitis: hepatitis A
  g. History of hepatitis B: delta hepatitis
  h. Homosexuals: all types of hepatitis
2. Clinical manifestations
  a. Anorexia, nausea, vomiting
  b. Generalized malaise, fever, myalgias
  c. Loss of taste for cigarettes and food
  d. Diarrhea, abdominal pain
  e. Dark urine, light colored stool
  f. Pruritus
  g. Patient may be asymptomatic
3. Physical exam
  a. Jaundice
  b. Tender hepatomegaly
  c. Splenomegaly in 20% of cases
  d. Posterior cervical adenopathy (rare)
  e. Rash with HBV
  f. Arthritis (rare)
  g. Physical exam may be normal

Table 23-10   Selected features of four cases of viral hepatitis *

	Type A Hepatitis	Type B Hepatitis	Non-A, Non-B Hepatitis*	Delta Hepatitis
Virus	27 nm, RNA	42 nm, DNA	30-60 nm RNA 27, 34 nm RNA and others	35 nm, RNA core: delta Ag surface: HB_sAg
Antigens	HA Ag	HB_sAg, HB_cAg, HB_eAg	Not identifiable by assay	Delta Ag
Antibodies	Anti-HAV	Anti-HB_s, anti-HB_c, anti-HB_e	Anti-HCV for hepatitis C	Anti-delta
Spread	Fecal-oral	Parenterally and sexually	Parenterally and sexually for hepatitis C; another form (?hepatitis E) is transmitted by fecal-oral route	Parenteral
Mean incubation (range)	30 days (15 to 45)	75 days (40 to 180)	50 days (15 to 150)	40 days (30 to 50)
Onset	Abrupt	Insidious	Insidious	Often abrupt
Severity of acute bout	Usually mild	Often severe	Often mild	Often severe
Jaundice	50%	33%	20%	Unknown
Chronicity	None	5-10%	20-40%	Unknown
Recovery	99%	85-90%	Variable	Unknown
Mortality	0.1%	1-3%	1-12%	Unknown
Treatment	Supportive	Supportive	Supportive	Supportive
Prophylaxis	ISG	HBIG, hepatitis B vaccine	?ISG	Unknown

*The term non-A, non-B hepatitis is used to represent at least two other viruses (HCV and ? HEV).

Modified from Gass MA, Cianflocco AJ: Resid Staff Physician 31(4):17PC, 1985.

4. Lab results
    a. Liver profile
        (1) Greatly increased ALT and AST (>500 IU/L)
        (2) Increased bilirubin (both direct and indirect)
        (3) Moderately elevated alkaline phosphatase
    b. Prothrombin time (PT), glucose are usually normal; increased PT or decreased glucose indicate severe liver damage
    c. Serologic tests: the nomenclature of the various serologic tests for infectious hepatitis is described in Table 23-11; Table 23-12 summarizes the interpretation of these tests

Diagnoses

1. Acute hepatitis A is diagnosed by
    a. Detection of immunoglobulin M antibodies to hepatitis A virus (HAV-IgM) in patient's serum
2. Acute hepatitis B is diagnosed by
    a. Detection of HB_sAg or
    b. Anti-HB_c–IgM
    NOTE: Anti-HB_c is particularly useful as a serologic marker of acute hepatitis during the "core antibody window" period, when both HB_sAg and anti-HB_s may be negative (see Fig. 23-4).
3. Hepatitis C: detection of anti-HCV in the serum
4. Delta hepatitis is diagnosed by the presence of delta antigen or antibody to delta antigen (anti-HDV) in the patient's serum; it can cause either acute or chronic hepatitis[22]
    a. Acute delta hepatitis can occur in two forms:
        (1) Coinfection: simultaneous occurrence of acute hepatitis B and acute delta infection; diagnosis is confirmed by the presence of anti-HDV and IgM anti-HB_c (marker of acute hepatitis B)
        (2) Superinfection: occurrence of acute delta infection in a chronic HBV carrier; diagnosis is made by presence of anti-HDV and HB_sAg in the serum; IgM anti-HB_c will be absent
    b. Chronic delta hepatitis is diagnosed by the presence in the serum of sustained high titers of anti-HDV and HB_sAg; liver biopsy will confirm the diagnosis by demonstrating HDVAg in liver tissue

Treatment

1. General measures
    a. Avoidance of strenuous activity and ingestion of excessive amounts of hepatotoxic agents (e.g., ethanol, acetaminophen); patients should be instructed on possible infectivity to others
    b. Correct any metabolic abnormalities (e.g., dextrose solutions for hypoglycemia, vitamin K 10-15 mg SQ prn for elevated PT)
    c. Pruritus can be treated with diphenhydramine 50 mg PO/IM q6h and cholestyramine 4 g bid
    d. Metoclopramide 10 mg 30 min ac is useful for treatment of nausea or vomiting
    e. A balanced high-carbohydrate diet is recommended

Table 23-11 Hepatitis nomenclature

Abbreviation	Term	Comments
Hepatitis A		
HAV	Hepatitis A virus	Etiologic agent of "infectious" hepatitis; a picornavirus; single serotype
Anti-HAV	Antibody to HAV	Detectable at onset of symptoms; lifetime persistence
IgM anti-HAV	IgM class antibody to HAV	Indicates recent infection with hepatitis A; positive up to 4-6 mo after infection
IgG anti-HAV	IgG antibody to HAV	Remote infection with hepatitis A
Hepatitis B		
HBV	Hepatitis B virus	Etiologic agent of "serum" or "long-incubation" hepatitis; also known as Dane particle
HB_sAg	Hepatitis B surface antigen	Surface antigen(s) of HBV detectable in large quantity in serum; several subtypes identified
HB_eAg	Hepatitis B_e antigen	Soluble antigen; correlates with HBV replication, high titer HBV in serum, and infectivity of serum
HB_cAg	Hepatitis B core antigen	No commercial test available
Anti-HB_s	Antibody to HB_sAg	Indicates past infection with and immunity to HBV, passive antibody from HBIG, or immune response from HBV vaccine
Anti-HB_e	Antibody to HB_eAg	Presence in serum of HB_sAg carrier suggests lower titer of HBV
Anti-HB_c	Antibody to HB_cAg	Indicates past infection with HBV at some undefined time
IgM anti-HB_c	IgM class antibody to HB_cAg	Indicates recent infection with HBV; positive from 4-6 months after infection

Reproduced with modifications from Immunization Practices Advisory Committee, Centers for Disease Control: Ann Intern Med 103:391, 1985.

Continued.

Table 23-11 Hepatitis nomenclature—cont'd

Abbreviation	Term	Comments
Hepatitis C		
HCV	Hepatitis C virus	Predominant etiologic agent of tranfusion associated hepatitis
Anti-HCV	Antibody to HCV	Detectable by 22 wk after transfusion or 15 wk after onset of clinical hepatitis[4]
Delta hepatitis		
δ virus	Delta virus	Etiologic agent of delta hepatitis; may only cause infection in presence of HBV
δ-Ag	Delta antigen	Detectable in early acute delta infection
Anti-δ	Antibody to delta antigen	Indicates past or present infection with delta virus
Non-A Non-B Hepatitis		
NANB	Hepatitis C virus and others	At least two candidate viruses (hepatitis C virus and others); epidemiology parallels that of hepatitis B
Epidemic Non-A, Non-B Hepatitis		
Epidemic NANB	Epidemic non-A, non-B hepatitis	Causes large epidemics in Asia, North Africa; fecal-oral or waterborne (? hepatitis E virus)
Immune Globulins		
IG	Immune globulin (previously ISG, immune serum globulin, or gamma globulin)	Contains antibodies to HAV, lower titer antibodies to HBV
HBIG	Hepatitis B immune globulin	Contains high titer antibodies to HBV

Table 23-12 Interpretation of hepatitis profiles

IgM Anti-HAV	HB$_s$Ag	IgM Anti-HB$_c$	Anti-HB$_s$	HB$_e$Ag	Anti-HB$_e$	Anti-HDV	Interpretation
−	−	−	−	−	−	−	Clinical acute hepatitis may be caused by non-A, non-B hepatitis, other viral infection, or liver toxin
+	−	−	−	−	−	−	Acute type A hepatitis
−	+	−	−	+	−	−	Late incubation period or early acute type B hepatitis
−	+	+	−	+	−	−	Acute type B hepatitis with persistent viral replication (HB$_s$Ag+) and high degree of infectivity (HB$_e$Ag+)
−	+	+	−	−	+	−	Acute type B hepatitis with favorable prognosis for resolution (seroconversion of HB$_e$Ag to anti-HB$_e$)
−	−	+	−	−	−/+	−	Acute infection nearly resolved (core window)
−	−	+/−	+	−	−/+	−	Convalescent phase of type B hepatitis with recovery and immunity

Continued.

Modified from Sass MA, Cianflocco AJ: Resid Staff Physician 31(4):17PC, 1985.

Table 23-12 Interpretation of hepatitis profiles—cont'd

IgM Anti-HAV	HB$_s$Ag	IgM Anti-HB$_c$	Anti-HB$_s$	HB$_e$Ag	Anti-HB$_e$	Anti-HDV	Interpretation
−	−	−	+	−	−	−	Past type B hepatitis long before with recovery and immunity, passive transfer of antibody (HBIG), or hepatitis-B vaccine
−	+	+	−	+/−	−	+	Acute hepatitis B with acute delta coinfection
−	+	−	−	−	−	+	Chronic hepatitis B with acute delta superinfection
−	+	−	−	−	−	++	Chronic hepatitis B with chronic delta hepatitis

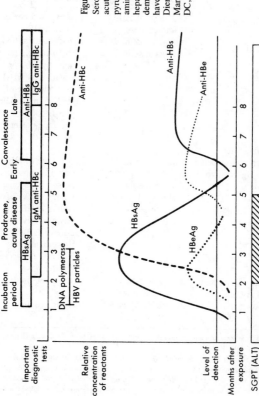

Figure 23-4
Serological and clinical patterns observed during acute HBV infection. (SGPT, Serum glutamic pyruvic transaminase; ALT, alanine aminotransferase.) Patients who do not resolve the hepatitis B infection (chronic carrier state) will demonstrate persistence of HBsAg and will not have an elevation of anti-HB$_s$. (From Hollinger FB, Dienstag JL: In Lennette EH, et al [editors]: Manual of clinical microbiology, ed 4, Washington DC, 1985, American Society for Microbiology.)

f. Hospitalization is rarely indicated except for severe volume depletion, encephalopathy, or intractable vomiting

2. Postexposure prophylaxis
    a. Hepatitis A: single IM dose of 0.02 ml/kg of immune globulin (IG)
    as soon as possible
    b. Hepatitis B: refer to Table 23-13 for recommendations after percuta-
    neous exposure
    c. Prophylaxis after sexual exposure to an HB$_s$Ag-positive partner is es-
    sentially the same as after percutaneous exposure and should be
    given within 14 days of sexual contact

Table 23-13   Recommendation for hepatitis B prophylaxis after
percutaneous exposure

Source	Exposed Person	
	Unvaccinated	Vaccinated
HB$_s$Ag positive	One dose of HBIG* immediately Initiate hepatitis B vaccine series†	Test exposed person for anti-HB$_s$ If inadequate antibody (<10 sample ratio units by RIA or negative by EIA), give one dose of HBIG* immediately plus hepatitis B vaccine booster dose
Known source High risk of being HB$_s$Ag positive	Initiate hepatitis B vaccine series† Test source for HB$_s$Ag; if positive, give one dose of HBIG* immediately	Test source of HB$_s$Ag only if exposed person is vaccine nonresponder; if source is HB$_s$Ag positive, give one dose of HBIG* immediately plus hepatitis B vaccine booster dose
Low risk of being HB$_s$Ag positive	Initiate hepatitis B vaccine series	Nothing required
Unknown source	Initiate hepatitis B vaccine series	Nothing required

Reproduced from Immunization Practices Advisory Committee, Centers for Disease Control: Ann
Intern Med 103:391, 1985.
*One dose of hepatitis B immune globulin (HBIG) is 0.06 ml/kg body weight IM. HB$_s$Ag,
hepatitis B surface antigen; RIA, radioimmunoassay; EIA, enzyme immunoassay; anti-HB$_s$Ag.
†Hepatitis B vaccine series is 20 µg IM for adults, 10 µg IM for infants or children under 10 yr
of age. The first dose is given within 1 wk of exposure, and the second and third doses, 1 and 6
mo later, respectively.

3. Preexposure prophylaxis for hepatitis B is recommended for IV drug users, prostitutes, homosexual/bisexual men, residents of correctional or long-term facilities, persons who have had multiple sex partners within the preceding 6 mo, persons seeking treatment for sexually transmitted disease, and health care workers[12]
   a. Both recombinant and plasma-derived vaccines are safe and effective; for dosage guidelines, refer to Table 23-13
   b. Prevaccination screening for antibody to hepatitis B is cost-effective only for groups at high risk of hepatitis B

Prognosis

1. Hepatitis A usually has a benign course, and virtually all previously healthy patients recover completely with no residual liver disease; fatalities can occur, but are rare
2. Approximately 10% of patients with hepatitis B develop a chronic carrier state
   a. Usually seen in patients with impaired immune response (e.g., immunosuppressive drugs, hemodialysis), infected neonates, and patients with a subclinical course (e.g., anicteric hepatitis)
   b. Chronic active hepatitis can develop into cirrhosis and is also associated with increased risk of hepatocellular carcinoma
3. Fulminant hepatic necrosis, manifested with hepatic encephalopathy, ascites, and severe prolongation of prothrombin time (>22 sec) is a rare complication of hepatitis B and less frequently non-A, non-B hepatitis; prognosis is poor; care is supportive only (e.g., control of bleeding, correction of hypoglycemia); liver transplantation may be indicated in otherwise healthy patients
4. Acute delta hepatitis coinfection is generally self-limited, whereas the majority of patients with acute delta superinfection develop chronic hepatitis with mortality rate of 5-20%
5. Use of alpha-interferon has resulted in improvement of liver function tests in patients with chronic hepatitis B, chronic hepatitis C, and delta hepatitis (while the drug is being used)

23.11 CIRRHOSIS

Etiology

1. Alcohol abuse
2. Secondary biliary cirrhosis, obstruction of common bile duct (stone, stricture, pancreatitis, neoplasm, sclerosing cholangitis)
3. Drugs (e.g., acetaminophen, isoniazid, methotrexate, methyldopa)
4. Hepatic congestion (e.g., CHF, constrictive pericarditis, tricuspid insufficiency, thrombosis of hepatic veins, obstruction to inferior vena cava)
5. Primary biliary cirrhosis
6. Hemochromatosis
7. Chronic active hepatitis
8. Wilson's disease
9. α-1-Antitrypsin deficiency

10. Infiltrative diseases (amyloidosis, glycogen-storage diseases, hemo-chromatosis)
11. Nutritional: jejunoileal bypass
12. Other: parasitic infections (schistosomiasis), idiopathic portal hypertension, congenital hepatic fibrosis, systemic mastocytosis, autoimmune chronic active hepatitis (lupoid hepatitis), hepatic steatosis

Diagnosis

History

1. Alcohol abuse: alcoholic liver disease
2. History of hepatitis B (chronic active hepatitis, primary hepatic neoplasm or hepatitis C)
3. History of inflammatory bowel disease (primary sclerosing cholangitis)
4. History of pruritus, hyperlipoproteinemia, and xanthomas in a middle-aged or elderly female (primary biliary cirrhosis)
5. Impotence, diabetes, hyperpigmentation (hemochromatosis), arthritis
6. Neurologic distrubances (Wilson's disease—hepatolenticular degeneration)
7. Family history of "liver disease" (hemochromatosis—positive family history in 25% of patients; α-1-antitrypsin deficiency)
8. History of recurrent episodes of RUQ pain (biliary tract disease)
9. History of blood transfusion (hepatitis C)
10. History of hepatotoxic drug exposure[30]

Physical exam

1. Skin: jaundice, palmar erythema (alcohol abuse), spider angiomata, ecchymosis (thrombocytopenia or coagulation factor deficiency), dilated superficial periumbilical veins (caput medusae), increased pigmentation (hemochromatosis), xanthomas (primary biliary cirrhosis), needle tracks (viral hepatitis)
2. Eyes: Kayser-Fleischer rings (corneal copper deposition seen in Wilson's disease, best diagnosed with slit-lamp exam), scleral icterus
3. Breath: fetor hepaticus (musty odor of breath and urine found in cirrhosis with hepatic failure)
4. Chest: gynecomastia in men may indicate chronic liver disease
5. Abdomen
   a. Tender hepatomegaly (congestive hepatomegaly)
   b. Small nodular liver (cirrhosis)
   c. Palpable, nontender gallbladder—Courvoisier's sign (neoplastic extrahepatic biliary obstruction)
   d. Palpable spleen (portal hypertension)
   e. Venous hum auscultated over periumbilical veins (portal hypertension)
   f. Ascites (portal hypertension, hypoalbuminemia)
6. Rectal exam
   a. Hemorrhoids (portal hypertension)
   b. Guaiac-positive stool (alcoholic gastritis, bleeding esophageal varices, PUD)

7. Genitalia: testicular atrophy in males (chronic liver disease)
8. Extremities
   a. Pedal edema (hypoalbuminemia, right-sided heart failure)
   b. Finger clubbing
9. Neurologic
   a. Flapping tremor—asterixis (hepatic encephalopathy)
   b. Choreoathetosis, dysarthria (Wilson's disease)

Lab results

1. Routine admission lab results
   a. Decreased hemoglobin/hematocrit (consider GI bleeding)
   b. Increased MCV (caused by RBC membrane abnormalities)
   c. Increased BUN, creatinine (prerenal azotemia, hepatorenal syndrome); the BUN can also be "normal" or low if the patient has severely diminished liver function
   d. Decreased sodium (dilutional hyponatremia)
   e. Decreased potassium (caused by secondary aldosteronism or urinary losses)
   f. Decreased glucose in a patient with liver disease indicates severe liver damage
2. Liver function studies[13]
   a. Serum transaminases
      (1) Alcoholic hepatitis and cirrhosis: mild elevations of ALT and AST, usually to <500 IU; AST > ALT (ratio >2:1)
      (2) Extrahepatic obstruction: moderate elevations of ALT and AST to levels <500 IU
      (3) Viral, toxic, or ischemic hepatitis: extreme elevations (>500 IU) of ALT and AST
      (4) Transaminases may be normal despite significant liver disease in patients with jejuno-ileal bypass operations, hemochromatosis, or following methotrexate injection
   b. Alkaline phosphatase is present in liver, bone, placenta, and intestine
      (1) Significant elevations of hepatic alkaline phosphatase occur in extrahepatic obstruction (calculi, strictures, neoplasm, pancreatitis), primary biliary cirrhosis, and primary sclerosing cholangitis
      (2) Measure serum 5'-nucleotidase or GGTP to determine if the elevated alkaline phosphatase is of hepatic origin; elevation of 5'-nucleotidase or GGTP implies a hepatobiliary source
      (3) A more reliable method to identify hepatic alkaline phosphatase is to fractionate the elevated alkaline phosphatase with polyacrylamide gel electrophoresis
   c. Serum lactate dehydrogenase (LDH) of hepatic origin (LDH$_5$ by isoenzyme determination) is significantly elevated in metastatic disease to the liver; lesser elevations are seen with hepatitis, cirrhosis, extrahepatic obstruction, and congestive hepatomegaly
   d. Serum γ-glutamyltranspeptidase (GGTP) is elevated in alcoholic liver disease but some heavy drinkers may not have GGTP elevation

  e. Serum bilirubin: refer to Section 6.21 for a listing of the major causes of conjugated and unconjugated hyperbilirubinemia
  f. Urine bilirubin: present in hepatitis, hepatocellular jaundice, and biliary obstruction
  g. Serum albumin: significant liver disease results in hypoalbuminemia; refer to Chapter 31 for a listing of the various causes of low serum albumin
  h. Prothrombin time (PT): reflects hepatic synthesis of Factors I, II, V, VII, X; an elevated PT in patients with liver disease indicates severe liver damage and poor prognosis; PT elevation may also be due to vitamin K deficiency secondary to cholestasis; in this case, parenteral administration of 10-15 mg of vitamin K will result in significant improvement (>30%) within 48 hr

3. Additional tests
  a. Presence of hepatitis B surface antigen (HB_sAg) implies acute or chronic active hepatitis B
  b. Presence of antimitochondrial antibody is suggestive of primary biliary cirrhosis or chronic active hepatitis
  c. Elevated serum copper, decreased serum ceruloplasmin, and elevated 24 hr urinary copper are diagnostic of Wilson's disease
  d. Protein immunoelectrophoresis
    (1) Decreased α-1-globulins (α-1 antitrypsin deficiency)
    (2) Increased IgA (alcoholic cirrhosis)
    (3) Increased IgM (primary biliary cirrhosis)
    (4) Increased IgG (chronic active hepatitis, cryptogenic cirrhosis)
  e. An elevated level of serum ferritin and increased transferrin saturation are suggestive of hemochromatosis
  f. An elevated blood ammonia level is suggestive of hepatocellular dysfunction; serial values are not useful in following patients with hepatic encephalopathy because there is poor correlation between blood ammonia level and the degree of hepatic encephalopathy[14]
  g. Serum cholesterol is elevated in cholestatic disorders
  h. Antinuclear antibodies (ANA): titers >1:150 may be found in autoimmune hepatitis
  i. Alpha-fetoprotein: levels >1000 pg/ml are highly suggestive of primary liver cell carcinoma
  j. Anti-HCV identifies patients with prior hepatitis C virus infection

Radiographic evaluation

1. Ultrasonography is the procedure of choice for detection of gallstones and dilation of common bile duct
2. CT scanning may be useful for
  a. Detecting mass lesions in liver and pancreas
  b. Assessing hepatic fat content[11]
  c. Identifying idiopathic hemochromatosis[23]
  d. Early diagnosis of Budd-Chiari syndrome[7]
  e. Dilation of intrahepatic bile ducts
3. Technetium-99m sulfur colloid scanning is useful for
  a. Diagnosing hepatic cirrhosis: there is a shift of colloid uptake to the spleen and sternal bone marrow

b. Identifying hepatic adenoma: "cold" defect is noted

c. Diagnosing of Budd-Chiari syndrome[50]: there is increased uptake by caudate lobe

4. Endoscopic retrograde cholangiopancreatography (ERCP) is the procedure of choice for diagnosing periampullary carcinoma and common duct stones[46]; it is also used for diagnosing primary sclerosing cholangitis

5. Percutaneous transhepatic cholangiography (PTC) is useful when evaluating patients with cholestatic jaundice and dilated intrahepatic ducts by ultrasonography[38]

6. Percutaneous liver biopsy is useful in

a. Evaluating hepatic filling defects

b. Undiagnosed hepatocellar disease/hepatomegaly

c. Persistently abnormal liver function tests

d. Diagnosing: hemochromatosis, primary biliary cirrhosis, Wilson disease, glycogen storage diseases, chronic hepatitis, type I Crigler-Najjar syndrome, infiltrative diseases (sarcoidosis, tuberculosis, amyloid), alcoholic liver disease, drug-induced liver disease, and primary or secondary carcinoma

Therapy

Eliminate causes of hepatic damage

1. Correct any mechanical obstruction to bile flow (e.g., calculi, strictures)

2. Avoid any hepatotoxins (e.g., ethanol); improve nutritional status

3. Therapy of underlying cardiovascular disorders in patients with cardiac cirrhosis

4. Remove excess body iron with phlebotomy and deferoxamine in patients with hemochromatosis

5. Remove copper deposits with D-penicillamine in patients with Wilson's disease

6. Liver transplantation may be indicated in otherwise healthy patients (age under 65) with sclerosing cholangitis, chronic hepatitis with cirrhosis, or primary biliary cirrhosis

Treatment of complications

1. Ascites: diagnostic paracentesis (see Chapter 30) may be necessary to exclude other disorders; Fig 23-5 describes the suggested management of ascites secondary to portal hypertension; total paracentesis plus IV albumin infusion to expand intravascular volume may be a convenient and cost-effective way to manage tense ascites refractory to fluid restriction and use of diuretics[51]; spontaneous bacterial peritonitis (SBP) is often associated with hepatic ascites; treatment of SBP is discussed in Section 25.13

2. Esophagogastric varices: bleeding is major cause of death in patients with cirrhosis and hypertension; following is a step-wise approach to management of bleeding esophageal varices:

a. Resuscitation (IV fluids and blood transfusion) and correction of any coagulation abnormalities (FFP)

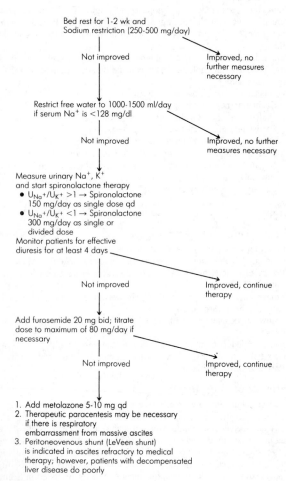

Bed rest for 1-2 wk and
Sodium restriction (250-500 mg/day)

Not improved → Improved, no further measures necessary

Restrict free water to 1000-1500 ml/day
if serum Na^+ is <128 mg/dl

Not improved → Improved, no further measures necessary

Measure urinary Na^+, K^+
and start spironolactone therapy
- U_{Na^+}/U_{K^+} >1 → Spironolactone 150 mg/day as single dose qd
- U_{Na^+}/U_{K^+} <1 → Spironolactone 300 mg/day as single or divided dose

Monitor patients for effective diuresis for at least 4 days

Not improved → Improved, continue therapy

Add furosemide 20 mg bid; titrate dose to maximum of 80 mg/day if necessary

Not improved → Improved, continue therapy

1. Add metolazone 5-10 mg qd
2. Therapeutic paracentesis may be necessary if there is respiratory embarrassment from massive ascites
3. Peritoneovenous shunt (LeVeen shunt) is indicated in ascites refractory to medical therapy; however, patients with decompensated liver disease do poorly

Figure 23-5
Algorithm for management of ascites secondary to portal hypertension.[43] Frequent monitoring of electrolytes, BUN, and creatinine is necessary.

b. IV vasopressin (see p. 287)

c. Emergency endoscopic sclerotherapy

d. Balloon tamponade (p. 287) may be necessary to control bleeding

e. Emergency mesocaval or selective distal portacaval or splenorenal shunt if above measures fail to stop bleeding

f. Beta blockers reduce portal pressure by decreasing cardiac output and splanchnic vasoconstriction; their use in prevention of initial or recurrent variceal bleeding remains controversial

NOTE: Endoscopic sclerotherapy should be undertaken even if bleeding is controlled with vasopressin or balloon tamponade because of the high recurrence rates of variceal hemorrhage when these measures are stopped.

Endoscopic sclerotherapy with surgical rescue for uncontrolled bleeding is the optimum therapy for patients with alcoholic cirrhosis and variceal bleeding. Survival is similar in non-alcoholic patients treated with either distal splenorenal shunt or endoscopic sclerotherapy, but shunting provides better control of variceal bleeding.[21]

3. Hepatic encephalopathy: abnormal mental status occurring in patients with severe impairment of liver function and consequent accumulation of toxic products not metabolized by the liver; management consists of

a. Identifying and treating precipitating causes (UGI bleeding, hypokalemia, hypomagnesemia, analgesic and sedative drugs, sepsis, alkalosis, increased dietary protein, and acute infections)

b. Reducing toxic protein metabolites
   (1) Restricting protein intake (30-40 g/day)
   (2) Reducing colonic ammonia production
      (a) Lactulose is a nonabsorbable synthetic disaccharide that acidifies the intestinal lumen; the increase in hydrogen ions facilitates the conversion of ammonia (NH_3) to ammonium (NH_4^+), which is then excreted in the stool; refer to Chapter 32 for dosage of lactulose
      (b) Neomycin is an antibiotic used to lower the concentration of urease-containing bacteria in the intestinal flora, thereby decreasing ammonia production; dosage is 1 g PO q4-6h or given as a 1% retention enema solution (1 g in 100 ml of isotonic saline)
      (c) A combination of lactulose and neomycin can be used when either agent is ineffective alone

c. Provide adequate calories to prevent protein catabolism

4. Hepatorenal syndrome (HRS) is a usually lethal complication of severe liver disease; it may occur following significant reduction of effective blood volume (e.g., paracentesis, GI bleeding, diuretics) or in the absence of any precipitating events; diagnosis is suspected when oliguria with concentrated urine and low urine sodium develop in a patient with severe liver disease; the hepatorenal syndrome must be differentiated from prerenal azotemia since renal function studies are similar in both conditions (urine sodium <10 mEq/L, U/P osm >1, U/P creatinine >30/1, usually normal renal sediment); acute tubular necrosis (ATN) must also be considered as a cause of renal failure; in patients with ATN urinary sodium excretion will be high and urinary osmolarity will be approximately 300 mOsm/kg; mortality exceeds 80% in HRS

HEPATIC FAILURE

Etiology

1. Progression of cirrhosis from any cause (see Section 23.11)
2. Drugs and toxins[30] (also refer to Table 23-14)

Isoniazid	Ethanol (males, 80 g/day for 10-20
Acetaminophen, diclofenac	yr; females, ?20-30 g/day
Halothane	[lower gastric alcohol dehydrog-
Valproic acid, phenytoin	enase activity] for 10-20 yr)
Methyldopa, labetalol	Carbon tetrachloride
Nitrofurantoin, sulfonamides	*Amanita phalloides* mushrooms
IV tetracycline	Vitamin A
Slow release nicotinic acid	Methotrexate, amiodarone

3. Acute fulminant viral hepatitis
4. Shock and/or sepsis
5. Reye's syndrome
6. Heat stroke
7. Metastatic carcinoma
8. Hepatocellular carcinoma
9. Sclerosing cholangitis
10. Fatty liver of pregnancy
11. Ischemic veno-occlusive disease (Budd-Chiari)
12. Autoimmune (steroid-responsive, [lupoid hepatitis])

Table 23-14   Examples of liver abnormalities secondary to adverse drug reactions*

Liver Abnormality	Agent
Acute hepatitis	Methyldopa, isoniazid, halothane
Acute necrosis	Carbon tetrachloride, acetaminophen
Cholestasis	
Canalicular	Sex hormones
Hepatocanalicular	Chlorpromazine, nitrofurantoin, erythromycin, azathioprine
Steatosis	
Microvesicular	Valproic acid, isoniazid
Macrovesicular	Methotrexate
Alcoholic hepatitis	Ethanol, amiodarone (+ fat)
Fibrosis	Methotrexate, vitamin A
Granulomatous	Sulfonamides, quinidine, allopurinol
Veno-occlusive	Cytotoxic agents, irradiation
Peliosis	Sex hormones
Neoplastic	
Adenoma	Sex hormones
Carcinoma	Sex hormones (rare)
Chronic hepatitis	Nitrofurantoin, INH, methyldopa

*A given drug may cause a variety of histologic abnormalities (e.g., methotrexate).
Modified from Reuben A: Department of Medicine, Yale University School of Medicine, 1990.

Pertinent history

1. Exposure to hepatitis, HIV, CMV
2. Ethanol intake
3. Drug history and exposure to toxins
4. IV drug abuse
5. History of cirrhosis
6. Heat exposure (heat stroke)
7. Measles, influenza with aspirin use (Reye's syndrome)
8. History of carcinoma (primary or metastatic)
9. Autoimmune disorders (autoimmune hepatitis)

Physical exam

1. Stigmata of cirrhosis (see Section 23.11) in patients with progression of cirrhosis to hepatic failure
2. Jaundice
3. Asterixis
4. Fetor hepaticus
5. Evidence of sepsis (fever, leukocytosis) and/or shock

Lab results

1. Liver function abnormalities
   a. Alcoholic hepatitis: mild elevation of AST and ALT (usually <500 U/L; AST > ALT [2:1])
   b. Bilirubin invariably elevated (except in Reye's syndrome); when >20 mg/dl, indicates poor prognosis
   c. Alkaline phosphatase only modestly elevated (markedly elevated in extrahepatic obstruction, primary biliary cirrhosis, and carcinoma of liver)
2. Anemia, leukocytosis
3. Hypoglycemia
4. Increased BUN, creatinine (prerenal azotemia, hepatorenal syndrome); BUN may be normal in end-stage liver disease
5. Elevated prothrombin time (poor prognosis if PT > 50 sec), elevated PTT, decreased platelets (if splenomegaly is present)
6. Decreased albumin
7. Decreased pH in acetaminophen overdose
8. Hepatitis markers (see Section 23.10)

Radiologic evaluation and therapy

Refer to Section 23.11

References

1. Allison JE, et al: Hemoccult screening in detecting colorectal neoplasm; sensitivity, specificity, and predictive value, Ann Intern Med 112:328, 1990.
2. Almy TP, Howell DA: Diverticular disease of the colon, N Engl J Med 302:324, 1980.
3. Almy TP, Naitove A: Diverticular disease of the colon. In Sleisinger MH, Fordtran JS (editors): Gastrointestinal disease, ed 3, Philadelphia, 1983, WB Saunders Co.

4. Alter HJ: Detection of antibody to hepatitis C virus in prospectively followed transfusion recipients with acute and chronic non-A, non-B hepatitis, N Engl J Med 321:1494, 1989.

5. Athanosoulis CA, et al: Mesenteric arterial infusions of vasopressin for hemorrhage from colonic diverticulosis, Am J Surg 129:212, 1975.

6. Azad Khan AK, et al: optimum dose of sulfasalazine for maintenance treatment of ulcerative colitis, Gut 12:232, 1980.

7. Baert AL, et al: Early diagnosis of Budd-Chiari syndrome by computed tomography and ultrasonography: report of five cases, Gastroenterology 84:587, 1983.

8. Banks PA: Clinical manifestations and treatment of pancreatitis. In Geokas MC (moderator): Acute pancreatis, Ann Intern Med 103:86, 1985.

9. Bradley EL III: Pancreatic pseudocysts. In Bradley EL III (editor): Complications of pancreatitis: medical and surgical management, Philadelphia, 1982, WB Saunders Co.

10. Brady PG: Endoscopic retrograde cholangiopancreatography; its role in diagnosis and therapy of pancreatitis, Postgrad Med 79:253, 1986.

11. Bydder G, et al: Accuracy of computed tomography in diagnosis of fatty liver, Br Med J 281:1042, 1980.

12. Centers for Disease Control: 1989 Sexually transmitted diseases; treatment guidelines, MMWR 38(5-8):37, 1989.

13. Chopra S, Griffin PH: Laboratory tests and diagnostic procedures in evaluation of liver disease, Am J Med 79:221, 1985.

14. Conn HO, Lieberthal MM: Blood ammonia determination. In Conn HO, Lieberthal MM (editors): The hepatic coma syndromes and lactulose, Baltimore, 1978, The Williams & Wilkins Co.

15. Dupont HL, et al: Prevention of traveler's diarrhea by the tablet formulation of bismuth subsalicylate, JAMA 257:1347, 1987.

16. Englert E Jr, et al: Cimetidine, antacid, and hospitalization in the treatment of benign gastric ulcer: a multicenter double blind study, Gastroenterology 74:416, 1978.

17. Ericsson CD, Dupont HL, et al: Treatment of traveler's diarrhea with sulfamethoxazole and trimethoprim and loperamide, JAMA 263:257, 1990.

18. Federle MP, Jeffrey RB: Computed tomography of pancreatic abscesses, AJR 136:879, 1981.

19. Go VL, Zacheck N: The role of tumor markers in the management of cancer, Cancer 50 (suppl):2618, 1982.

20. Goodman LT, Trenholme GM, et al: Empiric antimicrobial therapy of domestically acquired acute diarrhea in urban adults, Arch Intern Med 150:541, 1990.

21. Henderson JM, Kutner MH, et al: Endoscopic variceal sclerosis compared with distal splenorenal shunt to prevent recurrent variceal bleeding in cirrhosis, Ann Intern Med 112:262, 1990.

22. Hoofnagle JH: Type D (delta) hepatitis, JAMA 261:1321, 1989.

23. Howard JM, et al: Diagnostic efficacy of hepatic computed tomography in the detection of body iron overload, Gastroenterology 84:209, 1983.

24. Immunization Practices Advisory Committee, Centers for Disease Control: Recommendations for protection against viral hepatitis, Ann Intern Med 103:391, 1985.

25. Johnson HCL Jr, Block MA: Diverticular disease: current trends in therapy, Postgrad Med 78:75, 1985.

26. Karlson KB, et al: Percutaneous drainage of pancreatic pseudocysts and abscesses, Radiology 142:619, 1982.

27. Kolars JC, Ellis CJ, Levitt MD: Comparison of serum amylase pancreatic isoamylase and lipase in patients with hyperamylasemia, Dig Dis Sci 29:289, 1984.

28. Korman MG, et al: Ranitidine in duodenal ulcer: incidence of healing and effect of smoking, Dig Dis Sci 27:712, 1982.

29. Leppert M, Burt R, et al: Genetic analysis of an inherited predisposition to colon cancer in a family with a variable number of adenomatous polyps, N Engl J Med 322:904, 1990.

30. Ludwig J, Axelsen R: Drug effects on the liver, Dig Dis Sci 28:653, 1985.

31. Luk GD, Baylin SB: Ornithine decarboxylase as a biologic marker in familial colonic polyposis, N Engl J Med 311:80, 1984.

32. Lynch HT, Rozen P, Schuelke GS: Hereditary colon cancer: polyposis and nonpolyposis variants, CA 35:95, 1985.

33. Martin F, et al: Comparison of the healing capacities of sucralfate and cimetidine in the short-term treatment of duodenal ulcer: a double-blind randomized trial, Gastroenterology 82:401, 1982.

34. Moertel CG, Fleming TR, et al: Levimasole and fluorouracil for adjuvant therapy of resected colon carcinoma, N Engl J Med 322:252, 1990.

35. Moossa AR: Pancreatic pseudocysts in children, JR Coll Surg Edinb 19:149, 1974.

36. Moossa AR: The impact of computed tomography and ultrasonography on surgical practice, Bull Am Coll Surg 67:10, 1982.

37. Moossa AR: Diagnostic tests and procedures in acute pancreatitis, N Engl J Med 310:639, 1984.

38. Mueller PR, Van Sonnenberg E, Simeone JF: Fine needle transhepatic cholangiography: indications and usefulness, Ann Intern Med 95:567, 1982.

39. Orda R, et al: Lipase turbidimetric assay and acute pancreatitis, Dig Dis Sci 29:294, 1984.

40. Perkins JD, et al: Acute diverticulitis: comparison of treatment in immunocompromised patients, Am J Surg 148:745, 1984.

41. Ranson JHC: Etiological and prognostic factors in human pancreatitis, Am J Gastroenterol 77:633, 1982.

42. Richardson CT: Pathogenetic factors in peptic ulcer disease, Am J Med 79(suppl 2C):1, 1985.

43. Rocco VK, Ware AJ: Cirrhotic ascites: pathophysiology, diagnosis, and management, Ann Intern Med 105:573, 1986.

44. Sarver DK: Hepatitis in clinical practice, Postgrad Med 79:194, 1986.

45. Schuster DP, et al: Prospective evaluation of risk of upper gastrointestinal bleeding after admission to medical intensive care unit, Am J Med 76:623, 1984.

46. Siegal JH, Yatto RP: Approach to cholestasis: an update, Arch Intern Med 142:1897, 1982.

47. Silverstein W, et al: Diagnostic imagining of acute pancreatitis: prospective study using CT and sonography, AJR 137:497, 1981.

48. Sontag S, et al: Cimetidine, cigarette smoking, and recurrence of duodenal ulcer, N Engl J Med 311:690, 1984.

49. Spechler SJ, et al: Prevalence of normal serum amylase levels in patients with acute alcoholic pancreatitis, Dig Dis Sci 28:865, 1983.

50. Tavill AS, Wood EJ: The Budd-Chiari syndrome: correlation between hepatic scintigraphy and the clinical, radiological, and pathological findings in nineteen cases of hepatic venous outflow obstruction, Gastroenterology 68:509, 1975.

51. Tito L, et al: Total paracentesis plus IV albumin in management of ascites in cirrhotics, Gastroenterology 98:146, 1990.

52. Toskes PP: Bentiromide as a test of exocrine pancreatic function in adult patients with pancreatic exocrine insufficiency: determination of appropriate dose and urinary collection interval, Gastroenterology 85:565, 1983.

53. Waddell WR, Ganser GF, et al: Sulindac for polyposis of the colon, Am J Surg 157:175, 1989.

Hematology/Oncology

APPROACH TO THE PATIENT WITH ANEMIA
Robert Burd

Definition

Anemia can be defined as a reduction below normal limits in the amount of hemoglobin or in the volume of red blood cells (hematocrit) in a sample of peripheral venous blood.

Etiology

1. Decreased red blood cell production
   a. Deficiency of hematinic agents
   b. Bone marrow failure
2. Increased red cell destruction or loss
   a. Hemolysis
   b. Hemorrhage

Diagnosis

1. History
   a. Family and ethnic history: inquire about thalassemia, sickle cell anemia, splenectomy, cholelithiasis at an early age
   b. Drug and toxic exposures: e.g., chloramphenicol, methyldopa, quinidine, benzene, alkylating agents
   c. Obstetric and menstrual history: "excessive" menstrual bleeding is a frequent cause of iron deficiency anemia in menstruating women
   d. External blood loss: GI, GU (inquire about melena, hematochezia, gross hematuria)
   e. Dietary habits: poor dietary habits and alcohol intake may result in folic acid deficiency
   f. Rapidity of onset: gradual onset is suggestive of bone marrow failure or chronic blood loss whereas sudden onset of symptoms suggests hemolysis or acute hemorrhage
2. Physical exam
   a. General appearance: evaluate nutritional status
   b. Vital signs: hypotension, tachycardia (acute blood loss)

c. Skin: pallor of the conjunctivae, lips, oral mucosa, nail beds, and palmar creases; jaundice (hemolysis), petechiae, purpura (thrombocytopenia)

d. Mouth: glossitis (pernicious anemia, iron deficiency anemia)

e. Heart: listen for flow murmurs, prosthetic valves (increased RBC destruction)

f. Abdomen: splenomegaly (hemolysis, neoplasms, infiltrative disorders)

g. Rectum: examine stool for occult (or gross) blood

h. Lymph nodes: infiltrative lesions, infections

3. Lab results

a. Hemoglobin and hematocrit: provide a guide to diagnosis and severity of anemia; refer to Chapter 31 for normal values

b. Reticulocyte count

(1) Should be performed before any therapeutic maneuvers

(2) Reticulocyte counts below 1% indicate inadequate marrow production, counts above 4% indicate RBC destruction or acute blood loss

(3) However, the reticulocyte count should be considered in light of the degree of anemia and the shift of reticulocytes to the peripheral blood

(4) Further laboratory studies should be determined by the result of the reticulocyte count

c. Mean corpuscular volume (MCV): classifies anemia as normocytic, microcytic, or macrocytic

(1) Normocytic anemia: the reticulocyte count is used to distinguish excess destruction or blood loss (high reticulocyte count) from decreased production (low reticulocyte count); a bone marrow examination is of value in distinguishing the following causes of normocytic anemia and reticulocytopenia

(a) Marrow hypoplasia (toxic drugs, radiation)

(b) RBC aplasia

(c) Marrow infiltration (myeloma, lymphoma, leukemia)

(d) Myelofibrosis

(e) Renal insufficiency

(2) Microcytic anemia

(a) Iron deficiency is the most common cause

(b) Thalassemia, anemia of chronic disease, and sex-linked sideroblastic anemia are other causes

(c) The peripheral smear and RBC count may help distinguish iron deficiency from thalassemia minor (relatively high RBC count and basophilic stippling in the latter)

(d) Assess iron stores by determining the serum ferritin (or marrow iron stain if ferritin unavailable); if ferritin is low, iron deficiency is proved; but if normal or elevated, appropriate work-up for thalassemia (hemoglobin electrophoresis), sideroblastic anemia, and anemia of chronic disease (low serum iron, low TIBC, increased ferritin, decreased reticulocytes) should be obtained

(3) Macrocytic anemia

(a) Because reticulocytes have a large diameter, an elevated reticulocyte count will read out as an elevated MCV; if the reticulocyte count is elevated, hemolytic studies (haptoglobin, LDH, indirect bilirubin) are indicated

(b) If hemolysis is confirmed, determine the cause with Coombs' test; other studies (as suggested by RBC morphology) may be indicated (see p. 348)

(c) If the reticulocyte count is normal and RBCs are macrocytic, vitamin B_{12} or folate deficiency is possible, therefore RBC folate, serum vitamin B_{12}, and serum folate level should be obtained

(d) The presence of a megaloblastic bone marrow would enhance the diagnosis of vitamin B_{12} or folate deficiency; if the bone marrow exhibits dyserythropoiesis or WBC abnormalities, a myelodysplastic anemia is the cause of the macrocytic anemia

(e) A systematic and logical search, with avoidance of a "shotgun" diagnostic or therapeutic approach will yield the correct diagnosis

d. Review peripheral blood smear: red blood cell morphology should be evaluated for:

(1) Size
  (a) Normal RBCs have a diameter equal to that of the nucleus of a mature lymphocyte
  (b) Macrocytosis indicates megaloblastic anemia, liver disease, or refractory anemia
  (c) Microcytosis is seen with iron deficiency, hemoglobinopathies, and sideroblastic anemia

(2) Shape
  (a) Spherocytes (hereditary spherocytosis, immune, or other hemolytic states)
  (b) Tear drop cells (myeloproliferative diseases, pernicious anemia, thalassemia)
  (c) Helmet cells (microangiopathic hemolysis, severe iron deficiency)
  (d) Sickle cell (HbSS)

(3) Color
  (a) Hypochromasia (iron deficiency, sideroblastic anemias)
  (b) Hyperchromasia (megaloblastic anemia, spherocytosis)

e. Morphology of WBC and platelets should be noted and any abnormal cells identified; additional abnormalities of diagnostic value that may be present on peripheral smears are the following:

(1) Basophilic stippling: lead poisoning, thalassemia, hemolytic states

(2) Heinz bodies (denatured Hb): unstable hemoglobinopathies, some hemolytic anemias; identification of Heinz bodies requires supravital stain

(3) Howell-Jolly bodies (nuclear fragments): hemolytic and megaloblastic anemias, splenectomy

(4) Cabot ring (nuclear remnants): megaloblastic anemias
(5) Pappenheimer bodies: postsplenectomy, hemolytic, sideroblastic, and megaloblastic anemias
(6) Rouleaux formation: multiple myeloma, Waldenstrom's macroglobulinemia
(7) Presence of parasites: e.g., *Plasmodium* in malaria
(8) Nucleated RBCs: extramedullary hematopoiesis, hypoxia, hemolysis
(9) Target cells: hemoglobinopathies, iron deficiency, liver disease

24.2 MICROCYTIC ANEMIA

Etiology

1. Iron deficiency
2. Chronic disease
3. Sideroblastic anemia (sex-linked)
4. Thalassemia
5. Lead poisoning

Peripheral blood smear

1. Iron deficiency: microcytic, hypochromic RBCs with a wide area of central pallor; anisocytosis and poikilocytosis when severe
2. Chronic disease: normocytic or microcytic RBCs
3. Sideroblastic anemia: dimorphic population of cells (hypochromic cells and normochromic, normocytic cells); basophilic stippling may also be present
4. Thalassemia: basophilic stippling, target cells, high RBC count
5. Lead poisoning: basophilic stippling

Lab results

1. Serum ferritin: reflects the quantity of stored iron
   a. A low level is diagnostic of iron deficiency
   b. A normal or elevated level does not rule out iron deficiency because ferritin is an acute phase reactant and can be increased in the presence of infection, inflammation, or liver disease
2. A low serum iron and an elevated total iron-binding capacity indicate iron deficiency anemia (Table 24-1)

Table 24-1 Lab differentiation of microcytic anemias

Abnormality	Ferritin	Serum Iron	TIBC	RDW
Iron deficiency	↓	↓	↑	↑
Chronic disease	N/↑	↓	↓	N
Sideroblastic anemia	N/↑	↑	N	N
Thalassemia	N/↑	N/↑	N	N/↑

KEY: N, Normal; ↑, increased; ↓, decreased; TIBC, total iron binding capacity; RDW, red cell distribution width.

3. Reticulocyte count: should be viewed in relation to the degree of anemia; a frequently used correction method is the determination of the reticulocyte production index (RPI)[50]

$$RPI = \frac{\dfrac{(Measured\ hct/Normal\ hct)}{\times\ Reticulocyte\ count}}{Maturation\ factor}$$

The maturation factor (MF) equals 1 if the patient's hematocrit is 45. Each
10 point decrease in the patient's hematocrit will increase the maturation
factor by 0.5 (e.g., if the patient's hematocrit is 35, the MF is 1.5)

  a. The RPI subdivides anemias into two major classes:
    (1) RPI >3: proliferative anemia (hemolysis, hemorrhage, response
      to hematinic agents)
    (2) RPI <3: hypoproliferative anemia (marrow failure, iron defi-
      ciency, renal failure, endocrinopathies)

  Table 24-1 differentiates the causes of microcytic anemias based on the
initial lab evaluation.

Bone marrow exam (if indicated)

1. Iron deficiency
  a. Absent iron stores
  b. Absent sideroblasts
2. Chronic disease
  a. Normal or increased iron stores
  b. Absent or decreased sideroblasts
3. Sideroblastic anemia
  a. Normal or increased iron stores
  b. "Ringed" sideroblasts present
4. Thalassemia
  a. Normal or increased iron stores
  b. Normal or increased sideroblasts

Major causes of microcytic anemia

1. Iron deficiency anemia
  a. Lab results vary with the stage of deficiency
    (1) Absent iron marrow stores and decreased serum ferritin level are
      the initial abnormalities
    (2) Decreased serum iron and increased TIBC are the next abnor-
      malities
    (3) Hypochromic microcytic anemia is present with significant iron
      deficiency
  b. Anemia is usually secondary to excessive blood loss (GI, GU); addi-
    tional causes are iron malabsorption (postgastrectomy) and increased
    requirements (pregnancy)
  c. History may reveal melena, pagophagia (ice eating), or pica
  d. If the diagnosis of iron deficiency is made, it is mandatory to try to
    locate the site of iron loss (see Section 23.1)
  e. Treatment consists of ferrous sulfate 325 mg PO tid for at least 6 mo

2. Chronic disease states
   a. Anemia is often seen with chronic infection (e.g., TB, endocarditis), chronic inflammation (e.g., rheumatoid arthritis), or neoplasms
   b. It is caused by several mechanisms (e.g., decreased erythrocyte survival, inadequate transfer of iron from reticuloendothelial system)
   c. Treatment is aimed at identification and therapy of underlying disease
3. Sideroblastic anemia
   a. It is characterized by ineffective erythropoiesis as a result of enzymatic defects in the mitochondria of RBCs[9]
   b. Sideroblastic anemias can be hereditary or acquired (e.g., alcohol induced, lead intoxication, idiopathic, drug-induced [INH, hydralazine, chloramphenicol]); they are also associated with various malignant disorders (e.g., multiple myeloma, carcinomas, lymphomas, Di Guglielmo's disease) and hemochromatosis
   c. Elevated LDH and bilirubin may be present secondary to ineffective erythropoiesis
   d. If erythrocyte stippling is noted, a blood lead level should be done
   e. Management consists of treatment of underlying disorder, some primary sideroblastic anemias may respond to oral pyridoxine (vitamin B_6) 100 mg PO tid
4. Thalassemia
   a. Hereditary disorders characterized by defective hemoglobin synthesis, broadly classified into α- or β-thalassemias according to the affected globin chain
   b. The homozygous state of β-thalassemia (thalassemia major) is characterized by severe anemia and hepatosplenomegaly; patients with heterozygous β-thalassemia (thalassemia trait) have only mild anemia and microcytic indices without any significant clinical manifestations; splenomegaly may be present in about 20% of affected individuals
   c. The diagnosis of thalassemia trait is established by hemoglobin electrophoresis (elevation of HbA_2, from normal value of 2.5% to approximately 5% in β-thalassemia, or decreased HbA_2 in α-thalassemia)
   d. The major points in the management of homozygous β-thalassemia are:
      (1) Periodic transfusions to maintain Hb at approximately 10 g/dl
      (2) Chelation therapy with deferoxamine mesylate to achieve negative iron balance
      (3) Splenectomy age 5-10
      (4) Ancillary measures (folic acid, vitamin C)

24.3   NORMOCYTIC ANEMIA

Etiology

1. Hemolysis
2. Aplastic anemia
3. Acute hemorrhage (GI, GU) (see Section 23.1)
4. Renal failure (see Section 26.1)

5. Myelophthisis (marrow replacement by fibrosis, tumor, or granulomatous substance)
6. Combined microcytic and macrocytic anemia (e.g., iron and folate deficiency)
7. Endocrine disorders (hypothyroidism, gonadal dysfunction, adrenal insufficiency)
8. Chronic disease (connective tissue disorders, infection, cancer)
9. Bone marrow damage (e.g., ionizing radiation, benzene, drugs)

Peripheral blood smear

1. Hemolysis: the findings vary with the cause of the hemolysis:
   a. Helmet cells, schistocytes: microangiopathic hemolysis
   b. Sickle cells, Howell-Jolly bodies: sickle cell anemia
   c. RBC fragments in a patient with a mechanical heart valve: traumatic
      hemolysis
   d. Spherocytes: hereditary spherocytosis, autoimmune hemolytic ane-
      mias
   e. Spur cells (very irregular borders with thorny projections): hepatic
      cirrhosis
2. Aplastic anemia: neutropenia, thrombocytopenia (unless pure red cell
   aplasia is present)
3. Myelophthisis: the peripheral smear shows a leukoerythroblastic picture
   (normoblasts, granulocyte precursors) caused by premature release from
   bone marrow

Lab results

1. Reticulocyte count: elevated with RBC destruction (hemolysis), decreased with RBC underproduction (e.g., aplastic anemia, myelophthisis)
2. Coombs' test
   a. Direct: detects the presence of antibody or complement on the sur-
      face of RBCs
   b. Indirect: detects the presence of anti-RBC antibodies freely circulat-
      ing in the patient's serum
3. Lactate dehydrogenase (LDH): frequently elevated in patient with intravascular or extravascular hemolysis
4. Haptoglobin is a serum protein that binds hemoglobin, the hemoglobin-
   haptoglobin complex is then cleared by the liver; a low or absent haptoglobin indicates intravascular hemolysis
5. Indirect bilirubin: increased in both intravascular and extravascular hemolysis
6. Urine hemosiderin and urine hemoglobin: detected in moderate to severe intravascular hemolysis
7. Chromium-51 red cell survival: expensive and difficult test; it should
   not be done as part of the initial evaluation of hemolytic anemias
8. Additional studies depend on clinical presentation: BUN, creatinine (to
   rule out renal failure), and thyroid screening

Bone marrow exam

1. Aplastic anemia: scarcity or absence of erythropoietic and myelopoietic precursor cells; patients with pure red cell aplasia demonstrate only absence of RBC precursors in the marrow
2. Myelophthisis: replacement of normal marrow with fibrosis, granulomas, or tumor cells (lymphoma, leukemia, metastatic carcinoma)

Selected causes of normocytic anemia

1. Hemolytic anemia
   a. Classification: see box on the next page
   b. Additional evaluation of selected patients with hemolytic anemia includes ANA (to rule out connective tissue diseases) and CT scan of chest and abdomen (to rule out lymphoma)
   c. Patients with suspected PNH (history of voiding brown or red urine upon arising in AM) should be screened with sucrose lysis test (sugar water test) and acidified serum test (Ham test); Coombs' test is negative in these patients
   d. Treatment of hemolytic anemias varies with the cause
      (1) Drug induced
         (a) Discontinue drug
         (b) Immunosuppressive treatment with steroids (prednisone 60 mg/day) is indicated in symptomatic patients
         (c) Replace folic acid (folic acid 1 mg PO qd)
      (2) Hemolysis secondary to hereditary spherocytosis: splenectomy
      (3) Sickle cell anemia
      The abnormal hemoglobin (due to substitution of valine for glutamic acid in the sixth position of the β-globin chain) when exposed to low oxygen tension causes the red blood cells to assume a sickle shape, resulting in stasis of RBC in capillaries and causing pain.
         (a) Improve oxygenation (nasal O_2 to correct hypoxia)
         (b) Treat suspected infections; *Salmonella* osteomyelitis and pneumococcal infections occur more frequently in patients with sickle cell anemia because of splenic infarcts and atrophy
         (c) Maintain adequate hydration (PO or IV)
         (d) Pain relief during acute crisis
         (e) Replace folic acid; consider subcutaneous heparin
         (f) Avoid unnecessary transfusions
         (g) Hydroxyurea increases hemoglobin F production and reduces the rate of hemolysis and intracellular polymerization of hemoglobin S (investigational)[26]
      Exchange transfusion may be necessary for patients with acute neurologic signs or undergoing surgery.
      (4) Transfusion reaction
         (a) Stop transfusion immediately
         (b) Maintain urine flow greater than 100 ml/hr with adequate hydration plus mannitol and diuretics
         (c) Save suspected unit for analysis
      (5) Warm antibody autoimmune hemolytic anemia
         (a) Prednisone 1-1.5 mg/kg/day initially

Classification and Characteristics of Hemolytic Anemias

Acquired

1. Environmental factors
   a. Autoimmune; isohemagglutinins (e.g., transfusion reaction) or autoantibodies (e.g., warm [IgG] or cold [IgM])
      (1) Idiopathic
      (2) Drugs (three major mechanisms)
          (a) Antibody directed against Rh complex (e.g., methyldopa)
          (b) Antibody directed against RBC-drug complex (hapten-induced, e.g., penicillin)
          (c) Antibody directed against complex formed by drug and plasma proteins; the drug-plasma protein-antibody complex causes destruction of RBC (innocent bystander [e.g., quinidine])
      (3) Underlying diseases
          (a) Connective tissue diseases (e.g., SLE)
          (b) Non-Hodgkin's lymphoma, CLL
          (c) Infections (e.g., *Mycoplasma)*
   b. Nonimmune mediated
      (1) Microangiopathic (DIC, TTP, hemolytic-uremic syndrome, malignant hypertension)
      (2) Hypersplenism
      (3) Cardiac valve prosthesis
      (4) Giant cavernous hemangiomas
      (5) March hemoglobinuria
      (6) Physical agents (e.g., thermal injury)
      (7) Infections (e.g., malaria, *Clostridium welchii,* babesiosis, bartonellosis)
      (8) Drugs (e.g., nitrofurantoin, sulfonamides)
      (9) Chemicals (e.g., heavy metals)
2. Membrane defects
   a. Paroxysmal nocturnal hemoglobinuria (PNH)
   b. Spur-cell anemia (caused by lipid alterations secondary to liver disease)
   c. Wilson's disease

Congenital

1. Defects of cell interior
   a. Hemoglobinopathies (sickle cell disease, thalassemia, HbSC, HbCC)
   b. Enzymopathies (e.g., G_6PD deficiency)
2. Membrane defects: hereditary spherocytosis, elliptocytosis

        (b) Splenectomy in patients responding inadequately to corticosteroids when RBC sequestration studies indicate splenic sequestration

        (c) Danazol, usually used in conjunction with corticosteroids

        (d) Immunosuppressive drugs (azathioprine, cyclophosphamide) indicated only after both corticosteroids and splenectomy (unless surgery is contraindicated) have failed to produce an adequate remission

        (e) Transfuse only if absolutely necessary

    (6) Cold agglutinin disease

        (a) Avoid exposure to cold

        (b) Chlorambucil for severe cases

        (c) Corticosteroids are generally ineffective

        (d) Transfuse prn

    (7) Paroxysmal cold hemoglobinuria

        (a) Avoid exposure to cold

        (b) Corticosteroids may be used empirically; however, results are generally disappointing

        (c) Transfuse prn

1. Aplastic anemia
   a. Etiology
      (1) Toxins (e.g., benzene)
      (2) Drugs (e.g., busulphan and other myelosuppressive drugs, gold salts, chloramphenicol, sulfonamides, trimethadione, quinacrine, canthaxanthin [a synthetic carotenoid used for skin tanning[14]], phenylbutazone)
      (3) Ionizing radiation
      (4) Infections (e.g., hepatitis C)
      (5) Idiopathic
      (6) Inherited (Fanconi's anemia)
      (7) Associated with other disorders (e.g., leukemia, PNH)
   b. Diagnosis is confirmed by bone marrow exam, all patients should be screened for PNH since aplastic anemia associated with PNH has a better prognosis
   c. Treatment
      (1) Discontinue any offending drugs
      (2) Aggressive treatment and prevention of infections
      (3) Platelet and RBC transfusion prn; however, avoid transfusions in patients who are candidates for bone marrow transplantation (see below)
      (4) Immunosuppressive therapy with antithymocyte globulin (ATG) or antilymphocyte globulin
      (5) In patients with severe aplastic anemia who have HLA-matched donors, transplantation of allogeneic marrow is the treatment of choice; patients with severe aplastic anemia who have marrow transplants before the onset of transfusion-induced sensitization have an excellent probability of long-term survival and normal life[8]; age is a significant factor; the incidence of graft-versus-host disease (GVHD) increases with age and is over 90% in patients older than 30 yr

| 24.4 | **MACROCYTIC ANEMIA**

Etiology

1. Folate deficiency
2. Vitamin B_{12} deficiency
3. Chronic liver disease (the elevated MCV is multifactorial: ineffective erythropoiesis, hemolysis, acute blood loss)
4. Alcoholism (RBC membrane abnormalities)
5. Hypothyroidism (can also cause a normochromic, normocytic or hypochromic, microcytic anemia)
6. Elevated reticulocyte count (each increase in the reticulocyte count by 1% will increase the MCV by approximately 2 fL)
7. Some patients with aplastic anemia, myelodysplastic syndrome, or sideroblastic anemia may have macrocytic indices

Peripheral blood smear

Hypersegmented neutrophils (>6 lobes) are present in vitamin B_{12} and folate deficiency.

Lab results[48]

1. Serum vitamin B_{12} level: a low level indicates vitamin B_{12} deficiency; exceptions are falsely low levels seen in patients with severe folate deficiency or falsely high or normal levels when vitamin B_{12} deficiency coincides with severe liver disease or CLL
2. Serum folate, RBC folate: both tests should be ordered because serum folate alone is very labile and does not accurately reflect tissue folate levels, whereas RBC folate is a good indicator of tissue stores but may be reduced in severe cobalamin deficiency
3. Reticulocyte count
4. Thyroid and liver function studies

Bone marrow exam

Examination of the bone marrow will demonstrate megaloblastic erythroid hyperplasia.

Selected causes of macrocytic anemia

1. Folate deficiency
   a. Decreased intake (alcoholism, poor diet)
   b. Increased requirements (hemolysis, pregnancy, dialysis)
   c. Impaired absorption (e.g., sprue, IBD, ethanol)
   d. Drugs (e.g., phenytoin, methotrexate, ethanol, trimethoprim, antituberculous agents)
   e. Treatment: folic acid 1 mg PO qd
2. Vitamin B_{12} deficiency
   a. Etiology
      (1) Pernicious anemia (antibodies against intrinsic factor and gastric parietal cells)

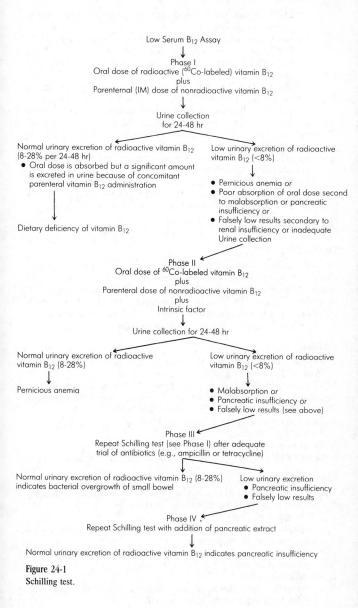

Low Serum B$_{12}$ Assay

Phase I
Oral dose of radioactive (^{60}Co-labeled) vitamin B$_{12}$
plus
Parenternal (IM) dose of nonradioactive vitamin B$_{12}$

Urine collection
for 24-48 hr

Normal urinary excretion of radioactive vitamin B$_{12}$
(8-28% per 24-48 hr)
• Oral dose is absorbed but a significant amount
  is excreted in urine because of concomitant
  parenteral vitamin B$_{12}$ administration

Dietary deficiency of vitamin B$_{12}$

Low urinary excretion of radioactive
vitamin B$_{12}$ (<8%)

• Pernicious anemia or
• Poor absorption of oral dose second
  to malabsorption or pancreatic
  insufficiency or
• Falsely low results secondary to
  renal insufficiency or inadequate
  Urine collection

Phase II
Oral dose of ^{60}Co-labeled vitamin B$_{12}$
plus
Parenteral dose of nonradioactive vitamin B$_{12}$
plus
Intrinsic factor

Urine collection for 24-48 hr

Normal urinary excretion of radioactive
vitamin B$_{12}$ (8-28%)

Pernicious anemia

Low urinary excretion of radioactive
vitamin B$_{12}$ (<8%)

• Malabsorption or
• Pancreatic insufficiency or
• Falsely low results (see above)

Phase III
Repeat Schilling test (see Phase I) after adequate
trial of antibiotics (e.g., ampicillin or tetracycline)

Normal urinary excretion of radioactive vitamin B$_{12}$ (8-28%)
indicates bacterial overgrowth of small bowel

Low urinary excretion
• Pancreatic insufficiency
• Falsely low results

Phase IV
Repeat Schilling test with addition of pancreatic extract

Normal urinary excretion of radioactive vitamin B$_{12}$ indicates pancreatic insufficiency

Figure 24-1
Schilling test.

   (2) Malabsorption (small bowel disease, pancreatic insufficiency, gastric abnormalities)
   (3) Inadequate dietary intake (rare, usually seen in strict vegetarians)
   (4) Interference with vitamin B_{12} absorption (fish tapeworm [e.g., sushi eaters], drugs, ileal transport defect [e.g., Crohn's disease])
   b. Clinical presentation: patients with severe deficiency can present with significant neurologic findings (paresthesias, ataxia, loss of position and vibration senses, memory impairment, depression, dementia); neuropsychiatric disorders due to cobalamin deficiency are common and may occur in the absence of anemia or an elevated MCV; elevated serum levels of methylmalonic acid and total hemocysteine are useful in the diagnosis of these patients[33] but are not routinely available in most laboratories
   c. Diagnostic approach: Schilling test (Fig. 24-1) if etiology not clear
   d. Therapy: 1000 μg of vitamin B_{12} (cyanocobalamin) IM every week for 6 wk followed by 500-1000 μg/mo indefinitely

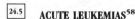

ACUTE LEUKEMIAS[58]

Definition

Acute leukemia is a disorder characterized by uncontrolled proliferation of abnormal immature white blood cell progenitors. Proliferation of abnormal immature lymphocytes and their progenitors is known as *acute lymphoblastic leukemia* (ALL). Proliferation of primitive myeloid cells (blasts) is called *acute nonlymphocytic leukemia* (ANLL). The distinction between the two types has therapeutic and prognostic significance.

Etiology

1. Previous use of antineoplastic agents (e.g., chemotherapy of NHL, Hodgkin's disease, ovarian cancer, myeloma)
2. Chromosomal abnormalities (e.g., Down's syndrome [twenty-fold increase in the risk of acute leukemia], C-group trisomy, neurofibromatosis, Klinefelter's syndrome [increased risk of ANLL])
3. Environmental factors (e.g., ionizing radiation)
4. Toxins (e.g., benzene)
5. Drugs (e.g., choramphenicol, phenylbutazone)
6. Others: CML, PNH, polycythemia vera, myelodysplastic syndromes

Classification

The distinction between ALL and ANLL and the classification of the various subtypes is based on the following factors:
1. Cell morphology
   a. Lymphoblasts: very high nucleus/cytoplasm ratio, usually cytoplasmic granules are not present
   b. Myeloblasts: abundant cytoplasm, cytoplasmic granules often present (Auer rods)
2. Histochemical stains
   a. Peroxidase and Sudan black stains: negative in ALL; useful to distinguish nonlymphoid from lymphoid cells

b. Chloracetate esterase: a pink cytoplasmic reaction identifies granulo-cytes; useful to distinguish granulocytes from monocytes in patients with ANLL

3. The French-American-British (FAB) cooperative study group has classi-fied ALL into three groups (L1 to L3) based on cell size, cytoplasmic appearance, nuclear shape, and chromatin pattern; the most common form is the L2 type; ANLL is diagnosed by the presence of at least 30% blast cells and positive peroxidase or Sudan black histochemical stain in the bone marrow aspirate; it is subdivided into seven categories (M1 to M7) based on the type and percentage of immature cells[12]; erythroleu-kemia (M6 or di Guglielmo's disease) and monocytic leukemia (M5) are forms of ANLL associated with poor prognosis; patients with acute pro-myelocytic leukemia (FABM3) frequently present with DIC

Characteristics and clinical presentation

1. ALL is primarily a disease of children (peak incidence ages 2-10) whereas ANLL usually affects adults (most patients are 30-60 yr old)
2. The patients generally come to medical attention because of the effects of the cytopenias:
   a. Anemia manifests with weakness and fatigue
   b. Thrombocytopenia can manifest with bleeding, petechiae, and ec-chymoses
   c. Neutropenia can result in fever and infections
3. The peripheral WBC varies from 5000/mm^3 to >100,000/mm^3
4. Occasionally patients may present with neurologic manifestations sec-ondary to meningeal leukemia (usually ALL) or cerebral leukostasis (in ANLL) secondary to very elevated WBC counts (>150,000/mm^3)
5. Additional systemic manifestations of acute leukemia are pneumonia (secondary to granulocytopenia), dysphagia (secondary to oropharyn-geal candidiasis), GI bleeding (secondary to thrombocytopenia), and acute prostatism (secondary to significant leukemic infiltration of the prostate)
6. Additional lab findings may include: elevated LDH and uric acid levels, decreased fibrinogen, and increased FDP secondary to DIC (more fre-quent in ANLL)
7. Cytogenetic abnormalities are very common
   a. Chromosome 8 is most frequently involved in ANLL
   b. Translocation (15→17) is characteristic of acute promyelocytic leu-kemia (FABM3)
   c. The presence of the Philadelphia (Ph^1) chromosome in ALL is a bad prognostic sign
   d. ANLL with the 5q- or 7q- genotype likewise has a poor prognosis
8. Physical exam may reveal petechiae and purpura (secondary to throm-bocytopenia), evidence of infections (e.g., oropharyngeal candidiasis), lymphadenopathy, infiltration (e.g., gingival hypertrophy in patients with acute monocytic leukemia), and hepatosplenomegaly
9. Lumbar puncture is indicated in patients with ALL because of the high incidence of CNS involvement

Treatment[30,17]

1. Emergency treatment is indicated in patients with intracerebral leuko-stasis; it consists of one or more of the following:
   a. Cranial irradiation
   b. Leukapheresis
   c. Oral hydroxyurea (requires 48-72 hr to significantly lower the cir-culating blast count)
2. Urate nephropathy can be prevented by lowering uric acid level with allopurinol and urine alkalinization with acetazolamide
3. Infections must be aggressively treated with broad-spectrum antibiotics
   a. Any febrile neutropenic patient must have cultures taken and be promptly treated with IV antibiotics (e.g., mezlocillin or ticarcillin plus an aminoglycoside to provide adequate coverage against gram-negative bacteria)
   b. If evidence of infection persists despite adequate treatment with an-tibiotics, amphotericin B may be added to provide coverage against fungal infections (*Candida, Aspergillus*)
   c. *Pneumocystis* pneumonia is common in patients with ALL
4. Correct significant thrombocytopenia (platelet counts $<20,000/mm^3$) with platelet transfusions
5. Bleeding secondary to DIC is treated with heparin
   a. Thrombocytopenia is not a contraindication to heparin therapy in these patients since bleeding from DIC is life-threatening
   b. Concomitant use of heparin and platelet transfusions is indicated in severely thrombocytopenic patients with DIC
6. Induction chemotherapy
   a. Intensive chemotherapy to destroy a significant number of leukemic cells and achieve remission; it usually consists of the following:
      (1) ALL: combination of vincristine (Oncovin), prednisone, L-as-paraginase (Elspar), and daunorubicin (Cerubidine)
      (2) ANLL: cytarabine (Cytosar) and daunorubicin (Cerubidine)
   b. It usually takes 28-32 days from the start of therapy to achieve re-mission
   c. The duration of remission is variable; the median duration of remis-sion in an adult with ANLL is 1 yr, but up to 50% of patients with ALL remain in remission for 2 or more yr
7. Consolidation therapy
   a. It consists of aggressive course of chemotherapy with or without ra-diotherapy shortly after complete remission has been obtained; its purpose is to prolong the remission period or cure
   b. Complications of consolidation therapy are usually secondary to se-vere bone marrow suppression (anemia, thrombocytopenia, granu-locytopenia)
   c. The risk of nonhematopoietic toxicity is also increased (e.g., GI tract ulceration and cardiac toxicity with use of daunorubicin)
8. Meningeal prophylactic therapy is indicated in patients with ALL
   a. Intrathecal methotrexate is used with or without cranial irradiation
   b. Meningeal prophylaxis in adults with ANLL is controversial be-cause meningeal leukemia is uncommon in these patients

9. Maintenance therapy
   a. Its goal is to maintain a state of remission
   b. The drugs used and the duration of therapy vary with the type of acute leukemia
      (1) ALL: intermittent therapy for at least 3 years with combination methotrexate and 6-mercaptopurine
      (2) ANLL: therapy is continued for at least 1 yr; cytarabine and 6-thioguanine are commonly used
10. Bone marrow transplantation (generally reserved for the first relapse)
    a. Allogeneic
       (1) The marrow from an HLA-matched sibling is transplanted into the patient after complete remission is achieved with chemotherapy
       (2) Because of a higher incidence of graft-versus-host disease with advancing age, allogeneic marrow transplants are usually performed only in patients less than 40 yr old
    b. Autologous
       (1) The patient's marrow is harvested after remission is achieved with chemotherapy
       (2) The patient is then irradiated and given high doses of cyclophosphamide to kill any residual leukemic cells
       (3) The previously harvested bone marrow is then returned to the patient; current research is directed at immunologic or chemotherapeutic manipulation of the marrow to destroy any residual leukemic cells before reimplantation

Complications of chemotherapy

The major complication is profound marrow depression with pancytopenia lasting 3-4 wk. Treatment is aimed at RBC and platelet replacement and aggressive monitoring and treatment of suspected infections. Some investigators have recommended prophylaxis with antifungal and antibacterial agents in patients with acute leukemia who are receiving remission induction treatment.[20] Prophylactic administration of quinolones (e.g., ciprofloxacin) in patients with acute leukemia and granulocytopenia may decrease the overall morbidity and frequency of gram-negative infections.[32]

24.6 CHRONIC LEUKEMIA

Chronic lymphocytic leukemia[15,44]

Definition

Chronic lymphocytic leukemia (CLL) is a lymphoproliferative disorder characterized by proliferation and accumulation of mature-appearing neoplastic lymphocytes.

Lab results

1. Peripheral lymphocytosis (generally ≥15,000/dl) of well-differentiated lymphocytes
2. Monotonous replacement of the bone marrow by small lymphocytes (marrow contains ≥30% well-differentiated lymphocytes)

3. Hypogammaglobulinemia and elevated LDH may be present at time of diagnosis
4. Anemia or thrombocytopenia, if present, indicate poor prognosis
5. Trisomy 12 is the most common chromosomal abnormality followed by 14q+, 13q, and 11q; these all indicate a poor prognosis

Characteristics and clinical manifestations

1. CLL generally occurs in middle-aged and elderly patients (median age is 60 yr); male to female ratio is 2:1
2. The abnormal lymphocytes are B-cells 90% of the time (B-cell monoclonal disorder)
3. Clinical presentation varies with the stage of the disease; many patients are diagnosed on the basis of a CBC obtained following routine physical exam, other patients may come to medical attention because of weakness or fatigue (secondary to anemia) or lymphadenopathy
4. Physical exam reveals lymphadenopathy, splenomegaly, and hepatomegaly in the majority of patients

Staging[29]

Rai et al.[45] divided chronic lymphocytic leukemia into five clinical stages based on the presence of lymphocytosis:
1. Stage 0—characterized by lymphocytosis only ($\geq$15,000/mm^3 on peripheral smear, bone marrow aspirate with $\geq$ 40% lymphocytes)
2. The coexistence of lymphocytosis and other factors increases the clinical stage
   a. Stage I—lymphadenopathy
   b. Stage II—splenomegaly/hepatomegaly
   c. Stage III—anemia: hemoglobin <11 g/mm^3
   d. Stage IV—thrombocytopenia: platelets <100,000/mm^3
   Another well-known staging system, developed by J.L. Binet, divides chronic lymphocytic leukemia into three stages:
1. Stage A: Hb $\geq$10 g/dl, platelets $\geq$ 100,000/mm^3, and less than three areas involved (the cervical, axillary, and inguinal lymph nodes [whether unilaterally or bilaterally], the spleen, and the liver)
2. Stage B: Hb $\geq$10 g/dl, platelets $\geq$100,000/mm^3, and three or more areas involved
3. Stage C: Hb < 10 g/dl or platelets < 100,000/mm^3, or both (independently of the areas involved)

Prognosis

The prognosis is directly related to the clinical stage. For example, the average survival for patients in the Rai Stage 0 or the Binet Stage A is greater than 120 mo whereas for the Rai Stage IV or Binet Stage C it is approximately 30 mo.

Treatment

The therapeutic approach varies with the clinical stage and presence or absence of symptoms.

Rai Stage 0, Binet Stage A: no treatment for asymptomatic
patients
Rai Stage I & II, Binet Stage B: symptomatic patients given
chlorambucil; local irradiation can be
used for isolated symptomatic
lymphadenopathy and lymph nodes
that interfere with vital organs
Rai Stage III & IV, Binet Stage C: chlorambucil chemotherapy with or
without prednisone
   a. Fludarabine used in patients who
      respond poorly to chlorambucil
   b. Splenic irradiation in selected
      patients with advanced disease[7]

Chronic granulocytic (myelogenous) leukemia[15,52]

Definition
Chronic granulocytic leukemia (CGL, CML) is a myeloproliferative disorder characterized by abnormal proliferation and accumulation of immature granulocytes.

Lab results
1. Elevated total leukocyte count (generally $>100,000/mm^3$) with wide spectrum of granulocytic forms
2. Bone marrow demonstrates hypercellularity with granulocytic hyperplasia
3. Philadelphia chromosome (shortening of long arms of chromosome G22, generally secondary to translocation of chromosomal material to the long arms of chromosome C9) is present in over 80% of patients with CGL; its presence is a major prognostic factor because the survival rate of patients with the Philadelphia chromosome is about eight times that of those without it
4. Leukocyte alkaline phosphatase (LAP) is markedly decreased (used to distinguish CGL from other myeloproliferative disorders)
5. Anemia and thrombocytosis are often present
6. Additional lab results are elevated vitamin B_{12} levels (caused by increased transcobalamin I from granulocytes) and elevated blood histamine levels (because of increased basophils)

Characteristics and clinical manifestations
1. CGL usually affects middle-aged patients
2. Common complaints at the time of diagnosis are weakness or discomfort secondary to an enlarged spleen (abdominal discomfort or pain)
3. CGL is characterized by a *chronic phase* lasting months to years, followed by an *accelerated myeloproliferative phase* manifested by poor response to therapy, worsening anemia, or decreased platelet count; this second phase then evolves into a terminal phase *(acute transformation)* characterized by elevated number of blast cells and numerous complications (e.g., sepsis, bleeding)
4. The median survival time from diagnosis of CGL is approximately 45 mo; the median duration of the terminal phase is 3 mo

5. Physical exam in the chronic phase usually reveals splenomegaly; hepatomegaly is not infrequent, but lymphadenopathy is very unusual and generally indicates the accelerated myeloproliferative phase of the disease

Treatment

The therapeutic approach varies with the clinical phase and the degree of hyperleukocytosis.

1. Symptomatic hyperleukocytosis (e.g., CNS symptoms are treated with leukapheresis and hydroxyurea); allopurinol should also be started to prevent urate nephropathy following rapid lysis of the leukemic cells
2. Cytotoxic chemotherapy usually includes either hydroxyurea or busulfan; the major complications associated with busulfan are its long-term toxic effect (aplasia) and pulmonary fibrosis
3. Severe persistent thrombocytosis may require treatment with thiotepa or melphalan
4. Allogeneic marrow transplantation (following intense chemotherapy and radiotherapy to destroy residual leukemic cells) is the only curative treatment for CGL
   a. It should be considered in young patients (increased survival in patients younger than 30) with compatible siblings
   b. Early transplantation is also very important for patient survival; a recent study demonstrated that the probability of long-term survival for allogeneic graft recipients was 49-58% for patients in the chronic phase, 15% in the accelerated phase, and 14% for patients in the blastic phase[55]

Hairy cell leukemia

Lymphoid neoplasm characterized by the proliferation of mature B-cells with prominent cytoplasmic projections (hairs); it occurs predominantly in men between 40 and 60 yr

1. Cells stain positively for tartrate-resistant acid phosphatase (TRAP) stain
2. Bone marrow may result in "dry tap" (due to increased marrow reticulin)
3. Anemia is usually present and varies from minimal to severe
4. Physical exam usually reveals splenomegaly secondary to tumor cell infiltration
5. Therapy is splenectomy in patients with massive splenomegaly; alpha interferon is effective and can result in complete remission (irrespective of prior splenectomy)
6. 2'Deoxycoformycin (DCF) is also effective but moderately myelotoxic; a newer agent, 2'chlorodeoxyadenosine, has been shown very effective at inducing stable remission and has fewer side effects[42]

24.7   HODGKIN'S DISEASE[18,43]

Definition

Hodgkin's disease is a malignant disorder of lymphoreticular origin, characterized histologically by the presence of multinucleated giant cells (Reed-Sternberg cells).

Characteristics and clinical manifestations

1. There is a bimodal age distribution (15-34 and over age 50)
2. The patient usually has painless lymphadenopathy, generally involving the cervical region; at times the disease is detected by the presence of mediastinal adenopathy on a routine chest x-ray
3. Symptomatic patients usually have the following manifestations:
   a. Fever and night sweats: when the fever has a cyclical pattern (days or weeks of fever alternating with afebrile periods), it is known as Pel-Ebstein fever
   b. Weight loss, generalized malaise
   c. Persistent, dry, nonproductive cough
   d. Pain associated with alcohol ingestion, often secondary to heavy eosinophil infiltration of the tumor sites
   e. Pruritus
   f. Others: superior vena cava syndrome and spinal cord compression are rare presentations
4. Initial lab evaluation generally reveals normochromic, normocytic/microcytic anemia, elevated sedimentation rate, and cutaneous anergy to common skin tests; elevated serum alkaline phosphatase, eosinophilia, lymphocytopenia, mild leukocytosis, and thrombocytosis may also be present

Histopathology

There are four main histologic subtypes, based on the number of lymphocytes and Reed-Sternberg cells and the presence of fibrous tissue: lymphocyte predominance, mixed cellularity, nodular sclerosis, and lymphocyte depletion. Nodular sclerosis is the most common type. Prognosis is generally best for lymphocyte predominance and worst for lymphocyte depletion. However, survival is more directly related to the pathologic and clinical stage rather than the histologic subtype.

Staging

1. The Ann Arbor staging classification[16] (Table 24-2) is commonly used; because of different therapeutic and prognostic implications, Stage III has been subdivided into III_1 (involvement of upper abdomen, spleen,

Table 24-2 Ann Arbor staging classification for Hodgkin's disease

Stage	Definition
I	Limited to one area
II	Involves two or more areas on the same side of the diaphragm
III	Involves two or more areas on both sides of the diaphragm
IV	Disseminated extralymphatic disease

KEY: A, Asymptomatic; B, symptomatic (fever, sweats, weight loss >10% of body weight); S, splenic involvement; E, extralymphatic site.
From Carbone PP, et al: Cancer Res 31:1860, 1971.

splenic and hilar nodes) and III_2 (involvement of lower abdominal nodes)

2. Proper staging requires the following:
   a. Detailed history and physical exam
   b. Surgical biopsy
   c. Lab evaluation (CBC, sedimentation rate, BUN, creatinine, alkaline phosphatase, liver function studies)
   d. Chest x-ray (PA and lateral)
   e. Bilateral bone marrow biopsy
   f. Computed tomography
      (1) Chest: indicated when abnormal findings are noted on chest x-ray
      (2) Abdomen and pelvis: to visualize the mesenteric, hepatic, portal, and splenic hilar nodes
   g. Exploratory laparotomy and splenectomy
      (1) Decision to perform staging laparotomy depends on the therapeutic plan; not indicated in patients who are to receive chemotherapy
      (2) It is generally recommended for patients with clinical Stage I-IIA and I-IIB
      (3) It is valuable in identifying patients who can be treated with radiation alone
      (4) Polyvalent pneumococcal vaccine should be given prophylactically to all patients before splenectomy (↑ risk of sepsis from encapsulated organisms in splenectomized patients)

Treatment

1. The main therapeutic modalities are radiotherapy and chemotherapy; the indications for each vary with the pathological stage and other factors
   a. Stages I and II: radiation therapy alone, unless a large mediastinal mass is present (mediastinal to thoracic ratio ≥ 1.3); in the latter case, a combination of chemotherapy and radiation therapy is indicated
   b. Stage IB or IIB: total nodal irradiation often used, though chemotherapy is performed at many centers
   c. Stage IIIA: treatment is controversial and varies with the anatomical substage after splenectomy
      (1) III_1A and minimum splenic involvement: radiation therapy alone may be adequate
      (2) III_2 or III_1A with extensive splenic involvement: there is disagreement whether chemotherapy alone or a combination of chemotherapy and radiotherapy is the preferred treatment modality
   d. Stages IIIB and IV: the treatment of choice is chemotherapy with or without adjuvant radiotherapy
2. Various regimens can be used for combination chemotherapy; some commonly used regimens are
   a. MOPP: mechlorethamine (nitrogen mustard), vincristine (Oncovin), procarbazine, prednisone
   b. MOPP-ABV (doxorubicin [Adriamycin], bleomycin, vinblastine)

3. Cure rates as high as 75-80% are now possible with appropriate initial therapy
4. Chemotherapy significantly increases the risk of leukemia
   a. The peak in the risk of leukemia is seen approximately 5 yr after initiation of chemotherapy
   b. The risk of leukemia is dose related and is greater for patients who undergo splenectomy and for patients with more advanced stages of Hodgkin's disease; the risk is unaffected by concomitant radiotherapy[31]

24.8   NON-HODGKIN'S LYMPHOMA[28,57]

Definition

Non-Hodgkin's lymphoma (NHL) is a heterogeneous group of malignancies of the lymphoreticular system.

Characteristics and clinical manifestations

1. The median age at time of diagnosis is 50 yr
2. Patients often have asymptomatic lymphadenopathy
   a. Involvement of extranodal sites can result in unusual presentations (e.g., GI tract involvement can simulate peptic ulcer disease)
   b. Pruritus is rare
   c. Fever, night sweats, and weight loss are less common than in Hodgkin's disease and their prognostic significance is less well defined
3. Initial lab evaluation may reveal only mild anemia

Histopathology and classification

Table 24-3 compares commonly used pathologic classifications of non-Hodgkin's lymphoma.

Staging

1. The Ann Arbor classification is also used to stage NHL (see Table 24-2)
2. Histopathology has greater therapeutic implications in NHL than in Hodgkin's disease
3. Proper staging usually requires the following:
   a. A thorough history and physical exam and an adequate biopsy
   b. Routine lab evaluation (CBC, sedimentation rate, urinalysis, BUN, creatinine, serum calcium, uric acid, liver function tests, serum protein electrophoresis)
   c. Chest x-ray (PA and lateral)
   d. Bone marrow evaluation (aspirate and four bone core biopsies)
   e. CT scan of abdomen and pelvis; CT scan of chest if chest x-ray is abnormal
   f. Bone scan (particularly in patients with histiocytic lymphoma)
   g. Depending on the histopathology, the results of the above studies, and the planned therapy, some other tests may be performed: gallium scan (e.g., in patients with high-grade lymphomas), liver-spleen scan, lymphangiography, lumbar puncture

Table 24-3 Comparison of pathological classifications of non-Hodgkin's lymphoma

Working Formulation of Non-Hodgkin's Lymphomas for Clinical Usage[40]	Rappaport[46]	Lukes and Collins[35]
Low Grade		
ML,* small lymphocytic	Diffuse lymphocytic, well differentiated	Small lymphocytic and plasmacytoid lymphocytic
ML, follicular, predominantly small cleaved cell	Nodular, poorly differentiated lymphocytic	Small cleaved FCC,† follicular only or follicular and diffuse
ML, follicular, mixed small cleaved and large cell	Nodular, mixed lymphocytic-histiocytic	Small cleaved FCC, follicular; large cleaved FCC, follicular
Intermediate Grade		
ML, follicular, predominantly large cell	Nodular histiocytic	Large cleaved or noncleaved FCC, follicular
ML, diffuse small cleaved cell	Diffuse lymphocytic, poorly differentiated	Small cleaved FCC, diffuse
ML, diffuse, mixed small and large cell	Diffuse mixed lymphocytic-histiocytic	Small cleaved, large cleaved, and/or large non-cleaved FCC, diffuse
ML, diffuse, large cell	Diffuse histiocytic	Large cleaved or noncleaved FCC, diffuse

High Grade

ML, large cell immunoblastic	Diffuse histiocytic	Immunoblastic sarcoma, T-cell or B-cell type
ML, lymphoblastic	Lymphoblastic convoluted/nonconvoluted	Convoluted T-cell
ML, small noncleaved cell	Undifferentiated, Burkitt and non-Burkitt	Small noncleaved FCC

Miscellaneous

Composite
Mycosis fungoides
Histiocytic
Extramedullary plasmacytoma
Unclassifiable

*ML, malignant lymphoma.
†FCC, follicular center cell.
Modified from the National Cancer Institute–sponsored study of the classifications of non-Hodgkin's lymphomas. Ultmann JE, Jacobs RH: CA 35:66, 1985.
Reproduced with permission of the American Cancer Society.

Treatment

The therapeutic regimen varies with the histological type and pathological stage. Following are the commonly used therapeutic modalities:

1. Low-grade NHL (e.g., nodular, poorly differentiated)
   a. Local radiotherapy for symptomatic obstructive adenopathy
   b. Deferment of therapy and careful observation in asymptomatic patients
   c. Single-agent chemotherapy with cyclophosphamide or chlorambucil
   d. Combination chemotherapy, alone or with radiotherapy, is generally indicated only when the lymphoma becomes more invasive, with poor response to less aggressive treatment
      (1) CVP: cyclophosphamide, vincristine, prednisone
      (2) CHOP: cyclophosphamide, doxorubicin, vincristine (Oncovin), prednisone
      (3) CHOP-Bleo: addition of bleomycin to CHOP
      (4) COPP: cyclophosphamide, vincristine, procarbazine, prednisone
      (5) BACOP: bleomycin, doxorubicin (Adriamycin), cyclophosphamide, vincristine, prednisone
2. Intermediate and high-grade lymphomas (e.g., diffuse histiocytic lymphoma)
   a. Combination chemotherapy, alone or with radiotherapy
      (1) Pro-MACE-MOPP[22]: prednisone, methotrexate, leucovorin, doxorubicin (Adriamycin), cyclophosphamide, epipodophyllotoxin (VP-16), mechlorethamine, vincristine, procarbazine, prednisone
      (2) COMLA: cyclophosphamide, vincristine, methotrexate, leucovorin, cytosine arabinoside (Ara-C)
      (3) M-BACOD: methotrexate, leucovorin, bleomycin, doxorubicin, cyclophosphamide, vincristine, dexamethasone
      (4) CHOP: cyclophosphamide, doxorubicin, vincristine, prednisone

Prognosis

Patients with low-grade lymphoma, despite their long-term survival, are rarely cured and the great majority (if not all) eventually die of the lymphoma, whereas patients with a high-grade lymphoma may achieve a cure with aggressive chemotherapy.

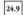 MULTIPLE MYELOMA[6,51]

Definition

Multiple myeloma is a malignancy of plasma cells characterized by overproduction of intact monoclonal immunoglobulin or free monoclonal kappa or lambda chains.

Characteristics and clinical manifestations

1. The median age at diagnosis is 60 yr; there is an increased incidence in blacks
2. The median survival is approximately 30 mo with standard therapy; the prognosis is much better in asymptomatic patients with indolent or

smoldering myeloma: median survival time approximately 10 yr in persons with no lytic bone lesions and a serum myeloma protein concentration <3.0 g/dl[5]

3. The patient usually comes to medical attention because of one or more of the following:

a. Bone pain (back, thorax) or pathological fractures caused by osteolytic lesions or osteoporosis

b. Fatigue or weakness because of anemia secondary to bone marrow infiltration with plasma cells

c. Recurrent infections as a result of multiple factors (deficiency of normal immunoglobulins, impaired neutrophil function, prolonged physical immobilization); common infecting organisms are *S. pneumoniae, S. aureus, H. influenzae, Pseudomonas, E. coli,* and *Klebsiella*

d. Nausea and vomiting caused by constipation and uremia (renal failure secondary to myeloma kidney, hypercalcemia, amyloidosis, hyperuricemia)

e. Confusion as a result of hypercalcemia from bone resorption secondary to osteoclast-activating factor (OAF) secreted by myeloma cells and lysis of bone due to tumor cell infiltration

f. Neurologic complications, such as spinal cord or nerve root compression, carpal tunnel syndrome secondary to amyloid infiltration, somnolence, blurred vision, or blindness from hyperviscosity

Lab results

1. Normochromic, normocytic anemia; rouleaux formation may be seen on peripheral smear

2. Hypercalcemia

3. Elevated BUN, creatinine, uric acid, and total protein

4. Proteinuria secondary to overproduction and secretion of free monoclonal kappa or lambda chains (Bence Jones protein)

5. Tall homogeneous monoclonal spike (M spike) is present on protein electrophoresis in approximately 75% of patients; decreased levels of normal immunoglobulins

a. The increased immunoglobulins are IgG, IgA, IgE, and rarely IgM

b. Some patients have no increase in immunoglobulins but increased light chains in the urine

c. A very small percentage (<2%) of patients have nonsecreting myeloma (no increase in immunoglobulins and no light chains in the urine), but have other evidence of the disease (e.g., positive bone marrow exam)

6. Reduced anion gap secondary to the positive charge of the M proteins and to the frequent presence of hyponatremia in myeloma patients

7. Bone marrow exam usually demonstrates nests or sheets of plasma cells; plasma cells usually comprise >30% of the bone marrow and ≥10% are immature

8. Serum hyperviscosity may be present (more common with production of IgA)

9. Serum β_2 microglobulin has little diagnostic value; it is useful for

prognosis since levels >8 mg/L indicate high tumor mass and aggressive disease

10. Elevated serum levels of LDH at the time of diagnosis define a subgroup of myeloma patients with very poor prognosis[10]

Radiologic evaluation

X-rays of painful areas usually will demonstrate punched out lytic lesions or osteoporosis. Bone scans are not useful since lesions are not blastic.

Diagnostic criteria

1. Presence of ≥10% immature plasma cells in the marrow
2. Presence of serum or urinary monoclonal protein
3. Osteolytic bone lesions
4. Plasmacytomas on tissue biopsy

Staging

Durie and Salmon[19] developed a clinical staging system correlated with tumor mass, response to treatment, and survival. It has been refined by Smith and Alexanian[51] to include the degree of marrow plasmacytosis, the level of serum β_2 microglobulin,[11] and the level of normal immunoglobulins (see box on the next page).

Treatment

1. Supportive measures
   a. Pain control with analgesics; radiation therapy and surgical stabilization may also be indicated
   b. Control hypercalcemia (see Section 22.8)
   c. Prompt diagnosis and treatment of any infection (see Section 25.5)
   d. Prevent renal failure by
      (1) Adequate hydration
      (2) Control of hypercalcemia
      (3) Control of hyperuricemia (allopurinol and urine alkalinization)
      (4) Avoid nephrotoxic agents
      (5) Avoid dye contrast studies (e.g., IVP and CT scans with contrast)
   e. Preserve ambulation and mobility
2. Chemotherapy is usually withheld until symptoms develop or complications are imminent; effective regimens include
   a. Melphalan and prednisone
   b. Vincristine, doxorubicin (Adriamycin), and methylprednisolone (VAMP) followed by high-dose melphalan and, when possible, autologous bone-marrow rescue[27]

24.10 POLYCYTHEMIA VERA[1,13]

Definition

Polycythemia vera is a chronic myeloproliferative disorder characterized mainly by erythrocytosis (increase in RBC mass).

Differential diagnosis

1. Smoking

Tumor Mass Staging of Multiple Myeloma*

1. High tumor mass
   a. Characterized by one of the following:
      (1) Hemoglobin <8.5 g/100 ml without renal failure or hypoferremia
      (2) Calcium >11.5 mg/100 ml† without bedridden status
   b. Supporting features often present
      (1) Marrow plasmacytosis >40% on flow cytometry or suspension smears in most patients
      (2) IgM <20 mg/100 ml or IgA <40 mg/100 ml or IgG <400 mg/100 ml in about half the patients
      (3) Serum β_2 microglobulin >8 mg/L without creatinine >1.8 mg/100 ml in about half the patients
2. Low tumor mass
   a. Characterized by all of the following:
      (1) Hemoglobin >10.5 g/100 ml, unless other factors are causing anemia
      (2) + Calcium <11 mg/100 ml†
      (3) + IgG or IgA peak <5.0 g/100 ml
      (4) + Serum β_2 microglobulin <4.5 mg/L
   b. Supporting features often present:
      (1) Marrow plasmacytosis <20% on flow cytometry or suspension smears in most patients
      (2) IgM >50 mg/100 ml and IgA >100 mg/100 ml and IgG >750 mg/100 ml in about half the patients
3. Intermediate tumor mass: all other patients

*IgM, IgG, and IgA are normal immunoglobulins.
†Corrected calcium (mg/100 ml) = Serum calcium (mg/100 ml) − Serum albumin (gm/100 ml) + 4.
From Smith L, Alexanian R: CA 35:214, 1985. Used with permission.

   a. Polycythemia is secondary to increased carboxyhemoglobin resulting in left shift in the hemoglobin dissociation curve
   b. Lab evaluation shows increased hematocrit, RBC mass, erythropoietin level, and carboxyhemoglobin
   c. Splenomegaly is not present on physical exam
2. Hypoxemia (secondary polycythemia): living for prolonged periods at high altitudes; pulmonary fibrosis, congenital cardiac lesions with right to left shunts
   a. Lab evaluation shows decreased arterial oxygen saturation and elevated erythropoietin level
   b. Splenomegaly is not present on physical exam
3. Erythropoietin-producing states: renal cell carcinoma, hepatoma, cerebral hemangioma, uterine fibroids, polycystic kidneys
   a. The erythropoietin level is elevated in these patients, the arterial oxygen saturation is normal
   b. Splenomegaly may be present with metastatic neoplasms

4. Stress polycythemia (Gaisböck's syndrome, relative polycythemia)
   a. Lab evaluation demonstrates normal RBC mass, arterial oxygen saturation, and erythropoietin level; plasma volume is decreased
   b. Splenomegaly is not present on physical exam
   c. These patients are at risk for thromboembolic events, particularly if they are smokers and are hypertensive
5. Hemoglobinopathies associated with high O_2 affinity: an abnormal oxyhemoglobin-dissociation curve (P50) is present

Characteristics and clinical manifestations

1. Polycythemia vera is slightly more common in men and in patients of Jewish descent
2. Average age at onset is 60 yr
3. The patient generally comes to medical attention because of symptoms associated with increased blood volume and viscosity or impaired platelet function
   a. Impaired cerebral circulation resulting in headache, vertigo, blurred vision, dizziness, TIA, CVA
   b. Fatigue, poor exercise tolerance
   c. Pruritus, particularly following bathing (due to overproduction of histamine)
   d. Bleeding: epistaxis, UGI bleeding (increased incidence of PUD)
   e. Abdominal discomfort secondary to splenomegaly; hepatomegaly may also be present
   f. Hyperuricemia may result in nephrolithiasis and gouty arthritis
4. Physical exam generally reveals facial plethora, enlargement and tortuosity of retinal veins, and splenomegaly

Lab results

1. Elevated RBC count (>6 million/mm^3), elevated hemoglobin (>18 g/dl in men, >16 g/dl in women), elevated hematocrit ($>54\%$ in men, $>49\%$ in women)
2. Increased WBC (often with basophilia), thrombocytosis is present in the majority of patients
3. Elevated leukocyte alkaline phosphatase, serum B_{12} level, and uric acid level are common

Diagnostic criteria

Diagnosis requires all three major criteria or the first two major criteria plus two minor criteria.
1. Major critera
   a. Increased RBC mass (≥36 ml/kg in men, ≥32 ml/kg in women)
   b. Normal arterial oxygen saturation ($\geq92\%$)
   c. Splenomegaly
2. Minor criteria
   a. Thrombocytosis ($>400,000$/mm^3)
   b. Leukocytosis ($>12,000$/mm^3)
   c. Elevated leukocyte alkaline phosphatase (>100)
   d. Elevated serum vitamin B_{12} (>900 pg/ml) or vitamin B_{12} binding protein (>2200 pg/ml)

Diagnostic step-wise approach

1. Measure RBC mass by isotope dilution using ^{51}Cr-labeled autologous RBCs; a high value eliminates stress polycythemia
2. Measure arterial saturation; a normal value eliminates polycythemia secondary to hypoxia
3. Measure carboxyhemoglobin; a normal value eliminates polycythemia secondary to smoking
4. Measure erythropoietin level; if elevated, obtain IVP and abdominal CT scan to rule out renal cell carcinoma
5. The diagnosis of hemoglobinopathy with high O_2 affinity is ruled out by a normal oxyhemoglobin dissociation curve

Treatment

1. Phlebotomy to keep Hb <15 mg/dl or hct ≤ 45%; the median survival time with phlebotomy is approximately 12 years
2. Diphenhydramine 25-50 mg q6h prn for pruritus
3. H_2 blockers to control gastric hyperacidity
4. Allopurinol may be necessary for hyperuricemia
5. Aspirin should be avoided because it may worsen bleeding associated with thrombocytosis
6. Radiophosphorus (^{32}P) produces hematologic remission in most patients, but it may result in an increased incidence of acute leukemia; therefore it should not be used routinely, but reserved for older patients responding poorly to the above measures
7. Hydroxyurea can be used in conjunction with phlebotomy and appears to be free of leukemogenic effect; indicated in elderly patients to decrease the incidence of thrombotic events

24.11 PLATELET DISORDERS

Thrombocytopenia

1. Definition: platelet count <100,000/mm^3
2. Clinical manifestations: ecchymoses, petechiae, purpura, menorrhagia, GI bleeding, epistaxes
3. Etiology
   a. Increased destruction
      (1) Immunological
         (a) Drugs: quinine, quinidine, digitalis, procainamide, thiazide diuretics, sulfonamides, phenytoin, aspirin, penicillin, heparin, gold
         (b) ITP: see next page
         (c) Transfusion reaction: transfusion of platelets with PLA-antigen in recipients without PLA-1 antigen
         (d) Fetal/maternal incompatibility
         (e) Vasculitis (e.g., SLE)
         (f) Autoimmune hemolytic anemia
         (g) Lymphoreticular disorders (e.g., CLL)
      (2) Nonimmunologic
         (a) Prosthetic heart valves
         (b) TTP

(c) Sepsis
(d) DIC: see Section 22.12
(e) Hemolytic-uremic syndrome
  b. Decreased production
    (1) Abnormal marrow
      (a) Marrow infiltration (e.g., leukemia, lymphoma, fibrosis)
      (b) Marrow suppression (e.g., chemotherapy, alcohol, radiation)
    (2) Hereditary disorders
      (a) Wiskott-Aldrich syndrome: X-linked disorder characterized by thrombocytopenia, eczema, and repeated infections
      (b) May-Hegglin anomaly: increased megakaryocytes but ineffective thrombopoiesis
    (3) Vitamin deficiencies (e.g., vitamin B_{12}, folic acid)
  c. Platelet sequestration and pooling
    (1) Splenomegaly
    (2) Cavernous hemangioma
  d. Dilutional, secondary to massive transfusion
4. Diagnostic approach to undetermined thrombocytopenia
  a. Thorough history (particularly drug history)
  b. Physical exam: evaluate for presence of splenomegaly (hypersplenism, leukemia, lymphoma)
  c. Examine peripheral blood smear; note platelet size and other abnormalities (e.g., fragmented RBCs may indicate TTP or DIC, increased platelet size suggests accelerated destruction and release of large young platelets into the circulation)
  d. Check PT, PTT, bleeding time, Coombs' test
  e. Bone marrow exam: increased megakaryocytes indicate thrombocytopenia secondary to accelerated destruction.

Idiopathic thrombocytopenic purpura (ITP)[37]

1. Definition: probable autoimmune disorder characterized by thrombocytopenia
2. Pathogenesis: Platelet destruction is believed to be mediated by autoantibodies or immune complexes triggered by an exposure to viral antigens
3. Characteristics and clinical manifestations
  a. ITP can be subdivided into acute and chronic forms: the acute form is generally seen in children following a viral infection; the chronic form occurs more frequently in young women (age 20-40)
  b. The clinical presentation is characterized by various manifestations of thrombocytopenia (petechiae, purpura, epistaxes, GI bleeding, menorrhagia); splenomegaly is generally not present on physical exam
4. Lab results
  a. Thrombocytopenia
  b. Anemia may be present in patients with significant hemorrhage
  c. Peripheral blood smear reveals a decreased amount of platelets, and normal or increased platelet size
  d. Bone marrow reveals increased number of megakaryocytes
  e. Increased platelet-associated IgG

5. Treatment
   a. Prednisone 1-2 mg/kg qd, continued until the platelet count is normalized, then slowly tapered off; prednisone improves platelet counts primarily by increasing platelet production
   b. Platelet transfusion only in case of life-threatening hemorrhage
   c. Have patient restrict physical activity and avoid any physical trauma
   d. Splenectomy (to prolong platelet survival) is indicated in patients not responding to steroids
   e. Immunosuppression with vincristine or cyclophosphamide may be necessary if significant thrombocytopenia persists despite steroids and splenectomy
   f. Gammaglobulins are effective primarily in children and in preparing patients for surgery and managing life-threatening bleeding; in adults, danazol, a synthetic attenuated androgen, is effective in chronic ITP and represents a good alternative to splenectomy in elderly patients[3,4]
6. Prognosis is excellent in children with the acute form (>90% recover within few months)

Thrombotic thrombocytopenic purpura[56]

1. Definition: rare disorder characterized by thrombocytopenia and microangiopathic hemolytic anemia
2. Characteristics and clinical manifestations
   a. Purpura (secondary to thrombocytopenia)
   b. Jaundice, pallor (secondary to hemolysis)
   c. Mucosal bleeding
   d. Fever
   e. Neurologic symptoms and signs (e.g., fluctuating levels of consciousness)
   f. Renal failure (secondary to renal cortical infarction and hypertension)
3. Lab results
   a. Severe anemia and thrombocytopenia
   b. Elevated BUN and creatinine
   c. Hematuria and proteinuria
   d. Peripheral blood smear shows severely fragmented RBCs (schistocytes)
   e. No lab evidence of DIC (normal FDP, fibrinogen)
4. Treatment[49]
   a. Plasmapheresis with fresh frozen plasma replacement
   b. Concomitant administration of corticosteroids and antiplatelet agents is often used
   c. Vincristine in patients refractory to plasmapheresis
   d. Splenectomy in refractory cases

24.12 DISSEMINATED INTRAVASCULAR COAGULATION

Definition

Disseminated intravascular coagulation (DIC) is characterized by generalized activation of the clotting mechanism

Etiology

1. Infections (e.g., gram-negative sepsis, viral infection)
2. Obstetric complications (e.g., dead fetus, amniotic fluid embolism, abruptio placentae)
3. Tissue trauma (e.g., burns)
4. Neoplasms (e.g., adenocarcinomas, acute promyelocytic leukemia)
5. Quinine

Clinical manifestations

DIC manifests with profuse bleeding (less commonly thrombosis) in association with any of the above clinical settings.

Lab results

1. Peripheral blood smear generally shows red blood cell fragments and low platelet count
2. Additional findings vary depending on whether the DIC is acute or chronic; Table 24-4 describes lab findings indicative of DIC
3. Coagulopathy secondary to DIC needs to be differentiated from that secondary to liver disease or vitamin K deficiency
   a. Vitamin K deficiency manifests with prolonged PT and normal PTT, TT, platelet, and fibrinogen level; PTT may be elevated in severe cases
   b. Patients with liver disease have abnormal PT and PTT; TT and fibrinogen are usually normal unless severe disease is present; platelets are usually normal unless splenomegaly is present
   c. DIC results in thrombocytopenia, decreased fibrinogen, and abnormal PT and TT; PTT may be normal or prolonged depending on the stage (acute vs chronic)

Table 24-4   Findings indicative of DIC

Test Parameter	Acute DIC	Chronic DIC
Fibrinogen (clottable)	↓↓ or ↓↓↓	N or ↑
Fibrinolytic activity	N rarely ↑	N rarely ↑
Fibrin breakdown products present	++	+
Soluble fibrin monomer complexes (protamine sulfate or ethanol gelation)	++	+
Platelet count	↓↓ to ↓↓↓	N to ↑
APTT (activated partial thromboplastin time)	↑ to ↑↑ to ↑↑↑	N
PT (prothrombin time)	↑	N
Thrombin time	↑↑	↑
RBC microangiopathy	—	↑

Therapy

1. Correct underlying cause (e.g., antimicrobial therapy for infection)
2. Replacement therapy with fresh-frozen plasma and platelets in patients with significant hemorrhage
3. Heparin therapy at a dose lower than that used in venous thrombosis may be useful in selected cases (e.g., DIC associated with acute promyelocytic leukemia)

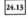 **CARCINOMA OF THE BREAST**
Joseph DiBenedetto, Jr.

Epidemiology

1. Most common malignant tumor in the western world (1 out of 12 women in the U.S. will develop breast cancer)
2. Increased incidence with age; two thirds of all cases develop after the age of 50
3. Breast cancer occurs overwhelmingly in women (less than 1% in men)
4. Women with first-degree relatives (mothers, sisters) who have had breast cancer are two to three times more likely to develop it
5. Increased incidence in women with previous history of breast cancer and those exposed to ionizing radiation
6. Some possible increase with high-fat diet and obesity
7. No definite link with oral contraceptives[39]

Histological classification

A number of pathological classifications of mammary carcinoma are used, with those presented by the Armed Forces Institute of Pathology and the World Health Organization the most common. Breast tumors usually originate from mammary epithelium and are either ductal or lobular corresponding to the ducts and lobules of the normal breast. Eighty percent of malignancies are infiltrating ductal carcinomas; less common are infiltrating lobular carcinoma, medullary carcinoma, and mucinous carcinoma. Medullary and mucinous carcinomas have a better survival rate than infiltrating ductal carcinoma. Inflammatory breast cancer is characterized by skin edema and an erysipeloid margin with induration of the surrounding tissue. Microscopically this is associated with involvement of dermal lymphatics by tumor and carries a poor prognosis.

All breast cancers should be tested for estrogen receptor (ER) and progesterone receptor (PR) proteins. Approximately a third of all premenopausal women will show receptors for estrogen and two thirds of postmenopausal patients will show receptors to estrogen.[41] ER positive tumors tend to be less virulent and are more likely to respond to hormonal manipulation by either drug therapy or surgical ablation. Tumors that contain both ERs and PRs have the greatest likelihood of responding after an endocrine maneuver, and the probability of a response increases directly with the titer of the receptor protein.

Diagnosis

1. Breast self-examination
   a. Most breast cancers (90%) are discovered first by the woman herself or her sexual partner

b. The American Cancer Society recommends monthly self-examination for all women over the age of 20
c. Premenopausal exams should be performed a week after the start of the menstrual period when the breasts are not swollen or tender
d. Postmenopausal exams usually are performed on the first of the month (or some easy-to-remember date)
e. Changes in contour, a swelling, or any dimpling or puckering of the skin, or a change in the nipple, may signal danger
f. Any mass that is new and persists for greater than a few weeks or is rapidly enlarging requires a physician's examination
g. Self-examination is without cost
2. Mammography (see Chapter 4)
3. About 50% of all breast cancers develop in the upper outer quadrant of the breast[53]
4. Diagnosis established only by biopsy

Staging

The staging of breast cancer reflects the anatomical extent of the tumor and is presented below:

1. Stage I—tumor less than 2 cm without skin involvement and with no clinically suspicious axillary nodes
2. Stage II—tumor less than 2 cm with clinically suspicious nodes; any tumor 2 to 5 cm with or without clinically suspicious nodes
3. Stage III—any tumor greater than 5 cm; skin involvement or chest wall attachment; any size of tumor with clinically fixed axillary nodes; arm edema; supraclavicular nodes; skin ulceration
4. Stage IV—metastatic disease
5. At time of diagnosis for white women:
   a. 50% Stage I or II
   b. 40% Stage III
   c. 10% Stage IV
6. At time of diagnosis for black women:
   a. 33% Stage I or II
   b. 50% Stage III
   c. 17% Stage IV
7. Stages correlate with survival and are important in treatment planning, but do not totally predict the clinical behavior of the tumor.
8. Staging work-up includes a history and physical, chest x-ray, a CBC, and liver chemistries. The value of bone scan, liver scan, and mammography has been a matter of controversy.[38] The carcinoembryonic antigen (CEA) may be of benefit as a marker; a rise following therapy may signify recurrent disease.[5]

Treatment

The ideal treatment of early cancer of the breast still generates controversy among physicians and patients, with such factors as age, estrogen receptor status, type of surgery, role of radiation therapy, need and type of chemotherapy, hormonal therapy, and length of treatment all contributing factors.

Some treatment recommendations include

1. Stage I & II—premenopausal (ER negative or ER positive)

   a. Modified radical mastectomy and 6 mo of adjuvant chemother-
      apy[2,36] or
   b. Lumpectomy with axillary dissection, local radiation,[22] and 6 mo
      of adjuvant chemotherapy[2,36]
2. Stage I & II—postmenopausal (ER negative)
   a. Modified radical mastectomy and 6 mo of adjuvant chemother-
      apy[23,36] or
   b. Lumpectomy with axillary dissection, local radiation,[22] and 6 mo
      of adjuvant chemotherapy[23,36]
3. Stage I & II—postmenopausal (ER positive)
   a. Modified radical mastectomy and tamoxifen therapy[2,24] or
   b. Lumpectomy with axillary dissection, local radiation,[22] and ta-
      moxifen therapy[2,10]
4. Stage III (locally advanced breast cancer)
   a. Induction chemotherapy followed by modified radical mastec-
      tomy followed by 1-2 additional yr of chemotherapy or
   b. Induction chemotherapy followed by primary radiation followed
      by 2 additional yr of chemotherapy
5. Stage IV disease
   a. Systemic chemotherapy and/or hormonal therapy depending upon
      several factors previously mentioned
6. The main chemotherapeutic agents used are cyclophosphamide,
   methotrexate, and 5-fluorouracil (CMF), or doxorubicin substituted
   for methotrexate (CAF); Other useful drugs include vinblastine, mitomycin C, L-phenylalanine mustard, and thiotepa; useful hormonal
   agents include tamoxifen, megestrol acetate, corticosteroids, aminoglutethimide, and androgens
7. Factors associated with increased probability of response
   a. Good performance status
   b. Ambulatory status
   c. Limited number of sites of disease
   d. High labeling indices
   e. High thymidine kinase levels
8. Factors associated with decreased probability of response
   a. Bone metastases
   b. Liver metastases
   c. Prior chemotherapy
   d. Prior radiotherapy
   e. Decreased lymphocyte count
   f. High levels of cathepsin D in node-negative patients[54]

References

1. Adamson JW: Polycythemia vera. In Petersdorf RG, et al (editors): Harrison's
   Principles of internal medicine, ed 10, New York, 1983, McGraw-Hill Book Co.
2. Adjuvant chemotherapy for breast cancer, JAMA 254:3461, 1985.
3. Ahm YS, et al: Danazol for the treatment of idiopathic thrombocytopenic purpura, N Engl J Med 308:1396, 1983.
4. Ahn YS, et al: Long-term danazol therapy in autoimmune thrombocytopenia: un-
   maintained remission and age-dependent response in women, Ann Intern Med
   111:723, 1989.

5. Alexanian R, et al: Prognosis of asymptomatic multiple myeloma, Arch Intern Med 148:1963, 1988.

6. Alexanian R, Dreicer R: Chemotherapy for multiple myeloma, Cancer 53:583, 1984.

7. Al-Mondhiry H, Stryker J, Kempin S: Splenic irradiation (SI) in chronic lymphocytic leukemia (CLL). Abstract, Proc Am Soc Clin Oncol 3:192, 1984.

8. Anasetti C, et al: Marrow transplantation for severe aplastic anemia, long-term outcome in fifty "untransfused" patients, Ann Intern Med 104:461, 1986.

9. Aoki Y: Multiple enzymatic defects in mitochondria in hematological cells of patients with primary sideroblastic anemia, J Clin Invest 66:43, 1980.

10. Barlogie B, et al: High levels of lactic dehydrogenase identify a high-grade lymphoma-like myeloma, Ann Intern Med 110:521, 1989.

11. Bataille R, Grenier J, Sany J: Beta-2-microglobulin in myeloma: optimal use for staging, prognosis, and treatment—a prospective study of 160 patients, Blood 63:468, 1984.

12. Bennett JM, Catovsky D, et al: Criteria for the diagnosis of acute leukemia of megakaryocyte lineage (M7), Ann Intern Med 103:460, 1985.

13. Berlin NI: Diagnosis and classification of the polycythemias, Semin Hematol 12:339, 1975.

14. Bluhm R, Branch R, et al: Aplastic anemia associated with canthaxanthin ingested for "tanning purposes," JAMA 264:1141, 1990.

15. Canellos GP: Chronic leukemias. In DeVita VT, Hellman S, Rosenberg SA (editors): Cancer: principles and practice of oncology, Philadelphia, 1985, JB Lippincott Co.

16. Carbone PP, et al: Report of the committee on Hodgkin's disease staging, Cancer Res 31:1860, 1971.

17. Cassileth PA: Adult acute nonlymphocytic leukemia, Med Clin North Am 68:675, 1984.

18. DeVita VT Jr, Jaffee ES, Hellman S: Hodgkin's disease and the non-Hodgkin's lymphomas. In DeVita VT, Hellman S, Rosenberg SA (editors): Cancer: principles and practice of oncology, Philadelphia, 1985, JB Lippincott Co.

19. Durie BGM, Salmon SE: A clinical staging system for multiple myeloma: correlation of measured myeloma cell mass with presenting clinical features, response to treatment, and survival, Cancer 36:842, 1975.

20. Estey E, et al: Infection prophylaxis in acute leukemia: comparative effectiveness of sulfamethoxazole and trimethoprim, ketoconazole, and a combination of the two, Arch Intern Med 144:1562, 1984.

21. Fehr J, Hofmann V, Kappeler U: Transient reversal of thrombocytopenic purpura by high dose intravenous gamma globulin, N Engl J Med 306:1254, 1982.

22. Fisher B, et al: Eight year results of a randomized clinical trial comparing total mastectomy and lumpectomy with or without irradiation in the treatment of breast cancer, N Engl J Med 320:822, 1989.

23. Fisher B, et al: A randomized clinical trial evaluating sequential methotrexate and fluorouracil in the treatment of patients with node-negative breast cancer who have estrogen receptor–negative tumors, N Engl J Med 320:473, 1989.

24. Fisher B, et al: A randomized clinical trial evaluating tamoxifen in the treatment of patients with node-negative breast cancer who have estrogen receptor–positive tumors, N Engl J Med 320:479, 1989.

25. Fisher RI, et al: Diffuse aggressive lymphomas: increased survival after alternating flexible sequences of ProMACE and MOPP chemotherapy, Ann Intern Med 98:304, 1983.

26. Goldberg MA, Brugnara C, et al: Treatment of sickle cell anemia with hydroxyurea and erythropoietin, N Engl J Med 323:366, 1990.

27. Gore ME, et al: Intensive treatment of multiple myeloma and criteria for complete remission, Lancet 2:879, 1989.

28. Haller DG: Non-Hodgkin's lymphomas, Med Clin North Am 68:741, 1984.

29. International workshop on chronic lymphocytic leukemia: Chronic lymphocytic leukemia: recommendations for diagnosis, staging, and response criteria, Ann Intern Med 110:236, 1989.

30. Jacobs AD, Gale RP: Recent advances in the biology and treatment acute lymphoblastic leukemia in adults, N Engl J Med 311:1219, 1984.

31. Kaldor JM, Day NE, et al: Leukemia following Hodgkin's disease, N Engl J Med 322:7, 1990.

32. Karp JE, et al: Oral norfloxacin for prevention of gram-negative bacterial infections in patients with acute leukemia and granulocytopenia, Ann Intern Med 106:1, 1987.

33. Lindenbaum J, et al: Neuropsychiatric disorders caused by cobalamin deficiency in the absence of anemia or macrocytosis, N Engl J Med 318:1720, 1988.

34. Loprinzi CL, et al: Prospective evaluation of the carcinoembryonic antigen levels and alternating chemotherapeutic regimens in metastatic breast cancer, J Clin Oncol 4:46, 1986.

35. Lukes RJ, Collins RD: Immunologic characterization of human malignant lymphomas, Cancer 34:1488, 1974.

36. Mansour EG, Gray R, Shatila AH, et al: Efficacy of adjuvant chemotherapy in high risk node-negative breast cancer, N Engl J Med 320:485, 1989.

37. McMillan R: Chronic idiopathic thrombocytopenic purpura, N Engl J Med 304:1135, 1981.

38. McNeil B, Pace PPD, Gray E: Pre-operative and follow-up bone scans in patients with primary carcinoma of the breast, Surg Gynecol Obstet 147:745, 1978.

39. McPherson K, Drife JO: The pill and breast cancer, why the uncertainty? Br Med J 293:709, 1986.

40. National Cancer Institutes–sponsored study on classification of non-Hodgkin's lymphoma: Summary and description of a working formulation for clinical usage. The non-Hodgkin's lymphoma pathological classification project, Cancer 49:2112, 1982.

41. Osborne CK: Receptors. In Harris JR, Hellman D, et al (editors): Breast diseases, Philadelphia, 1987, JB Lippincott Co, pp 210-232.

42. Piro LD, Carrera CJ, et al: Lasting remission in hairy-cell leukemia induced by a single infusion of 2-chlorodeoxyadenosine, N Engl J Med 322:117, 1990.

43. Portlock CS: Hodgkin's disease, Med Clin North Am 68:729, 1984.

44. Rai KR, et al: Chronic lymphocytic leukemia, Med Clin North Am 68:697, 1984.

45. Rai KR, et al: Clinical staging of chronic lymphocytic leukemia, Blood 46:219, 1975.

46. Rappoport H: Tumors of the hematopoietic system. In Atlas of tumor pathology. Section 3, Fascicle 8, Washington DC, 1966, Armed Forces Institute of Pathology.

47. Schreeder MT, Prchal JT: Successful treatment of thrombotic thrombocytopenic purpura by vincristine, Am J Hematol 14:75, 1983.

48. Schrier SL: Anemia: production defects. In Rubenstein E, Federman DD (editors): Scientific American medicine, New York, 1985, Scientific American Inc, Chapter 9, Section 5.

49. Sennett ML, Conrad ME: Treatment of thrombotic thrombocytopenic purpura: plasmapheresis, plasma transfusion, and vincristine, Arch Intern Med 146:266, 1986.

50. Skihne BS: A practical approach to the initial diagnosis of anemia, Med Times 114:63, 1986.

51. Smith L, Alexanian R: Treatment strategies for plasma cell myeloma, CA 35:214, 1985.

52. Spiers ASD: Chronic granulocytic leukemia, Med Clin North Am 68:713, 1984.

53. Spratt JS, Donegan WL: Cancer of the breast, Philadelphia, 1967, WB Saunders Co.

54. Tandon AK, et al: Cathepsin D and prognosis in breast cancer, N Engl J Med 322:297, 1990.

55. Thomas ED, Clift RA: Marrow transplantation for the treatment of chronic myelogenous leukemia, Ann Intern Med 104:155, 1986.
56. Thompson HN, McCarthy LJ: Thrombotic thrombocytopenic purpura, Arch Intern Med 143:2117, 1983.
57. Ultmann JE, Jacobs RH: The non-Hodgkin's lymphomas, CA 35:66, 1985
58. Wiernik PH: Acute leukemias of adults. In DeVita VT, Hellman S, Rosenberg SA (editors): Cancer: principles and practice of oncology, Philadelphia, 1985, JB Lippincott Co.

Infectious Diseases

NOSOCOMIAL INFECTIONS
Joseph Herbin

Definition

A nosocomial infection is one that was not present or incubating when the patient entered the hospital. It includes any infection acquired during hospitalization and manifested clinically after hospital discharge (e.g., hepatitis B).

Predisposing factors

1. Surgery or other invasive procdures
2. Urinary or intravenous catheters
3. Immunocompromised host because of underlying disease (e.g., leukemia) or treatments (e.g., immunosuppressive agents)

Clinical manifestations

1. Fever; its absence does not rule out infection (particularly in elderly patients)
2. Change in mental status, delirium
3. Unexplained hypotension, tachycardia, tachypnea

Lab results

1. Alterations of WBC ranging from neutropenia to marked leukocytosis with shift to left
2. Metabolic acidosis
3. Hypernatremia, elevated BUN, creatinine (secondary to dehydration)

Common sites of infections

1. Urinary tract
2. Surgical wounds
3. Intravascular devices
4. Respiratory tract

Control of nosocomial infection

General principles

Consistent with universal precautions, disposable gloves should be worn if contact with blood or body fluids of any patient is anticipated.

1. Handwashing is the single most important procedure for prevention of nosocomial infections[9]
   a. In the absence of a true emergency, personnel should *always* wash their hands:
      (1) Before performing invasive procedures
      (2) Before taking care of particularly susceptible patients (e.g., immunocompromised patients, newborns)
      (3) After removing gloves
      (4) After touching inanimate sources that are likely to be contaminated with virulent or epidemiologically important microorganisms (e.g., urine measuring devices or secretion collection apparatus)
      (5) After caring for an infected patient or one likely to be colonized with microorganisms of special clinical or epidemiologic significance (e.g., bacteria resistant to multiple antibiotics)
      (6) Between contacts with different patients in high-risk units
   b. Most routine, brief patient care activities other than those above (e.g., measuring blood pressure) do not require handwashing
   c. Most routine hospital activities involving indirect patient contact (e.g., handling medication, food, or other objects) do not require handwashing

Selected nosocomial infections

1. Urinary tract infections (UTIs) are the most common nosocomial occurrence
   a. Manifestations: most patients are asymptomatic, but 1% may develop bacteremia (chills, fever) and localized symptoms (dysuria, frequency, urgency, CVA tenderness)
   b. Contributing factors: Foley catheters, cystoscopy or surgery, obstruction with ureteral reflux
   c. Common organisms: gram-negative bacilli, *Escherichia, Pseudomonas aeruginosa, Proteus*/Providencia, group D streptococci, *Staphylococcus aureus,* and *Candida*
   d. Prevention
      (1) Insert Foley catheter only if absolutely necessary
      (2) Insert with aseptic technique
      (3) Keep system closed
      (4) Remove catheter as soon as possible
      (5) Treat "positive" cultures only if the patient is symptomatic
   e. Management of suspected UTI
      (1) Patient without Foley catheter
         (a) Insert a Foley catheter and record residual urine volume; if volume >250 ml, leave catheter in
         (b) Obtain urinalysis and culture
         (c) Perform Gram stain of urine sediment
         (d) Treat symptomatic patients on the basis of Gram stain results

- Gram-positive cocci: treat for enterococci and *S. aureus*
- Gram-negative bacilli: treat for presumed *Pseudomonas*

  (2) Patient with Foley catheter
- (a) Rule out other sources of infection
- (b) If no other sources are found and urine culture is positive, treat symptomatic patient based on culture results
- (c) If urine culture is negative, perform Gram stain of urine sediment and treat as described above

2. Surgical wound infection: a wound is considered infected if purulent material drains from it, even if cultures reveal no growth; most infections are confined to the incisional wound, the deep tissues are rarely involved
   a. Contributing factors: impaired host resistance (e.g., malnourished patient), poor surgical technique, surgery involving contaminated or potentially contaminated areas (e.g., traumatic lacerations), virulence, and number of organisms that contaminate the wound
   b. Common organisms: *S. aureus* is the most common pathogen isolated; other frequent pathogens include streptococci, gram-negative bacilli, and anaerobes
   c. Prevention: good surgical technique is the most important measure in the prevention of a wound infection; additional recommendations are as follows[10]:
      (1) In elective surgery, the preoperative hospital stay should be as short as possible
      (2) If the patient is malnourished and surgery is not urgent, the patient should receive enteric or parenteral hyperalimentation before surgery
      (3) In elective surgery, all bacterial infections, except that for which the operation is performed, should be treated before surgery
      (4) When indicated (e.g., endocarditis prophylaxis), prophylactic antibiotics should be given just before surgery and discontinued promptly afterwards
      (5) If hair removal is necessary, clipping is preferable to shaving
      (6) The common accepted preoperative, intraoperative, and postoperative procedures should be strictly followed
      (7) Personnel should wash their hands before and after taking care of a surgical wound
      (8) Fresh or open wounds should be touched only with sterile gloves
      (9) Dressings should be removed or changed if wet or if the patient has signs suggestive of infection; wound drainage should be Gram stained and cultured
      (10) Patients with infected wounds should be placed on isolation precautions according to the hospital's infection control guidelines
   d. Management of infected surgical wounds
      (1) Inspect the wound thoroughly
      (2) If the wound is sutured or closed but shows signs of infection (erythema, foul smell, drainage), surgical evaluation is indicated with possible removal of sutures and exploration of the wound for presence of pus
      (3) If purulence is present, Gram stain and aerobic and anaerobic cultures should be obtained

        (4) Consider necrotizing cellulitis or fasciitis if symptoms are severe or if local findings are extensive; urgent surgical evaluation is indicated

        (5) If deep infection is suspected, obtain ultrasound or CT scan to rule out abscess formation

        (6) The choice of antibiotics depends on the Gram stain results; if no organisms are seen, treat for *S. aureus*

3. Intravascular device infection can result in septicemia, endocarditis, suppurative thrombophlebitis, tract infection, and local site infection

    a. Common organisms: *S. aureus* and *Staphylococcus epidermidis* are the most frequent infecting organisms; other organisms include gram-negative bacilli, *Candida*, enterococci, and diphtheroids

    b. Prevention

        (1) All major intravascular devices (e.g., CVP lines, arterial lines) should be inserted using sterile technique and should be sutured to the skin to prevent movement

        (2) Whenever possible, use peripheral rather than central lines, percutaneous rather than cut-down insertion, and upper rather than lower extremities

    c. When a device is inserted using unsterile technique (i.e., in an emergency situation) consider removal within 24 hr and replacement, using sterile technique

        (1) Remove all intravascular devices as soon as possible (increased risk of infection after 72 hr); culture catheter tip

    d. Management

        (1) If catheter-related infection is suspected, obtain blood cultures from a peripheral site, through an intravascular catheter, or both

        (2) Remove the catheter, obtain Gram stain and culture of any purulent drainage, and culture the catheter tip (preferably by quantitative technique)

        (3) Antibiotic choice depends upon the Gram stain results; if no organism is seen, treat for *S. aureus*

4. Respiratory tract infection: pneumonia is the leading cause of death of all nosocomial infections

    a. Manifestations

        (1) Fever, dyspnea, cough, increased sputum production

        (2) Decreased arterial Po_2, leukocytosis

        (3) New or worsening infiltrate on chest x-ray

        (4) Purulent sputum

    b. Risk factors

        (1) Severity of underlying disease (e.g., COPD, cancer, leukemia)

        (2) Surgery (thoracic or thoracoabdominal surgery)

        (3) Intubation or tracheostomy

        (4) Hospitalization in an intensive care unit (ICU)

        (5) Atelectasis

        (6) Excessive sedation

        (7) Immunosuppressive medication (e.g., steroids)

        (8) Antibiotic therapy

        (9) Advanced age

    c. Common organisms: *S. aureus* and gram-negative bacilli are the most common infecting organisms; less common are *Haemophilus influenzae, Streptococcus pneumoniae,* anaerobes, *Legionella,* viruses, and fungi *(Candida, Aspergillus)*

d. Prevention is difficult; measures include the following:

  (1) Prevention of atelectasis in postoperative patients by encouraging deep breathing and coughing in addition to incentive spirometry

  (2) Minimize excessive sedation to prevent aspiration

  (3) Avoid (if possible) the use of steroid immunosuppressive therapy

  (4) Minimize continuous ventilatory support

  (5) Use sucralfate instead of antacids or H_2 blockers for prevention of stress ulcers in intubation patients (↑ risk of gram-negative pneumonia in patients with ↑ gastric pH)

e. Diagnosis of suspected respiratory tract infection

  (1) Chest x-ray: look for new or changing pulmonary infiltrates

  (2) Obtain a sputum specimen for Gram stain and culture; consider transtracheal aspiration if necessary to obtain an adequate sputum specimen

  (3) Obtain two or three blood cultures from different sites (not through an intravascular device)

  (4) Check arterial blood gases and WBC

f. Management: the choice of antibiotics depends on the clinical setting, the sputum Gram stain, and the chest x-ray film

  (1) Gram-positive cocci: treat for *S. aureus*

  (2) Gram-negative bacilli; treat for *Pseudomonas aeruginosa*

  (3) Inconclusive Gram stain and

    (a) Localized infiltrate: consider gram-negative bacilli or *S. aureus;* treat with third generation cephalosporin plus aminoglycoside

    (b) Diffuse infiltrates: consider *Legionella* (treat with erythromycin) or *Pneumocystis carinii* in immunocompromised host (treat with IV trimethoprim/sulfamethoxazole); aerobic gram-negative bacilli, gram-positive bacteria, anaerobes, and fungal pneumonia should also be considered in patients with diffuse infiltrates

  (4) If there is no significant clinical response to the initial antibiotics, fiberoptic bronchoscopy should be strongly considered

Additional recommendations

1. Immunization of house staff: hepatitis vaccine, DT, measles, influenza

2. Zidovudine (AZT) prophylaxis following exposure to HIV infected blood/body fluids (refer to Section 25.4)

25.2 PRINCIPLES OF ANTIBIOTIC USE

Characteristics of commonly used antimicrobial agents

Cephalosporins (see Table 33-20)

Cephalosporins are subdivided into three generations based on their gram-negative enteric bacillary activity:

1. First-generation: excellent broad-spectrum activity against gram-positive

cocci *(Staphylococcus aureus, Streptococcus pneumoniae);* limited activity against gram-negative bacilli, except *E. coli, Proteus mirabilis,* and *Klebsiella;* poor coverage of *Enterococcus*
2. Second-generation: more effective against gram-negative bacilli than first generation cephalosporins
   a. Cefoxitin and cefotetan have excellent activity against *Bacteroides fragilis* and *Serratia* sp
   b. Cefuroxime crosses the blood-brain barrier (useful in the treatment of some forms of bacterial meningitis)
   c. Cefamandole and cefotetan can prolong bleeding time
3. Third-generation: broader activity against most enteric gram-negative bacilli
   a. Cefotaxime, ceftriaxone, and moxalactam demonstrate good CSF penetration and are useful in the treatment of gram-negative meningitis
   b. Ceftazidime is active against *Pseudomonas* sp
   c. Moxalactam can cause bleeding by prolonging prothrombin time and inhibiting platelet function

Aminoglycosides

Aminoglycosides are bactericidal by virtue of irreversible inhibition of protein synthesis. Elimination is by glomerular filtration; therefore dosage must be adjusted in renal failure, and monitoring of aminoglycoside peaks and troughs and serum creatinine levels should be performed.
1. Common preparations: gentamicin, tobramycin, amikacin, kanamycin, neomycin, netilmicin, streptomycin
2. Comments
   a. Aminoglycosides have excellent activity against aerobic gram-negative rods; however, they are ineffective against anaerobic organisms and streptococci
   b. Amikacin has the broadest spectrum of activity; it is useful in the treatment of gentamicin- or tobramycin-resistant bacteria
   c. Netilmicin is a new aminoglycoside similar to gentamicin but less nephrotoxic and ototoxic
   d. Kanamycin is infrequently used because of a high degree of bacterial resistance
   e. Neomycin is used orally to reduce intestinal bacteria in patients with hepatic encephalopathy
   f. Gentamicin is the drug of choice against sensitive strains because of its lower cost and extensive clinical experience

Penicillins

Can be subdivided into four generations based on an increasing spectrum of activity (see Tables 33-12 and 33-14).
1. First-generation
   a. Penicillin G (aqueous, procaine, benzathine), phenoxymethyl penicillin (penicillin V), methicillin, oxacillin, dicloxacillin, nafcillin
   b. Comments
      (1) Penicillins G and V are useful against streptococci, most anaerobes found in the oral cavity, *Treponema pallidum, Clostridium,* non–penicillinase-producing staphylococci, most *Neisseria* and

   Bacteroides sp (except *B. fragilis), Listeria,* and *Pasteurella multocida*
  (2) Methicillin, nafcillin, oxacillin, and dicloxacillin are effective against penicillinase-producing strains of *S. aureus*
2. Second-generation
 a. Ampicillin and amoxicillin
 b. Comments
  (1) Broader spectrum against gram-negative organisms *(E. coli, Proteus mirabilis,* and *H. influenzae)*
  (2) Ineffective against penicillinase-producing bacteria, *Klebsiella,* and *Pseudomonas* strains
3. Third-generation
 a. Carbenicillin and ticarcillin
 b. Comments
  (1) Increased activity against *P. aeruginosa, Enterobacter* sp, *Morganella morgagni,* and *Proteus* sp
  (2) Ineffective against penicillinase-producing bacteria
  (3) Less active against enterococci than ampicillin
  (4) Often used in combination with an aminoglycoside to treat *P. aeruginosa* infections
4. Fourth-generation
 a. Azlocillin, mezlocillin, and piperacillin
 b. Comments
  (1) Broader spectrum of activity than third generation penicillins
  (2) More active against enterococci
  (3) Greater activity against *P. aeruginosa* and *Klebsiella* strains
  (4) Inactive against penicillinase-producing staphylococci or ampicillin-resistant *Haemophilus influenzae*

Erythromycin

1. Active against most gram-negative cocci
2. Effective against *Mycoplasma pneumoniae, Legionella* sp, pneumococci, group A streptococci, *Chlamydia,* and *Campylobacter jejuni*
3. Inactive against most gram-negative bacilli

Metronidazole

1. Effective against anaerobes (*B. fragilis, Clostridium, Fusobacterium,* anaerobic cocci); useful for intraabdominal and pelvic infections
2. Good CSF penetration; useful in the treatment of meningitis or brain abscess secondary to *B. fragilis*
3. Effective in the treatment of pseudomembranous colitis secondary to *Clostridium difficile*
4. Antiprotozoal useful for therapy for *Trichomonas* and *Entamoeba histolytica*

Trimethoprim/sulfamethoxazole

1. Indicated for *Pneumocystis carinii* pneumonia
2. Useful for treatment of outpatient UTIs
3. Effective in otitis media (in penicillin-allergic patients) and in exacerbation in COPD

Vancomycin

1. Excellent activity against gram-positive bacteria (including methicillin-resistant staphylococci)
2. Useful in enterococcal infections in patients allergic to penicillin
3. Effective orally for pseudomembranous colitis secondary to *C. difficile*
4. Used in combination with gentamicin and rifampin for prosthetic valve endocarditis caused by methicillin-resistant *Staphylococcus*
5. Intraperitoneal vancomycin is used for *S. epidermidis* peritonitis in patients on peritoneal dialysis

Clindamycin

1. Effective against anaerobes *(B. fragilis)* and gram-positive cocci
2. Useful for intraabdominal infections and for infections secondary to gram-positive cocci in patients allergic to penicillin

Imipenem

1. New class of broad-spectrum antibiotics (Carbapenem); administered in combination with cilastin (Primaxin) to prevent rapid renal metabolism
2. Comments
   a. Imipenem/cilastin (Primaxin) has the broadest antibacterial spectrum of any available antibiotic
   b. Effective against most bacterial pathogens, including anaerobes, *Listeria,* and *Nocardia*
   c. Ineffective against *Streptococcus faecalis* and some *Pseudomonas* sp *(P. cepacia, P. maltophilia),* some methicillin-resistant staphylococci, *C. difficile,* and *Legionella* species
   d. Indicated only in life-threatening intraabdominal/pelvic infections or mixed soft tissue infections of the extremities in patients with occlusive arterial disease when the organisms are resistant to other antibiotics or when multiple antibiotics may be necessary

Monobactams

1. Narrow spectrum of activity, limited to aerobic gram-negative organisms
2. Aztreonam (Azactam) is very useful in the treatment of complicated and uncomplicated urinary tract infections

Beta-lactamase inhibitors

1. Clavulanate can be administered in combination with amoxicillin (Augmentin) or ticarcillin (Timentin)
   a. Augmentin has a spectrum similar to second generation cephalosporins and is active against enterococci; it is useful for otitis media and sinusitis
   b. Timentin has a spectrum similar to third generation cephalosporins
2. Sulbactam is available in combination with ampicillin (Unasyn) for parenteral use; it is useful in mixed aerobic-anaerobic soft tissue infection and in gynecological and intraabdominal infections

Quinolones (see Table 33-32)

1. New class of antimicrobial agents structurally related to nalidixic acid but with greater potency and a broader spectrum of activity; they exert their action by inhibiting bacterial DNA replication
2. Quinolone agents available in the USA or pending FDA approval are ciprofloxacin, norfloxacin, enoxacin, ofloxacin, and pefloxacin
   a. Ciprofloxacin (Cipro) is well absorbed from the GI tract and achieves excellent serum and tissue concentrations; it is useful in nosocomial UTI as well as infections of the skin, soft tissue, bone, and joints and in lower respiratory infections and infectious diarrhea; it offers an economical alternative to parenteral therapy in many infections
   b. Norfloxacin (Noroxin) is useful in nosocomial urinary tract infection.
3. Concomitant administration of antacids must be avoided since the absorption of all quinolones is significantly reduced by antacids containing magnesium and/or aluminum; quinolones (particularly enoxacin) also interfere with theophylline metabolism (via inhibition of cytochrome P-450) and can result in theophylline toxicity; the simultaneous administration of sucralfate will impair absorption of ciprofloxacin and norfloxacin[37]

Rifampin

1. Semisynthetic antibiotic derivative of rifamycin B
2. Indicated in all forms of tuberculosis
3. Used to eliminate meningococci from the nasopharynx
4. May be useful as an addition to erythromycin for poorly responsive *Legionella* pneumonia

Antibiotic susceptibility testing[13]

1. MIC (minimum inhibitory concentration): lowest antibiotic concentration that inhibits visible growth of a standardized inoculum after overnight incubation
2. MBC (minimum bactericidal concentration): lowest concentration of an antibiotic necesssary to kill 99.9% of bacterial cells when a mixture of bacteria and antibiotic have been incubated together
3. SBT (serum bactericidal titer): determined by inoculating dilutions of the patient's serum with the infecting bacterial isolate; dilutes with no growth after 24 hr are then cultured without antibiotic (the SBT is the highest titer with a 99.9% kill)

Antibiotics in renal failure

Table 33-4 describes antibiotic dosage reduction necessary in patients with impaired renal function.

25.3 FEVER OF UNKNOWN ORIGIN

Definition[37]

A fever is considered to be of unknown origin (FUO) when it has been present for at least 3 wk, with temperature elevations of 101° F (38.3° C), and of undetermined etiology after 1 wk of investigation in a hospital.

Etiology

1. Neoplasm*
   a. Lymphomas, Hodgkin's disease
   b. Leukemias
   c. Hepatic neoplasms (primary or metastatic)
   d. Hypernephroma
   e. Carcinoma of lung
   f. Other: carcinoma of colon, prostate, thyroid
2. Infectious diseases
   a. Tuberculosis
   b. Bacterial endocarditis
   c. Intraabdominal infections (liver, subphrenic, renal, splenic, or perinephric abscess)
   d. Other: cholangitis, hepatitis, infectious mononucleosis, fungal infections, malaria, brucellosis, babesiosis, Lyme disease, AIDS, ARC
3. Collagen-vascular diseases
   a. Allergic vasculitis
   b. Polymyalgia rheumatica and temporal arteritis
   c. SLE
   d. Rheumatoid arthritis
   e. Other; polyarteritis nodosa, juvenile rheumatoid arthritis, Wegener's granulomatosis, polymyositis
4. Drugs
   a. Barbiturates
   b. Antibiotics (sulfonamides, penicillins, nitrofurantoin, amphotericin B, INH, cephalosporins, rifampin, PAS, vancomycin, tetracyclines)
   c. Antihypertensives (methyldopa, diuretics, hydralazine)
   d. Antidysrhythmics (procainamide, quinidine)
   e. Phenytoin
   f. Other: antihistamines, salicylates, cimetidine, bleomycin, allopurinol
5. Miscellaneous
   a. Factitious fever
   b. Pulmonary emboli
   c. Periodic fever
   d. Inflammatory bowel disease
   e. Other: subacute thyroiditis, familial Mediterranean fever (FMF), retroperitoneal hematoma, alcoholic hepatitis

Diagnostic approach

When attempting to diagnose a FUO, think of unusual presentations of common diseases rather than rare diseases

History

1. Occupational history
   a. Rule out idiosyncratic reaction to fumes, dusts, chemicals (e.g., zinc or nickel)
   b. Consider diseases of animals (e.g., brucellosis, leptospirosis) in veterinarians, butchers, trappers, and workers in meat packing plants

---

*Neoplasms have replaced infections as the commonest cause of FUO.[29]

2. Travel history: inquire about travel to areas endemic with malaria, babesiosis, histoplasmosis, coccidioidomycosis, Lyme disease, or enteric diseases

3. Duration of fever and associated symptoms
   a. Prolonged fever and significant weight loss: consider neoplasm
   b. History of myalgias, arthralgias: collagen-vascular diseases
   c. Dyspnea, cough: tuberculosis, multiple pulmonary emboli, sarcoidosis, lung neoplasm
   d. Abdominal pain: intraabdominal abscess, neoplasm
   e. Look for fever patterns: temperature elevation for several days alternating with normal temperature (Pel-Ebstein fever) can be seen in patients with Hodgkin's disease and *Borrelia* infections; patients with malaria may have fever every second or third day early in the disease associated with synchronized release of parasites into the bloodstream

4. Family history of episodic or periodic fever: consider FMF, periodic fever

5. Current or recent drug use: rule out drug fever

6. IV drug addict: consider SBE, AIDS, ARC

7. Recent abdominal surgery: possible intraabdominal abscess

8. History of multiple hospitalizations and numerous diagnostic tests without elucidation of cause of fever: consider factitious fever

9. Homosexual patient, history of IV drug abuse: consider ARC and AIDS

Physical exam

1. Temperature: measure temperature rectally; if elevated and factitious fever is suspected, remeasure temperature immediately without leaving the room or measure urine temperature immediately after voiding (usually 2° F lower than rectal temperature)

2. Pulse: each increase in temperature of 1° F generally increases the pulse by 10 beats/minute
   a. Exceptions are typhoid fever (relative bradycardia), some viral infections, and use of beta adrenergic blockers
   b. A significant discrepancy between pulse and temperature indicates possible factitious fever

3. Skin
   a. Look for evidence of internal malignancy (see Table 21-5)
   b. Skin lesions (SLE, vasculitis, chronic meningococcemia, Lyme disease, erythema nodosum, Kaposi's sarcoma, rheumatic fever)
   c. Jaundice indicates hepatitis or neoplastic hepatic involvement
   d. Cool skin in a patient with "high temperature" is suggestive of factitious fever
   e. Examine skin for evidence of infection and insect or animal bites and ECM in Lyme disease (see Plate 3)

4. Lymph nodes: generalized lymphadenopathy is suggestive of lymphoma, Hodgkin's disease, AIDS, or ARC

5. Head: tenderness and nodularity over the temporal artery is suggestive of temporal arteritis

6. Eyes: perform careful funduscopic exam to rule out presence of choroid tubercles (indicative of tuberculosis), Roth's spots (infectious endocarditis), CMV retinitis (AIDS), *Candida* infections

7. Neck: rule out presence of thyroid nodules (suggestive of carcinoma); a tender thyroid suggests subacute thyroiditis
8. Heart: the presence of new murmurs or variation of an existing cardiac murmur is suggestive of bacterial endocarditis
9. Abdomen: rule out presence of any palpable masses (neoplasm, abscess), hepatosplenomegaly (hepatitis, miliary TB, neoplasms)
10. Rectum
    a. Enlarged, hard, nodular prostate is suggestive of carcinoma
    b. Guaiac-positive stool is suggestive of colon carcinoma, IBD
11. Joints: evidence of arthritis
12. Neurologic: presence of focal neurologic deficits is suggestive of cerebral neoplasm (primary or metastatic) or cerebral abscess

Lab results

1. CBC; examine peripheral smear for presence of parasites
2. Urinalysis, urine culture and sensitivity
3. Obtain three sets of paired blood cultures from different sites both aerobic and anaerobic
4. Sedimentation rate (nonspecific, generally not helpful)
5. PPD, anergy panel, histoplasmin, coccidioidin
6. Obtain sputum for cytology, cultures, and AFB; stain and culture if chest x-ray is abnormal
7. Liver function studies
8. ANA, rheumatoid factor
9. Mononucleosis test, CMV and other viral titers, ASLO and streptozyme titers
10. Serum calcium, thyroxine level
11. CK
12. HIV titer
13. Stool cultures in patients with diarrhea

Radiographic evaluation

1. Chest x-rays: look for evidence of TB, mediastinal adenopathy (sarcoidosis, neoplasm), cardiomegaly, failure (decompensation secondary to valvular lesions)
2. Abdominal x-rays: indicated in patients with a history of abdominal pain; look for evidence of calcifications (calculi, TB), obstruction (neoplasms), abdominal abscess
3. CT of the abdomen to detect adenopathy, abscess

Additional diagnostic tests

Additional tests are indicated if the initial tests are nondiagnostic or if the history and physical exam suggest a particular diagnosis.

1. Focal neurologic deficits: CT scan of head to rule out cerebral abscess, neoplasm
2. Lethargy, confusion: lumbar puncture to rule out meningitis, encephalitis, meningeal carcinomatosis
3. Lymphadenopathy: lymph node biopsy to rule out lymphoma or neoplasm, HIV titer

4. Cough, dyspnea: bronchoscopy to rule out TB or neoplasm if chest x-ray shows abnormalities; consider gastric aspirate for acid-fast culture to rule out TB; consider ventilation/perfusion scan to rule out pulmonary embolism
5. Hepatosplenomegaly or abdominal pain: CT scan of abdomen
6. Cardiac murmur: echocardiogram may show valve vegetation in SBE
7. Headache, tenderness over temporal area: temporal artery biopsy to rule out temporal arteritis
8. Bone pain: bone scan, metastatic bone series, protein immunoelectrophoresis
9. Guaiac-positive stool: colonoscopy or barium enema plus sigmoidoscopy
10. Hematuria: renal ultrasound, IVP, cystoscopy
11. Liver biopsy: useful in patients with hepatic dysfunction to rule out granulomatous liver disease
12. Bone marrow exam: useful in suspected lymphoma, myeloma, or miliary TB
13. Gallium scan: used to detect occult infection or neoplasm, but it is rarely helpful
14. Exploratory laparotomy: indicated only rarely and when other tests (CT scan of abdomen, liver-spleen scan, or ultrasound) are nondiagnostic and an abdominal source of fever is suspected
15. Naproxen has been reported to have selective antipyretic activity against neoplastic fever; complete lysis of fever and sustained normal temperature during a trial of naproxen 375 mg bid for three doses ("naproxen test") is suggestive of neoplastic fever[12]

25.4 | ACQUIRED IMMUNE DEFICIENCY SYNDROME—AIDS: CLINICAL AND EPIDEMIOLOGICAL ISSUES
Powel H. Kazanjian

1. Clinical manifestations of HIV infection
   a. Acute infection
      (1) Mononucleosis-like syndrome may appear 2-6 wk after infection in half of patients
         (a) Common: fever, myalgia, arthralgia, headache, photophobia, diarrhea, sore throat, lymphadenopathy, and maculopapular rash
         (b) Less common: Acute meningoencephalitis and peripheral neuropathy
         (c) Serological markers: P-24 antigen positive, HIV ELISA negative
   b. Early infection
      (1) Asymptomatic: average 1-8 yr
      (2) Dermatologic manifestations
         (a) Molluscum contagiosum
         (b) Recurrent herpes zoster, persistent mucocutaneous herpes simplex, seborrheic dermatitis resistant to therapy
      (3) Serological markers: P-24 antigen negative, HIV ELISA positive
      (4) Total T_4 lymphocyte count >400

c. Middle stage
   (1) Persistent generalized lymphadenopathy; presence of two or more extrainguinal sites of lymphadenopathy for a minimum of 3-6 mo without an alternate cause; common sites: anterior cervical, axillary; nontender, nonadherent, 1-2 cm in size
   (2) Oral lesions
      (a) Thrush: painful whitish plaques removable by tongue blade on soft palate, tonsils, buccal mucosa
      (b) Hairy leukoplakia: oftentimes painless, raised, white, nonremovable lesion on the tongue, associated with EBV
      (c) Aphthous ulcers: extremely painful, viral cultures negative
      (d) Idiopathic thrombocytopenic purpura: asymptomatic most often and discovered upon routine clinical examination
      (e) Total T_4 lymphocyte count 100-400
d. Late stage, AIDs-defining illnesses
   (1) Infections and therapy
      (a) Fungal
         • *Cryptococcus* extrapulmonic: amphotericin B or fluconazole
         • Candidiasis of esophagus, trachea, bronchi, or lungs: nystatin, clotrimazole, ketoconazole for localized disease, amphotericin B for disseminated candidiasis or unresponsive esophagitis
         • Disseminated histoplasmosis or coccidioidomycosis
      (b) Mycobacterial
         • Extrapulmonic *Mycobacterium tuberculosis:* standard antituberculous chemotherapy
         • *Mycobacterium avium* or *M. kansasii:* 4 to 6 antituberculous drugs, ciprofloxacin, and clofazimine
      (c) Bacterial
         • Recurrent nontyphoidal *Salmonella* bacteremia: ampicillin, third-generation cephalosporin
      (d) Viral
         • Herpes simplex virus causing a mucocutaneous ulcer that persists longer than 1 mo or involving the lung, bronchus, or esophagus: acyclovir
         • Cytomegalovirus involving the retina, GI tract, or lung: ganciclovir (DHPG)
         • Progressive multifocal leukoencephalopathy: papovavirus
         • HIV encephalopathy, HIV wasting syndrome
      (e) Parasitic infections
         • *Pneumocystis carinii:* trimethoprim/sulfamethoxazole or pentamidine, or dapsone/trimethoprim plus prednisone
         • *Toxoplasma gondii:* pyrimethamine with sulfadiazine
         • *Isospora belli:* TMP/SMX (Bactrim)
         • *Cryptosporidium*
   (2) Neoplasia
      (a) Kaposi's sarcoma in a patient less than 60 yr old
         • Current outbreak involves a much younger population

- Distribution of cutaneous lesions is not predominantly in the lower extremity; head, neck, trunk, GI tract are involved
    - Current outbreak involves a much more aggressive lymphadenopathic form of the disease than that seen previously
    - Therapy is under investigation, observation; recombinant interferon—alpha or standard chemotherapy (e.g., vinblastine, VP-16, Adriamycin) are the current options
  - (b) Non-Hodgkin's lymphoma
    - B-cell tumor often with EBV DNA present
    - Less frequent than Kaposi's sarcoma
    - Often involves intraabdominal sites or the CNS
    - Combination chemotherapy used, but response rate is poor
- e. Evaluation of pulmonary symptoms
  - (1) Observe if examination, chest x-ray, and diffusion of carbon monoxide normal
  - (2) Sputum induction if chest x-ray or diffusion of carbon monoxide abnormal
  - (3) If specific diagnosis not made, bronchoscopy with lavage
  - (4) Most opportunistic infections diagnosed by this method; if not, transbronchial biopsy may reveal noninfectious causes such as lupoid interstitial pneumonia or Kaposi's sarcoma
  - (5) Open lung biopsy rarely necessary
- f. Evaluation of neurologic symptoms
  - (1) If nonfocal examination and no papilledema, lumbar puncture
  - (2) If papilledema or focal examination, head CT prior to lumbar puncture
2. Human T-lymphotropic virus (HTLV)
  - a. HTLV-I: associated with adult T-cell leukemia in Japan, and the Caribbean, with sporadic cases worldwide; T4 tropic (but not T4 restricted) infection results in transformation and immortalization of target cells
  - b. HTLV-II: isolated from two cases of T-cell hairy cell leukemia and from IV drug addicts in the U.S.A. and Great Britain
  - c. Human immunodeficiency virus (HIV) (also known as LAV or HTLV-III): isolated from patients with, and at risk for, AIDS; infection results in lysis of target cell; closely related to visna, a lentivirus of sheep
  - d. HIV-2, HTLV-IV, LAV-2: first of what is likely to be a series of retroviral agents that differ from HIV-1 sufficiently to be partially missed by current HIV-1 serologic tests; first isolated in West Africa; can cause disease indistinguishable from HIV-1–induced AIDS
3. HIV serology
  - a. Methods for serological testing
    - (1) ELISA: using disrupted viral particles relatively sensitive for screening, and for patients with AIDS related complex; less sensitive with AIDS per se; simple to perform; quality of antigen critical; second-generation ELISAs using recombinant antigens have decreased false-positives

      (2) Western blot: more sensitive than ELISA; much more laborious; too labor intensive for screening

      (3) Polymerase chain reaction: same attributes as Western blot

    b. Pitfalls in HIV antibody testing by ELISA

      (1) False-negatives

        (a) HIV-infected individuals in early stage of infection

        (b) HIV-infected individuals who fail to make antibody

        (c) Subgroup of patients with AIDS

      (2) False-positives

        (a) Multiparous women

        (b) Transfusion or organ allograft recipients

        (c) Occasional members of general population

4. Antiretroviral therapy

    a. Nucleoside analogs; interfere with reverse transcription or viral RNA to DNA

      (1) Azidothymidine (AZT, zidovudine)

        (a) To be recommended for patients with CD4 cells $< 200/mm^3$, as it prolongs survival and delays the onset of opportunistic infection; duration of benefit unknown; it is also to be offered for early infected patients with T cells < 500 and patients in the middle or late stage of infection

        (b) Toxicity: common; marrow suppression, headache

        (c) Resistance may develop; AZT does not eliminate the virus but only suppresses its growth

      (2) Experimental: dideoxyinosine (ddI)

        (a) Protocols to assess utility in patients who are intolerant of AZT or who develop opportunistic infections while on AZT

        (b) Toxicity: peripheral neuropathy, pancreatitis

    b. Others: soluble CD4, dextran sulfate, ribavirin, castanospermine

5. Therapeutic difficulties in patients with AIDS

    a. Relatively high frequency of baseline organ system dysfunction

    b. Increased frequency of adverse drug effects, especially sulfonamides

    c. Chronicity of immunoincompetence resulting in

      (1) Little immunologic help in dealing with infections

      (2) Requirement for simultaneous use of several agents for concurrent problem

      (3) Limitations in use of cytotoxic chemotherapeutic agents for malignancy

    d. Need for ongoing decisions about degree of intervention

6. Role of corticosteroids[7]

    a. Early adjunctive treatment with corticosteroids reduces the risk of respiratory failure and death in patients with AIDS and moderate to severe PCP

    b. Dosage regimens

      (1) Methylprednisolone: 40 mg IV q6h × 7 days

      (2) Prednisone: 40 mg PO bid × 5 days followed by 20 mg qd for the duration of antipneumocystis therapy

7. AIDS patients by risk group

Risk Group	Adult (%)	Pediatric (%)
Homosexual/bisexual men	66	
IV drug abusers	17	
Homosexual male and IV drug abusers	8	
Hemophilia/coagulation disorders	1	6
Heterosexual contact	4	
Transfusion associated	2	13
Other/unknown	3	3
Parents with or at increased risk for AIDS		79

8. Epidemiological intervention to prevent spread of HTLV-III

a. Gay men	Decrease number of sexual partners; reliance on "safe" sexual partners; use of condoms may decrease risk
b. IV drug abusers	Drug counseling and prevention programs; cessation of use of contaminated paraphernalia
c. Infants	Slowing of spread of IV drug abusing population; HIV antibody screening of mothers at high risk for HIV infection or who are sexual partners of high-risk men
d. Hemophiliacs	Use of heat-inactivated Factor VIII
e. Transfusion recipients	Self-deferral of high-risk donors; HIV antibody screening of donated units; autologous transfusion
f. Heterosexuals	Decreased number of intimate sexual partners; avoidance of prostitutes; use of condoms may decrease risk
g. Hospital personnel	Routine utilization of prudent infection control measures

9. Prophylaxis
   a. Prophylaxis after HIV exposure[23]
      (1) The risk of HIV infection through an occupational exposure (percutaneously or through mucous membranes) is <1%
      (2) The risk/benefit ratio of AZT prophylaxis is unclear
      (3) If a decision to start AZT prophylaxis is made, informed consent from the worker affirming that the decision to undergo chemo-prophylaxis rests with the worker is advisable

(4) Chemoprophylaxis should be started as soon after exposure as possible (preferably within 24 hr)

(5) The duration of prophylaxis and optimal dose of AZT are unknown; currently there are two alternatives:

    (a) NIH method—AZT 200 mg q4h for 42 days

    (b) San Francisco General Hospital—AZT 200 mg q4h with omission of 4 AM dose and duration of 28 days

b. Guidelines for prophylaxis against PCP in persons infected with HIV[11] (in addition to AZT)

  (1) Indications

    (a) HIV-infected patients with prior episode of PCP (even if the patient has been receiving AZT)

    (b) HIV-infected patients who have never had an episode of PCP, whose CD4+ cell count is $<200/mm^3$, or whose CD4+ cells are $<20\%$ of total lymphocytes

  (2) Choice of prophylactic agent

    (a) Trimethoprim/sulfamethoxazole: 160 mg of trimethoprim and 800 mg of sulfamethoxazole bid with 5 mg leucovorin qd; this form of prophylaxis should not be given to patients with a history of type I hypersensitivity (angioedema or anaphylaxis) or prior episodes of Stevens-Johnson syndrome associated with sulfonamides or trimethoprim; the efficacy of leucovorin in preventing toxicity is unknown

    (b) Aerosol pentamidine: dose is 300 mg q4wk via the Respirgard II jet nebulizer; the dose should be diluted in 6 ml of sterile water and delivered at 6 L/min from a 50 psi compressed air source until the reservoir is dry; pretreatment with a bronchodilator is useful for patients who develop cough or wheezing while receiving aerosol pentamidine

    (c) Since neither aerosol pentamidine nor oral trimethoprim/sulfamethoxazole prophylaxis is known to be safe in association with pregnancy, it is inadvisable to give either agent to HIV-infected pregnant women

25.5　INFECTIONS IN THE IMMUNOCOMPROMISED HOST

Definition

An immunocompromised host is one whose resistance to infection is impaired by an underlying disease or by immunosuppressive therapy.

Diagnostic considerations

1. The list of potential pathogens in the immunocompromised host is quite extensive and includes organisms commonly affecting normal hosts in addition to those usually found in compromised individuals; specific immune deficits predispose to infection with specific microorganisms; thus the type of infection present in the immunocompromised host can often be predicted by the immune defect observed (Table 25-1)

2. The clinical manifestations may be greatly modified or masked by the underlying illness:

  a. The patient may not be able to mount a fever response or a leukocytosis

Table 25-1 Infections in immunocompromised hosts

Underlying Disorder	Likely Infecting Organism
Splenectomy Chronic lymphocytic leukemia (CLL) Sickle cell anemia	Encapsulated organism *(S. pneumoniae, H. influenzae)*
Acute nonlymphocytic leukemia (ANLL) Acute lymphocytic leukemia Cancer chemotherapy	Gram-negative bacilli *(Pseudomonas, Klebsiella, E. coli)* *Staphylococcus aureus, S. epidermidis* *Pneumocytis carinii* Fungi *(Candida, Aspergillus)*
Lesions of skin barrier (burns, penetrating trauma)	*Staphylococcus aureus* *S. epidermidis, Pseudomonas*
Multiple myeloma	Encapsulated organisms *Pseudomonas, E. coli, Klebsiella, S. aureus*
AIDS	Refer to Section 25.4

Complement   C3
  deficiencies
            C5b-C9
	S. aureus, Pseudomonas, S. pneumoniae, Proteus
	Neisseria sp

   b. Pulmonary infiltrates in pulmonary infections may be absent or slow to develop because of leukopenia

   c. The clinical findings may be minimal (e.g., mild headache without meningismus in patients with cryptococcal meningitis, deep-seated abscesses without evidence of inflammation)

3. For infections in AIDS patients refer to Section 25.4

General approach to neutropenic patients with suspected infection

1. History
   a. Inquire about recent use of antibiotics, steroids, chemotherapeutic agents, and radiotherapy
   b. History of recurrent infections, recent travel, and exposure to contagious diseases
2. Physical exam
   a. Presence of skin lesions
      (1) Ecthyma gangrenosum: embolic skin manifestations of gram-negative bacilli; usually begins as a red macule (0.5-3 cm in diameter) then becomes more papular with central necrosis of vesicle formation surrounded by erythema
      (2) Mucormycosis: usually seen in diabetics; manifested as a black eschar on the palate and nasal passages

   b. Evidence of fungal colonization (oropharynx, rectum, vagina)
   c. Evaluate mental status, look for evidence of meningism or focal deficits
   d. Auscultate the heart for presence of new murmurs or accentuation of an existing murmur (suggestive of bacterial endocarditis) particularly in IV drug addicts and patients with central lines
   e. Evidence of respiratory infection (decreased breath sounds, rales, rhonchi); the lungs are the most frequent site of infection in immunocompromised patients
3. Initial lab results
   a. CBC with differential count
   b. Urinalysis, urine culture, sensitivity, and Gram stain
   c. Blood cultures
   d. Sputum Gram stain, acid-fast stain, and cultures
   e. Culture, sensitivity, and Gram stain of any skin lesions
   f. Lumbar puncture, if indicated
4. Chest x-ray: look for infiltrates, lobar consolidation, cavitary lesions

Therapy of the febrile neutropenic patient (<500 PMNs/mm^3)

1. Consider gram-negative organisms *(Pseudomonas, Klebsiella, E. coli)* and initiate IV antibiotic therapy with combination of
   a. Aminoglycoside (amikacin, tobramycin, gentamicin) plus
   b. β-Lactam (azlocillin, mezlocillin) or selected cephalosporins with antipseudomonal activity (e.g., ceftazidime); preliminary reports indicate that the combination of IV ciprofloxacin and azlocillin avoids potential ototoxicity and nephrotoxicity associated with aminoglycoside usage and represents an effective alternative to combination therapy of aminoglycoside and cephalosporins (e.g., amikacin and ceftazidime) in febrile neutropenic patients[18]
2. In centers where gram-positive organisms are frequently encountered, it is reasonable to add nafcillin, cefazolin, or vancomycin to provide additional gram-positive coverage
3. If fever persists and there is no clinical improvement in a patient with suspected pulmonary infection, add erythromycin to provide coverage against *Legionella*[14]
4. If there is no improvement after 4 days and all cultures are negative, the addition of amphotericin B for therapy of possible fungal infections may be beneficial
5. If progressive pulmonary involvement occurs, consider open lung biopsy

25.6   BACTEREMIA AND SEPSIS

Definitions[41]

1. Bacteremia: presence of viable bacteria in the blood as evidenced by a positive blood culture; bacteremia can be:
   a. Transient (e.g., dental extractions)
   b. Continuous or sustained (e.g., bacterial endocarditis)
   c. Intermittent (e.g., intermittent biliary tract obstruction)

2. Septicemia: bacteremia with clinical manifestations (fever, chills)
3. Septic shock: Life-threatening manifestations of bacteremia caused by the effects of bacteria cell wall substances (activation of the complement, coagulation, and kallikrein-kinin systems, ACTH/endorphin release)[36]

Septic shock

1. Etiology
   a. Gram-negative bacilli (*Escherichia coli, Pseudomonas, Proteus, Klebsiella, Enterobacter, Serratia, Meningococcus*)
   b. Gram-positive organisms (*Staphylococcus aureus*, pneumococci, streptococci)
   c. Fungal infections
2. Sites of infection
   a. GU tract (most common site of sepsis in the elderly)
   b. GI tract
   c. Respiratory tract
   d. Wounds, infected IV lines
   e. Meninges
3. Predisposing factors: malnutrition, instrumentation or other invasive procedures, advanced age, immunosuppressive therapy, neoplastic diseases
4. Clinical manifestations
   a. Early phase
      (1) Hypotension
      (2) Hyperventilation (respiratory alkalosis)
      (3) Skin warm, dry
      (4) Fever (may not be present in elderly or chronically ill patients; some of these patients may actually manifest hypothermia)
      (5) Chills generally occur approximately 1 hour after the acute episode of bacteremia,[4] at a time when the host has cleared the bloodstream of bacteria; the highest yield for blood cultures is before the onset of chills
      (6) Lab results: leukocytosis with shift to left or neutropenia
      (7) Hemodynamic monitoring: decreased PCWP and SVR, and increased CO
   b. Late phase
      (1) Significant hypotension
      (2) Skin cool and clammy
      (3) Oliguria
      (4) Metabolic acidosis (secondary to lactic acidosis)
      (5) Hemodynamic monitoring: decreased PCWP and CO, and increased SVR
5. Management
   a. Treat hypotension with saline infusion; aggressive volume resuscitation with hemodynamic monitoring is one of the first critical steps
      (1) Colloid plus crystalloid solutions may be necessary in selected patients
      (2) Vasopressors are indicated only when previous measures fail to correct the hypotension and PCWP has been raised to 15-18 mm Hg; dopamine should be titrated to raise the mean BP to at least 60 mm Hg

b. IV antibiotic therapy: early treatment is crucial for patient survival, (do not wait until all blood cultures have been obtained); use broad antibiotic coverage with a combination of
   (1) Aminoglycoside (amikacin, gentamicin, tobramycin)
   (2) Additional agents depending on suspected site of infection and predisposing factors:
      (a) Neutropenic patient: add a β-lactam (ticarcillin, mezlocillin) to provide additional coverage against *Pseudomonas*
      (b) Suspected skin infection: add anti-staphylococcal agent (nafcillin, oxacillin)
      (c) Suspected intraabdominal focus: add cefotetan, cefoxitin, clindamycin, or metronidazole to cover anaerobic organisms, plus ampicillin to cover enterococci
      (d) Suspected pulmonary infection: add a cephalosporin (e.g., cefuroxime, cefazolin)
      (e) Suspected UTI: add ampicillin to cover enterococci
c. Monitor with a pulmonary artery catheter and arterial line
d. Low-dose dopamine (1-4 μg/kg/min) is useful to maintain renal perfusion
e. Drain any septic foci; necrotic bowel should be treated surgically
f. Monitor blood gases, electrolytes, and renal function
g. Measure hourly urine output
h. Measure mixed venous Po_2 to determine tissue oxygenation
i. Correct acid/base and electrolyte disturbances and hypoxia
j. Correct hypocalcemia if present
k. Administer IV hydrocortisone 100 mg q4h only if adrenal insufficiency is suspected (elevated K^+ and/or refractory shock)

25.7   CELLULITIS

Definition

Cellulitis is a superficial inflammatory condition of the skin. It is characterized by erythema, warmth, and tenderness of the area involved.

General approach

1. Lab tests
   a. Gram stain and culture (aerobic and anaerobic) of
      (1) Aspirated material from
         (a) Advancing of edge of cellulitis
         (b) Any vesicles
      (2) Swab of any drainage material
      (3) Punch biopsy (in selected patients)
   b. Blood cultures
   c. ASLO titer (in suspected streptococcal disease)
2. Despite the above measures, the cause of cellulitis remains unidentified in most patients[25]; in these patients initial antimicrobial therapy should cover both staphylococcal and streptococcal cellulitis (e.g., first-generation cephalosporin or penicillinase-resistant penicillin)

Identification and therapy[32]

1. Erysipelas
   a. Superficial spreading, warm, erythematous lesion distinguished by its indurated, elevated margin; lymphatic involvement and vesicle formation are common
   b. Generally secondary to group A beta-hemolytic streptococci
   c. Commonly involves face and legs
   d. Gram stain reveals small gram-positive cocci in chains
   e. Therapy
      (1) PO: penicillin V, 250-500 mg qid
      (2) IM: penicillin G (procaine), 600,000 U bid
      (3) IV: penicillin G (aqueous), 4-6 million U/day
      NOTE: Use erythromycin, cephalosporins, clindamycin, or vancomycin in patients allergic to penicillin
2. Staphylococcal cellulitis
   a. Area involved is erythematous, hot, and swollen; differentiated from erysipelas by nonelevated, poorly demarcated margins
   b. Local tenderness and regional adenopathy are common
   c. Gram stain shows clusters of large gram-positive cocci
   d. Therapy
      (1) PO: dicloxacillin 250-500 mg qid
      (2) IV: oxacillin or nafcillin 1-2 g q4-6h
      (3) Use vancomycin in patients allergic to penicillin
      (4) Cephalosporins (cephalotin, cephalexin, cephradine) also provide adequate antistaphylococcal coverage
3. *Haemophilus influenzae* cellulitis
   a. Area involved has a blue red–purple red color
   b. Occurs mainly in children; it generally involves the face in children and the neck or upper chest in adults
   c. Gram stain shows pleomorphic gram-negative rods; blood cultures are frequently positive
   d. Therapy
      (1) PO: amoxicillin, cefaclor, cefixime, or cefuroxime
      (2) IV: cefuroxime or ampicillin; trimethoprim/sulfamethoxazole or chloramphenicol may be used in patients allergic to penicillin
      (3) Amoxicillin is ineffective in ampicillin-resistant strains; IV cefuroxime is indicated in severely ill patients
4. *Vibrio vulnificus*
   a. Most patients (75%) have preexisting liver disease
   b. History of exposure to salt water or eating raw seafood
   c. Large hemorrhagic bullae, lymphadenitis, myositis, DIC, septic shock occur frequently
   d. Mortality is >50% in septic shock
   e. Treatment: aminoglycoside plus tetracycline or chloramphenicol
5. *Borrelia burgdorferi:* erythema chronicum migrans (see Section 25.11)

| 25.8 | **URINARY TRACT INFECTIONS** |

Definitions

1. Pyuria: presence of >10 leukocytes/ml of uncentrifuged urine
2. Bacteriuria
   a. "Significant" bacteriuria has been generally defined as the presence of $>100,000$ bacteria/ml of urine (in urine cultures)
   b. Counts between 10,000-100,000/ml can also be indicative of infection, especially in the presence of pyuria; the growth of $\geq 10^3$ colony-forming units/ml of a single or predominant species reliably indicates true bacteriuria in male patients, whereas counts $\leq 10^3$, or growth in any amount of three or more species, with none being predominant, nearly always represents specimen contamination[31]
   c. The presence of bacteria on urinalysis implies bacterial counts $>30,000$/ml

Diagnostic methods

1. Urinalysis (clean-catch specimen)
2. Gram stain of urine
3. Urine culture
4. Blood cultures: indicated only in suspected pyelonephritis or sepsis
5. IVP/cystoscopy/ultrasound: indicated in men with UTI and women with recurrent UTI; done to rule out obstruction, calculi, and papillary necrosis

Major risk factors

1. Indwelling Foley catheters and other instrumentation
2. Obstruction to urine flow (strictures, calculi, neurogenic bladder, prostatic hypertrophy)
3. Pregnancy
4. Female sex
5. Immunocompromised host
6. Frequent sexual intercourse

Common infecting organisms

1. *Escherichia coli*
2. *Proteus*
3. *Klebsiella*
4. Enterococci
5. *Pseudomonas*
6. *Staphylococcus* (diabetics)

Classification of dysuria

Dysuria (pain or discomfort on voiding) affects approximately 25% of all women yearly. Recognizing that dysuria can be caused by several disease entities, Komaroff[27,28] has categorized "acute dysuria" into seven entities, based on clinical and lab findings:

1. Acute pyelonephritis
2. Subclinical pyelonephritis
3. Chlamydial urethritis

4. Urethritis secondary to gonococci (also *Candida albicans, Trichomonas vaginalis,* herpes simplex)
5. Vaginitis
6. Lower urinary tract bacterial infection
7. No apparent infectious pathogen

Diagnosis and therapy[27,28]

The diagnostic and therapeutic approach to acute dysuria varies with the suspected cause. The salient points to each cause are described below:

1. Acute pyelonephritis
   a. Symptoms
      (1) Fever, frequency, dysuria, urgency
      (2) Flank pain or tenderness
      (3) Malaise, myalgias, anorexia
   b. Lab results
      (1) Urinalysis shows pyuria, bacteriuria
      (2) Gram stain of urine shows presence of bacteria and leukocytes
      (3) Urine culture counts generally >100,000 bacteria/ml of urine
      (4) Gram-negative rods are most commonly seen
      (5) Blood cultures are indicated in patients suspected of acute pyelonephritis
   c. Treatment: IV antibiotic therapy based on Gram stain of urine
      (1) If gram-negative rods or gram-positive cocci are present, the patient should be started on an aminoglycoside (gentamicin, tobramycin) plus ampicillin or cefazolin; aztreonam is useful in gram-negative infections
      (2) In case of penicillin allergy and gram-positive cocci, use vancomycin plus an aminoglycoside; vigorous hydration is also indicated
2. Subclinical pyelonephritis
   a. Diagnosis
      (1) Clinical presentation undistinguishable from "lower tract" UTI (dysuria, frequency, urgency)
      (2) Increased incidence in diabetics, the immunosuppressed, and patients with recurrent UTI or history of childhood UTIs
      (3) Urinalysis shows pyuria, bacteriuria
      (4) Urine culture colony counts generally >100,000/ml
   b. Therapy
      (1) Preferred initial treatment is single-dose amoxicillin 3 g, PO
         (a) Therapy with single-dose amoxicillin is also useful to differentiate bladder infection from subclinical pyelonephritis, since persistent infection on another culture 48 hr after treatment, or relapse within a few weeks of treatment, indicates subclinical pyelonephritis which would dictate a 2 wk course of therapy
         (b) Male patients, pregnant females, immunosuppressed hosts, and any patient with underlying obstruction should be treated initially with 7-14 days of therapy
      (2) A follow-up urine culture (posttreatment) may be indicated following single-dose amoxicillin therapy[47]

3. Chlamydial urethritis
   a. Diagnosis
      (1) Dysuria present in a young, sexually active patient
      (2) Urinalysis shows pyuria without bacteriuria
      (3) Mucopurulent endocervical secretions and edema of exocervix noted on pelvic exam
      (4) Diagnosis can be easily made with use of commercially available monoclonal antibodies[51]
   b. Treatment
      (1) Tetracycline 500 mg or erythromycin 250 PO qid for 10 days
      (2) In pregnant women, use erythromycin 250 mg PO qid for 7 days
      (3) Both patient and sexual partner should be treated
4. Gonococcal urethritis
   a. Diagnosis
      (1) Dysuria and urethral or cervical os discharge in a sexually active patient
      (2) Urinalysis shows pyuria without bacteriuria
      (3) Gram stain of urethral discharge shows polymorphonuclear leukocytes with intracellular gram-negative diplococci
   b. Treatment: see Section 25.9
5. Vaginitis must be considered in any young woman presenting with symptoms of "dysuria", vaginal discharge, and pruritus; there are 3 major etiological agents[34]:
   a. *Gardnerella vaginalis* (bacterial vaginosis)
      (1) Moderate homogenous vaginal discharge with "fishy" odor when mixed with two drops of 10% potassium hydroxide (positive sniff test).
      (2) pH of vaginal discharge >4.5
      (3) Microscopic exam of wet mount reveals "clue cells"; high-dry magnification reveals adherence of bacteria to epithelial cells, resulting in granulated surface and indistinct cell margins
      (4) Treatment is metronidazole 500 mg bid for 7 days
   b. *Trichomonas vaginalis*
      (1) Protozoan parasite; it can cause both vaginitis and urethritis
      (2) Diagnosis can be made by microscopic vaginal discharge mixed with drops of saline
      (3) Treatment (both patient and sexual partners) is metronidazole 2 g PO given as a single dose
   c. *Candida* vulvovaginitis
      (1) Can be caused by *C. albicans* or *C. glabrata*
      (2) Vaginal exam reveals white clumps adherent to inflamed mucosa; diagnosis is confirmed by Gram stain or 10% potassium hydroxide preparation of the vaginal discharge
      (3) Treatment is clotrimazole vaginal tablets 100 mg qhs for 1 wk
6. "Lower tract" UTI (cystitis, acute urethral syndrome)
   a. Diagnosis
      (1) Dysuria, frequency, urgency, suprapubic pain or fullness
      (2) Pyuria and bacteriuria seen on urinalysis
      (3) Urine culture is not cost effective[8] and should not be routinely obtained in suspected lower tract UTI

b. Treatment: for otherwise healthy female patients, single-dose trimethoprim/sulfamethoxazole (TMP/SMX)[49] 320 mg/1600 mg (e.g., Bactrim DS—two tablets) or amoxicillin 3 g PO; male patients, pregnant females, diabetics, or any patient with underlying obstruction will require 7-14 days of therapy (e.g., TMP/SMX 160 mg/800 mg PO bid or ampicillin 250-500 mg qid)

7. No apparent infectious pathogen
   a. These patients have dysuria but not pyuria
   b. The dysuria may be secondary to urethral trauma, interstitial cystitis, chemical agents, or estrogen deficiency (postmenopausal women)
   c. Antibiotic treatment is not indicated

Management of asymptomatic bacteriuria

The management of asymptomatic bacteriuria varies with the age of the patient and with the presence of associated conditions (pregnancy, immunosuppression).

1. Elderly patients
   a. Bacteriuria is common in the elderly
   b. It appears related to functional status and is generally transient
   c. Antibiotic treatment is generally not indicated[6]
2. Nonpregnant adults
   a. Antimicrobial therapy is controversial
   b. Single-dose treatment with trimethoprim/sulfamethoxazole (320/1600 mg) is generally indicated in diabetics, patients undergoing urological manipulation, and immunocompromised patients
3. Pregnant women
   a. Treat pregnant patients; if untreated, they have a higher incidence of acute pyelonephritis and low–birth weight infants
   b. The choice of antibiotic depends on the results of urine culture and sensitivity; however, avoid antibiotics contraindicated in pregnancy

Management of recurrent UTI

1. Determine reason for recurrence:
   a. Superinfection: common in patients with indwelling catheters
   b. Reinfection: generally associated with sexual intercourse
   c. Resistant organism
2. Repeated infections with the same pathogen is an indication for cystoscopy and IVP to rule out underlying urinary tract disease
3. Prophylactic therapy with TMP/SMX (e.g., ½ tab qhs or nitrofurantoin 50 mg qhs) may be effective in some patients
4. Female patients with recurring UTI following intercourse may benefit from postcoital prophylaxis (e.g., ½ tab TMP/SMX after coitus)[50]

| 25.9 | **TREATMENT GUIDELINES FOR SELECTED SEXUALLY TRANSMITTED DISEASES*** |

DISEASES CHARACTERIZED BY GENITAL ULCERS OR INGUINAL LYMPHADENOPATHY

In the United States most patients with genital ulcers have genital herpes, syphilis, or chancroid. Inguinal lymphadenopathy is common in these infections. More than one of these diseases may be present in a patient. Patients who have genital ulcers may be at increased risk for HIV infection.

Diagnosis based only on history and physical examination is often inaccurate. Thus, evaluation of most persons with genital ulcers should include one or more of the following:

Dark-field examination or direct immunofluorescence test for *T. pallidum*
Serologic test(s) for syphilis
Culture or antigen test for HSV
Culture for *Haemophilus ducreyi*

Chancroid

Because of recent spread of *H. ducreyi*, chancroid has become an important STD in the United States. Its importance is enhanced by the knowledge that outside the United States chancroid has been associated with increased infection rates for HIV. Chancroid must be considered in the differential diagnosis of any patient with a painful genital ulcer. Painful inguinal lymphadenopathy is present in about half of all chancroid cases.

Recommended regimen

Erythromycin base 500 mg orally qid for 7 days
or
Ceftriaxone 250 mg intramuscularly (IM) in a single dose

Alternative regimens

Trimethoprim/sulfamethoxazole 160/800 mg (one double-strength tablet) orally bid for 7 days
Comment: The susceptibility of *H. ducreyi* to this combination of antimicrobial agents varies throughout the world; clinical efficacy should be monitored, preferably in conjunction with monitoring of susceptibility patterns.
or
Amoxicillin 500 mg plus clavulanic acid 125 mg orally tid for 7 days
Comment: Not evaluated in the U.S.
or
Ciprofloxacin 500 mg orally bid for 3 days
Comment: Although a regimen of 500 mg orally once was effective outside the U.S., based on pharmacokinetics and susceptibility data, 2- or 3-day regimens of the same dose may be prudent, especially for patients coinfected with HIV. Quinolones, such as ciprofloxacin, are contraindicated during pregnancy and in children 16 yr of age or younger.

Management of sex partners

Sex partners, within the 10 days preceding onset of symptoms in an infected patient, whether symptomatic or not, should be examined and treated with a recommended regimen.

*From MMWR 38(S-8):1, 1989.

Follow-up

If treatment is successful, ulcers due to chancroid symptomatically improve within 3 days and objectively improve (evidenced by resolution of lesions and clearing of exudate) within 7 days after institution of therapy. Clinical resolution of lymphadenopathy is slower than that of ulcers and may require needle aspiration (through healthy, adjacent skin), even during successful therapy. Patients should be observed until the ulcer is completely healed. Because of the epidemiologic association with syphilis, serological testing for syphilis should be considered within 3 months after therapy.

Treatment failures

If no clinical improvement is evident by 7 days after therapy, the clinician should consider whether (1) antimicrobials were taken as prescribed, (2) the *H. ducreyi* causing infection is resistant to the prescribed antimicrobial, (3) the diagnosis is correct, (4) coinfection with another STD agent exists, or (5) the patient is also infected with HIV. Preliminary information indicates that patients coinfected with HIV do not respond to antimicrobial therapy as well as patients not infected with HIV, especially when single-dose treatment is used. Antimicrobial susceptibility testing should be performed on *H. ducreyi* isolated from patients who do not respond to recommended therapies.

Syphilis

Serologic tests

Dark-field examinations and direct fluorescent antibody tests on lesions or tissue are the definitive methods for diagnosing early syphilis. Presumptive diagnosis is possible by using two types of serologic tests for syphilis: (1) treponemal (e.g., fluorescent treponemal antibody absorbed [FTA-ABS] microhemagglutination assay for antibody to *T. pallidum* [MHATP]) and (2) nontreponemal (e.g., Venereal Disease Research Laboratory [VDRL], rapid plasma reagin [RPR]). Neither test alone is sufficient for diagnosis. Treponemal antibody tests, once positive, usually remain so for life, regardless of treatment of disease activity. Treponemal antibody titers do not correlate with disease activity and should be reported as positive or negative. Nontreponemal antibody titers do tend to correlate with disease activity, usually rising with new infection and falling after treatment. Nontreponemal antibody test results should be reported quantitatively and titered out to a final end point rather than reported as greater than an arbitrary cutoff (e.g., $>1:512$). With regard to changes in nontreponemal test results, a fourfold change in titers is equivalent to a two-dilution change—e.g., from $1:16$ to $1:4$, or from $1:8$ to $1:32$.

For sequential serological tests, the same test (e.g., VDRL or RPR) should be used, and it should be run by the same laboratory. The VDRL and RPR are equally valid, but RPR titers are often slightly higher than VDRL titers and therefore are not comparable.

Neurosyphilis cannot be accurately diagnosed from any single test. Cerebrospinal fluid (CSF) tests should include cell count, protein, and VDRL (not RPR). The CSF leukocyte count is usually elevated (>5 WBC/mm^3) when neurosyphilis is present and is a sensitive measure of the efficacy of therapy. VDRL is the standard test for CSF; *when positive* it is considered *diagnostic* of neurosyphilis. However, it may be negative when neurosyphilis is present and cannot be used to rule out neurosyphilis. Some experts also order an FTA-ABS; this may be less specific (more false-positives) but is highly sensitive. The positive predictive value of the CSF FTA-ABS is lower; but *when negative,* this test provides evidence against neurosyphilis.

Penicillin therapy

Penicillin is the preferred drug for treating patients with syphilis. Penicillin is the only proven therapy that has been widely used for patients with neurosyphilis, congenital syphilis, or syphilis during pregnancy. For patients with penicillin allergy, skin testing—with desensitization, if necessary—is optimal.

Jarisch-Herxheimer reaction

The Jarisch-Herxheimer reaction is an acute febrile reaction, often accompanied by headache, myalgia, and other symptoms, that may occur after any therapy for syphilis, and patients should be so warned. Jarisch-Herxheimer reactions are more common in patients with early syphilis. Antipyretics may be recommended, but no proven methods exist for preventing this reaction. Pregnant patients, in particular, should be warned that early labor may occur.

Persons exposed to syphilis (epidemiologic treatment)

Persons sexually exposed to a patient with early syphilis should be evaluated clinically and serologically. If the exposure occurred within the previous 90 days, the person may be infected yet seronegative and therefore should be presumptively treated. It may be advisable to presumptively treat persons exposed more than 90 days previously if serologic test results are not immediately available and follow-up is uncertain.) Patients who have other STD may also have been exposed to syphilis and should have a serologic test for syphilis. The dual therapy regimen currently recommended for gonorrhea (ceftriaxone and doxycycline) is probably effective against incubating syphilis. If a different, nonpenicillin antibiotic regimen is used to treat gonorrhea, the patient should have a repeat serologic test for syphilis in 3 mo.

Early syphilis

Primary and secondary syphilis and early latent syphilis of less than 1 yr duration

Recommended regimen

Benzathine penicillin G, 2.4 million units IM, in one dose.

Alternative regimens for penicillin-allergic patients (nonpregnant)

Doxycycline, 100 mg orally bid for 2 wk
   or
Tetracycline, 500 mg orally qid for 2 wk

   Doxycycline and tetracycline are equivalent therapies. There is less clinical experience with doxycycline, but compliance is better. In patients who cannot tolerate doxycycline or tetracycline, three options exist:

1. If follow-up or compliance cannot be ensured, the patient should have skin testing for penicillin allergy and be desensitized if necessary.
2. If compliance and follow-up are ensured, erythromycin, 500 mg orally qid for 2 wk, can be used.
3. Patients who are allergic to penicillin may also be allergic to cephalosporins; therefore, caution must be used in treating a penicillin-allergic patient with a cephalosporin. However, preliminary data suggest that ceftriaxone, 250 mg IM qd for 10 days, is curative—but careful follow-up is mandatory.

Follow-up

Treatment failures can occur with any regimen. Patients should be re-examined clinically and serologically at 3 mo and 6 mo. If nontreponemal antibody titers have not declined fourfold by 3 mo with primary or secondary syphilis, or by 6 mo in early latent syphilis, or if signs or symptoms persist and reinfection has been ruled out, patients should have a CSF examination and be retreated appropriately.

HIV-infected patients should have more frequent follow-up, including serologic testing at 1, 2, 3, 6, 9, and 12 mo. In addition to the above guidelines for 3 and 6 mo, any patient with a fourfold increase in titer at any time should have a CSF examination and be treated with the neurosyphilis regimen unless reinfection can be established as the cause of the increased titer.

Lumbar puncture in early syphilis

CSF abnormalities are common in adults with early syphilis. Despite the frequency of these CSF findings, very few patients develop neurosyphilis when the treatment regimens described above are used. Therefore, unless clinical signs and symptoms of neurologic involvement exist, such as optic, auditory, cranial nerve, or meningeal symptoms, lumbar puncture is not recommended for routine evaluation of early syphilis. This recommendation also applies to immunocompromised and HIV-infected patients, since no clear data currently show that these patients need increased therapy.

HIV testing

All syphilis patients should be counseled concerning the risks of HIV and be encouraged to be tested for HIV.

Late latent syphilis of more than 1 yr duration, gummas, and cardiovascular syphilis

All patients should have a thorough clinical examination. Ideally, all patients with syphilis of more than 1 yr duration should have a CSF examination; however, performance of lumbar puncture can be individualized. In older asymptomatic individuals, the yield of lumbar puncture is likely to be low; however, CSF examination is clearly indicated in the following specific situations:

Neurologic signs or symptoms

Treatment failure
Serum nontreponemal antibody titer $\geq 1:32$
Other evidence of active syphilis (aortitis, gumma, iritis)
Nonpenicillin therapy planned
Positive HIV antibody test

NOTE: If CSF examination is performed and reveals findings consistent with neurosyphilis, patients should be treated for neurosyphilis (see next section). Some experts also treat cardiovascular syphilis patients with a neurosyphilis regimen.

Recommended regimen

Benzathine penicillin G, 7.2 million units total, administered as 3 doses of 2.4 million units IM, given 1 wk apart for 3 consecutive wk

Alternative regimens for penicillin-allergic patients (nonpregnant)

Doxycycline, 100 mg orally bid for 4 wk
    or
Tetracycline, 500 mg orally qid for 4 wk

If patients are allergic to penicillin, alternate drugs should be used only after CSF examination has excluded neurosyphilis. Penicillin allergy is best determined by careful history taking, but skin testing may be used if the major and minor determinants are available

Follow-up

Quantitative nontreponemal serologic tests should be repeated at 6 mo and 12 mo. If titers increase fourfold, if an initially high titer ($\geq 1:32$) fails to decrease, or if the patient has signs or symptoms attributable to syphilis, the patient should be evaluated for neurosyphilis and retreated appropriately.

HIV testing

All syphilis patients should be counseled concerning the risks of HIV and be encouraged to be tested for HIV antibody.

Neurosyphilis

Central nervous system disease may occur during any stage of syphilis. Clinical evidence of neurologic involvement (e.g., optic and auditory symptoms, cranial nerve palsies) warrants CSF examination.

Recommended regimen

Aqueous crystalline penicillin G, 12-24 million units administered 2-4 million units q4h IV for 10-14 days

Alternative regimen (if outpatient compliance can be ensured)

Procaine penicillin, 2-4 million units IM qd
    and
Probenecid, 500 mg orally qid, both for 10-14 days

Many authorities recommend addition of benzathine penicillin G, 2.4 million units IM weekly for three doses after completion of these neurosyphilis treatment regimens. No systematically collected data have evaluated therapeutic alternatives to penicillin. Patients who cannot tolerate penicillin should be skin tested and desensitized, if necessary, or managed in consultation with an expert.

Follow-up

If an initial CSF pleocytosis was present, CSF examination should be repeated every 6 mo until the cell count is normal. If it has not decreased at 6 mo, or is not normal by 2 yr, retreatment should be strongly considered.

HIV Testing

All syphilis patients should be counseled concerning the risks of HIV and be encouraged to be tested for HIV antibody.

Syphilis in pregnancy

Screening

Pregnant women should be screened early in pregnancy. Seropositive pregnant women should be considered infected unless treatment history and sequential serologic antibody titers are showing an appropriate response. In populations in which prenatal care utilization is not optimal, patients should be screened, and if necessary, treatment provided at the time pregnancy is detected. In areas of high syphilis prevalence, or in patients at high risk, screening should be repeated in the third trimester and again at delivery.

Treatment

Patients should be treated with the penicillin regimen appropriate for the woman's stage of syphilis. Tetracycline and doxycycline are contraindicated in pregnancy. Erythromycin should not be used because of the high risk of failure to cure infection in the fetus. Pregnant women with a history of penicillin allergy should first be carefully questioned regarding the validity of the history. If necessary, they should then be skin tested and either treated with penicillin or referred for desensitization. Women who are treated in the second half of pregnancy are at risk for premature labor and/or fetal distress if their treatment precipitates a Jarisch-Herxheimer reaction. They should be advised to seek medical attention following treatment if they notice any change in fetal movements or have any contractions. Stillbirth is a rare complication of treatment; however, since therapy is necessary to prevent further fetal damage, this concern should not delay treatment.

Follow-up

Monthly follow-up is mandatory so retreatment can be given if needed. The antibody response should be the same as for nonpregnant patients.

HIV testing

All syphilis patients should be counseled concerning the risks of HIV and be encouraged to be tested for HIV antibody.

Lymphogranuloma venereum

Lymphogranuloma venereum (LGV) is caused by *Chlamydia trachomatis* (LGV serovars). Inguinal lymphadenopathy is the most common clinical manifestation. Diagnosis is often made clinically and may be confused with chancroid. LGV is not a common cause of inguinal lymphadenopathy in the United States.

Treatment: Genital, inguinal, or anorectal

Recommended regimen

Doxycycline 100 mg orally bid for 21 days

Alternative regimen

Tetracycline 500 mg orally qid for 21 days
    or
Erythromycin 500 mg orally qid for 21 days
    or
Sulfisoxazole 500 mg orally qid for 21 days or equivalent sulfonamide course

Genital herpes simplex virus infections

Genital herpes is a viral disease that may be chronic and recurring and for which no known cure exists. Systemic acyclovir treatment provides partial control of the symptoms and signs of herpes episodes; it accelerates healing but does not eradicate the infection nor affect the subsequent risk, frequency, or severity of recurrences after the drug is discontinued. Topical therapy with acyclovir is substantially less effective than therapy with the oral drug.

First clinical episode of genital herpes

Recommended regimen

Acyclovir 200 mg orally 5 times daily for 7-10 days or until clinical resolution occurs

First clinical episode of herpes proctitis

Recommended regimen

Acyclovir 400 mg orally 5 times daily for 10 days or until clinical resolution occurs

Inpatient therapy

For patients with severe disease or complications necessitating hospitalization

Recommended regimen

Acyclovir 5 mg/kg body weight IV q8h for 5-7 days or until clinical resolution occurs

Recurrent episodes

Most episodes of recurrent herpes do not benefit from therapy with acyclovir. In severe recurrent disease, some patients who start therapy at the beginning of the prodrome or within 2 days after onset of lesions may benefit from therapy, although this has not been proven.

Recommended regimen

Acyclovir 200 mg orally 5 times daily for 5 days
  or
Acyclovir 800 mg orally bid for 5 days

Daily suppressive therapy

Daily treatment reduces frequency of recurrences by at least 75% among patients with frequent (more than six per year) recurrences. Safety and efficacy have been clearly documented among persons receiving daily therapy for up to 3 yr. Acyclovir-resistant strains of HSV have been isolated from persons receiving suppressive therapy, but they have not been associated with treatment failure among immunocompetent patients. After 1 yr of continuous daily suppressive therapy, acyclovir should be discontinued so that the patient's recurrence rate may be reassessed.

Recommended regimen

Acyclovir 200 mg orally 2 to 5 times daily

Acyclovir 400 mg orally 2 times daily

Gonococcal infections

Because of the wide spectrum of antimicrobial therapies effective against *Neisseria gonorrhoeae*, these guidelines are *not* intended to be a comprehensive list of all possible treatment regimens.

Treatment of adults

Uncomplicated urethral, endocervical, or rectal infections

Single-dose efficacy is a major consideration in choosing an antibiotic regimen to treat persons infected with *N. gonorrhoeae*. Another important concern is coexisting chlamydial infection, documented in up to 45% of gonorrhea cases in some populations. Until universal testing for chlamydia with quick, inexpensive, and highly accurate tests becomes available, persons with gonorrhea should also be treated for presumptive chlamydial infections. Generally, patients with gonorrhea infections should be treated simultaneously with antibiotics effective against both *C. trachomatis* and *N. gonorrhoeae*. Simultaneous treatment may lessen the possibility of treatment failure due to antibiotic resistance.

Recommended regimen

Ceftriaxone 250 mg IM once
  plus
Doxycycline 100 mg orally bid for 7 days
  Some authorities prefer a dose of 125 mg ceftriaxone IM because it is less expensive and can be given in a volume of only 0.5 ml, which is more

easily administered in the deltoid muscle. However, the 250 mg dose is recommended because it may delay the emergence of ceftriaxone-resistant strains. At this time, both doses appear highly effective for mucosal gonorrhea at all sites.

Alternative regimens

For patients who cannot take ceftriaxone, the preferred alternative is spectinomycin 2 g IM, in a single dose (followed by doxycycline).

Other alternatives, for which experience is less extensive, include ciprofloxacin* 500 mg orally once; norfloxacin* 800 mg orally once; cefuroxime axetil 1 g orally once with probenecid 1 g; cefotaxime 1 g IM once; and ceftizoxime 500 mg IM once. All of these regimens are followed by doxycycline 100 mg orally, twice daily for 7 days. If infection was acquired from a source proven *not* to have penicillin-resistant gonorrhea, a penicillin such as amoxicillin 3 g orally with 1 g probenecid followed by doxycycline may be used for treatment.

Doxycycline or tetracycline alone is no longer considered adequate therapy for gonococcal infections but is added for treatment of coexisting chlamydial infections. Tetracycline may be substituted for doxycycline; however, compliance may be worse since tetracycline must be taken at a dose of 500 mg qid between meals, whereas doxycycline is taken at a dose of 100 mg bid without regard to meals. Moreover, at current prices, tetracycline costs only a little less than generic doxycycline.

For patients who cannot take a tetracycline (e.g., pregnant women), erythromycin may be substituted (erythromycin base or stearate at 500 mg orally qid for 7 days or erythromycin ethylsuccinate, 800 mg orally qid for 7 days). See "Chlamydial Infections" for further information on management.

Special considerations

All patients with gonorrhea should have a serological test for syphilis and should be offered confidential counseling and testing for HIV infection. Most patients with incubating syphilis (those who are seronegative and have no clinical signs of syphilis) may be cured by any of the regimens containing β-lactams (e.g., ceftriaxone) or tetracyclines.

Spectinomycin and the quinolones (ciprofloxacin, norfloxacin) have not been shown to be active against incubating syphilis. Patients treated with these drugs should have a serological test for syphilis in 1 mo.

Patients with gonorrhea and documented syphilis and gonorrhea patients who are sex partners of syphilis patients should be treated for syphilis (see "Syphilis") as well as for gonorrhea.

Some practitioners report that mixing 1% lidocaine (without epinephrine) with ceftriaxone reduces the discomfort associated with the injection (see package insert). No adverse reactions have been associated with use of lidocaine diluent.

---

*Quinolones, such as ciprofloxacin and norfloxacin, are contraindicated during pregnancy and in children 16 yr of age or younger.

Management of sex partners

Persons exposed to gonorrhea within the preceding 30 days should be examined, cultured, and treated presumptively.

Follow-up

Treatment failure following combined ceftriaxone/doxycycline therapy is rare; therefore, a follow-up culture ("test-of-cure") is not essential. A more cost-effective strategy may be a reexamination with culture 1-2 mo after treatment ("rescreening"); this strategy detects both treatment failures and reinfections. Patients should return for examination if symptoms persist after treatment. Because there is less long-term experience with drugs other than ceftriaxone, patients treated with regimens other than ceftriaxone/doxycycline should have follow-up cultures obtained for 4-7 days after completion of therapy.

Treatment failures

Persistent symptoms after treatment should be evaluated by culture for *N. gonorrhoeae*, and any gonococcal isolate should be tested for antibiotic sensitivity. Symptoms of urethritis may also be caused by *C. trachomatis* and other organisms associated with nongonococcal urethritis (see "Nongonococcal Urethritis"). Additional treatment for patients with gonorrhea should be ceftriaxone, 250 mg, followed by doxycycline. Infections occurring after treatment with one of the recommended regimens are commonly due to reinfection rather than to treatment failure and indicate a need for improved sex-partner referral and patient education.

Pharyngeal gonococcal infection

Patients with uncomplicated pharyngeal gonococcal infection should be treated with ceftriaxone 250 mg IM once. Patients who cannot be treated with ceftriaxone should be treated with ciprofloxacin 500 mg orally as a single dose. Since experience with this regimen is limited, such patients should be evaluated with repeat culture 4-7 days after treatment.

Disseminated gonococcal infection

Hospitalization is recommended for initial therapy of patients with DGI, especially those who cannot reliably comply with treatment, have uncertain diagnoses, or have purulent synovial effusions or other complications. Patients should be examined for clinical evidence of endocarditis or meningitis.

Recommended regimens—DGI inpatient

Ceftriaxone 1 g IM or IV q24h
    or
Ceftizoxime 1 g IV q8h
    or
Cefotaxime 1 g IV q8h
Patients who are allergic to β-lactam drugs should be treated with spectinomycin 2 g IM q12h.

When the infecting organism is proved to be penicillin-sensitive, parenteral treatment may be switched to ampicillin 1 g q6h (or equivalent). Patients treated for DGI should be tested for genital *C. trachomatis* infection.

If chlamydial testing is not available, patients should be treated empirically for coexisting chlamydial infection.

Reliable patients with uncomplicated disease may be discharged 24-48 hr after all symptoms resolve and may complete the therapy (for a total of 1 wk of antibiotic therapy) with an oral regimen of cefuroxime axetil 500 mg bid *or* amoxicillin 500 mg with clavulanic acid tid *or,* if not pregnant, ciprofloxacin 500 mg bid.

Meningitis and endocarditis

Meningitis and endocarditis caused by *N. gonorrhoeae* require high-dose IV therapy with an agent effective against the strain causing the disease, such as ceftriaxone 1-2 g IV q12h. Optimal duration of therapy is unknown, but most authorities treat patients with gonococcal meningitis for 10-14 days and with gonococcal endocarditis for at least 4 wk. Patients with gonococcal nephritis, endocarditis or meningitis, or recurrent DGI should be evaluated for complement deficiencies. Treatment of complicated DGI should be undertaken in consultation with an expert.

Adult gonococcal ophthalmia

Adults and children over 20 kg with nonsepticemic gonococcal ophthalmia should be treated with ceftriaxone 1 g IM once. Irrigation of the eyes with saline or buffered ophthalmic solutions may be useful adjunctive therapy to eliminate discharge. All patients must have careful ophthalmologic assessment, including slit-lamp examination for ocular complications. Topical antibiotics alone are insufficient therapy and are unnecessary when appropriate systemic therapy is given. Simultaneous ophthalmic infection with *C. trachomatis* has been reported and should be considered for patients who do not respond promptly.

Chlamydial infections

Culture and nonculture methods for diagnosis of *C. trachomatis* are now available. Appropriate use of these diagnostic tests is strongly encouraged, especially for screening asymptomatic high-risk women in whom infection would otherwise be undetected. However, in clinical settings where testing for *Chlamydia* is not routine or available, treatment often is prescribed on the basis of clinical diagnosis or as cotreatment for gonorrhea (see "Gonococcal Infections"). In clinical settings, periodic surveys should be performed to determine local chlamydial prevalence in patients with gonorrhea. Priority groups for *Chlamydia* testing, if resources are limited, are high-risk pregnant women, adolescents, and women with multiple sexual partners.

Results of chlamydial tests should be interpreted with care. The sensitivity of all currently available laboratory tests for *C. trachomatis* tests is substantially less than 100%; thus, false-negative tests are possible. Although the specificity of nonculture tests has improved substantially, false-positive results still occur with nonculture tests. Persons with chlamydial infections may remain asymptomatic for extended periods.

Treatment of uncomplicated urethral, endocervical, or rectal *C. trachomatis* infections

Recommended regimen

Doxycycline 100 mg orally bid for 7 days
> or

Tetracycline 500 mg orally qid for 7 days

Alternative regimens

Erythromycin base 500 mg orally qid or equivalent salt for 7 days
> or

Erythromycin ethylsuccinate 800 mg orally qid for 7 days
If erythromycin is not tolerated because of side effects, the following regimen may be effective:
Sulfisoxazole 500 mg orally qid for 10 days or equivalent

Test of cure

Because antimicrobial resistance of *C. trachomatis* to recommended regimens has not been observed, test-of-cure evaluation is not necessary when treatment has been completed.

Treatment of *C. trachomatis* in pregnancy

Pregnant women should undergo diagnostic testing for *C. trachomatis, N. gonorrhoeae,* and syphilis, if possible, at their first prenatal visit and, for women at high risk, during the third trimester. Risk factors for chlamydial disease during pregnancy include young age (<25 yr), past history or presence of other STD, a new sex partner within the preceding 3 mo, and multiple sex partners. Ideally, pregnant women with gonorrhea should be treated for chlamydia on the basis of diagnostic studies, but if chlamydial testing is not available, treatment should be given because of the high likelihood of coinfection.

Recommended regimen

Erythromycin base 500 mg orally 4 times a day for 7 days.
If this regimen is not tolerated, the following regimens are recommended:

Alternative regimens,

Erythromycin base 250 mg orally qid for 14 days
Erythromycin ethylsuccinate 800 mg orally qid for 7 days
> or

Erythromycin ethylsuccinate 400 mg orally qid for 14 days

Alternative if erythromycin cannot be tolerated

Amoxicillin 500 mg orally tid for 7 days (limited data exist concerning this regimen)
Erythromycin estolate is contraindicated during pregnancy, since drug-related hepatoxicity can result

Sex partners of patients with *C. trachomatis* infections

Sex partners of patients who have *C. trachomatis* infection should be tested and treated for *C. trachomatis* if their contact was within 30 days of onset of symptoms. If testing is not available, they should be treated with the appropriate antimicrobial regimen.

Nongonococcal urethritis

Among men with urethral symptoms, nongonococcal urethritis (NGU) is diagnosed by Gram stain demonstrating abundant polymorphonuclear leukocytes without intracellular gram-negative diplococci. *C. trachomatis* has been implicated as the cause of NGU in about 50% of cases. Other organisms that cause 10-15% of cases include *Ureaplasma urealyticum, T. vaginalis,* and herpes simplex virus. The cause of other cases is unknown.

Recommended regimen

Doxycycline 100 mg orally bid for 7 days
    or
Tetracycline 500 mg orally qid for 7 days

Alternative regimens

Erythromycin base 500 mg orally qid or equivalent salt for 7 days
    or
Erythromycin ethylsuccinate 800 mg orally qid for 7 days
    If high-dose erythromycin schedules are not tolerated, the following regimen is recommended:
Erythromycin ethylsuccinate 400 mg orally qid for 14 days
    or
Erythromycin base 250 mg orally qid or equivalent salt for 14 days

Management of sex partners

Sex partners of men with NGU should be evaluated for STD and treated with an appropriate regimen based on the evaluation.

Recurrent NGU unresponsive to conventional therapy

Recurrent NGU may be due to lack of compliance with an initial antibiotic regimen, to reinfection due to failure to treat sex partners, or to factors currently undefined. If noncompliance or reinfection cannot be ruled out, repeat doxycycline (100 mg orally bid for 7 days) *or* tetracycline (500 mg orally qid for 7 days).

If compliance with the initial antimicrobial agent is likely, treat with one of the above listed regimens.

If objective signs of urethritis continue after adequate treatment, these patients should be evaluated for evidence of other causes of urethritis and referred to a specialist.

Epididymitis

Among sexually active heterosexual men <35 yr of age, epididymitis is most likely caused by *N. gonorrhoeae* or *C. trachomatis.* Specimens should be obtained for a urethral smear for Gram stain and culture for *N.*

gonorrhoeae and *C. trachomatis* and for a urine culture. Empiric therapy based on the clinical diagnosis is recommended before culture results are available.

Recommended regimen

Ceftriaxone 250 mg IM once
 and
Doxycycline 100 mg orally bid for 10 days
 or
Tetracycline 500 mg orally qid for 10 days

Pelvic inflammatory disease

Treatment guidelines

Pelvic inflammatory disease (PID) comprises a spectrum of inflammatory disorders of the upper genital tract in women. PID may include endometritis, salpingitis, tubo-ovarian abscess, and pelvic peritonitis. Sexually transmitted organisms, especially *N. gonorrhoeae* and *C. trachomatis,* are implicated in most cases; however, endogenous organisms, such as anaerobes, gram-negative rods, streptococci, and *Mycoplasma,* may also be etiologic agents of disease.

A confirmed diagnosis of salpingitis and more accurate bacteriologic diagnosis is made by laparoscopy. Since laparoscopy is not always available, the diagnosis of PID is often based on imprecise clinical findings and culture or antigen detection tests of specimens from the lower genital tract.

Guidelines for the treatment of patients with PID have been designed to provide flexibility in therapeutic choices. PID therapy regimens are designed to provide empiric, broad-spectrum coverage of likely etiologic pathogens. Antimicrobial coverage should include *N. gonorrhoeae, C. trachomatis,* gram-negatives, anaerobes, Group B streptococcus, and the genital mycoplasmas. Limited data demonstrate that effective treatment of the upper genital tract pyogenic process will decrease the incidence of long-term complications such as tubal infertility and ectopic pregnancy.

Ideally, as for all intraabdominal infections, hospitalization is recommended whenever possible, and particularly when (1) the diagnosis is uncertain; (2) surgical emergencies such as appendicitis and ectopic pregnancy cannot be excluded; (3) a pelvic abscess is suspected; (4) the patient is pregnant; (5) the patient is an adolescent (the compliance of adolescent patients with therapy is unpredictable, and the long-term sequelae of PID may be particularly severe in this group); (6) severe illness precludes outpatient management; (7) the patient is unable to follow or tolerate an outpatient regimen; (8) the patient has failed to respond to outpatient therapy; or (9) clinical follow-up within 72 hr of starting antibiotic treatment cannot be arranged. Many experts recommend that all patients with PID be hospitalized so treatment with parenteral antibiotics can be initiated.

Selection of a treatment regimen must consider institutional availability, cost-control efforts, patient acceptance, and regional differences in antimicrobial susceptibility.

These treatment regimens are recommendations only and the specific antibiotics named are examples. Treatments used for PID will continue to be broad spectrum and empiric until more definitive studies are performed.

Inpatient treatment

One of the following:

Recommended regimen A

Cefoxitin 2 g IV q6h *or* cefotetan* IV 2 g q12h
  plus
Doxycycline 100 mg q12h orally or IV

The above regimen is given for at least 48 hr after the patient clinically improves

Following discharge from hospital, continuation of doxycycline 100 mg orally bid for a total of 10-14 days

Recommended regimen B

Clindamycin IV 900 mg q8h
  plus
Gentamicin loading dose IV or IM (2 mg/kg) *followed by* a maintenance dose (1.5 mg/kg) q8h

The above regimen is given for at least 48 hr after the patient improves. After discharge from hospital, continuation of:
Doxycycline 100 mg orally bid for 10-14 days total

Continuation of clindamycin, 450 mg orally, 5 times daily, for 10 to 14 days, may be considered as an alternative. Continuation of medication after hospital discharge is important for the treatment of possible *C. trachomatis* infection. Clindamycin has more complete anaerobic coverage. Although limited data suggest that clindamycin is effective against *C. trachomatis* infection, doxycycline remains the treatment of choice for patients with chlamydial disease. When *C. trachomatis* is strongly suspected or confirmed as an etiologic agent, doxycycline is the preferable alternative. In such instances, doxycycline therapy may be started during hospitalization if initiation of therapy before hospital discharge is thought likely to improve the patient's compliance.

Rationale

Clinicians have extensive experience with both the cefoxitin/doxycycline and the clindamycin/aminoglycoside combinations. Each provides broad coverage against polymicrobial infection. Cefotetan has properties similar to those of cefoxitin and requires less frequent dosing. Clinical data are limited on third-generation cephalosporins (ceftizoxime, cefotaxime, ceftriaxone), although many authorities believe they are effective. Doxycycline administered orally has bioavailability similar to that of the IV formulation and may be given if normal gastrointestinal function is present.

Experimental studies suggest that aminoglycosides may not be optimal treatment for gram-negative organisms within abscesses, but clinical studies suggest that they are highly effective in the treatment of abscesses when administered in combination with clindamycin.

*Other cephalosporins such as ceftizoxime, cefotaxime, and ceftriaxone, which provide adequate gonococcal, other facultative gram-negative aerobic, and anaerobic coverage, may be utilized in appropriate doses.

Although short courses of aminoglycosides in healthy young women usually do not require serum-level monitoring, many practitioners may elect to monitor levels.

Ambulatory management of PID

Recommended regimen

Cefoxitin 2 g IM *plus* probenecid, 1 g orally concurrently *or* ceftriaxone 250 mg IM, *or* equivalent cephalosporin
   plus
Doxycycline 100 mg orally bid for 10-14 days
   or
Tetracycline 500 mg orally qid for 10-14 days

Alternative for patients who do not tolerate doxycycline

Erythromycin, 500 mg orally qid for 10-14 days may be substituted for doxycycline/tetracycline.

This regimen, however, is based on limited clinical data.

Rationale

These empirical regimens provide broad-spectrum coverage against the common etiologic agents of PID. Parenteral β-lactam antibiotics are recommended in all cases. The cephalosporins are effective in the treatment of gram-negative organisms, including enteric rods, anaerobic organisms, and gonococci. Although decreased susceptibility of gonococci to cefoxitin has been recently noted, treatment failure has not yet been a clinical problem. Patients who do not respond to therapy within 72 hr should be hospitalized for parenteral therapy. Doxycycline provides definitive therapy for chlamydial infections. Patients treated on an ambulatory basis need to be monitored closely and reevaluated in 72 hr.

Management of sex partners

Sex partners of women with PID should be evaluated for STD and, after evaluation, should be empirically treated with regimens effective against *N. gonorrhoeae* and *C. trachomatis* infections.

Intrauterine device

The intrauterine device (IUD) is a risk factor for the development of pelvic inflammatory disease. Although the exact effect of removing an IUD on the response of acute salpingitis to antimicrobial therapy and on the risk of recurrent salpingitis is unknown, removal of the IUD is recommended soon after antimicrobial therapy has been initiated. When an IUD is removed, contraceptive counseling is necessary.

25.10   INFECTIOUS ARTHRITIS

Etiology

The type of infecting organism varies with the age of the patient and predisposing factors:

1. *Neisseria gonorrhoeae* is the most common organism in the 15-40 year old age group

2. *Staphylococcus aureus* is the most common cause of nongonococcal bacterial arthritis in adults; very common in patients with underlying rheumatoid arthritis
3. Streptococci (group A, nongroup A) is common in all age groups; they represent approximately 25% of cases of nongonococcal bacterial arthritis
4. Gram-negative bacilli are common in compromised hosts (e.g., malignancy, immunosuppression, chronic debilitating diseases) and IV drug addicts
5. *Haemophilus influenzae* is common in pediatric patients
6. *Staphylococcus epidermidis* is common in prosthetic joint infections
7. Lyme disease is caused by a spirochete *(Borrelia burgdorferi)* transmitted via the bite of a tick *(Ixodes dammini* and related species)
8. Viral arthritis is associated with viral hepatitis, rubella infection or immunization, mumps, HIV, infectious mononucleosis, herpesvirus
9. Others: *Mycobacterium tuberculosis,* atypical mycobacteria, fungal infections *(Candida,* coccidioidomycosis, sporotrichosis), *Meningococcus*

Predisposing factors

1. Septicemia
2. Immunosuppression (neoplasm, steroids)
3. Rheumatoid arthritis
4. IV drug abuse
5. Joint prosthesis
6. Penetrating wounds
7. Prior site of inflammation or damage
8. Other: deficiency of C_7, C_8 (increased risk of gonococcal and meningococcal arthritis), hypogammaglobulinemia, inherited disorders of chemotaxis

Diagnostic approach

1. History and physical exam
   a. Classical presentation: fever, erythema, pain, swelling, and limited motion of involved joint; however, these signs and symptoms may be absent or minimal, particularly in patients with rheumatoid arthritis or immunosuppression
   b. Nongonococcal arthritis is generally monoarticular; the knee is the joint most commonly involved
   c. Gonococcal arthritis usually presents with a migratory polyarthralgia and is often accompanied by tenosynovitis (inflammation of the tendon sheath) and erythematous pustular skin lesions (see Fig. 21-1)
   d. Lyme disease: refer to Section 25.11 for diagnosis and treatment
   e. *Pseudomonas aeruginosa* septic arthritis is usually associated with IV drug abuse and often involves the sternoclavicular or sacroiliac joints
   f. Tuberculous arthritis is generally monoarticular and usually involves large joints
2. Arthrocentesis with analysis of joint fluid: refer to Section 30.4 for procedure and interpretation of results
3. X-rays of the involved joints: indicated initially (as well as often following therapy), to rule out osteomyelitis; in septic arthritis, x-rays early in the course generally reveal only the presence of joint effusion

4. Lab results
   a. WBC: peripheral leukocytosis is usually present
   b. Blood cultures (aerobic and anaerobic): indicated in all patients
   c. Skin cultures: should be done on any skin lesions
   d. Genitourinary, pharyngeal, and rectal cultures: indicated in suspected gonococcal arthritis
   e. Sedimentation rate: generally not helpful; if initially elevated, it may be useful in following response to therapy (progressive decrease of sedimentation rate with successful treatment)
   f. Serologic testing: antibody titers against *Borrelia burgdorferi* are useful in suspected Lyme arthritis

Therapy[20,43]

1. IV antibiotic therapy: based on results of Gram stain of synovial fluid
   a. Gram-negative cocci
      (1) In an adult patient consider *N. gonorrhoeae* see treatment guidelines for sexually transmitted diseases (Section 25.9)
      (2) In a young child consider *H. influenzae* and treat with ampicillin IV 200 mg/kg/day in divided doses q6h; if allergic to penicillin, consider chloramphenicol or cefuroxime
   b. Gram-positive cocci: consider *S. aureus* and treat with oxacillin or nafcillin IV 9-12 g/day for at least 3 wk; in patients allergic to penicillin, use vancomycin or cefazolin
   c. Gram-negative bacilli: consider *Pseudomonas* or *Escherichia coli*
      (1) Initial IV treatment consists of an aminoglycoside plus mezlocillin or azlocillin
      (2) Suggested duration of treatment is 6-8 wk, followed by 2-4 wk of PO therapy in severe cases
   d. Inconclusive Gram stain: treat according to presumed organism (based on age and risk factors)
      (1) In a compromised host use an aminoglycoside plus mezlocillin to cover for *P. aeruginosa*
      (2) In a young, otherwise healthy adult use ceftriaxone to cover for *N. gonorrhoeae*
      (3) For treatment of patients with suspected Lyme disease, refer to Section 25.11
2. Drainage of infected joint: generally accomplished with needle aspiration; open drainage is generally reserved for prosthetic joint infections, inaccessible joints (e.g., hip), or inadequate drainage with needle aspiration
3. Joint immobilization: indicated in symptomatic patients; weight bearing by the infected joint should also be limited

25.11   LYME DISEASE

Definition

Multisystem disease caused by a spirochete *(Borrelia burgdorferi)* transmitted via the bite of a tick *(Ixodes dammini* and related species)

Table 25-2 Manifestations of Lyme disease by stage*

System†	Early Infection Localized (Stage 1)	Disseminated (Stage 2)	Late Infection Persistent (Stage 3)
Skin	Erythema migrans	Secondary annular lesions, malar rash, diffuse erythema or urticaria, evanescent lesions, lymphocytoma	Acrodermatitis chronica atrophicans, localized scleroderma-like lesions
Musculoskeletal system		Migratory pain in joints, tendons, bursae, muscle, bone; brief arthritis attacks; myositis‡; osteomyelitis‡; panniculitis‡	Prolonged arthritis attacks, chronic arthritis, peripheral enthesopathy, periostitis or joint subluxations below lesions of acrodermatitis
Neurologic system		Meningitis, cranial neuritis, Bell's palsy, motor or sensory radiculoneuritis, subtle encephalitis, mononeuritis multiplex, myelitis,‡ chorea,‡ cerebellar ataxia‡	Chronic encephalomyelitis, spastic parapareses, ataxic gait, subtle mental disorders, chronic axonal polyradiculopathy, dementia‡

Lymphatic system	Regional lymphadenopathy	Regional or generalized lymphadenopathy, splenomegaly
Heart		Atroventricular nodal block, myopericarditis, pancarditis
Eyes		Conjunctivitis, iritis,‡ choroiditis,‡ retinal hemorrhage or detachment,‡ panophthalmitis‡	Keratitis
Liver		Mild or recurrent hepatitis
Respiratory system		Nonexudative sore throat, nonproductive cough, adult respiratory distress syndrome‡
Kidney		Microscopic hematuria or proteinuria
Genitourinary system		Orchitis‡
Constitutional symptoms	Minor	Severe malaise and fatigue	Fatigue

*The classification by stages provides a guideline for the expected timing of the illness's manifestations, but this may vary from case to case.
†Systems are listed from the most to the least commonly affected.
‡The inclusion of this manifestation is based on one or a few cases.
From Steere AC: N Engl J Med 321:586, 1989. Reproduced with permission.

History and physical exam

The clinical manifestations of Lyme disease vary with the stage of the disease (Table 25-2) and include several presentations:

1. Stage I (localized early infection): usually manifested by a characteristic expanding annular skin lesion (erythema chronicum migrans, see Plate 3)
2. Stage II (disseminated infection): follows Stage I by days or weeks; patients may experience attacks of joint swelling and pain in large joints, neurologic complications (aseptic meningitis, encephalitis, cranial neuritis), cardiac abnormalities (AV block, myocarditis), and various other multisystem manifestations
3. Stage III (persistent infection): follows Stage II by 1 or more yr and is manifested by inflammatory arthritis affecting large joints (particularly the knee) and chronic cutaneous and neurologic sequelae; chronic Lyme arthritis is associated with HLA-DR4 and HLA-DR2 alleles

Diagnosis

Diagnosis is made primarily on clinical grounds and confirmed by serological testing.

1. Only one third of patients remember a tick bite
2. Greater than 80% of symptomatic patients will develop the rash of erythema chronicum migrans
3. Serological testing is performed with enzyme-linked immunoassay (ELISA), immunofluorescence assay (IFA), or Western blot analysis; false-negatives may be seen in the initial 2-4 wk of infection; false-positive results can occur with other spirochetal infections; in addition, there is significant lack of standardization among laboratories or test kits

Therapy

Treatment varies with the stage and clinical manifestations of the disease. The recommended therapeutic regimens are described in Table 25-3.

Table 25-3   Treatment regimens for Lyme disease

Manifestation	Regimen*
Early infection*	
Adults	Tetracycline, 250 mg orally 4× daily, 10-30 days†
	Doxycycline, 100 mg orally 2× daily, 10-30 days†‡
	Amoxicillin, 500 mg orally 4× daily, 10-30 days†‡

*Treatment failures have occurred with all these regimens, and retreatment may be necessary.
†The duration of therapy is based on clinical response.
‡The antibiotic has not yet been tested systematically for this indication in Lyme disease.
§The appropriate duration of therapy is not yet clear for patients with late neurologic abnormalities, and it may be longer than 2 wk.
From Steere AC: N Engl J Med 321:586, 1989. Reproduced with permission.

Table 25-3   Treatment regimens for Lyme disease—cont'd

Manifestation	Regimen*
Children (≤8 yr)	Amoxicillin or penicillin V, 250 mg orally 3× daily or 20 mg/kg body weight/day in divided doses, 10-30 days
	In case of penicillin allergy:
	Erythromycin, 250 mg orally 3× daily or 30 mg/kg/day in divided doses, 10-30 days‡
Neurologic abnormalities (early or late)*	
General	Ceftriaxone, 2 g intravenously 1× daily, 14 days§
	Penicillin G, 20 million U intravenously, 6 divided doses daily, 14 days§
	In case of ceftriaxone or penicillin allergy:
	Doxycycline, 100 mg orally 2× daily, 30 days‡
	Chloramphenicol, 250 mg intravenously 4× daily, 14 days‡
Facial palsy alone	Oral regimens may be adequate
Cardiac abnormalities	
First-degree atrioventricular block (PR interval <0.3 sec)	Oral regimens, as for early infection
High-degree atrioventricular block	Ceftriaxone, 2 g intravenously 1× daily, 14 days‡
	Penicillin, 20 million U intravenously, 6 divided doses daily, 14 days‡
Arthritis (intermittent or chronic)†	Doxycycline, 100 mg orally 2× daily, 30 days
	Amoxicillin and probenecid, 500 mg each orally 4× daily, 30 days
	Ceftriaxone, 2 g intravenously 1× daily, 14 days
	Penicillin, 20 million U intravenously, 6 divided doses daily, 14 days
Acrodermatitis	Oral regimens for 1 mo usually adequate

OSTEOMYELITIS

Definition

Osteomyelitis is an infection involving the bones and bone marrow.

Etiology

1. *Staphylococcus aureus* is the most common causative agent
2. Gram-negative bacilli: *Salmonella, Escherichia coli, Pseudomonas, Klebsiella*
   a. *Salmonella* is often seen in patients with sickle cell disease
   b. *Pseudomonas* is more frequent in IV drug addicts
   c. There is an increased incidence of gram-negative osteomyelitis in immunocompromised or chronically debilitated patients
3. *Haemophilus influenzae:* generally seen in infants and children
4. *Staphylococcus epidermidis:* often associated with prosthetic joints
5. Anaerobes often involve the sacrum (associated with infected decubitus ulcers), skull, and hands (following human bites)
6. Others: streptococci, *Mycobacterium tuberculosis* (generally involves spine and results in compression fractures), fungi (*Candida albicans, histoplasmosis*)

Major predisposing factors

1. Sickle cell disease (bone infarcts, marrow thrombosis)
2. Compound fractures, open reduction of fractures
3. IV drug abuse
4. Peripheral vascular disease (atherosclerosis, diabetes mellitus)
5. Contiguous focus of infection (septic arthritis, otitis media, infected decubitus ulcer)
6. Trauma (particularly in children)
7. Recent complete joint arthroplasty

Diagnostic approach

1. History and physical exam
   a. Classical presentation consists of bone pain, fever, chills, and generalized malaise
      (1) There is significant tenderness over the bone and limitations of movement of the involved extremity
      (2) Osteomyelitis can also present with minimal, vague symptoms (e.g., vertebral osteomyelitis)
   b. History and physical exam often reveal one or more preexisting factors (see above)
2. Lab results
   a. Blood cultures
   b. WBC: peripheral leukocytosis is usually present
   c. Sedimentation rate: a normal value does not rule out osteomyelitis; an initially elevated sedimentation rate may be useful in following the course of the disease
   d. Aspirate and culture any joint effusions: refer to Section 30.4 for arthrocentesis and interpretation of results; bone biopsy may be necessary to establish diagnosis

3. Radiographic evaluation
   a. Initial x-rays may be normal because radiologic changes lag behind the clinical manifestations
   b. Initial changes consist of subperiosteal elevation and soft tissue swelling; these are then followed by lytic changes generally 3-4 wk after the onset of disease
   c. Radionuclide scanning (technetium-99 pyrophosphate) can detect osteomyelitis early in its course; however, neoplasms, trauma, and other inflammatory processes may also produce positive radionuclide scans

Treatment

1. IV antibiotics
   a. The choice of antibiotic depends on the suspected likely pathogen (e.g., adult with suspected *S. aureus* osteomyelitis should be initially treated with IV oxacillin or nafcillin); the fluoroquinolones are playing an increasing role in the treatment of bone infections; ciprofloxacin is very useful in cases of hematogenous and vertebral osteomyelitis
   b. Antibiotics are generally continued for 8-12 wk following resolution of tenderness and local signs of swelling
2. Surgical debridement of all devitalized bone
3. Immobilization of affected bone (plaster, traction)
4. Radiographic surveillance during and after treatment

25.13 SPONTANEOUS BACTERIAL PERITONITIS

Definition

Spontaneous bacterial peritonitis (SBP) is defined as the onset of bacterial peritonitis without an evident source of infection.

Pathogenesis

SBP usually occurs as a complication of hepatic ascites. The following mechanisms may account for bacterial seeding of the ascitic fluid:
1. Hematogenous transmission
2. Direct transmural passage following mucosal damage (ischemia, edema)
3. Bowel perforation following paracentesis (uncommon)[36]

Infecting organisms

1. *Escherichia coli*
2. *Streptococcus* group D, *S. pneumoniae,* and *S. viridans*
3. Others: *Enterobacter, Pseudomonas, Klebsiella*

Clinical manifestations

1. Fever
2. Abdominal pain and tenderness
3. Jaundice and encephalopathy
4. Hypoactive bowel sounds
5. Diarrhea
6. Sudden deterioration of mental status or renal function

Ascitic fluid analysis (see Section 30.3)[19,24,45]

1. Polymorphonuclear (PMN) cell count >250/mm³ in ascitic fluid; this is the most sensitive and specific test for SBP if >500/mm³
2. Presence of bacteria on initial Gram stain of ascitic fluid
3. Lactic acid (lactate) >32 mg/dl[22]
4. pH <7.31 or arterial/ascitic fluid pH >0.1
5. Protein <1 g/dl
6. Glucose >50 mg/dl
7. Lactate dehydrogenase <225 mU/ml

Major distinguishing factors between SBP and secondary peritonitis (perforation of bowel wall)[45]

1. Presence of free air on abdominal x-rays in secondary peritonitis
2. Common presence of multiple organisms and anaerobes in ascitic fluid in secondary peritonitis
3. Analysis of ascitic fluid in secondary peritonitis generally reveals: leukocyte count >10,000/mm³, LDH >225 mU/ml, protein >1 g/dl, and glucose <50 mg/dl
4. Repeat paracentesis after 48 hr of appropriate antibiotic therapy will reveal a significant decrease in ascitic fluid polymorphonuclear leukocyte count in patients with SBP, and no decrease in patients with a secondary bacterial peritonitis[1]

Therapy of SBP[16]

Cefotaxime 2 g IV q4h (in patients with normal renal function). The combination of an aminoglycoside and ampicillin is also effective; however, nephrotoxicity is a major problem.

25.14   BACTERIAL MENINGITIS

Etiology

The type of infecting organism varies with the age of the patient and several predisposing factors:

1. *Streptococcus pneumoniae* is common in adults and elderly patients; predisposing factors include blunt head trauma, otitis media, pneumonia, and CSF leaks; mortality is 30%; permanent neurologic sequelae occur in 50% of survivors
2. *Neisseria meningitidis* is common in young adults and children
3. *Haemophilus influenzae* is usually seen in preschool age children; predisposing factors in adults include head trauma, otitis media, and sinusitis
4. *Listeria monocytogenes* is common in immunosuppressed patients (lymphoma, organ transplant recipients)
5. *Gram-negative bacilli* are usually seen in neonates (acquired in passage through birth canal) and in elderly debilitated patients
6. *Staphylococcus aureus* is seen in diabetics, patients with *S. aureus* pneumonia, or cancer

Diagnostic approach

1. History and physical exam
   a. The classic presentation consists of fever, headache, lethargy, confusion, and nuchal rigidity; these manifestations are not always present, particularly in infants, elderly, and immunocompromised patients
   b. Physical exam
      (1) Kernig's sign: resistance to knee extension following flexion of the patient's hips and knees by the examiner
      (2) Brudzinski's sign: rapid flexion of the neck elicits involuntary flexing of the knees in a supine patient
      (3) Altered mental status (confusion, lethargy)
      (4) Bulging fontanelle in infants
      (5) Petechial or purpuric rash generally involving the trunk or extremities; the rash is suggestive of meningococcal meningitis but can also be present in viral meningitis, other bacterial meningitis, bacterial endocarditis, and bacteremia secondary to staphylococci and other organisms
      (6) Papilledema is unusual and should raise the suspicion of brain abscess or mass lesion
2. Lab results
   a. WBC usually reveals leukocytosis with shift to the left; however, leukopenia can also be present; peripheral lymphocytosis is usually suggestive of a viral etiology (aseptic meningitis)
   b. Blood cultures are appropriate; however, antibiotic therapy should not be delayed until all cultures are obtained if patient is very ill
3. Lumbar puncture: refer to Section 30.1 for procedure, diagnostic studies, and interpretation of results; in bacterial meningitis, the classic findings on CSF examination are: elevated WBC (predominantly PMNs), decreased glucose, elevated protein, and positive Gram stain
4. *Limulus* lysate assay (for gram-negative endotoxin), latex agglutination and staphylococcal coagglutination (for bacterial antigen detection) are useful in patients with suspected bacterial meningitis and a negative Gram stain

Treatment

IV antibiotic therapy should be based on the results of the Gram stain and consideration of predisposing factors for specific organisms (e.g., age, head trauma, immunosuppression). Tables 25-4 to 25-6 describe suggested initial treatment of bacterial meningitis in adults.

Suggested duration of therapy in bacterial meningitis

The duration of treatment varies with the infecting organism and the patient's clinical course. Guidelines are listed in Table 25-7.

Prophylaxis of bacterial meningitis[48]

1. Indications
   a. Meningococcal meningitis and *H. influenzae* meningitis (type B)
      (1) Members of the same household
      (2) Individuals who have had close contact with the index case (e.g., babysitter, boyfriend, girlfriend)

Table 25-4 Antimicrobial Therapy for Bacterial Meningitis

Organism	Standard Therapy	Alternative Therapies
Neisseria meningitidis	Penicillin G, or ampicillin	Third-generation cephalosporin*; cefuroxime; chloramphenicol
Streptococcus pneumoniae	Penicillin G or ampicillin	Third-generation cephalosporin*; cefuroxime; chloramphenicol
Haemophilus influenzae (beta-lactamase-negative)	Ampicillin	Third-generation cephalosporin*; cefuroxime; chloramphenicol
H. influenzae (beta-lactamase-positive)	Third-generation cephalosporin*	Chloramphenicol; cefuroxime
Enterobacteriaceae	Third-generation cephalosporin*	Extended spectrum penicillin† plus an aminoglycoside; aztreonam‡; quinolones‡
Pseudomonas aeruginosa	Ceftazidime (plus an aminoglycoside)	Extended spectrum penicillin† plus an aminoglycoside; aztreonam‡; imipenem‡; quinolones‡

Streptococcus agalactiae	Penicillin G or ampicillin (plus an aminoglycoside)	Third-generation cephalosporin*; chloramphenicol
Listeria monocytogenes	Ampicillin or penicillin G (plus an aminoglycoside)	Trimethoprim-sulfamethoxazole
Staphylococcus aureus (methicillin-sensitive)	Nafcillin or oxacillin	Vancomycin
Staphylococcus aureus (methicillin-resistant)	Vancomycin	Trimethoprim-sulfamethoxazole; quinolones‡
Staphylococcus epidermidis	Vancomycin (plus rifampin)	Teicoplanin ‡; daptomycin ‡

*Cefotaxime, ceftizoxime, and ceftriaxone have received the most scrutiny and are recommended. Cefoperazone and moxalactam are not indicated. Ceftazidime should be reserved for suspected or proven Pseudomonas aeruginosa meningitis.

†Piperacillin or azlocillin.

‡The effectiveness of these antibiotics in bacterial meningitis has not been clearly documented.

Reproduced with permission from Tunkel AR, Wispelwey B, Scheld WM: Ann Intern Med 112:610, 1990.

Table 25-5 Empirical Therapy for Purulent Meningitis*

Age	Common Microorganisms	Therapy
0 to 4 wk	Escherichia coli, group B streptococci, Listeria monocytogenes	Ampicillin plus a third-generation cephalosporin,[†] or ampicillin plus an aminoglycoside
4 to 12 weeks	E. coli, group B streptococci, L. monocytogenes, Haemophilus influenzae, Streptococcus pneumoniae	Ampicillin plus a third-generation cephalosporin
3 mo to 18 yr	H. influenzae, Neisseria meningitidis, S. pneumoniae	Third-generation cephalosporin; or ampicillin plus chloramphenicol
18 to 50 yr	S. pneumoniae, N. meningitidis	Penicillin G or ampicillin
Older than 50 yr	S. pneumoniae, N. meningitidis, L. monocytogenes, gram-negative bacilli	Ampicillin plus a third-generation cephalosporin

*Patients without underlying illness.
[†]Cefotaxime, ceftizoxime, or ceftriaxone (most studies have evaluated only cefotaxime or ceftriaxone).
Reproduced with permission from Tunkel AR, Wispelwey B, Scheld WM: Ann Intern Med 112:610, 1990.

Table 25-6 Recommended Doses of Antibiotics for Bacterial Meningitis in Adults with Normal Renal Function

Antibiotic	Daily Dose (per 24 hr)	Dosing Interval (hr)
Penicillin G	20 to 24 million U	4
Ampicillin	12 g	4
Nafcillin, oxacillin	9-12 g	4
Chloramphenicol	4 to 6 g*	6
Cefotaxime	12 g	4
Ceftizoxime	6 to 9 g†	8
Ceftriaxone	4 to 6 g‡	12
Ceftazidime	6 to 12 g§	8
Vancomycin	2 g	12
Gentamicin, tobramycin	3 to 5 mg/kg BW	8
Amikacin	15 mg/kg BW	8

*Higher dose recommended if used for pneumococcal meningitis.
†Limited data exist; higher dose recommended pending further study.
‡Actual dose studied was 50 mg/kg body weight every 12 hr.
§Not enough patients studied to make firm recommendations.
Reproduced with permission from Tunkel AR, Wispelwey B, Scheld WM: Ann Intern Med 112:610, 1990.

Table 25-7 Suggested duration of therapy in bacterial meningitis[5, 21, 30, 53]

Infecting Organism	Suggested Duration of Therapy
N. meningitidis	10 days
S. pneumoniae	12-14 days
H. influenzae, type B	14 days
Gram-negative bacilli	10-14 days after negative repeat CSF culture
L. monocytogenes	4-6 wk
S. aureus	4-6 wk

    (3) Hospital personnel who performed mouth-to-mouth resuscitation on the patient
    (4) Contacts at day care, school, or chronic care facilities should be considered on an individual basis
2. Prophylaxis
   a. Meningococcal meningitis
    (1) Adults: rifampin 600 mg PO bid for 2 days
    (2) Children: rifampin 10 mg/kg PO bid for 2 days
   b. *H. influenzae* meningitis
    (1) Adults: rifampin 600 mg PO qd for 4 days
    (2) Children: rifampin 20 mg/kg (maximum 600 mg) PO qd for 4 days

25.15   **INFECTIVE ENDOCARDITIS**

Etiology

1. Streptococci
   a. *S. viridans* the most common organism, except for those causing right-sided and prosthetic-valve endocarditides
   b. Enterococci (group D streptococci), often occurring in elderly males with genitourinary disorders
   c. *S. bovis* and other streptococci
2. Staphylococci
   a. *Staphylococcus aureus* is the most common organism in right-sided endocarditis
   b. *Staphylococcus epidermidis* is the most common organism in prosthetic valve endocarditis
3. Others: fungi (IV drug abusers, immunocompromised patients), gram-negative bacilli, gonococci, pneumococci

Risk factors

1. Rheumatic valvulitis
2. IV drug abuse
3. Bicuspid aortic valve
4. Aortic stenosis (AS)
5. Aortic insufficiency
6. Mechanical heart valves
7. Mitral insufficiency
8. Coarctation of aorta, VSD, PDA
9. Mitral valve prolapse
10. Marfan syndrome
11. Myxomas associated with calcification of the valves
12. Previous endocarditis
13. Mitral stenosis
14. Male gender
15. Black race
16. Pulmonary artery catheterization

Diagnosis

1. History and physical exam
   a. Presence of any risk factors (see above)
   b. Physical exam
      (1) Heart murmur is usually present in subacute bacterial endocarditis (SBE), but may be absent in acute bacterial endocarditis and right-sided endocarditis
      (2) Fever is generally present; may be absent in elderly or immunocompromised patients
      (3) Flame-shaped retinal hemorrhages with pale centers (Roth spots)
      (4) Painless erythematous papules and macules on the palms of the hands and soles of the feet (Janeway lesions)
      (5) Painful erythematous subcutaneous papules (Osler nodes)
      (6) Petechiae
      (7) Subungual splinter hemorrhages

(8) Splenomegaly

(9) Other: headaches, backache, arthralgias, confusion

2. Lab results

   a. Blood cultures: positive in 85-95% of patients; negative cultures are usually secondary to[52]:

      (1) Prior antibiotic therapy (in preceding 2 wk)

      (2) Fastidious organisms with special growth requirements (anaerobes, *Coxiella burnetti, Chlamydia psittaci, Brucella, Neisseria, Corynebacterium*)

      (3) Slow-growing organisms (*Haemophilus, Actinobacillus*)

      (4) Fungi (*Candida, Aspergillus, Histoplasma, Cryptococcus*)

      (5) Improper collection of blood and cultures

   b. Decreased hemoglobin/hematocrit: usually secondary to decreased RBC production caused by inflammatory state

   c. Normal, elevated, or decreased WBC, usually with shift to left

   d. Assay of teichoic acid antibody: can aid in the diagnosis of *S. aureus* endocarditis (e.g., IV drug addicts); an assay should be obtained on admission and repeated in 1-2 wk in patients with suspected *S. aureus* endocarditis

   e. Urinalysis: may show hematuria with associated RBC casts

   f. Rheumatoid factor: positive in approximately 50% of cases after 6 wk; its significance is unclear

   g. Sedimentation rate: generally elevated, not helpful

3. Echocardiography

   a. Useful to demonstrate valvular vegetations and to evaluate valvular damage and left ventricular function; however, a normal echocardiogram does not rule out endocarditis; if normal, should be repeated in 1 wk

   b. Two-dimensional echocardiography is preferred over M-mode because of increased sensitivity (can detect 80-85% of vegetations)[31]; transesophageal echo further enhances sensitivity

   c. The incidence of complications (e.g., heart failure, embolization) is directly related to the size of the vegetation[60]

   d. Echocardiographically documented vegetations ≥1 cm in patients with right-sided infective endocarditis are associated with a lower response rate to appropriate medical therapy[44]

Special diagnostic considerations

1. Right-sided endocarditis

   a. Usually seen in IV drug addicts

   b. Physical exam may reveal a murmur of tricuspid regurgitation (holosystolic, heard at left lower sternal border, increased by inspiration, decreased by expiration and Valsalva maneuver); evidence of right-sided heart failure may also be present (neck vein distention, congestive hepatomegaly)

   c. Blood cultures reveal *S. aureus* (50% of cases), streptococci and enterococci (20% of all cases), and gram-negative bacilli (approximately 10% of cases)

   d. Chest x-ray may demonstrate peripheral wedge-shaped infiltrates with cavitation (septic pulmonary emboli)

2. Prosthetic valve endocarditis[58]

a. Overall frequency is approximately 2%
b. Overall mortality is 59%
c. The microbiological agent involved and the mortality are releated to the time of onset of endocarditis after cardiac valve implantation
    (1) Early onset prosthetic valve endocarditis (within 2 mo of implantation)
        (a) Frequency of endocarditis (0.78%)
        (b) Usually resulting from surgical infection
        (c) Staphylococci are the most common organisms (*S. epidermidis* the predominant one); they are usually resistant to cephalosporins and semisynthetic penicillinase-resistant penicillins
        (d) Mortality (77%)
    (2) Late-onset prosthetic valve endocarditis (occurring more than 2 mo postoperatively)
        (a) Frequency of endocarditis (1.1%)
        (b) Usually community-acquired infection
        (c) Streptococci are the predominant organisms
        (d) Overall mortality (46%)
3. *Streptococcus bovis* endocarditis
    a. Often associated with a gastrointestinal lesion
    b. A GI work-up should be undertaken

Major complications of infective endocarditis

1. CHF caused by valvular destruction or associated myocarditis
2. Embolism
    a. CNS: hemiplegia, sensory loss, aphasia, meningeal irritation, mycotic aneurysm, brain abscesses, seizures, headaches
    b. Kidneys: hematuria secondary to focal glomerulonephritis, renal failure secondary to diffuse proliferative glomerulonephritis, renal emboli, and infarction
    c. Coronary arteries: heart failure, angina, MI
    d. Spleen: splenic infarct
3. Dysrhythmias
4. Pericarditis, myocardial abscess, myocarditis

Management

1. Medical
    a. Tables 25-8 to 25-13 describe antibiotic treatment in adults, based on positive blood culture results
        (1) Antibiotic therapy (upon identification of the organism) should be guided by susceptibility testing (MIC, MBC)[59]
        (2) Peak serum bactericidal titers $\geq 1:64$ and trough bactericidal titers $\geq 1:32$ are recommended[55]
    b. Initial IV antibiotic therapy (before culture results) is aimed at the most likely organism
        (1) In patients with prosthetic valves or patients with native valves but allergic to penicillin: vancomycin plus rifampin and gentamicin
        (2) In IV drug addicts: penicillinase-resistant penicillin (oxacillin or nafcillin) plus gentamicin

(3) In native valve endocarditis: combination of penicillin and gentamicin; a penicillinase-resistant penicillin should be added if acute bacterial endocarditis is present or if *Staphylococcus aureus* is suspected as one of the possible causative organisms

2. Surgical: indications for cardiac surgery in patients with active infective endocarditis are listed in the box below.

Indications for Cardiac Surgery in Patients with Active Infective Endocarditis

Indications for Urgent Cardiac Surgery in Patients with Active Infective Endocarditis

1. Hemodynamic compromise
   a. Severe heart failure
   b. Valvular obstruction
2. Uncontrolled infection
   a. Fungal endocarditis
   b. Persistent bacteremia
   c. No effective antimicrobial agent available
3. Unstable prosthesis

Relative Indications for Cardiac Surgery in Active Native Valve Endocarditis

1. Etiological bacteria other than "susceptible" streptococci
2. Relapse
3. Evidence for intracardiac extension of the infection
   a. Ruptured chordae tendineae or papillary muscle
   b. Rupture of sinus of Valsalva or ventricular septum
   c. Heart block
   d. Abscess demonstrated by echocardiography or catheterization
4. Two or more emboli (controversial)
5. Usually large and mobile vegetations demonstrated by echocardiography
6. Mitral valve preclosure by echocardiography, indicating severe aortic regurgitation

Relative Indications for Cardiac Surgery in Active Prosthetic Valve Endocarditis

1. Early prosthetic valve endocarditis
2. Nonstreptococcal late prosthetic valve endocarditis
3. Periprosthetic leak
4. Two or more emboli
5. Relapse
6. Evidence for intracardiac extension of infection

Modified from Alsip SG, Blackstone MD, et al: Am J Med 78(suppl 6B):138, 1985. Reproduced with permission.

Table 25-8 Suggested regimens of therapy for endocarditis due to penicillin-susceptible *Streptococcus viridans* and *S. bovis* (MIC, ≤0.1 μg/ml)*

Antibiotic	Adult Dose and Route†	Pediatric Dose and Route	Duration (wk)
1. Aqueous crystalline penicillin G‡	10-20 million U/24 hr IV either continuously or in 6 equally divided doses	150,000-200,000 U/kg per 24 hr IV (not to exceed 20 million U/24 hr) either continuously or in 6 equally divided doses	4
2. Aqueous crystalline penicillin G§	10-20 million U/24 hr IV either continuously or in 6 equally divided doses	150,000-200,000 U/kg per 24 hr IV (not to exceed 20 million U/24 hr) either continuously or in 6 equally divided doses	2
With streptomycin‖	7.5 mg/kg IM (not to exceed 500 mg) every 12 hr	15 mg/kg IM (not to exceed 500 mg) every 12 hr	2
or With gentamicin‖	1 mg/kg IM or IV (not to exceed 80 mg) every 8 hr	2.0-2.5 mg/kg IV (not to exceed 80 mg) every 8 hr	2

3. Aqueous crystalline penicillin G§	10-20 million U/24 hr IV either continuously or in 6 equally divided doses	150,000-200,000,000 U/kg per 24 hr IV (not to exceed 20 million U/24 hr) either continuously or in 6 equally divided doses	4
With streptomycin||	7.5 mg/kg IM (not to exceed 500 mg) every 12 hr	15 mg/kg IM (not to exceed 500 mg) every 12 hr	2
or With gentamicin||	1 mg/kg IM or IV (not to exceed 80 mg) every 8 hr	2.0 to 2.5 mg/kg IV (not to exceed 80 mg) every 8 hr	2

*Therapy for penicillin-allergic patients; antibiotic doses for patients with impaired renal function should be modified appropriately. MIC is minimum inhibitory concentration.

†IV indicates intravenously; and IM, intramuscularly.

‡Preferred in most patients older than 65 yr of age and in those with impairment of the eighth nerve or of renal function.

§Or, procaine penicillin G, 1.2 million U IM every 6 hr. Procaine penicillin G is not recommended for treatment of endocarditis due to *S. viridans* in children.

||Should be given in addition to penicillin. If regimen 3 is selected, streptomycin or gentamicin should be given for the first 2 wk. Peak streptomycin levels of approximately 20 μg/ml and peak gentamicin levels of approximately 3 μg/ml are desirable. Dosing of aminoglycosides on a milligram per kilogram basis will produce higher serum concentrations in obese than in lean patients. Relative contraindications to use of aminoglycosides are age greater than 65 yr or renal or eighth nerve impairment.

Reproduced courtesy the ad hoc writing group of the Committee on Rheumatic Fever, Endocarditis, and Kawasaki Disease of the American Heart Association's Council on Cardiovascular Disease in the Young, Dallas Tex. (Bisno AL, Dismukes WE, et al: JAMA 261:1471, 1989.)

Table 25-9 Therapy for endocarditis due to penicillin-susceptible *Streptococcus viridans* and *S. bovis* (MIC, ≤0.1 µg/ml) in patients allergic to penicillin*

Antibiotic	Adult Dose and Route†	Pediatric Dose and Route†	Duration (wk)
1. Cephalothin‡§	2 g IV every 4 hr	100-150 mg/kg per 24 hr IV (not to exceed 12 g/24 hr) in equally divided doses every 4 to 6 hr	4
or Cefazolin‡§	1 g IM or IV every 8 hr	80-100 mg/kg per 24 hr IM or IV (not to exceed 3.0 g/24 hr) in equally divided doses every 8 hr	4
2. Vancomycin‖	30 mg/kg per 24 hr in 2 or 4 equally divided doses, not to exceed 2 g/24 hr unless serum levels are monitored	40 mg/kg per 24 hr IV in 2 or 4 equally divided doses, not to exceed 2 g/24 hr unless serum levels are monitored	4

*Vancomycin dose should be reduced in patients with renal dysfunction; cephalosporin dose may need to be reduced in patients with moderate to severe renal dysfunction. MIC is minimum inhibitory concentration.

†IV indicates intravenously; and IM, intramuscularly.

‡Streptomycin or gentamicin may be added to cephalothin or cefazolin for first 2 wk in doses recommended in Table 25-8.

§There is potential cross-allergenicity between penicillins and cephalosporins. Cephalosporins should be avoided in patients with Immediate-type hypersensitivity to penicillin.

‖Peak serum concentrations of vancomycin should be obtained 1 hr after infusion and should be in the range of 30 to 45 µg/ml for twice daily dosing and 20 to 35 µg/ml for four times daily dosing. Vancomycin or aminoglycosides given on a milligram per kilogram basis will produce higher serum concentrations in obese than in lean patients. Each dose of vancomycin should be infused over 1 hr.

Reproduced courtesy the ad hoc writing group of the Committee on Rheumatic Fever, Endocarditis, and Kawasaki Disease of the American Heart Association's Council on Cardiovascular Disease in the Young, Dallas, Tex. (Bisno AL, Dismukes WE, et al: JAMA 261:1471, 1989.)

Table 25-10 Therapy for endocarditis due to strains of *Streptococcus viridans* and *S. bovis* relatively resistant to penicillin G (MIC, >0.1 µg/ml and <0.5 µg/ml)*

Antibiotic	Adult Dose and Route†	Pediatric Dose and Route	Duration (wk)
Aqueous crystalline penicillin G	20 million U/24 hr IV either continuously or in 6 equally divided doses	200 000 to 300 000 U/kg per 24 hr IV (not to exceed 20 million U/24 h) given continuously or in 6 equally divided doses	4
With streptomycin‡	7.5 mg/kg IM (not to exceed 500 mg) every 12 hr	15 mg/kg IM (not to exceed 500 mg) every 12 hr	2
or With gentamicin‡	1 mg/kg IM or IV (not to exceed 80 mg) every 8 hr	2.0 to 2.5 mg/kg IM or IV (not to exceed 80 mg) every 8 hr	2

*Cephalothin or cefazolin (with an aminoglycoside for the first two weeks) or vancomycin alone can be used in patients whose penicillin hypersensitivity is not of the immediate type. Vancomycin also can be used in patients with immediate penicillin allergy. Antibiotic doses should be modified appropriately for patients with impaired renal function. MIC is minimum inhibitory concentration.

†IV indicates intravenously; and IM, intramuscularly.

‡Streptomycin or gentamicin should be given in addition to penicillin for the first 2 wk. Peak streptomycin levels of approximately 20 µg/ml and peak gentamicin levels of about 3 µg/ml are desirable. For the rare *S. viridans* with minimum inhibitory concentration greater than or equal to 0.5 µg/ml of penicillin G, aminoglycoside therapy should be continued for 4 wk with appropriate monitoring of serum levels of streptomycin or gentamicin. Aminoglycosides given on a milligram per kilogram basis will produce higher serum concentrations in obese than in lean patients.

Reproduced courtesy the ad hoc writing group of the Committee on Rheumatic Fever, Endocarditis, and Kawasaki Disease of the American Heart Association's Council on Cardiovascular Disease in the Young, Dallas Tex. (Bisno AL, Dismukes WE, et al: JAMA 261:1471, 1989.)

Table 25-11 Therapy for endocarditis due to enterococci (or to *Streptococcus viridans*) (MIC, ≥0.5 μg/ml)*

Antibiotic	Adult Dose and Route†	Pediatric Dose and Route	Duration (wk)
Regimen for Non-Penicillin-Allergic Patients			
1. Aqueous crystalline penicillin G	20 to 30 million U/24 hr IV given continuously or in 6 equally divided doses	200,000 to 300,000 U/kg per 24 hr IV (not to exceed 30 million U/24 h) given continuously or in 6 equally divided doses	4-6
With gentamicin‡§‖	1 mg/kg IM or IV (not to exceed 80 mg) every 8 hr	2.0 to 2.5 mg/kg IM or IV (not to exceed 80 mg) every 8 hr	4-6
or With streptomycin‡‖¶	7.5 mg/kg IM (not to exceed 500 mg) every 12 hr	15 mg/kg IM (not to exceed 500 mg) every 12 hr	4-6
2. Ampicillin	12 g/24 hr IV given continuously or in 6 equally divided doses	300 mg/kg per 24 hr IV (not to exceed 12 g/24 hr) in 4 to 6 equally divided doses	4-6
With gentamicin‡§‖	1 mg/kg IM or IV (not to exceed 80 mg) every 8 hr	2.0 to 2.5 mg/kg IM or IV (not to exceed 80 mg) every 8 hr	4-6
or With streptomycin‡‖¶	7.5 mg/kg IM (not to exceed 500 mg) every 12 hr	15 mg/kg IM (not to exceed 500 mg) every 12 hr	4-6

Regimen for Penicillin-Allergic Patients
(Desensitization Should Be Considered; Cephalosporins Are Not Satisfactory Alternatives)

Vancomycin#	30 mg/kg per 24 hr IV in 2 or 4 equally divided doses, not to exceed 2 g/24 hr unless serum levels are monitored	40 mg/kg per 24 hr IV in 2 or 4 equally divided doses, not to exceed 2 g/24 hr unless serum levels are monitored	4-6
With gentamicin‡§||	1 mg/kg IM or IV (not to exceed 80 mg) every 8 hr	2.0 to 2.5 mg/kg IM or IV (not to exceed 80 mg) every 8 hr	4-6
or With streptomycin‡||¶	7.5 mg/kg IM (not to exceed 500 mg) every 12 hr	15 mg/kg IM (not to exceed 500 mg) every 12 hr	4-6

*Antibiotic doses should be modified appropriately in patients with impaired renal function. MIC is minimum inhibitory concentration.

†IV indicates intravenously; and IM, intramuscularly.

‡Choice of aminoglycoside depends on resistance level of infecting strain (see text). Enterococci should be tested for high-level resistance (minimum inhibitory concentration, ≥2000 μg/ml).

§Serum concentration of gentamicin should be monitored and dose adjusted to obtain a peak level of approximately 3 μg/ml.

||Dosing of aminoglycosides and vancomycin on a milligram per kilogram basis will give higher serum concentrations in obese than in lean patients.

¶Serum concentration of streptomycin should be monitored if possible and dose adjusted to obtain a peak level of approximately 20 μg/ml.

#Peak serum concentrations of vancomycin should be obtained 1 hr after infusion and should be in the range of 30 to 45 μg/ml for twice daily dosing and 20 to 35 μg/ml for four times daily dosing. Each dose should be infused over 1 hr.

Reproduced courtesy the ad hoc writing group of the Committee on Rheumatic Fever, Endocarditis, and Kawasaki Disease of the American Heart Association's Council on Cardiovascular Disease in the Young, Dallas Tex. (Bisno AL, Dismukes WE, et al: JAMA 261:1471, 1989.)

Table 25-12 Therapy for endocarditis due to staphylococci in the absence of prosthetic material*

Antibiotic	Adult Dose and Route†	Pediatric Dose and Route	Duration (wk)
Methicillin-Susceptible Staphylococci			
Regimen for Non–Penicillin-Allergic Patients			
Nafcillin	2 g IV every 4 hr	150-200 mg/kg per 24 h IV (not to exceed 12 g/24 hr) in 4 to 6 equally divided doses	4-6
or Oxacillin	2 g IV every 4 hr	150-200 mg/kg per 24 h IV (not to exceed 12 g/24 hr) in 4 to 6 equally divided doses	4-6
With optional addition of gentamicin‡§	1 mg/kg IM or IV (not to exceed 80 mg) every 8 hr	2.0-2.5 mg/kg IV (not to exceed 80 mg) every 8 hr	3-5 days
Regimen for Penicillin-Allergic Patients			
1. Cephalothin‖	2 g IV every 4 hr	100-150 mg/kg per 24 hr IV (not to exceed 12 g/24 h) in equally divided doses every 4 to 6 h	4-6
or Cefazolin‖	2 g IV every 8 hr	80-100 mg/kg per 24 hr IV (not to exceed 6 g/24 h) in equally divided doses every 8 h	4-6

With optional addition of gentamicin‡	Same as for non–penicillin-allergic patients		· · ·
2. Vancomycin‡¶	30 mg/kg per 24 hr IV in 2 or 4 equally divided doses, not to exceed 2 g/24 hr unless serum levels are monitored	Same as for non–penicillin-allergic patients	40 mg/kg per 24 hr IV in 2 or 4 equally divided doses, not to exceed 2 g/24 hr unless serum levels are monitored	4-6
Methicillin-Resistant Staphylococci			
Vancomycin‡¶	30 mg/kg per 24 hr IV in 2 or 4 equally divided doses, not to exceed 2 g/24 hr unless serum levels are monitored		40 mg/kg per 24 hr IV in 2 or 4 equally divided doses, not to exceed 2 g/24 hr unless serum levels are monitored	4-6

*Antibiotic doses should be modified appropriately for patients with impaired renal function. For treatment of endocarditis due to penicillin-susceptible staphylococci (minimum inhibitory concentration, ≤0.1 μg/ml), aqueous crystalline penicillin G (Table 25-8, first regimen) should be used for 4-6 wk instead of nafcillin or oxacillin. Shorter antibiotic courses have been effective in some drug addicts with right-sided endocarditis due to *Staphylococcus aureus*. See text for comments on use of rifampin.

†IV indicates intravenously; and IM, intramuscularly.

‡Dosing of aminoglycosides and vancomycin on a milligram per kilogram basis will give higher serum concentrations in obese than in lean patients.

§Benefit of additional aminoglycoside has not been established. Risk of toxic reactions due to these agents is increased in patients who are older than age 65 yr or who have renal or eighth nerve impairment.

‖There is potential cross-allergenicity between penicillins and cephalosporins. Cephalosporins should be avoided in patients with immediate-type hypersensitivity to penicillin.

¶Peak serum concentration of vancomycin should be obtained 1 hr after infusion and should be in the range of 30 to 45 μg/ml for twice daily dosing and 20 to 35 μg/ml for four times daily dosing. Each dose of vancomycin should be infused over 1 hr. See text for consideration of optional addition of gentamicin.

Reproduced courtesy the ad hoc writing group of the Committee on Rheumatic Fever, Endocarditis, and Kawasaki Disease of the American Heart Association's Council on Cardiovascular Disease in the Young, Dallas Tex. (Bisno AL, Dismukes WE, et al: JAMA 261:1471, 1989.)

Table 25-13 Treatment of staphylococcal endocarditis in the presence of a prosthetic valve or other prosthetic material*

Antibiotic	Adult Dose and Route†	Pediatric Dose and Route	Duration, (wk)
Regimen for Methicillin-Resistant Staphylococci			
Vancomycin‡,§	30 mg/kg per 24 hr IV in 2 or 4 equally divided doses, not to exceed 2 g/24 hr unless serum levels are monitored	40 mg/kg per 24 hr IV in 2 or 4 equally divided doses, not to exceed 2 g/24 hr unless serum levels are monitored	≥6
With rifampin‖	300 mg PO every 8 hr	20 mg/kg per 24 hr PO (not to exceed 900 mg/24 hr) in 2 equally divided doses	≥6
and With gentamicin§‖#	1.0 mg/kg IM or IV (not to exceed 80 mg) every 8 hr	2.0-2.5 mg/kg per 24 hr IV (not to exceed 80 mg) every 8 hr	2

Regimen for Methicillin-Susceptible Staphylococci

Nafcillin or oxacillin**	2 g IV every 4 hr	150-200 mg/kg per 24 hr IV (not to exceed 12 g/24 hr) in 4 to 6 equally divided doses	≥6
With rifampin‖	300 mg PO every 8 hr	20 mg/kg per 24 hr PO (not to exceed 900 mg/24 hr) in 2 equally divided doses	≥6
and With gentamicin§‖#	1.0 mg/kg IM or IV (not to exceed 80 mg) every 8 hr	2.0-2.5 mg/kg IV (not to exceed 80 mg) every 8 hr	2

*Vancomycin and gentamicin doses must be modified appropriately in patients with renal failure.

†IV indicates intravenously; PO, orally; and IM, intramuscularly.

‡Peak serum concentrations of vancomycin should be obtained 1 hr after infusion and should be in the range of 30 to 45 µg/ml for twice daily dosing and 20 to 35 µg/ml for four times daily dosing. Each dose should be infused over 1 hr.

§Aminoglycosides or vancomycin given on a milligram per kilogram basis will produce higher serum concentrations in obese than in lean patients.

‖Rifampin is recommended for therapy of infections due to coagulase-negative staphylococci. Its use in coagulase-positive staphylococcal infections is controversial. Rifampin increases the amount of warfarin sodium required for antithrombotic therapy.

¶Serum concentration of gentamicin should be monitored and dose should be adjusted to obtain a peak level of approximately 3 µg/ml.

#Use during initial 2 wk. See text on alternative aminoglycoside therapy for organisms resistant to gentamicin.

**First-generation cephalosporins or vancomycin should be used in penicillin-allergic patients. Cephalosporins should be avoided in patients with immediate-type hypersensitivity to penicillin and in patients infected with methicillin-resistant staphylococci.

Reproduced courtesy the ad hoc writing group of the Committee on Rheumatic Fever, Endocarditis, and Kawasaki Disease of the American Heart Association's Council on Cardiovascular Disease in the Young, Dallas Tex. (Bisno AL, Dismukes WE, et al: JAMA 261:1471, 1989.)

Prophylaxis for infective endocarditis

Cardiac conditions and procedures for which endocarditis prophylaxis is recommended are described in the adjacent box. Suggested antibiotic regimens for prophylaxis of bacterial endocarditis are listed in Table 25-14.[15,35]

Table 25-14   Recommendations for prophylaxis of endocarditis in adults*

Standard Regimen	
For dental procedures and oral or upper respiratory tract surgery	Amoxicillin 3 g PO 1 hr before, then 1.5 g 6 hr later
Special Regimens	
Parenteral regimen for high-risk patients; also for GI or GU tract procedures	Ampicillin 2 g IM or IV plus gentamicin 1.5 mg/kg† IM or IV, 30 min before; then amoxicillin 1.5 g PO 6 hr later, or repeat parenteral regimen 8 hr after initial dose
Parenteral regimen for patients allergic to penicillin	Vancomycin 1 g IV slowly over 1 hr, starting 1 hr before; add gentamicin 1.5 mg/kg IM or IV if GI or GU tract involved
Oral regimen for patients allergic to penicillin (oral and respiratory tract only)	Erythromycin ethylsuccinate 800 mg or erythromycin stearate 1 g PO 2 hr before, then half the dose 6 hr later; clindamycin can also be used, dosage 300 mg PO 1 hr before and 150 mg 6 hr later
Oral regimen for minor GI or GU tract procedures	Amoxicillin 3 g PO 1 hr before, then 1.5 g 6 hr later
Cardiac surgery, including implantation of prosthetic valves	Cefazolin 2 g IV at induction of anesthesia, repeated 8 and 16 hr later

*These regimens are empirical suggestions; no regimen has been proved effective for prevention of endocarditis; failures may occur with any regimen. These regimens are not intended to cover all clinical situations; the practitioner should evaluate safety and cost-benefit issues in each case. One or two additional doses may be given if the period of risk for bacteremia is prolonged.
†Not to exceed 80 mg

From (1) Durack DT, et al (editors): Principles and practice of infectious disease, ed 3, New York, 1990, Churchill-Livingstone Inc, p 716; (2) Med Lett Drugs Ther 31:112, 1989; and (3) American Heart Association recommendations for prevention of bacterial endocarditis, JAMA 264:299 1990.

Indications for Endocarditis Prophylaxis

Procedures

1. Oral cavity and respiratory tract
   a. All dental procedures likely to induce gingival bleeding (not simple adjustment of orthodontic appliances or shedding of deciduous teeth)
   b. Tonsillectomy or adenoidectomy
   c. Surgical procedures or biopsy involving respiratory mucosa
   d. Bronchoscopy, especially with a rigid bronchoscope*
   e. Incision and drainage of infected tissue
2. Genitourinary and gastrointestinal tracts
   a. Cystoscopy
   b. Prostatic surgery
   c. Urethral catheterization (especially in the presence of infection)
   d. Urinary tract surgery
   e. Vaginal hysterectomy
   f. Gallbladder surgery
   g. Colonic surgery
   h. Esophageal dilation
   i. Sclerotherapy for esophageal varices
   j. Colonoscopy
   k. Upper gastrointestinal tract endoscopy with biopsy
   l. Proctosigmoidoscopic therapy

Cardiac Conditions

1. Endocarditis prophylaxis recommended
   a. Prosthetic cardiac valves (including biosynthetic valves)
   b. Most congenital cardiac malformations
   c. Surgically constructed systemic-pulmonary shunts
   d. Rheumatic and other acquired valvular dysfunction
   e. Idiopathic hypertrophic subaortic stenosis
   f. Previous history of bacterial endocarditis
   g. Mitral valve prolapse with insufficiency†
   h. Pulmonic stenosis
2. Endocarditis prophylaxis not recommended
   a. Isolated secundum atrial septal defect
   b. Secundum atrial septal defect repaired without a patch 6 or more months earlier
   c. Patent ductus arteriosus ligated and divided 6 or more months earlier
   d. Postoperatively after coronary artery bypass graft surgery

Adapted from Shulman ST, et al: Circulation 70:1123A, 1984. Used with permission.
*The risk with flexible bronchoscopy is low, but the necessity for prophylaxis is not yet defined.
†Definitive data to provide guidance in management of patients with mitral valve prolapse are particularly limited. In general, such patients are clearly at low risk of development of endocarditis, but the risk-benefit ratio of prophylaxis in mitral valve prolapse is uncertain.

References

1. Akriviadis EA, Runyon BA: Utility of an algorithm in differentiating spontaneous from secondary bacterial peritonitis, Gastroenterology 98:127, 1990.

2. Armstrong D, et al: Treatment of infections in patients with the acquired immunodeficiency syndrome, Ann Intern Med 103:738, 1985.

3. Baumgartner JD, et al: Prevention of gram-negative shock and death in surgical patients by antibody to endotoxin core glycolipid, Lancet 2:59, 1985.

4. Bennet IV Jr, Beeson PB: Bacteremia: a consideration of some experimental and clinical aspects, Yale J Biol Med 26:241, 1954.

5. Bolan G, Barza M: Acute bacterial meningitis in children and adults, Med Clin North Am 69:236, 1986.

6. Boscia JA, et al: Epidemiology of bacteriuria in an elderly ambulatory population, Am J Med 80:208, 1986.

7. Bozzette SA, Sattler FR, et al: A controlled trial of early adjunctive treatment with corticosteroids for PCP in AIDS, N Engl J Med 323: 1451, 1990.

8. Carlson KJ, Mulley AG: Management of acute dysuria: a decision-analysis model of alternative strategies, Ann Intern Med 102:244, 1985.

9. Centers for Disease Control, U.S. Department of Health and Human Services: CDC guideline for handwashing and hospital environmental control, Atlanta, 1985, The Centers.

10. Centers for Disease Control, U.S. Department of Health and Human Services: CDC guideline for prevention of surgical wound infections, Atlanta, 1985, The Centers.

11. Centers for Disease Control, U.S. Department of Health and Human Services: Guidelines for prophylaxis against Pneumocystis carinii pneumonia for persons infected with human immunodeficiency virus, MMWR 38(S-5):1, 1989.

12. Chang JC: Neoplastic fever; a proposal for diagnosis, Arch Intern Med 149:1728, 1989.

13. Cohen SH, Jordan GW: Clinical use of antimicrobial susceptibility data, Hosp Physician 88:11, 1986.

14. Cordonnier C, et al: Legionnaire's disease and hairy-cell leukemia: an unfortuitous association? Arch Intern Med 144:2373, 1984.

15. Durack DT, Mandell GL, et al (editors): Principles and practice of infectious disease, ed 3, New York, 1990, Churchill Livingstone Inc, p 716.

16. Felisart J, et al: Cefotaxime is more effective than ampicillin-tobramycin in cirrhotics with severe infections, Hepatology 5:457, 1985.

17. Fischinger PJ: Acquired immune deficiency syndrome: the causative agent and the evolving perspective, Curr Probl Cancer 9(1):4, 1985.

18. Flaherty JP, et al: Multicenter, randomized trial of ciprofloxacin plus azlocillin versus ceftazidime plus amikacin for empiric treatment of febrile neutropenic patients, Am J Med 87(suppl 5A):278S, 1989.

19. Garcia-Tsao G, Conn HO, Lerner R: The diagnosis of bacterial peritonitis: comparison of pH, lactate concentration, and leukocyte count, Hepatology 5:91, 1985.

20. Goldenberg DL, Reed JI: Bacterial arthritis, N Engl J Med 312:764, 1985.

21. Gordon JJ, Harter DH, Phair JP: Meningitis due to Staphylococcus aureus, Am J Med 78:965, 1985.

22. Guyton BJ, Achord JL: The rapid determination of ascitic fluid L-lactate for the diagnosis of spontaneous bacterial peritonitis, Am J Gastroenterol 78:231, 1983.

23. Henderson DK, Gerberding JL: Prophylactic zidovudine after occupational exposure to the human immunodeficiency virus: an interim analysis, J Infect Dis 160:321, 1989.

24. Hoefs JC, Runyon BA: Spontaneous bacterial peritonitis. DM 31:9, 1985.

25. Hook EW, Hooton TM: Microbiologic evaluation of cutaneous cellulitis in adults, Arch Intern Med 146:295, 1986.

26. Kiehn TE, et al: Infections caused by *Mycobacterium avium* complex in immuno-compromised patients: diagnosis by blood culture and fecal examination, antimicrobial susceptibility tests, and morphological and seroagglutination characteristics, J Clin Microbiol 21:168, 1985.

27. Komaroff AL: Acute dysuria in women, N Engl J Med 310:368, 1984.

28. Komaroff AL: Urinalysis and urine culture in women with dysuria, Ann Intern Med 104:212, 1986.

29. Larson EB, Featherstone HJ: Fever of unknown origin: diagnosis and follow-up of 105 cases, 1970-1980, Medicine 61:269, 1982.

30. Levitz R, Quintiliani R: Trimethoprim-sulfamethoxazole for bacterial mengenitis, Ann Intern Med 100:881, 1984.

31. Lipsky BA: Urinary tract infections in man. Epidemiology, pathophysiology, diagnosis, and treatment, Ann Intern Med 110:138, 1989.

32. Magnussen CR: Skin and soft tissue infections. In Reese RE, Douglas RG (editors): A practical approach to infectious diseases, Boston, 1983, Little Brown & Co.

33. Martin RP, et al: Clinical utility of two-dimensional echocardiography in infective endocarditis, Am J Cardiol 46:379, 1980.

34. McCue JD: Evaluation and management of vaginitis: an update for primary care physicians, Arch Intern Med 149:565, 1989.

35. Parker MM, et al: Profound but reversible myocardial depression in patients with septic shock, Ann Intern Med 100:483, 1984.

36. Petersdorf RG, Wallace JF: Fever of unknown origin. In Barondess JA (editor): Diagnostic approaches to presenting syndromes, Baltimore, 1971, The Williams & Wilkins Co.

37. Polk RE: Drug-drug interactions with ciprofloxacin and other fluoroquinolones, Am J Med 87(suppl 5A):76, 1989.

38. Prevention of bacterial endocarditis, Med Lett Drugs Ther 31:112, 1989.

39. Recommendations for preventing transmission of infection with human T-lymphotropic virus type III/lymphadenopathy-associated virus in the work place, MMWR 34:45, 1985.

40. Redfield RR, Markham PD, Solahuddin SZ: Heterosexually acquired HTLV-III/LAV disease (AIDS-related complex with AIDS), JAMA 254:2094, 1985.

41. Reese RE: Bacteremias and sepsis. In Reese RE, Douglas RG Jr (editors): A practical approach to infectious diseases, Boston, 1983, Little Brown & Co.

42. Revision of the case definition of acquired immunodeficiency syndrome for national reporting: United States, MMWR 34:373, 1985.

43. Roberts NJ Jr: Joint infections. In Reese RE, Douglas RG Jr (editors): A practical approach to infectious diseases, Boston, 1983, Little Brown & Co.

44. Robbins MJ, et al: Influence of vegetation size on clinical outcome of right-sided infective endocarditis, Am J Med 80:165, 1986.

45. Runyon BA, Hoefs JC: Ascitic fluid analysis in the differentiation of spontaneous bacterial peritonitis from gastrointestinal tract perforation into ascitic fluid, Hepatology 4:447, 1984.

46. Sangadharan MG, et al: Antibodies reactive with human T-lymphotropic retrovirus (HTLV III) in the serum of patients with AIDS, Science 224:506, 1984.

47. Savard-Fenton M, et al: Single-dose amoxicillin therapy with follow-up urine culture, Am J Med 73:808, 1982.

48. Shapiro E: Prophylaxis for bacterial meningitis, Med Clin North Am 69:269, 1985.

49. Stamm WE: Management of recurrent urinary tract infections with patient administered single dose therapy, Ann Intern Med 102:302, 1985.

50. Stapleton A, Latham RH, et al: Postcoital antimicrobial prophylaxis for recurrent urinary tract infection, JAMA 264:703, 1990.

51. Tam MR, et al: Culture-independent diagnosis of *Chlamydia trachomatis* using monoclonal antibodies, N Engl J Med 310:1146, 1984.

51a. Tunkel AR, Wispelwey B, Scheld WM: Bacterial meningitis: recent advances in pathophysiology and treatment, Ann Intern Med 112:610, 1990.

52. Van Scoy RE: Culture negative endocarditis, Mayo Clin Proc 57:149, 1982.

53. Van Voris LP, Roberts NL Jr: Central nervous system infections. In Reese RE, Douglas RG Jr (editors): A practical approach to infectious diseases, Boston, 1983, Little Brown & Co.

54. Volberding PA, et al: Vinblastine therapy for Kaposi sarcoma in the acquired immunodeficiency syndrome, Ann Intern Med 103:335, 1985.

55. Weinstein MP, Stratton CW: Multicenter collaborative evaluation of a standardized serum bactericidal test as a prognostic indicator in infective endocarditis, Am J Med 78:262, 1985.

56. Weiss SH, et al: Screening test for HTLV III (AIDS agent) antibody: specificity, sensitivity, and applications, JAMA 253:221, 1985.

57. Weiss SH, Saxinger WC, Richtman D: HTLV-III infection among health care workers, JAMA 254:2089, 1985.

58. Wilson WR, Danielson GK, Giuliani ER, Ceraci JE: Prosthetic valve endocarditis, Mayo Clin Proc 57:155, 1982.

59. Wilson WR, Giuliani ER, Geraci JE: General consideration in the diagnosis and treatment of infective endocarditis, Mayo Clin Proc 57:81, 1982.

60. Wong DH, et al: Clinical implications of large vegetations in infectious endocarditis, Arch Intern Med 143:1874, 1983.

Nephrology

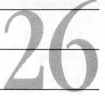

RENAL FAILURE
James Grant

Classification

1. Prenatal: secondary to decreased renal perfusion, volume contraction, CHF, and altered renal hemodynamics
2. Renal: associated with acute or chronic intrinsic renal disease (e.g., ATN, glomerulonephritis, vasculitis, interstitial disease)
3. Postrenal: obstructive uropathy (e.g., prostatic hypertrophy, bilateral ureteral obstruction, neurogenic bladder)

Prerenal failure

Etiology

1. Volume deficits: including extrarenal losses (e.g., hemorrhage, GI bleeding, inadequate fluid intake), third-spacing, and urinary losses secondary to diuretics or osmotically obligatory urine volumes
2. Low output states: including CHF, dysrhythmias, and pericardial disease
3. Decreased systemic vascular resistance as seen in sepsis, pancreatitis, pharmacologic resistance circuit unloaders, and cirrhosis
4. Decreased oncotic vascular volume support: nephrosis, severe catabolic states
5. Reversible prerenal insufficiency secondary to decreased renal blood flow can be seen with the use of prostaglandin inhibitors (NSAIDs)
   Additional effects include
   Sodium retention
   Hyperkalemia
   Blunting of diuretic response to furosemide
   These reversible changes not to be confused with the occasional development of allergic interstitial nephritis with NSAIDs after prolonged use
6. Inhibition of intrinsic renal vascular modulation (autoregulation) with ACE inhibitors; occasionally acute renal failure can develop in patients

457

with renal artery stenosis; this effect on efferent arteriolar tone has been used to diagnose renal artery stenosis employing radioisotopic renographic measurements (captopril renogram)

7. Hepatorenal syndrome: labeled "prerenal" because when the involved kidney is transplanted to a normal host it functions normally; the syndrome is associated with severe oliguria, a falling GFR with rising creatinine, but a persistently low urinary sodium level

Characteristics of prerenal failure

1. Decreased renal perfusion results in increased sodium and water reabsorption at the proximal tubule (in an attempt to reexpand circulating blood volume)
   a. Oliguria
   b. Decreased urine sodium (<20 mEq/L)
2. Serum sodium that reflects relative sodium-water losses and/or gains
3. Decreased distal tubular flow results in increased urea absorption and decreased K^+ secretion, but marginal effect on creatinine
   a. BUN/Cr increased ($>15:1$)
   b. U/P Cr >40
   c. FE_{Na} is considered the most sensitive differentiation test ($< 1 =$ prerenal; $> 1 =$ renal)
4. Increased renal "threshold" for plasma ions
   a. Increased HCO_3^- absorption: contraction alkalosis
   b. Increased uric acid absorption: hyperuricemia
5. Increased ADH secretion: increased water absorption; urine osmolarity greater than serum osmolarity
6. Hyponatremia with free water loading until volume is restored
7. Increased BUN, with blood in the GI tract

Treatment

1. Appropriate volume challenge in contracted patients
2. Maximize cardiac function
3. Discontinue offending drugs

Intrinsic renal failure

Etiology

1. Acute tubular necrosis
2. Acute allergic interstitial nephritis
3. Acute glomerular syndromes
4. Drug-induced nephrotoxicity
5. Chronic (sclerotic) established renal disease
6. Vascular disorders
7. Myeloma kidney
8. Functional tubular disorders
9. Atheromatous emboli

Characteristics of specific causes of intrinsic renal failure

1. Acute tubular necrosis (ATN) is the most common form of acute renal failure in the hospital setting
   a. Precipitating factors

   (1) Severe and protracted decrease in renal perfusion: prolonged prerenal failure, shock, hypovolemia, sepsis and low-output states, CABG surgery, aortic aneurysm repair
   (2) Pigment toxicity: transfusion reactions, rhabdomyolysis (seizures, crush injury), surgery in hyperbilirubinemic states
   (3) Aminoglycoside antibiotics
   (4) Radiographic dyes (arteriography, CT scan, pyelography)[2]
   b. Diagnostic features
   (1) Serial increases in creatinine and BUN vary with catabolic rate and protein intake
   (2) Oliguria or nonoliguria, but relatively fixed outputs
   (3) Variable response to high dose furosemide, may convert oliguria to nonoliguria but does not change the underlying lesion
   (4) Pulmonary vascular congestion and hyperkalemia represent the most important parameters to follow; PA catheter may be necessary to monitor fluid status
   (5) Urine sodium is high, generally >30
   (6) Urine osmolarity is less than 350 mOsm/kg and generally fixed (±300 mOsm/kg)
   (7) Urine creatinine is low in relation to urine volume, leading to a U/P creatinine less than 20
   (8) Fractional excretion of sodium[13] (FE_{Na}) is greater than 1 (see Table 26-1)
   (9) Urine sediment contains "muddy-brown" renal tubular casts
   (10) Myoglobinuria and serum CPK elevations in rhabdomyolysis
   (11) Polyuric phase often heralds healing
2. Acute allergic interstitial nephritis
   a. Drug-induced: β-lactams, trimethoprim/sulfamethoxazole, NSAIDs, cimetidine, rifampin, azathioprine, diuretics, anticonvulsants
   b. Differentiated from ATN by: presence of a putative drug, rash, absence of polyuric phase, eosinophils on stained urine sediment preparations, pyuria, lymphocyturia; positive gallium (Ga) scan may be helpful
   c. Biopsy may be necessary for diagnosis
   d. Course of the disease may be shortened by steroids
3. Acute glomerular syndromes
   a. Acute glomerulonephritis (GN)
   (1) Etiology
      (a) Prototypically poststreptococcal glomerulonephritis (PSGN)
         • Occurs 3-4 wk after a streptococcal infection; pharyngitis or impetigo common
         • Manifested by hypertension, gross or microscopic hematuria, periorbital edema
         • Positive throat culture
         • Lab results: 1-3 g/24 hr protein excretion, low C3, elevated antibodies to streptococcal antigens (ASLO, antihyaluronidase, ANADase), low urinary sodium, active urinary sediment including RBC casts

- Progressive resolution is usually the case, with normalization of C3 and clearing of urinary findings
- Proteinuria can last 6-8 mo
- Microhematuria can last 1-2 yr

(b) Other glomerular and systemic diseases may present as acute, nonprogressive, or slowly progressive glomerulonephritis although they can present with a rapidly progressive course; three important examples are:

- Mesangiocapillary GN (hypocomplementemic GN): predominant in young females, insidious onset, and persistently low complement (C3)
- Lupus nephritis with focal involvement: positive ANA, anti-ds DNA, and anti-Sm, together with elements of the total clinical complex
- IgA nephropathy (Berger's disease): usually presenting with recurrent hematuria following URIs
- Membranous nephropathy
- Systemic or localized vasculitis
- Often ANCA is positive

(2) Diagnosis post-streptococcal glomerulonephritis (PSGN) possible on clinical grounds

(a) Alternative diagnoses require renal biopsy

(b) Biopsy is mandatory if immunotherapy is considered

(c) Light immunofluorescence and electron microscopy are used to identify deposits (IgA, IgG, IgM, complement) and distinguish their location within the glomerulus (mesangial, subepithelial, and subendothelial)

(3) Treatment

(a) If self-limited (e.g., PSGN), treatment consists of blood pressure control and symptomatic measures

(b) With biopsy-proven diagnosis of a potentially progressive disease, immunosuppressive therapeutic measures are of value:

- Alternate day steroids in mesangiocapillary GN
- Pulse cyclophosphamide (Cytoxan) in lupus GN, Wegener's granulomatosis, systemic vasculitis
- Ponticelli regimen for membranous nephropathy

b. Rapidly progressive glomerulonephritis (RPGN)

(1) Definition: rapidly progressive renal failure, with BUN and creatinine rising incrementally over the course of days to weeks, in association with an active urinary sediment (including RBC casts); pathologically RPGN is characterized by the presence of crescents (usually over 80%) on light microscopy; it represents the fulminating end of many acute progressive glomerulonephritides

(2) Etiology

(a) PSGN, in rare cases; more likely severe RPGN in adults

(b) Associated with chronic infectious processes (infective endocarditis, abdominal sepsis, hepatitis B)

      (c) Associated with systemic vasculitis (SLE, Wegener's granulomatosis, hypersensitivity angiitis, polyarteritis)

      (d) Antiglomerular basement membrane syndromes (Goodpasture's syndrome with lung hemorrhage)

      (e) Idiopathic

    (3) Clinical manifestations

      (a) May be dominated by the systemic manifestations of the associated disorder (e.g., pulmonary findings in Wegener's granulomatosis)

      (b) Renal manifestations: hypertension, hematuria, proteinuria, active sediment (including RBC casts and broad tubular casts) indicating widespread renal damage, progressive increases in BUN and creatinine

    (4) Diagnosis: The above clinical manifestations require a renal biopsy to confirm the diagnosis and exclude unusual presentations of alternative diseases (including interstitial nephritis, ATN, and multiple myeloma)

    (5) Serological lab studies (ANA, C3, C4, ANCA [antineutrophil cytoplasmic antibody]) may support diagnosis of Wegener's granulomatosis or vasculitis

    (6) Treatment: aggressive therapy with immunosuppressive regimens is indicated

      (a) Plasmapheresis and immunosuppression in early cases of Goodpasture's syndrome

      (b) Pulse steroids or cyclophosphamide for SLE and vasculitic syndromes

  c. Nephrotic syndrome

    (1) Definition: protein excretion exceeding 3 g/24 hr, associated with edema, hypoalbuminemia, hypercoagulopathy, and hyperlipidemia, with or without the findings of acute glomerular diseases

    (2) Etiology

      (a) Children: 90% nil disease, with steroid responsiveness

      (b) Adults: idiopathic membranous nephropathy, focal sclerosis, amyloid disease, underlying malignancy, DM, drug-induced (penicillamine, gold, NSAID, captopril, anticonvulsants, probenemid, chlorpropamide), and in addition, nephrotic range proteinuria can be part of all the "acute glomerular syndromes"

4. Drug-induced nephropathy

  a. Aminoglycosides

    (1) Latent period 7-10 days; shorter with advanced age, volume depletion, previous treatment

    (2) Nonoliguric

    (3) Magnesium and potassium depletion

  b. Tetracycline

    (1) Antianabolic rise in the BUN

    (2) Significant if superimposed on a high baseline

  c. Chemotherapeutic agents

    (1) Cisplatin and mithramycin are common examples

     (2) Magnesium wasting

     (3) Avoidable with vigorous concomitant hydration

  d. Lithium

     (1) Reversible nephrogenic diabetes insipidus

     (2) ?Mild chronic interstitial nephritis

  e. Heroin abuse

     (1) Focal sclerosis

     (2) Amyloid disease in "skin poppers"

  f. Toxic obstructive nephropathies

     (1) Oxalate

       • Following ethylene glycol ingestion

       • Increased absorption with short bowel syndromes and IBD

       • Diagnostic crystals in the urine

     (2) Uric acid

       • Following lysis of hematological malignancies

       • Treated with hydration and alkalinization; occasionally anuria will require dialysis

     (3) Methotrexate

     (4) Sulfonamides

  g. Chronic tubulointerstitial nephritis

     (1) Analgesic nephropathy

       • Large cumulative doses needed

       • Variable worldwide incidence

       • Combinations of phenacetin implicated

       • Associated with papillary necrosis

     (2) Lead

       • Occupational exposure or "moonshine" whiskey preparation

       • Hyperuricemia with actual gout

  h. Drug-induced nephrotic syndromes

     (1) Penicillamine

     (2) Gold

     (3) Captopril (rare)

5. Chronic (sclerotic) established renal disease

  a. Etiology

     (1) May represent the later stages of any acute glomerulonephritis that has progressed to a predominantly sclerotic or "burned out" phase

     (2) Nephrosclerosis secondary to longstanding hypertension

     (3) Diabetic glomerulosclerosis

       (a) Usually follows a 12-15 yr latent period

       (b) More common in type I DM but more cases of type II are seen because of its increased prevalence

       (c) Preceded by proteinuria

       (d) There is parallel development of retinopathy

     (4) Hereditary renal disease

       (a) Polycystic kidney disease

       (b) Alport's syndrome (initially a hematuric syndrome)

  b. Diagnostic characteristics of renal failure

     (1) Generally small renal outlines on ultrasound

      (2) Stable (over short periods) BUN and creatinine

      (3) Urine volumes that remain greater than 1 L until end stage

      (4) Potassium levels that remain normal with stable urine volumes despite substantial elevations of creatinine

      (5) Evidence of retained uremic poisons (see p. 468)

      (6) Hypertension frequently present

      (7) Evidence of osteodystrophy

      (8) Metabolic acidosis, non-gap initially due to decreased NH_3 production, developing into mixed non–anion-gap and anion-gap acidosis as the GFR falls

  c. Treatment

      (1) Before dialysis is necessary

          (a) Low-protein diet (40 g/day) may prolong remaining renal life

          (b) Avoid dehydration with overuse of diuretics

          (c) Strict control of hypertension; emphasis should be on vasoactive drugs with judicious diuretic use

          (d) Adjust drug doses to correct for prolonged half-lives (particularly digoxin and aminoglycosides)

          (e) Start PO_4^{-3} binder and 1,25 dihydrocholecalciferol (Rocaltrol) therapy when serum calcium and phosphorus levels become abnormal

          (f) Consider starting erythropoietin before dialysis

          (g) Consider using ACE inhibitors to reduce glomerular hyperfiltration

      (2) Initiation of dialysis

          (a) Urgent indications: pericarditis, neuropathy, and neuromuscular abnormalities (asterixis, CHF, hyperkalemia, seizures)

          (b) Judgmental indications: creatinine clearance below 10-15 ml/min; progressive anorexia, weight loss, reversal of sleep pattern, pruritus, uncontrolled fluid gains with hypertension and signs of congestive failure

6. Acute or chronic renal failure secondary to vascular disorders

  a. Atheromatous emboli

      (1) Most commonly seen following aortic catheterization, but can occur spontaneously

      (2) Characteristic livedo reticularis pattern seen in the lower extremities

      (3) Likely acute and progressive

  b. Major renal vascular occlusive disease

      (1) Associated with renal vascular hypertension

      (2) Bruits likely to be present

      (3) Susceptibility to acute renal failure with captopril

      (4) Arteriography needed for definitive diagnosis

      (5) In selected cases, vascular repair or percutaneous angioplasty has slowed the progressive course

  c. Disseminated coagulopathy with acute renal failure

      (1) Hemolytic/uremic syndrome

      (2) Thrombotic thrombocytopenic purpura

(3) Malignant hypertension

   d. Nephrosclerosis secondary to chronic essential hypertension: characteristic benign sediment and minimum proteinuria

7. Myeloma of the kidney
   a. Tubular light chain deposition with acute renal failure
   b. Monoclonal light chains in the urine
   c. Must be differentiated from hypercalcemic nephropathy, ATN, and amyloid disease

8. Functional tubular disorders (when to suspect renal tubular acidosis):
   a. Electrolyte picture on non-anion gap acidosis without renal insufficiency and in the absence of respiratory alkalosis
   b. Hypokalemia or hyperkalemia depending on the nature of the tubular defect
   c. Finding unexplained osteomalacia even to the point of acute muscle weakness (Type I RTA)
   d. Finding nephrocalcinosis
   e. In paraproteinemic states
   f. After implicatable drug administration (amphotericin)
   g. Finding proximal amino acid and glucose urinary losses
   h. Urine pH and P_{CO_2}
      (1) pH never below 6 in distal RTA; HCO_3^- wasting in proximal RTA
      (2) Urinary P_{CO_2} low in distal RTA when HCO_3^- is given

Diagnostic methods

1. Determine if renal failure is acute or chronic (Tables 26-1 and 26-2)
   a. Rate of rise in BUN and creatinine
   b. Urine/plasma creatinine ratios
   c. Renal size by ultrasonography
   d. Historical lab data if available
   e. Anemia can occur early in renal failure and correlates poorly with the duration of the disease

2. Clinical correlates from history and physical exam
   a. Purpura: Henoch-Schoenlein purpura, vasculitis
   b. Pulmonary disease: Wegener's granulomatosis, Goodpasture's syndrome, SLE, vasculitis
   c. Connective tissue abnormalities: SLE, scleroderma, mixed connective tissue disease (MCTD)
   d. Heart murmur: SBE with glomerulonephritis
   e. Fever and abdominal pain: consider abdominal sepsis with glomerulonephritis
   f. Drug abuse: focal sclerosis, amyloidosis
   g. Amyloidosis: chronic infection, enteritis, rheumatoid arthritis
   h. Diabetes: glomerulosclerosis, pyelonephritis, papillary necrosis
   i. Sickle cell disease: papillary necrosis, type IV RTA
   j. Chemotherapy: lysis with uric acid nephropathy
   k. Hearing loss: Alport's syndrome
   l. AIDS nephropathy: life-style

TABLE 26-1 Serum and radiographic abnormalities in renal failure

	Prerenal	Postrenal (Acute)	Intrinsic Renal (Acute)	Intrinsic Renal (Chronic)
BUN	$\uparrow$ 10:1 > Cr	$\uparrow$ 20-40/day	$\uparrow$ 20-40/day	Stable, $\uparrow$ varies with protein intake
Serum creatinine	N/Moderate $\uparrow$	$\uparrow$ 2-4/day	$\uparrow$ 2-4/day	Stable $\uparrow$ (production = excretion)
Serum potassium	N/Moderate $\uparrow$	$\uparrow$ varies with urine volume	$\uparrow$ $\uparrow$ (particularly when patient is oliguric) $\uparrow$ $\uparrow$ with rhabdomyolysis	Normal until endstage, unless tubular dysfunction (type IV RTA)
Serum phosphorus	N/Moderate $\uparrow$	Moderate $\uparrow$ $\uparrow$ $\uparrow$ with rhabdomyolysis	$\uparrow$ Poor correlation with duration of renal disease	Becomes significantly elevated when serum creatinine surpasses 3 mg/100 ml
Serum calcium	N	N/$\downarrow$ with PO_4^{-3} retention	$\downarrow$ (poor correlation with duration of renal failure)	Usually $\downarrow$
Renal size By ultrasound	N/$\uparrow$	$\uparrow$ and dilated calyces	N/$\uparrow$	$\downarrow$ and with $\uparrow$ echogenicity
FE_{Na}*	<1	<1 $\rightarrow$ >1	>1	>1

KEY: $\uparrow$, increase; $\downarrow$, decrease; N, normal; $\uparrow$ $\uparrow$, large increase; U, urine; P, plasma; Na, sodium; Cr, creatinine

*$FE_{Na} = \dfrac{U_{Na}/P_{Na}}{U_{Cr}/P_{Cr}} \times 100$.

Table 26-2 Urine abnormalities in renal failure

	Prerenal	Postrenal (Acute)	Intrinsic Renal (Acute)	Intrinsic Renal (Chronic)
Urine volume	↓	Absent-to-wide fluctuation	Oliguric or nonoliguric	1000 ml + until end stage
Urine creatinine	↑ (U/P Cr >40)	↓ (U/P Cr >20)	↓ (U/P Cr <20)	↓ (U/P Cr <20)
Osmolarity	↑ (>400 mOsm/kg)	(<350 mOsm/kg)	(<350 mOsm/kg)	(<350 mOsm/kg)
Degree of proteinuria	Minimum	Absent	Varies with etiology of renal failure: Modest with ATN Nephrotic range common with acute glomerulopathies, usually < 2 g/24 hr with interstitial disease*	Varies with etiology of renal disease (from 1-2 g/day to nephrotic range)
Urine sediment	Negative, or occasional hyaline cast	Negative or hematuria with stones or papillary necrosis Pyuria with infectious prostatic disease	ATN: muddy brown Interstitial nephritis: lymphocytes, eosinophils (in stained preparations), and WBC casts RPGN: RBC casts Nephrosis: oval fat bodies	Broad casts with variable renal "residual" acute findings

KEY: ↑, increased; ↓, decreased; U/P, urine/plasma; Clearance = $\dfrac{\text{Urine concentration} \times \text{Urine volume}}{\text{Plasma concentration}}$; Cr, creatinine

*Except NSAID-induced allergic interstitial nephritis with concomitant "nil disease."

3. Diagnostic supports from serum analysis
   a. Consider SLE if positive ANA, along with positive anti-Sm and anti-ds DNA
   b. C3: if decreased, suspect infectious etiology (post-streptococcal infection, infective endocarditis, visceral sepsis, primary mesangiocapillary disease)
   c. C4: decreased in SLE
   d. Hepatitis B$_S$Ag positive: consider nephritis with vasculitis, membranous nephropathy
   e. Cryoglobulins present: consider SLE, systemic vasculitis, postinfectious streptococcal infection, visceral sepsis, myeloma, Waldenstrom's macroglobulinemia, hepatitis B infection, mixed essential cryoglobulinemia
   f. Abnormal protein immunoelectrophoresis: myeloma
   g. Abnormal immunoelectrophoresis: myeloma, IgA nephropathy (Berger's disease), Waldenstrom's macroglobulinemia
   h. Rheumatoid factor positive: polyarteritis, connective tissue disease
   i. ASLO titer: post-streptococcal (acute) glomerulonephritis
4. Major diagnoses established by renal biopsy
   a. Differential diagnosis of the nephrotic syndrome: all primary and secondary glomerulopathies, amyloid, focal sclerosis, membranous glomerulopathy, or diabetes (if not otherwise established)
   b. Separation of lupus vasculitis from other vasculitis (employing EM deposit pattern) and of lupus membranous from idiopathic membranous
   c. Confirmation of hereditary nephropathies on the basis of their ultrastructure
   d. Diagnosis of RPGN (crescenteric) with the finding of extracapillary crescent formation
   e. Separation of allergic interstitial nephritis from ATN in cases of prolonged acute renal failure
   f. Separation of the primary glomerulonephritis syndromes: poststreptococcal infection, mesangiocapillary types 1-4, membranous, focal vs diffuse, IgG or IgA (done by using immunofluorescence and electron microscopy to visualize varying deposit patterns)
   g. Finding focal segmental necrosis to suggest an underlying vasculitis not otherwise apparent

Postrenal failure

1. Etiology
   a. Urethral obstruction (prostatic hypertrophy, urethral stricture)
   b. Bladder calculi or neoplasms
   c. Pelvic or retroperitoneal neoplasms
   d. Bilateral ureteral obstruction (neoplasm, calculi)
   e. Retroperitoneal fibrosis
2. Diagnosis
   a. History of dysuria
   b. Evidence of prostatic hypertrophy in men and pelvic pathology in women
   c. Catheterization after voiding to assess residual volume
   d. Ultrasound of abdomen, pelvis, and kidney

3. Therapy: catheter drainage, ureteral stents, percutaneous nephrostomy following urological consultation

Effects of retained uremic toxins and the uremic milieu

1. General
   a. Anorexia, early satiety
   b. Nausea and vomiting
   c. Pruritus
   d. Fatigue, weakness
2. Cardiovascular
   a. Cardiomyopathy: with chronic fluid overload; concentric hypertrophy is common
   b. Pericarditis: the clinical presentation varies from small pericardial effusions to acute pericarditis with tamponade
   c. Accelerated atherogenesis: elevated triglycerides, decreased HDL
   d. Hypertension: multifactorial (sodium retention, disturbances of renin-angiotension axis)
3. CNS: Abnormalities range from neuromuscular irritability (e.g., "restless legs") to asterixis and coma (metabolic encephalopathy)
4. Endocrine
   a. Abnormal glucose metabolism secondary to
      (1) Increased insulin resistance
      (2) Prolonged insulin half-life
      (3) Decreased gluconeogenesis with lower amino acid pool
      (4) Increased renal threshold for glucose
   b. Decreased T_4: secondary to decreased protein binding; normal free T_4
5. Hematopoietic
   a. Anemia: usually normochromic, normocytic; multifactorial:
      (1) Chronically depressed erythropoietin levels
      (2) Hemolysis
      (3) Blood loss
      (4) Folate deficiency
   Epoetin alfa, a recombinant human erythropoietin, is effective for treating anemia of chronic renal failure; hypertension is a potential serious adverse effect
   b. Iron overload from transfusions
   c. Coagulopathy
      (1) Platelet count is normal, but thromboasthenia is present with decreased platelet aggregation and adhesiveness
      (2) Prolonged bleeding time improved with DDAVP or cryoprecipitate
6. Gastrointestinal
   a. Increased incidence of duodenitis (increased gastrin levels)
   b. Increased incidence of angiodysplasia of stomach and proximal intestine[3]
   c. Autonomic neuropathy in diabetics

7. Divalent ion disturbances
   a. Increased PTH: measurement is complicated by inactive fragments present in the assay; the midportion the C-terminal or N-terminal is most reflective of the active compound
   b. Decreased production of calcitriol
   c. High phosphorus, low calcium, and bone disease: osteitis fibrosa cystica, osteomalacia
   d. Retained aluminum: from prolonged phosphorus binder therapy or dialysate levels; it can lead to bone disease and CNS abnormalities
8. Miscellaneous
   a. Trace metal deficiency: zinc-hypogeusia
   b. Increased incidence of carpal tunnel syndrome: amyloid deposits
   c. Acquired cystic degeneration in remnant kidneys with hemorrhage and rarely neoplastic transformation
   d. Renal oxalate deposition

Indications for dialysis in acute or chronic renal failure

1. Progressive metabolic encephalopathy
2. Uncontrolled hyperkalemia
3. Pericarditis
4. Intractable fluid overload
5. BUN/Creatinine levels arbitary; but it is generally advisable to keep BUN <100 mg/dl

Considerations in evaluating the patient on chronic hemodialysis

1. Fluid overload caused by excessive interdialytic weight gain
2. Acute hyperkalemia
3. Pericarditis with tamponade
4. Spontaneous hypoglycemia
5. Hyperosmolarity and hyperkalemia (frequent in diabetics)
6. Infection and sepsis (vascular access site, infective endocarditis)
7. Subdural hematoma secondary to heparin use during dialysis
8. Seizures secondary to osmotic shifts produced by dialysis
9. Dysrhythmias caused by electrolyte shifts
10. GI bleeding secondary to coagulopathy, duodenitis, angiodysplasia
11. Hypercalcemia caused by excessive vitamin D replacement
12. Bone fractures secondary to osteodystrophy
13. Dementia possibly caused by elevated CNS aluminum concentrations
14. Rupture of a berry or aortic aneurysm in patients with polycystic kidneys
15. Higher incidence of pancreatitis, diverticular disease, carpal tunnel syndrome
16. Psychosocial disturbances (depression, loss of independence, denial)
17. Hepatitis and carrier state

26.2 **DISORDERS OF SODIUM HOMEOSTASIS**

Hyponatremia[1,6,7,10]

Definition: plasma sodium concentration <134 mEq/L
1. Etiology and classification
    a. Hypotonic hyponatremia
        (1) Isovolemic
            (a) SIADH
            (b) Water intoxication (e.g., schizophrenic patients)
            (c) Renal failure
            (d) Reset osmostat (e.g., chronic active TB, carcinomatosis)
            (e) Glucocorticoid deficiency (hypopituitarism)
            (f) Hypothyroidism
            (g) Thiazide diuretics, NSAIDs
        (2) Hypovolemic
            (a) Renal losses (diuretics, partial urinary tract obstruction, salt-losing renal disease)
            (b) Extrarenal losses: GI (vomiting, diarrhea), extensive burns, third spacing (peritonitis, pancreatitis)
            (c) Adrenal insufficiency
        (3) Hypervolemic
            (a) CHF
            (b) Nephrosis
            (c) Cirrhosis
    b. Isotonic hyponatremia (normal serum osmolality)
        (1) Pseudohyponatremia (increased serum lipids and serum proteins)
        (2) Isotonic infusion (e.g., glucose, mannitol)
    c. Hypertonic hyponatremia (increased serum osmolality)
        (1) Hyperglycemia: each 100 ml/dl increment in blood sugar above normal decreases plasma sodium concentration by 1.6 mEq/L[8]
        (2) Hypertonic infusions (e.g., glucose, mannitol)
3. Clinical manifestations of hyponatremia vary with the degree of hyponatremia and the rapidity of onset
    a. Moderate hyponatremia or gradual onset: confusion, muscle cramps, lethargy, anorexia, nausea
    b. Severe hyponatremia or rapid onset: seizures, coma
4. Diagnostic approach: refer to Fig. 26-1
5. Management
    a. Isovolemic hyponatremia
        (1) SIADH: fluid restriction (refer to Section 22.6)
        (2) Acute symptomatic water intoxication: hypertonic 3% or 5% saline infusion; give 200-500 ml slowly, followed by fluid restriction to 750 ml/day for 24-48 hr
        (3) Generally the serum sodium should be corrected only halfway to normal in the initial 24 hr to prevent complications from rapid correction (cerebral edema, pontine myelinolysis, seizures)

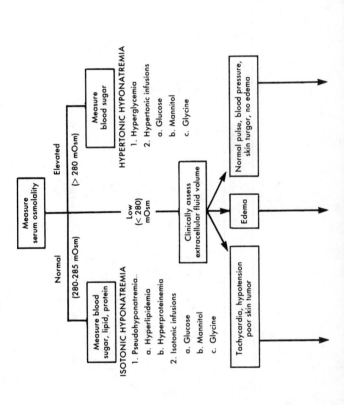

Continued.

Figure 26-1
For legend see p. 472.
For legend see p. 472.

Hypovolemic hypotonic hyponatremia

Causes	BUN/Creat	Uric acid	Urinary Osm.	(Na)
GI losses	↑↑/↑	↑	↑↑	↓↓
Skin losses	↑↑/↑	↑	↑↑	↓↓
Lung losses	↑↑/↑	↑	↑↑	↓↓
Third space	↑↑/↑	↑	↑↑	↓↓
Renal losses				
Diuretics	↑↑/↑	↑	ISO	↑
Renal damage	↑↑/↑↑	↑	ISO	↑
Partial urinary tract obstruction	↑↑/↑	↑	ISO	(↓) ↑
Adrenal insufficiency	↑↑/↑	↑	↑	↑

Hypervolemic hypotonic hyponatremia

Causes	BUN/Creat	Uric acid	Urinary Osm.	(Na)
CHF	↑↑/↑	↑	↑	↓
Liver damage	↑↑/↑	↑	↑	↓
Nephrosis	↑↑/↑ (↑↑/↑↑)	↑	↓	(ISO↑)

Isovolemic hypotonic hyponatremia

Causes	BUN/Creat	Uric acid	Urinary Osm.	(Na)
H₂O intoxication	↓/↓	↓	↑,(↓)	↓
Renal failure	↑↑/↑↑	↑	ISO	↑
K⁺ loss	↑/↑(N)	↑	↑	↑
SIADH	↓/↓	↓↓	↑	↑
Reset osmostat	N	N	V	V

Figure 26-1, cont'd

Diagnostic approach to hyponatremia. ↑, Increases; ↓, decreases; N, normal; V, variable. (From Narins RG, et al: Am J Med 72:496, 1982.)

b. Hypovolemic hyponatremia: 0.9% saline infusion

NOTE: In symptomatic patients with hyponatremia an increase in the serum sodium concentration of 2 mEq/L/hr to a level of 120-130 mEq/L is considered adequate by most experts[9]; however, less rapid correction may be indicated in patients with severe hyponatremia

c. Hypervolemic hyponatremia: sodium and water restriction

NOTE: The combination of captopril and furosemide is effective in patients with hyponatremia secondary to CHF

Hypernatremia[1,7,10]

1. Definition: plasma sodium concentration >144 mEq/L
2. Etiology and classification
   a. Isovolemic (decreased total body water [TBW], normal total body sodium [TBNa] and extracellular fluid [ECF])
      (1) Diabetes insipidus (neurogenic and nephrogenic)
      (2) Skin loss (hyperthermia), iatrogenic, reset osmostat
   b. Hypervolemic (increased TBW, markedly increased TBNa and ECF)
      (1) Iatrogenic (administration of hypernatremic solutions)
      (2) Mineralocorticoid excess (Conn's syndrome, Cushing's syndrome)
      (3) Salt ingestion
   c. Hypovolemic: loss of H_2O and Na^+ (H_2O loss >Na^+)
      (1) Renal losses (e.g., diuretics, glycosuria)
      (2) GI, respiratory, skin losses
      (3) Adrenal deficiencies
3. Clinical manifestations vary with degree of hypernatremia and rapidity of onset; they range from confusion and lethargy to seizures and coma
4. Diagnostic approach (refer to Fig. 26-2)
5. Management
   a. Isovolemic hypernatremia
      (1) Fluid replacement with D_5W
         (a) Correct only half of estimated volume deficit in initial 24 hr
         (b) The rate of correction of serum sodium should not exceed 1 mEq/L/hr in acute hypernatremia, 0.5 mEq/L/hr in chronic hypernatremia
      (2) Water deficit in liters = $0.6 \times$ Body weight (kg) $\times \left(\dfrac{\text{Measured serum sodium}}{\text{Normal serum sodium}} - 1 \right)$
   b. Hypovolemic hypernatremia
      (1) Fluid replacement with hypotonic saline
      (2) The rate of correction of plasma osmolarity should not exceed 2 mOsm/kg/hr
   c. Hypervolemic hypernatremia: fluid replacement with D_5W (to correct hypertonicity) is instituted following use of loop diuretics (to increase sodium excretion)

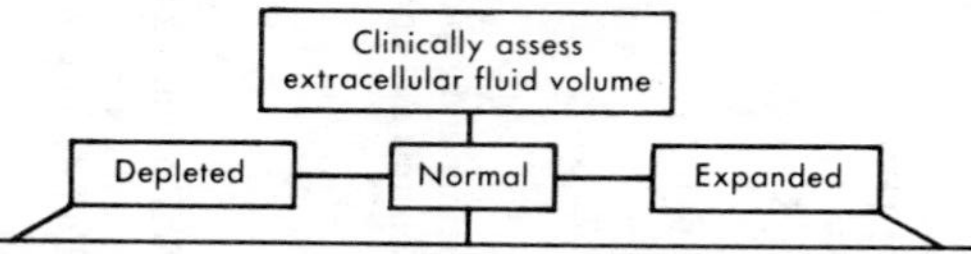

Clinically assess extracellular fluid volume → Depleted | Normal | Expanded

	Hypovolemic hypernatremia — Loss of water + Na (H_2O loss > Na) [Depleted]			Isovolemic hypernatremia — Loss of water [Normal]			Hypervolemic hypernatremia — Gain water + Na (Na gain > H_2O) [Expanded]		

Hypovolemic hypernatremia — Loss of water + Na (H_2O loss > Na)

Causes	BUN/Creat	Urinary (Na)	Urinary Osm
Renal			
Diuretics	↑↑/↑	↑	↓
Glycosuria	↑/N,↑	↑	↓
Urea diuresis	↑↑/N,↑	↑	↓
Acute/chronic renal failure	↑↑/↑	↑	↓
Partial obstruction	↑↑/↑↑	↑	↑
Adrenal			
Congenital or acquired deficiencies	↑↑/↑	↑	±↑
GI losses	↑↑/↑	↓	↑
Respiratory losses	↑↑/↑	↓	↑
Skin losses	↑↑/↑	↓	↑

Isovolemic hypernatremia — Loss of water

Causes	BUN/Creat	Urinary (Na)	Urinary Osm
Diabetes insipidus			
Central	↑/N	N	↓
Nephrogenic	↑/N	N	↓
Reset osmostat	N/N	N	↑
Skin loss	↑/N	N→↑	↑
Iatrogenic	N/N	V	↑

Hypervolemic hypernatremia — Gain water + Na (Na gain > H_2O)

Causes	BUN/Creat	Urinary (Na)	Urinary Osm
Iatrogenic	V	↑,(V)	>
Mineralocorticoid excess	V	↑	>
First-degree aldosteronism	N	N	>
Cushing's syndrome	N	N	>
Congenital adrenal hyperplasia	N	N	>
Exogenous	N	N	>

Figure 26-2

Diagnostic approach to hypernatremia. ↑, Increases; ↓, decreases; N, normal; V, variable. (From Narins RG, et al: Am J Med 72:496, 1982.)

26.3 **DISORDERS OF POTASSIUM HOMEOSTASIS**

Hypokalemia[1,4,10]

1. Definition: plasma potassium concentration <3.3 mEq/L
2. Etiology and classification
   a. Cellular shift (redistribution) and undetermined mechanisms
      (1) Alkalosis (each 0.1 increase in pH decreases serum potassium by 0.4-0.6 mEq/L)
      (2) Insulin administration
      (3) Vitamin B_{12} therapy for megaloblastic anemias, acute leukemias
      (4) Hypokalemic periodic paralysis: rare familial disorder manifested by recurrent attacks of flaccid paralysis and hypokalemia
      (5) Beta adrenergic agonists (e.g., terbutaline)
      (6) Barium poisoning, toluene intoxication
      (7) Correction of digoxin intoxication with digoxin antibody fragments (Digibind)
   b. Increased renal excretion
      (1) Drugs
         (a) Diuretics, including carbonic anhydrase inhibitors (e.g., acetazolamide)
         (b) Amphotericin B
         (c) High-dose sodium penicillin or carbenicillin
         (d) Cisplatin
         (e) Aminoglycosides
         (f) Corticosteroids
      (2) Renal tubular acidosis (RTA): distal (Type I) or proximal (Type II)
      (3) DKA, ureteroenterostomy
      (4) Magnesium deficiency
      (5) Postobstruction diuresis, diuretic phase of ATN
      (6) Osmotic diuresis (e.g., mannitol)
      (7) Bartter's syndrome: hyperplasia of JG cells leading to increased renin and aldosterone, metabolic alkalosis, hypokalemia, muscle weakness, and tetany (seen in young adults)
      (8) Interstitial nephritis
      (9) Increased mineralocorticoid activity (primary or secondary aldosteronism), Cushing's syndrome
      (10) Chronic metabolic alkalosis from loss of gastric fluid (increased renal potassium secretion)
   c. GI loss
      (1) Vomiting, nasogastric suction
      (2) Diarrhea
      (3) Laxative abuse
      (4) Villous adenoma
      (5) Fistulae
   d. Inadequate dietary intake (e.g., anorexia nervosa)
   e. Cutaneous loss (excessive sweating)

6. Clinical manifestations
   a. Depending on the level of hypokalemia and the rate of decrease, manifestations range from mild muscle weakness to overt paralysis (including respiratory paralysis) and rhabdomyolysis
   b. Atrial and ventricular dysrhythmias may develop (particularly in patients receiving digitalis); ventricular dysrhythmias are one of the leading causes of death in patients with anorexia nervosa and severe potassium deficiency
7. ECG manifestations
   a. Mild hypokalemia: flattening of T waves, ST segment depression, PVCs, prolonged QT interval
   b. Severe hypokalemia: prominent U waves, AV conduction disturbances, ventricular tachycardia or fibrillation
8. Diagnostic approach
   a. Distinguish true hypokalemia from redistribution (e.g., alkalosis, insulin administration)
   b. Measure 24-hour urinary potassium excretion while patient is on a regular dietary sodium intake
      (1) <20 mEq: consider extrarenal potassium loss
      (2) >20 mEq: renal potassium loss
   c. If renal potassium wasting is suspected, the following steps are indicated:
      (1) Measure 24 hr urine chloride
         (a) >10 mEq: diuretics, Bartter's syndrome, mineralocorticoid excess (chloride unresponsive)
         (b) <10 mEq: vomiting, gastric drainage (chloride responsive)
      (2) Measure blood pressure; if elevated, consider mineralocorticoid excess (see Section 22.9)
      (3) Measure serum bicarbonate (HCO_3^-): a low level is suggestive of RTA
9. Management
   a. Potassium replacement; Table 33-2 describes commonly available products
      (1) PO potassium replacement is preferred
      (2) IV infusion should not exceed 40 mEq/hour
   b. Monitor ECG and urine output
   c. Identify underlying cause and treat accordingly[1]
   d. IV NS in chloride responsive hypokalemia

Hyperkalemia[1,4,5,10]

1. Definition: plasma potassium concentration >4.9 mEq/L
2. Etiology and classification
   a. Pseudohyperkalemia
      (1) Hemolyzed specimen
      (2) Severe thrombocytosis (platelet count >10^6/ml)
      (3) Severe leukocytosis (WBC >10^5/ml)
      (4) Fist clenching during phlebotomy
   b. Excessive potassium intake
      (1) Potassium replacement therapy

    (2) High-potassium diet
    (3) Salt substitutes with potassium
    (4) Potassium salts of antibiotics
  c. Decreased renal excretion
    (1) Potassium-sparing diuretics (e.g., spironolactone, triamterene, amiloride)
    (2) Renal insufficiency
    (3) Mineralocorticoid deficiency
    (4) Hyporeninemic hypoaldosteronism (DM)
    (5) Tubular unresponsiveness to aldosterone (e.g., SLE, multiple myeloma, sickle cell disease)
    (6) Type IV RTA
    (7) ACE inhibitors
    (8) Heparin administration
    (9) NSAIDs
  d. Redistribution (excessive cellular release)
    (1) Acidemia (each 0.1 decrease in pH increases the serum potassium by 0.4-0.6 mEq/L)
    (2) Insulin deficiency
    (3) Drugs (e.g., succinylcholine, markedly increased digitalis level, arginine, beta adrenergic blockers)
    (4) Hypertonicity
    (5) Hemolysis
    (6) Tissue necrosis, rhabdomyolysis, burns
    (7) Hyperkalemic periodic paralysis
3. Clinical manifestations: weakness (generalized), irritability, paresthesias, decreased DTR, paralysis, cardiac dysrhythmias (ventricular ectopy, bradycardia, asystole)
4. ECG manifestations
  a. Mild hyperkalemia: peaking or tenting of T waves, PVCs
  b. Severe hyperkalemia: peaking of T waves, widening of QRS complex, depressed ST segments, prolongation of PR interval, sinus arrest, deep S wave, PVCs, ventricular tachycardia, fibrillation, and cardiac arrest
5. Diagnostic and therapeutic approach
  a. Rule out pseudohyperkalemia or lab error
    (1) Obtain ECG; in patients with pseudohyperkalemia secondary to hemolyzed specimen or thrombocytosis, the ECG will not show any manifestations of hyperkalemia
    (2) Repeat serum potassium level
    (3) In patients with thrombocytosis or severe leukocytosis, an accurate serum potassium can be determined by drawing a heparinized sample
  b. Stop all potassium intake (IV and PO)
  c. In patients with true hyperkalemia and ECG or clinical manifestations, immediate intervention is indicated with one or more measures depending on the severity of hyperkalemia (see Table 26-3)
  d. Monitor ECG
  e. Check pH, correct acidosis (if present)

Table 26-3   Therapy of acute hyperkalemia associated with ECG changes or clinical manifestations

Treatment Options	Onset of Action	Duration of Action
Glucose 50 g IV bolus or IV infusion of 500 ml of 10% dextrose solution, *plus* insulin 10 U regular insulin IV	Approximately 30 min	3 hr
Calcium gluconate* (10% solution) 5-10 ml IV over 3 min	5 min	Less than 1 hr
Dialysis (hemodialysis or peritoneal)	5 min after start of dialysis	3 hr after end of dialysis
Sodium bicarbonate ($NaHCO_3$) 1 amp (44 mEq) over 5 min	Approximately 30 min	3 hr
Sodium polystyrene sulfonate (Kayexalate) PO or via NG tube:	1-2 hr	3 hr
20-50 g Kayexalate plus 100-200 ml of 20% sorbitol		
Retention enema: 50 g Kayexalate in 200 ml of 20% sorbitol		

*Use with caution in patients receiving digitalis.

   f. Check calcium, magnesium, electrolytes, BUN, creatinine levels
   g. Identify underlying cause of hyperkalemia and treat if possible
      (1) Dialysis for renal failure
      (2) Exogenous mineralocorticoids in mineralocorticoid deficiency
      (3) Stop any potassium-sparing diuretics

26.4   **DISORDERS OF MAGNESIUM METABOLISM**

Hypomagnesemia[1,11]

1. Definition: plasma magnesium concentration <1.8 mg/dl
2. Etiology
   a. Gastrointestinal and nutritional
      (1) Defective GI absorption (malabsorption)
      (2) Inadequate dietary intake (e.g., alcoholics)
      (3) Parenteral therapy without magnesium
   b. Excessive renal losses
      (1) Diuretics
      (2) Renal tubular acidosis

(3) Diuretic phase of ATN

(4) Endocrine disturbances (DKA, hyperaldosteronism, hyperthyroidism, hyperparathyroidism)

(5) Cisplatin, alcohol, cyclosporine

(6) Antibiotics (gentamycin, ticarcillin, carbenicillin)

3. ECG manifestations: prolonged QT interval, T wave flattening, prolonged PR interval, atrial fibrillation, torsade de pointes

4. Clinical and lab manifestations

   a. Neuromuscular: weakness, hyperreflexia, fasciculations, tremors, convulsions, delirium, coma

   b. Cardiovascular: cardiac dysrhythmias

   c. Hypokalemia refractory to potassium replacement

   d. Hypocalcemia refractory to calcium replacement

5. Management

   a. Correct magnesium deficiency

      (1) Mild: 600 mg magnesium oxide PO provides 35 mEq of magnesium; dosage is 1-2 tab qd

      (2) Moderate: 50% solution magnesium sulfate (each 2 ml ampul contains 8 mEq or 96 mg of elemental magnesium); dosage is one 2 ml ampule of 50% magnesium solution q6h prn

      (3) Severe (serum magnesium level <1.0 mg/dl) and symptomatic patient (seizures, tetany): 2 g magnesium in 20 ml D_5W IV over 60 minutes; monitor ECG, blood pressure, pulse, respiration, deep tendon reflexes, and urine output

   b. Identify and correct underlying disorder

Hypermagnesemia

1. Definition: plasma magnesium concentration >2.3 mg/dl

2. Etiology

   a. Renal failure (decreased GFR)

   b. Decreased renal excretion secondary to salt depletion

   c. Abuse of antacids and laxatives containing magnesium in patients with renal insufficiency

   d. Endocrinopathies (deficiency of mineralocorticoid or thyroid hormone)

   e. Increased tissue breakdown

3. ECG manifestations: shortened QT interval, heart block, peaked T waves

4. Clinical manifestations: paresthesias, hypotension, confusion, decreased DTR, paralysis, apnea, acute hypermagnesemia suppresses PTH secretion and can produce hypocalcemia

5. Management

   a. Identify and correct underlying disorder

   b. Intracardiac conduction abnormalities can be treated with IV calcium gluconate

   c. Dialysis for severe hypermagnesemia

References

1. Arieff AI, DeFronzo RA: Fluid, electrolyte, and acid base disorders, New York, 1985, Churchill-Livingstone Inc.
2. Berkseth RO, Kjellstrandt CM: Radiologic contrast induced nephropathy, Med Clin North Am 68:351, 1984.
3. Clouse RE, et al: Angiodysplasia as a cause of upper gastrointestinal bleeding. Arch Intern Med 145:458, 1985.
4. Cox M: Potassium homeostasis, Med Clin North Am 65:363, 1981.
5. DeFronzo RA, et al: Clinical disorders of hyperkalemia, Ann Rev Med 33:531, 1982.
6. DeFronzo RA, Thier SO: Pathophysiologic approach to hyponatremia, Arch Intern Med 140:897, 1980.
7. Goldberg MP Hyponatremia, Med Clin North Am 65:251, 1981.
8. Katz MA: Hyperglycemia-induced hyponatremia: calculation of expected serum sodium depression, N Engl J Med 289:843, 1973.
9. Narins RG: Therapy of hyponatremia: does haste make waste? N Engl J Med 314:1574, 1986.
10. Narins RG, et al: Diagnostic strategies in disorders of fluid, electrolyte, and acid-base homeostasis, Am J Med 72:496, 1982.
11. Reinhart R: Magnesium metabolism, Arch Intern Med 148:2415, 1988.
12. Zarich S, Fang LS, Diamond JR: Fractional excretion of sodium: exceptions to its diagnostic value, Arch Intern Med 145:108, 1985.

Neurology

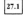 **GENERALIZED TONIC-CLONIC SEIZURES**
Kenneth Siegel

General approach

1. The diagnosis of a seizure disorder is made on clinical grounds
   a. Most seizures stop in 30-90 sec
   b. The most important diagnostic tool is an adequate history obtained from the patient and other observers of the event
   c. A telephone call is frequently the most important diagnostic tool
2. History
   a. Recent head trauma
   b. Alcohol ingestion, anxiolytics, and other drugs
   c. Diabetic patient on insulin or sulfonylureas: consider drug-induced hypoglycemia
   d. Previous neurologic insults (e.g., CVA)
   e. History of meningitis or encephalitis
   f. Were others present during the seizure?
   g. Were eyes tonically deviated during the seizure (e.g., eye deviation to the left during the seizure implies a lesion in the right hemisphere)
3. Approach varies with clinical presentation (e.g., alert patient after single convulsive episode vs patient with continuing seizure activity)

Evaluation of patient with single convulsive episode

1. Draw routine studies when an IV line is started
   a. Serum electrolytes: to rule out hyponatremia/hypernatremia
   b. Glucose: to rule out hypoglycemia
   c. Calcium: to rule out hypocalcemia/hypercalcemia
   d. Magnesium: to rule out hypomagnesemia
   e. CBC: to rule out an infectious process (e.g., sepsis, meningitis, encephalitis), thrombocytopenia, and hemoglobinopathy
   f. BUN and creatinine: to rule out renal failure
   g. Toxicology screen (blood and urine): to rule out suspected drug ingestion; HIV (in selected patients)
   h. ANA, ESR in suspected CNS vasculitis, SLE cerebritis

481

2. If the patient has stopped convulsing, therapy with IV diazepam should not be instituted, nor should the patient be rushed into the CT scanner before being fully stabilized

3. Obtain a CT scan or MRI scan to rule out CNS hemorrhage/infarct, mass lesions, AVM, aneurysms, cysticercosis, toxoplasmosis

4. An electroencephalogram (EEG) is indicated in any patient with new-onset generalized tonic-clonic seizures

5. Perform lumbar puncture (if indicated) only after visualizing the intracranial structures (CT scan or MRI scan) and in the absence of a demonstrable lesion

6. If there is suspicion of meningitis or encephalitis, perform lumbar puncture immediately after ruling out increased intracranial pressure with a funduscopic exam (without waiting for CT or MRI scan)

Treatment of the patient with a single tonic-clonic convulsive episode

1. Correct treatment is still very controversial

2. Focal abnormalities on neurologic exam, CT scan or MRI scan, or EEG serve as a guide; spike activity 24 hr after a seizure or a focal cerebral lesion on CT scan or MRI scan are reasons to institute therapy, since the risk of recurrence varies from 50-90%

3. In the absence of abnormal EEGs, CT scan, or MRI scan, observe patient; the chance of recurrence varies from 20-30%

4. Pharmacologic therapy
   a. Oral anticonvulsants can achieve therapeutic levels in a short period of time in most patients
      (1) 24-28 hr with high dosages of phenytoin (Dilantin) 15-18 mg/kg PO in the first 24 hr or
      (2) 3-5 days with carbamazepine (Tegretol) 600 mg qd
   b. A single anticonvulsant should be tried and pushed to clinical toxicity level (if necessary) before considering a second drug
   c. The drug of choice in IV therapy is phenytoin 18 mg/kg at no more than 50 mg/min (with ECG monitoring)

Management of status epilepticus

1. Aggressive treatment is required for patients with continuing seizures lasting 10 min or seizures without intervening consciousness

2. Seizure activity continuing for 30 min or intermittently over a 30 min period without the patient's regaining consciousness is termed *status epilepticus*[7]

3. Management of status epilepticus[5,7]
   a. Insert oral airway
   b. Start IV with normal saline solution
   c. Draw samples to evaluate ABG, electrolyte, glucose, BUN, creatinine, calcium, magnesium, toxicology screen, and anticonvulsant levels
   d. Institute electrocardiographic, respiratory, and blood pressure monitoring
   e. Give 100 mg of thiamine IM
   f. Give 50 ml bolus injection of a 50% glucose solution

g. Give diazepam (Valium) 2 mg IV push/min to a maximum of 20 mg total dose
   (1) Monitor closely for respiratory depression and hypotension
   (2) Emergency intubation may be required
   (3) Increase saline infusion if the patient becomes hypotensive
h. Give phenytoin (Dilantin) simultaneously at a rate of 50 mg/min until a loading dose of 18 mg/kg is reached

4. Above measures will control 90% of all patients within 30-40 min; if seizures continue, *intubate patients* and proceed with the following measures.
   a. Give phenobarbital 100 mg/min IV, to a maximum of 20 mg/kg, or
   b. Give diazepam (100 mg in 500 ml of D_5W) infused at 40 ml/hr; this will result in diazepam serum levels of 0.2-0.8 μg/ml
   c. If seizure activity persists longer than 60 min, institute general anesthesia with isoflurane and neuromuscular blockade

27-2 TRANSIENT ISCHEMIC ATTACK

Definition

Transient ischemic attack (TIA) is a sudden or rapid onset of neurologic deficit caused by cerebral ischemia. It may last for a few minutes or up to 24 hr and clears without residual signs.

Etiology[1,26]

1. Cardiac emboli
   a. Atrial fibrillation, sick sinus syndrome (SSS)
   b. Mitral valve disease (MS, MR, MVP)
   c. Prosthetic heart valves
   d. Bacterial and marantic endocarditis
   e. After MI, ventricular wall aneurysm (mural thrombus)
   f. Calcific aortic stenosis, calcification of mitral annulus
   g. Atrial myxoma
   h. Cardiomyopathies
   i. Intracardiac defects with paradoxical embolism (patent foramen ovale, atrial septal defect, Eisenmenger's)
2. Carotid or vertebral artery disease
   a. Arteriosclerosis
   b. Artery-to-artery embolism
   c. Anterograde extension of embolus into cerebral arteries
   d. Fibromuscular hyperplasia
   e. Dissecting aortic aneurysm
   f. Arteritis (Takayasu's, giant cell)
   g. Vasculitis
   h. Other: traumatic and spontaneous carotid and vertebrobasilar artery dissection, granulomatous angiitis, vasculopathy from drug abuse, arteriolar spasm
3. Hematologic causes
   a. RBC disorders
      (1) Increased sludging (polycythemia vera, sickle cell anemia, erythrocytosis)

(2) Decreased cerebral oxygenation (severe anemia)
    b. Platelet disorders: thrombocytosis and thrombocytopenia
    c. Myeloproliferative disorders, leukemias with white cell counts >150,000
    d. Increased viscosity (e.g., Waldenstrom's macroglobulinemia)
4. Other: transient hypotension, compression of neck vessels by osteophytes, kinking of neck vessels during rotation of the head, cocaine abuse, hypoglycemia, blood protein defects (protein C or S deficiency, lupus anticoagulant, antithrombin III deficiency, plasminogen deficiency)

Risk factors

Hypertension   Hyperlipidemias
Smoking   Advanced age
Obesity

The risk for stroke is highest in months immediately following the initial TIA and decreases thereafter.

General approach

1. Determine if the TIA involves the carotid or vertebrobasilar territory
    a. Prognosis and therapeutic approach depend on the vascular territory involved; the boxes below describe the various characteristics of carotid and vertebrobasilar insufficiency

---

Characteristics of Carotid Artery Syndrome

1. Ipsilateral monocular vision loss (amaurosis fugax); the patient often feels as if "a shade" has come down over one eye
2. Episodic contralateral arm, leg, and face paresis and paresthesias
3. Slurred speech, transient aphasia
4. Ipsilateral headache of vascular type
5. Carotid bruit may be present over the carotid bifurcation
6. Microemboli, hemorrhages, and exudates may be noted in the ipsilateral retina

---

Characteristics of Vertebrobasilar Artery Syndrome

1. Binocular visual disturbances (blurred vision, diplopia, total blindness)
2. Vertigo, nausea, vomiting, tinnitus
3. Sudden loss of postural tone of all four extremities (drop attacks) with no loss of consciousness
4. Slurred speech, ataxia, numbness around lips or face

b. In approximately 5-10% of TIAs, patients experience symptoms that reflect abnormalities in both carotid and vertebrobasilar territories[1]

2. Initial lab evaluation should include the following: CBC, platelet count, PT, PTT, glucose, VDRL, sedimentation rate, lipid profile, electrolytes, BUN, creatinine, ANA

3. Chest x-ray: evaluate heart size and configuration; check for any lung masses (lung neoplasm can initially manifest only with neurologic findings secondary to cerebral metastases)

4. ECG: evaluate patient's baseline rhythm, rule out atrial fibrillation, rule out recent MI (mural thrombi)

5. CT of the head: rule out hemorrhage/infarct and subdural hematoma; as many as 20% of patients with TIAs that resolve within 24 hr have evidence of cerebral infarction on CT scan of the head[26]

6. Echocardiography is indicated in any patients with cardiac murmurs to rule out an embolic focus from the heart

7. A 24 hr Holter monitor is indicated in any patient with suspected dysrhythmias

8. Duplex ultrasonography is the preferred noninvasive study in symptomatic patients with TIAs in the anterior circulation who are candidates for carotid endarterectomy; it is safe, has 85% sensitivity and 90% specificity, and is useful in identifying hemodynamically significant carotid stenosis; it distinguishes high-grade stenosis from occlusion and can detect ulcers, plaques, and plaque hemorrhages[10]

9. Carotid Doppler, alone or combined with periorbital Doppler, is useful when duplex ultrasonography is not available[10]

10. Cerebral arteriography should be done only in patients whose symptoms suggest involvement of the carotid circulation and the patient is a candidate for carotid endarterectomy; the morbidity associated with the retrograde femoral technique in patients with reasonable risk ranges from 0.2% to as much as 14%, and the incidence of serious complications (e.g., aortic dissection, embolic stroke) with permanent injury or even death is 0.5-1.2%[26]

Treatment

1. Medical therapy
    a. Anticoagulation: initially with heparin, then followed by warfarin
       (1) Indications
          (a) TIA due to emboli arising from mural thrombi after MI
          (b) TIA from suspected emboli in patients with mitral stenosis (with or without atrial fibrillation)
          (c) TIA in patients with prosthetic heart valves
          (d) Recurrent TIAs despite platelet antiaggregant agents
       (2) Duration of treatment
          (a) TIA secondary to mitral valve disease: prolonged treatment (years)
          (b) TIA secondary to mural thrombus: 2-6 mo of anticoagulant therapy followed by an additional 6-12 mo of aspirin therapy

(3) General contraindications to oral anticoagulants: history of GI bleeding, bleeding tendencies, severe hypertension, elderly patients with frequent falls, uncooperative patients

b. Antiplatelet therapy is indicated in patients who are not candidates for surgery or warfarin therapy (e.g., frequent falls, severe hypertension)

   (1) Aspirin decreases the risk of subsequent stroke by 15-30% in patients with TIA; doses ≤325 mg/day are as effective as higher ones and are associated with fewer side effects

   (2) Ticlopidine inhibits platelet aggregation, blocks the platelet-release action, and prolongs bleeding time; it has been reported effective in reducing the risk of subsequent stroke in both men and women with recent thromboembolic events[12]

2. Surgical therapy in patients with carotid distribution TIAs: carotid endarterectomy is indicated in the following settings[2]:

   a. High-grade (≥70%) isolateral stenosis and surgery can be done early and at low risk

   b. Greater than 50% stenosis associated with a large carotid artery ulcer

   c. Multiple TIAs despite medical therapy, in the setting of high-grade or ulcerative ipsilateral disease, and surgery can be done at low to medium risk

   d. Crescendo attacks in the setting of high-grade or ulcerative ipsilateral disease and surgery can be done at low to medium risk

      Patient preference and the experience of the surgical team should be considered whenever surgery is contemplated.

27.3   STROKE

Definition

Stroke can be defined as the rapid onset of a neurologic deficit involving a certain vascular territory and lasting longer than 24 hr.

Etiology and risk factors

The etiology and risk factors for stroke are the same as those given for TIA. Cocaine-related stroke is increasing in frequency. A thorough history focusing on the use of cocaine and toxicological screening of urine and serum should be part of the evaluation of any young patient with a stroke.[19]

Classification

Ischemic stroke

1. Etiology: thrombosis or embolism; although the clinical distinction between them is often impossible, the major distinguishing factors are described in Table 27-1

2. Clinical presentation varies with the cerebral vessel involved (see Table 27-2 for description of common stroke syndromes)

3. Management of ischemic stroke[6]

   a. CT scan of the head

Table 27-1 Characteristics of cerebral thrombosis and embolism

	Thrombosis	Embolism
Onset of symptoms	Progression of symptoms over hours to days	Very rapid (seconds)
History of prior TIA	Common	Uncommon
Time of presentation	Often during night hours while the patient is sleeping	Patient is usually awake and involved in some type of activity
	Classically the patient awakes with a slight neurologic deficit that gradually progresses in a step-wise fashion	
Predisposing factors	Atherosclerosis, hypertension, diabetes, arteritis, vasculitis, hypotension, trauma to head and neck	Atrial fibrillation, mitral stenosis and regurgitation, endocarditis, mitral valve prolapse

    (1) Indications
        (a) To rule out cerebral hemorrhage when considering anticoagulation
        (b) When signs and symptoms cannot be explained by one lesion
        (c) Any patient on anticoagulant therapy presenting with a stroke
        (d) To rule out brain abscess, tumor, and subdural hematoma
    (2) Diagnosis: cerebral infarction is seen on CT scan as an area of decreased density; initial CT scan may be negative and infarct may not be evident for 2-3 days after the infarction
  b. Blood pressure control[18]
    (1) Lowering systemic blood pressure in patients with acute cerebral infarction is contraindicated since it may produce clinical deterioration (secondary to spontaneous fluctuations in blood pressure and impaired cerebral autoregulation) unless
      • Diastolic pressure is $\geq$130 mm Hg
      • Hypertensive encephalopathy is present
      • Vital organs (heart, kidney) are compromised
    (2) Blood pressure generally should not drop below 150/100 since cerebral perfusion could be impaired

Table 27-2   Selected stroke syndromes

Artery Involved	Neurologic Deficit
Middle cerebral artery	Hemiplegia (upper extremity and face are usually more involved than lower extremities)
	Hemianesthesia (hemisensory loss)
	Hemianopia (homonymous)
	Aphasia (if dominant hemisphere is involved)
Anterior cerebral artery	Hemiplegic (lower extremities more involved than upper extremities and face)
	Primitive reflexes (e.g., grasp and suck)
	Urinary incontinence
Vertebral and basilar arteries	Ipsilateral cranial nerve findings
	Contralateral (or bilateral) sensory or motor deficits
Deep penetrating branches of major cerebral arteries (lacunar infarction)	Usually seen in elderly hypertensive patients and diabetics
	Four characteristic syndromes are possible[26]
	1. Pure motor hemiplegia (66%)
	2. Dysarthria—clumsy hand syndrome (20%)
	3. Pure sensory stroke (10%)
	4. Ataxic hemiplegia syndrome with pyramidal tract signs

   c. Anticoagulation: initially with heparin followed by warfarin
     (1) Indications
       (a) Worsening neurologic deficits (stroke in evolution)
       (b) Suspected cerebral embolism from
         • Mural thrombus, after MI
         • Mitral stenosis (with or without atrial fibrillation)
         • Atrial fibrillation
     (2) Contraindications
       (a) Absolute: CT scan or lumbar puncture evidence of cerebral hemorrhage, tumor, abscess, subdural or epidural hematoma
       (b) Relative: history of GI bleeding, bleeding tendencies, severe hypertension
       (c) Completed stroke, unless embolization is determined to be the cause
   d. Rehabilitation should be a combined effort by the attending physi-

cian, physical therapist, speech therapist, nursing staff, social service, and the patient's family

e. Carotid endarterectomy may be indicated for patients after atherothrombotic stroke whose surgery can be delayed at least 1 mo and who have minor deficits, high-grade ipsilateral stenosis or large ulcerative lesions, and low to medium surgical risk[2]

Hemorrhagic stroke

1. Subarachnoid hemorrhage (SAH)[26]
   a. Etiology: ruptured congenital aneurysm or AV malformation
   b. Clinical manifestations
      (1) Generalized excruciating headache that radiates into the posterior neck region, and is worsened by neck and head movements
      (2) Coma
      (3) Diplopia, dilated pupil, pain above or behind an eye, neck stiffness
   c. Physical exam
      (1) Focal neurologic signs usually are absent
      (2) Level of consciousness varies from normal to deeply comatose
      (3) Fever and nuchal rigidity are present or usually develop with 24 hours
      (4) Fundi may show papilledema and/or retinal hemorrhage
      (5) Cranial nerve abnormalities may be noted (e.g., pupillary dilation secondary to oculomotor nerve dysfunction)
   d. Diagnosis
      (1) CT scan of head confirms the presence of subarachnoid blood localized to the basal cisterns or extending intracerebrally or in the ventricles; a fresh hemorrhage produces an area of increased density; the scan may be normal if done more than 48 hr after the SAH or if the hemorrhage is small
      (2) Lumbar puncture is indicated if a CT scan of the head is not available or if CT is negative and the index of suspicion is high
         (a) A good funduscopic exam to rule out papilledema must be done before LP
         (b) In SAH the CSF will be uniformly grossly bloody, whereas in a traumatic LP the number of RBCs decreases progressively from tube 1 to tube 4
         (c) More reliable is the presence of xanthochromia in the CSF (see Section 30.1)
      (3) Angiography is necessary to determine the best therapeutic approach (medical vs surgical)
   e. Management of SAH varies with the patient's clinical status and the location and surgical accessibility of the aneurysm
      (1) Medical management
         (a) Strict bed rest in a quiet darkened private room with cardiac monitoring (frequent dysrhythmias)
         (b) Control of headache with acetaminophen and codeine
         (c) Have the patient avoid all forms of straining (stool softeners and mild laxatives are indicated to prevent constipation)
         (d) Maintain systolic pressure in the range of 140-160 mm Hg

Table 27-3   Grading of surgical risks in patients with aneurysms

Grade	Criteria
0	Unruptured aneurysm
I	Minimal headache or nuchal rigidity, or asymptomatic
Ia	Fixed neurologic deficit without acute meningeal or brain reaction
II	Absence of neurologic deficit with moderate to severe headache or nuchal rigidity
III	Drowsiness, confusion, or mild focal deficit
IV	Stupor, moderate or severe hemiparesis, possible early decerebrate rigidity or vegetative disturbances
V	Deep coma, decerebrate rigidity or moribund state

From Hunt WE, Hess RM: J Neurosurg 28:14, 1968.

     (e) Reduce cerebral edema with mannitol

     (f) Nimodipine, a calcium channel blocker, is useful in the treatment of cerebral blood vessel spasm following subarachnoid hemorrhage from ruptured congenital intracranial aneurysms in patients who are in good neurologic condition postictus (e.g., Hunt and Hess grades I-II, see Table 27-3); it has been shown to decrease the incidence of permanent neurologic damage and death; therapy should be initiated within 96 hr of the onset of hemorrhage; dosage is 60 mg q4h for 21 days; it may be administered via NG tube; dosage reduction is necessary in patients with liver disease

  (2) Surgical management: the indications for surgery and the patient's prognosis depend on the size of the aneurysm, the patient's age and clinical condition, and the neurosurgeon; Table 27-3 describes the grading of surgical risks in patients with aneurysms; the chance of survival is excellent in grades 0-II, very poor in grade V

  (3) Heavy particle radiation: this represents a reasonable alternative for symptomatic surgically inaccessible intracranial arteriovenous malformations[25]

  f. Prognosis of cerebral AVMs: the rate of rebleeding for cerebral arteriovenous malformations in patients with hemorrhage is about 6% in the first 6 mo after the hemorrhage; thereafter, it is approximately 4% per year, a rate identical to the yearly risk of a first hemorrhage in patients with malformations that have never bled; therefore surgery is much more desirable in a younger patient[14a]

2. Intracerebral hemorrhage

  a. Etiology: generally associated with hypertension

  b. Clinical manifestations

    (1) The hemorrhage usually occurs during periods of activity, often manifesting with headache, vomiting, and sudden onset of neu-

rologic deficits that can rapidly progress to coma and death; the neurologic deficits vary with the area involved

(2) The box on p. 492 describes localizing signs in patients with intracerebral hemorrhage

(3) In addition to the focal deficits, the patient may also show signs of increased ICP (e.g., bradycardia, decreased respiratory rate, third nerve palsy)

c. Diagnosis: on a CT scan of the head, the area of hemorrhagic infarct appears as a zone of increased density; shifts of intracranial contents and compression of the ventricles may be present

d. Management

   (1) Medical therapy

      (a) Control of severe hypertension: lower blood pressure may reduce cerebral edema, but it risks promoting border zone ischemia[18]; blood pressure reduction if indicated, should not exceed 20%[16] and should be achieved with short-acting agents (e.g., sodium nitroprusside)

      (b) Treatment of cerebral edema; mannitol, 1-1.5 g/kg of a 20% solution given IV over 30 min is generally effective

      (c) Maintain a clear airway

      (d) Supportive measures

        • Careful IV fluid administration; excessive fluid administration can worsen cerebral edema

        • Phenytoin if seizure activity is noted

        • Frequent turning of comatose patients to prevent decubitus ulcers

        • Nutritional support

        • Physical therapy

   (2) Surgical evacuation of hematomas is indicated in the following situations[28]:

      (a) Noncomatose patients with cerebellar hemorrhage

      (b) Patients with surgically accessible cerebral hematomas that produce progressive signs of temporal lobe herniation

27.4 CEREBRAL NEOPLASMS

Classification and prevalence[3,30]

1. Primary CNS neoplasms
   a. Gliomas (33-42%)
   b. Meningiomas (13-18%)
   c. Pituitary adenoma (8-17.8%)
   d. Acoustic neuroma (7.6-8.7%)
   e. Craniopharyngioma (2.5-4.6%)
   f. Miscellaneous (17.9-18.2%)
2. Metastatic CNS neoplasms (4-4.2%): lung, breast, melanoma, kidney, thyroid (other tumors metastasize to brain less frequently)

Localizing Signs in Patients with Intracerebral Hemorrhage[11]

Location of Intracerebral Hemorrhage	Common Neurologic Signs	Examples
Putamen	Both eyes deviate conjugately to the side of the lesion (away from hemiparesis)	Left putaminal hemorrhage
	Pupils normal in size and react normally	
	Contralateral hemiplegia present	
	Hemisensory defect noted	
Thalamus	Both eyes deviate downward and look at the nose	Thalamic hemorrhage
	Impairment of vertical eye movements present	
	Pupils small (approximately 2 mm) and nonreactive	
	Contralateral hemisensory loss present	
Pons	Both eyes in mid-position	Pontine hemorrhage
	No doll's eye movements	
	Pupils are pinpoint but reactive (use magnifying glass)	
	Coma is common	
	Flaccid quadriplegia noted	
Cerebellum	Ipsilateral paresis of conjugate gaze (inability to look toward side of lesion)	Cerebellar hemorrhage
	Pupils normal in size and react normally	
	Inability to stand or walk	
	Vertigo and dysarthria present	

Clinical manifestations

Clinical manifestations depend on
1. Type of tumor (more than 60% of pituitary adenomas are hypersecretory): e.g., patients with an ACTH-secreting pituitary adenoma will have symptoms of Cushing's disease (see Section 22.9)
2. Location of tumor: e.g., a tumor compressing the optic chiasm will result in bitemporal hemianopia; Fig. 27-1 shows the visual field defects produced by lesions along the optic pathway

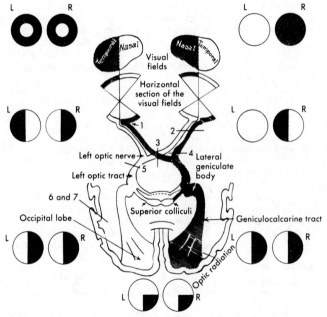

Figure 27-1

Visual field defects associated with lesions of the visual system. **1,** Circumferential blindness ("tubular vision") may be caused by hysteria, or optic or retrobulbar neuritis. **2,** Total blindness of right eye caused by complete lesion of right optic nerve, such as trauma. **3,** Bitemporal hemianopia because of chiasmal lesions, such as pituitary tumors. **4,** Right nasal hemianopia resulting from a lesion involving perichiasmal area, such as calcified right internal carotid artery. **5,** Right homonymous hemianopia caused by lesion of left parietal or temporal lobes with pressure on left optic tract. **6,** Right homonymous inferior quadrarantanopia because of partial involvement of optic radiation (upper portion of left optic radiation in this case). **7,** Right homonymous hemianopia with no pupillary change as a result of complete involvement of the left optic radiation. (From Chusid JG: Correlative neuroanatomy and functional neurology, ed 19, Los Altos Calif, 1985, Lange Medical Publications.)

3. Size of tumor: large tumors often present with signs of increased ICP (headache, nausea, vomiting, bradycardia, papilledema, third nerve palsy, and hypoventilation)

Diagnosis

1. History
   a. Inquire about symptoms of visual disturbances, hearing loss, localized weakness, headaches, seizures, behavioral changes
   b. Duration of symptoms
   c. Family history of "brain tumors" (MEN)
2. Physical exam: perform careful neurologic exam; note any signs of increased ICP or evidence of focal motor or sensory deficits
3. Lab results: an elevated prolactin level is suggestive of a pituitary tumor; in addition to prolactin level, endocrine evaluation of pituitary neoplasms should include urine free cortisol, T_4, T_3RU, TSH, and somatomedin C levels; LH, FSH, and estradiol levels should also be checked in amenorrheic women; and testosterone levels in men
4. Radiographic evaluation
   a. CT scan of head or MRI scan
      (1) CT identifies approximately 90% of intraparenchymal lesions[13]
      (2) MRI is superior to CT in identifying cerebral neoplasms, particularly in the diagnosis of posterior fossa tumors
   b. Angiography is indicated in the following[17]:
      (1) Detection of vascular lesions (AVM, meningioma)
      (2) Preoperative evaluation of surgically relevant tumor vasculature
      (3) Differentiation of hemorrhage secondary to tumor from hemorrhage due to aneurysm
      (4) Aid in diagnosis of poorly visualized lesions by CT or MRI
   c. EEG: Nonspecific; useful in the evaluation of new onset seizure activity in a patient with suspected cerebral neoplasm
   d. Skull x-ray: limited value; may show bone erosion, abnormal calcifications, or abnormalities in the size and shape of the sella turcica

Treatment

1. Medical management
   a. Phenytoin (Dilantin) is indicated for prevention and treatment of seizures
   b. Reduction of cerebral edema[4]
      (1) Mannitol: 1-1.5 g/kg as a 20% solution infused over 30 min is indicated in an emergency situation
      (2) Dexamethasone: 10 mg IV loading dose followed by 4 mg IV 6qh until the effects of cerebral edema are controlled, then change to PO dexamethasone; the cerebral edema–reducing effect of dexamethasone is generally delayed for several hours
2. Surgery, radiotherapy, and chemotherapy: the use of these modalities depends on the type of tumor (benign vs. malignant), location (surgically accessible), and radiosensitivity (e.g., medulloblastomas are generally radiosensitive)

27.6   **PARKINSON'S DISEASE**

Definition

Parkinson's disease is a progressive neurologic disorder. It is characterized pathologically by cytoplasmic eosinophilic inclusions (Lewy bodies) in neurons of the substantia nigra and locus ceruleus and by depigmentation of the brainstem nuclei. Parkinson's disease is part of the clinical syndrome of parkinsonism, an extrapyramidal disorder characterized by rigidity, tremor at rest, bradykinesia, and loss of postural reflexes.

Classification of parkinsonism[9]

1. Primary (Parkinson's disease)
2. Secondary (acquired parkinsonism)
    a. Iatrogenic (e.g., phenothiazines, butyrophenones)
    b. Postencephalitic (sequela of encephalitis lethargica)
    c. Toxins (e.g., MPTP [a neurotoxic meperidine analog used by drug addicts], manganese, carbon monoxide)
    d. Hypoparathyroidism (e.g., postparathyroidectomy)
    e. Vascular insufficiency (e.g, after CVA)
3. Parkinsonism-plus: symptoms and signs of parkinsonism occurring in association with other multisystem degenerative diseases (e.g., Wilson's disease, Alzheimer's disease, NPH)

Clinical manifestations

The disease often begins insidiously and can manifest itself with a slight loss of motor dexterity, generalized slowness, or a decrease in overall motor activity. Table 27-4 describes the various initial presentations of Parkinson's disease. The classical manifestations of Parkinson's disease are:

1. Rigidity: increased muscle tone
    a. It involves both agonist and antagonist muscle groups
    b. The resistance to passive movement is widespread and more prominent at large joints ("cog-wheeling" rigidity is noted)
2. Tremor: resting tremor, with a frequency of 4-7 movements/sec
    a. The tremor is usually noted in the hands and often involves the thumb and forefinger ("pill-rolling" tremor)
    b. Parkinsonian tremor is often confused with essential senile tremor; their major distinguishing characteristics are described in Table 27-5

Table 27-4   Initial symptoms in Parkinson's disease[29]

Symptoms	Percent of Cases
Tremor	70
Stiffness or slowness of movement	20
Loss of dexterity or handwriting disturbance	13
Gait disturbance	12
Muscle pain, cramps, aching	8
Other: depression, nervousness, psychiatric disturbance, speech disturbances, drooling	1-5

Table 27-5 Distinguishing characteristics of parkinsonian tremor and essential senile tremor

Type of Tremor	Family History	Characteristics	Effect of Ethanol	Therapy
Parkinsonian tremor	Negative	Present at rest Improves or disappears with purposeful function Supination/pronation type	No effect	Levodopa Anticholinergics Bromocriptine
Essential senile tremor	Positive	Present during maintenance of posture (postural tremor) and aggravated by stressful situations Flexion/extension type	Decreases tremor	Propranolol 60-240 mg/day in 3-4 divided doses is effective in approximately 50% of patients Primidone 25 mg tid initially, titrated prn to maximum of 250 mg tid, may be effective in patients refractory to propranolol

3. Akinesia: inability to initiate or execute a movement
   a. The patient often sits immobile since even the simple task of getting up from a chair becomes impossible
   b. The face shows a marked absence of movement (masked facies); the mouth is usually open and the patient drools
4. Gait disturbance
   a. The patient assumes a stooped posture (head bowed, trunk bent forward, shoulders dropped, knees and arms flexed)
   b. There is difficulty initiating the first step and this is followed by small shuffling steps that increase in speed (festinating gait), as if the patient is chasing his or her center of gravity (the patient's steps become progressively faster and shorter while the trunk inclines further forward)
5. Abnormal reflexes
   a. Palmomental reflex: stroking the palm of the hand near the base of the thumb results in contraction of the ipsilateral mentalis muscle, causing wrinkling of the skin of the chin
   b. Glabellar reflex: repeated gentle tapping on the glabella evokes blinking of both eyes
6. Dementia: occurs in approximately 50% of patients
7. Others: orthostatic hypotension, micrographia

Management

1. General principles: physical therapy, encouragement, reassurance, and treatment of possible associated conditions (e.g., depression)
2. Avoidance of drugs that can induce or worsen Parkinson's disease:
   a. Neuroleptic agents (especially haloperidol)
   b. Certain antiemetics (e.g., prochlorperazine, trimethobenzamide); these drugs will block dopamine receptors; diphenidol (Vontrol) may be used for nausea
   c. Metoclopramide (Reglan)
   d. Nonselective MAO inhibitors (may induce hypertensive crisis)
   e. Certain antihypertensives (reserpine, methyldopa)
3. Drug therapy should be delayed until symptoms significantly limit the patient's daily activities, since tolerance and side effects to parkinsonian agents are common.
   a. Anticholinergic agents can be used alone or in combination with levodopa
      (1) Trihexyphenidyl (Artane): initial dosage is 1 mg PO tid pc
      (2) Benztropine (Cogentin): the usual dosage is 0.5-1 mg PO qd or bid
   b. Amantadine (Symmetrel): antiviral agent with antiparkinsonian effect; dosage is 100 mg PO qd or bid initially
   c. Levodopa therapy: often started when the above agents fail to control the parkinsonian symptoms or if the patient develops significant side effects; levodopa is commonly used with a peripheral dopa decarboxylase inhibitor (carbidopa) to minimize side effects (nausea, mood changes, cardiac dysrhythmias, postural hypotension)

(1) The combination of the two drugs is marketed under the trade name Sinemet
(2) Carbidopa/levodopa is available in tablets (10/100 mg, 25/100 mg, 25/250 mg)
(3) Therapy can be started with 25-100 mg PO tid
(4) The best therapeutic approach is to minimize the patient's symptoms with the lowest possible dose.
(5) Common side effects of long-term levodopa therapy are
    (a) "on-off" effect: sudden fluctuation of clinical status from good mobility to stiffness
    (b) Dyskinesia: chronic movements, more frequently seen when higher doses are used
    (c) Development of tolerance: loss of efficacy, requiring higher doses to achieve the therapeutic effect
  d. Dopamine receptor agonists
    (1) Bromocriptine (Parlodel): initial dosage is 1.25 mg hs for several days; usual range is 10-40 mg daily
    (2) Pergolide (Permax): initial dosage is 0.05 mg for first 2 days, increased by 0.1 mg every third day over the next 12 days; maximum daily dosage is 5 mg (usually given in three divided doses)
  e. Selegine (Deprenyl, Eldepryl): selective MAO type B inhibitor; it is useful in delaying the requirement for L-dopa therapy and for minimizing the "wearing off" effect; dosage is 5 mg bid with breakfast and lunch

27.6 | MULTIPLE SCLEROSIS

Definition

Multiple sclerosis is a chronic demyelinating disease of unknown cause. It is characterized pathologically by zones of demyelinization (plaques) scattered throughout the white matter.

Clinical manifestations

The clinical signs vary with the location of plaques. The more common manifestations are
1. Weakness: usually involving the lower extremities; the patient may complain of difficulty ambulating, tendency to drop things, easy fatigability
2. Sensory disturbances: numbness, tingling, "pins and needles" sensation
3. Visual disturbances: diplopia, blurred vision, visual loss
4. Incoordination: gait impairment, clumsiness of upper extremities
5. Other: vertigo, incontinence, loss of sexual function, slurred speech

Physical exam

1. Visual abnormalities
   a. Paresis of medial rectus muscle on lateral conjugate gaze (internuclear ophthalmoplegia) and horizontal nystagmus of the adducting eye

    b. Central scotoma, decreased visual acuity (optic neuritis)

    c. Nystagmus

2. Abnormalities of reflexes

    a. Increased deep tendon reflexes

    b. Positive Hoffman's sign, positive Babinski's sign

    c. Decreased abdominal skin reflex, decreased cremasteric reflex

3. Lhermitte's phenomenon: flexion of the neck while the patient is lying down elicits an electrical sensation extending bilaterally down the arms, back, and lower trunk

4. Charcot's triad: nystagmus, scanning speech, and intention tremor

Diagnostic evaluation

1. Lumbar puncture

    a. In multiple sclerosis the CSF may show increased gamma globulin (mostly IgG, but often IgA and IgM)

    b. Agarose electrophoresis discloses separate discrete "oligoclonal" bands in the gamma region in approximately 90% of patients, including some with normal IgG levels

    c. Other possible CSF abnormalities: increased total protein, increased mononuclear white cells, presence of myelin basic protein (elevated in acute attacks, indicates active myelin destruction)

2. Measurement of visual evoked response (VER) is useful to assess nerve fiber conduction (myelin loss or destruction will slow conduction velocity)

3. CT may demonstrate hypodense areas; however, it is usually normal

4. MRI is more sensitive than CT; it can identify lesions as small as 3-4 mm and is frequently diagnostic in suspected cases

Therapy

1. Specific treatment: there is no proved treatment that will significantly alter the course of multiple sclerosis; severe attacks in patients with the relapsing-remitting form of the disease may respond to plasma exchange in conjunction with ACTH and cyclophosphamide[27]

2. Supportive measures

    a. Control of spasticity: diazepam (Valium) or baclofen (Lioresal) may be useful

    b. Control of paresthesias: carbamazepine (Tegretol)

    c. Control of action tremor: isoniazid may be of value[23] (controversial)

    d. Physical therapy, social counseling, and psychiatric support

Clinical course

The majority of patients experience clinical improvement in weeks to months following the initial manifestations. The disease may be of the exacerbating-remitting type or may follow a chronic progressive course. The average interval from initial clinical presentation to death is 35 yr. Premature death is usually secondary to infection.[25]

27.7   **PERIPHERAL NERVE DYSFUNCTION**

Definitions[24]

1. Peripheral neuropathy: any disorder involving the peripheral nerves
2. Polyneuropathy (symmetric polyneuropathy): generalized process resulting in widespread and symmetric effects on the peripheral nervous system
3. Focal or multifocal neuropathy (mononeuropathy, mononeuropathy multiplex): local involvement of one or more individual peripheral nerves
4. Paresthesia: spontaneous aberrant sensation (e.g., pins and needles)

Classification and characteristics[21]

1. Hereditary neuropathies
   a. Charcot-Marie-Tooth syndrome
      (1) Most common familial motor and sensory abnormality
      (2) Foot deformity is common
      (3) Braces for correction of foot drop are useful
      (4) Surgical management is generally necessary for stability and cosmetic appearance of the feet[8]
   b. Others: Dejerine-Sottas disease, Refsum's disease, Riley-Day syndrome
2. Acquired neuropathies
   a. Neuropathy associated with systemic disease
      (1) Diabetes mellitus (see Section 22.1)
      (2) Myxedema: distal sensory neuropathy manifested by burning sensation and paresthesias of the limbs; delayed relaxation phase of DTR is common
      (3) Uremia: symmetrical distal mixed motor and sensory disturbances
      (4) Sarcoidosis: cranial nerve palsies (most common is facial nerve), polyneuropathy
      (5) Alcohol: pain, numbness, and weakness of extremities
      (6) Neoplasms: sensory and sensorimotor neuropathies
      (7) Nutritional deficiencies: thiamine, folic acid, vitamin B_{12}; vitamin B_{12} deficiency affects the posterior and lateral columns of the spinal cord; it manifests with numbness and paresthesias of the extremities, weakness, ataxia, and loss of vibration sense
      (8) Other: collagen vascular diseases, amyloidosis, multiple myeloma
   b. Guillain-Barré neuropathy (see Section 27.8)
   c. Toxic neuropathies[24]
      (1) Drugs: chloramphenicol, lithium, isoniazid, pyridoxine, nitrofurantoin, disulfiram, dapsone, ethionamide, cisplatin, vincristine, metronidazole, gold, hydralazine, amiodarone, phenytoin
      (2) Toxic chemicals: lead, arsenic, cyanide, thallium, carbon disulfide, mercury, organophosphates, trichloroethylene

d. Neuropathies associated with infection: leprosy, herpes zoster, diphtheria, Lyme disease (see Section 25.11), HIV. There are two major forms of neuropathy associated with HIV:
   (a) Distal symmetrical polyneuropathy, manifested by paresthesias of the feet and distal weakness in the legs
   (b) Inflammatory demyelinating neuropathy, manifested by progressive weakness in the legs, pain involving the feet, and gradual loss of ankle and knee reflexes; it is usually seen in ARC patients
e. Entrapment neuropathy (e.g., carpal tunnel syndrome, see Section 29.3)

Approach to the patient with a peripheral neuropathy

1. History
   a. Family history of neuropathies: to rule out hereditary neuropathies
   b. Current and past employment: to rule out exposure to toxic agents
   c. Current or recent medications: to rule out neuropathy secondary to drugs
   d. Any systemic disease, such as diabetes, renal failure, hypothyroidism
   e. Ethanol abuse: alcoholic neuropathy
   f. Any special diets (e.g., food faddists): to rule out nutritional deficiencies
   g. History of trauma: to rule out compression entrapment neuropathies
   h. Duration and progression of symptoms
   i. Risk factors for AIDS (see Section 25.4)
   j. History of tick bite or ECM (see Fig. 21-3): Lyme disease
2. Physical exam
   a. Define the type of neuropathy present
      (1) Sensory vs motor vs mixed
      (2) Number of nerves involved (e.g., mononeuropathy, polyneuropathy, mononeuropathy multiplex)
   b. Determine the territory of neurologic deficit (see Figs. 3-4 and 3-5 for segmental distribution of cutaneous nerves)
   c. Evaluate DTRs; they are decreased in root and peripheral nerve disease
3. Initial lab evaluation
   a. CBC, electrolytes, BUN, creatinine, glucose, LFTs, calcium, magnesium, phosphorus; HIV in patients with risk factors, Lyme titer in patients with a suggestive history
   b. If toxic neuropathy is suspected, heavy metal screening should be ordered; in suspected lead poisoning, blood lead concentration, urinary tests for coproporphyrin and δ-aminolevulinic acid, and bone marrow aspirates (to evaluate the presence of basophilic stippling in normoblasts) are indicated
   c. TSH level in suspected hypothyroidism
   d. Vitamin B_{12} and folate levels in suspected nutritional deficiencies
   e. Chest x-ray to rule out sarcoidosis
   f. LP in suspected Guillain Barré syndrome

   g. X-ray in suspected trauma or peripheral nerve compression
4. Electromyography: in neurogenic lesions there are spontaneous fibrillation potentials and positive sharp waves at rest
5. Nerve conduction studies

Treatment

1. Specific treatment (e.g., combination with BAL-CaEDTA in patients with lead poisoning, plasmapheresis followed by low-dose prednisone in AIDS/ARC patients with inflammatory demyelinating neuropathy)
2. Supportive measures (e.g., physical therapy, emotional support)

 GUILLAIN-BARRÉ SYNDROME

Definition

Guillain-Barré syndrome is an acute rapidly progressing symmetrical polyradiculoneuropathy, predominantly affecting motor function[15]

Incidence

There are bimodal peaks of occurrence in the 15-35 yr and 50-75 yr age groups.

Clinical manifestations

1. Rapid progression of symmetrical weakness manifested initially in the lower extremities
   a. The patient often reports difficulty in ambulating, getting up from a chair, or climbing stairs
   b. In some patients the initial manifestations may involve the cranial musculature or the upper extremities (e.g., tingling of the hands)
2. Two thirds of all patients give a history of respiratory or gastrointestinal illness within 30 days of onset of neurological symptoms[22]

Physical exam

1. Symmetrical weakness, involving both proximal and distal muscles
2. Depressed or absent reflexes bilaterally
3. Minimum to moderate glove and stocking anesthesia
4. Ataxia and pain in a segmental distribution may be seen in some patients (caused by involvement of posterior nerve roots)
5. Autonomic abnormalities (bradycardia/tachycardia, hypotension/hypertension)
6. Respiratory insufficiency (caused by weakness of intercostal muscles)
7. Facial paresis, difficulty swallowing (secondary to cranial nerve involvement)

Diagnostic evaluation

1. Rule out other causes of neuropathy (e.g., metabolic, toxic, or nutritional deficiencies, spinal cord lesions, infections, porphyria, collagen-vascular disease)
2. Lumbar puncture

   a. Typical findings include elevated CSF protein (especially IgG) and presence of few mononuclear leukocytes

   b. Normal values may be seen at beginning of illness

   c. If the diagnosis is strongly suspected, repeat lumbar puncture is indicated

3. Electromyography reveals slowed conduction velocities; prolonged motor, sensory, and F wave latencies are also present

Therapy

1. Supportive measures
   a. Close monitoring of respiratory function (frequent measurements of vital capacity and pulmonary toilet) because respiratory failure is the major potential problem in Guillain-Barré syndrome; approximately 10-20% of patients will require respiratory support[22]
   b. Frequent repositioning of patient to minimize formation of pressure sores
   c. Prevention of thrombophlebitis with antithrombotic stockings and SC heparin (5000 U q12h)
   d. Active physical therapy program
   e. Emotional support and social counseling
2. Plasmapheresis: results from the Guillain-Barré Study Group[14] show that although plasmapheresis is not effective for all patients, it is particularly effective for patients who receive this treatment within 7 days of onset of symptoms and for patients who require mechanical ventilation
3. Use of corticosteroids is controversial, major studies have shown that there is no benefit from corticosteroid therapy

References

1. Barnett HJM: Cerebrovascular diseases. In Wyngaarden JB, Smith LH (editors): Cecil Textbook of medicine, ed 17, Philadelphia, 1985, WB Saunders Co, vol 1.
2. Cebul RD, Whisnant JP: Indications for carotid endoarterectomy, Ann Intern Med 111:675, 1989.
3. Cushing H: Intracranial tumors: notes upon a series of two thousand verified cases with surgical mortality percentages pertaining thereto, Springfield Ill, 1932, Charles C Thomas Publisher.
4. Cutler RWP: Neoplastic disorders. In Rubenstein E, Federman DD (editors): Scientific American medicine, New York, 1985, Scientific American Inc, Chapter 11, Section 6.
5. Dalessio DJ: Seizure disorders and pregnancy, N Engl J Med 312:559, 1985.
6. Dawson DM: Stroke and TIA: solutions to the Dx and Rx dilemmas, Modern Medicine, vol 53, p 30, 1985.
7. Delgado-Escueta AV, et al: Management of status epilepticus, N Engl J Med 306:1337, 1982.
8. Drennan J: Orthopedic management of neuromuscular disorders, Philadelphia, 1983, JB Lippincott Co.
9. Fahn S: The extrapyramidal disorders. In Wyngaarden JB, Smith LH (editors): Cecil Textbook of medicine, ed 17, Philadelphia, 1985, WB Saunders Co, vol 2.
10. Feussner JR, Matchar DB: Diagnostic evaluation of the carotid arteries. Health and Public Policy Committee, American College of Physicians, Ann Intern Med 109:835, 1988.

11. Fisher CM: Some neuro-ophthalmological observations, J Neurol Neurosurg Psychiatry 30:383, 1967.

12. Gent M, et al: The Canadian American Ticlopidine Study (CATS) in thromboembolic stroke, Lancet 1:1215, 1989.

13. Greitz T: Computer tomography for diagnosis of intracranial tumors compared with other neuroradiological procedures. In Lindgren T (editor): Computer tomography of brain lesions, Acta Radiol 346(suppl):14, 1975.

14. The Guillain-Barré Syndrome Study Group: Plasmapheresis and acute Guillain-Barré syndrome, Neurology 35:1096, 1985.

14a. Heros RC, Korosue K: Radiation treatment of cerebral arteriovenous malformations, N Engl J Med 323:127, 1990.

15. Jones HJ Jr: Diseases of the peripheral motor-sensory unit. Clinical symposia, New York, 1985, CIBA-Geigy Corporation, vol 37, no 2.

16. Kaneko T, Swada T, Niimi T: Lower limit of blood pressure in treatment of acute hypertension intracranial hemorrhage (AHCH), J Cereb Blood Flow Metabol 3(suppl 1):S51, 1983.

17. Kornblith PL, Walker MD, Cassady JR: Neoplasms of the central nervous system. In DeVita CT Jr, Hellman S, Rosenberg SA (editors): Cancer: principles and practice of oncology, ed 2, Philadelphia, 1985, JB Lippincott Co, vol 2.

18. Lavin P: Management of hypertension in patients with acute stroke, Arch Intern Med 146:66, 1986.

19. Levine SR, Brust JCM, et al: Cerebrovascular complications of the use of the "crack" form of alkaloidal cocaine, N Engl J Med 323:699, 1990.

20. Deleted in proofs.

21. Pleasure DE, Schotland DL: Peripheral nerve disorders. In Rowland LP (editor): Merritt's Textbook of neurology, ed 7, Philadelphia, 1984, Lea & Febiger.

22. Riggs JE: Adult-onset muscle weakness: how to identify the underlying cause, Postgrad Med 78:217, 1985.

23. Sabra AF, et al: Treatment of action tremor in multiple sclerosis with isoniazid, Neurology 39:912, 1982.

24. Schaumburg H: Diseases of the peripheral nervous system. In Wyngaarden JB, Smith LH (editors): Cecil Textbook of medicine, ed 17, Philadelphia, 1985, WB Saunders Co, vol 1.

25. Steinberg GK, Fabrikant JI: Stereotactic heavy charged particle Bragg-peak radiation for intracranial arteriovenous malformations, N Engl J Med 323:96, 1990.

26. Toole JF: Cerebrovascular disorders, ed 3, New York, 1984, Raven Press.

27. Weiner HL, et al: Double-blind study of true vs sham plasma exchange in patients treated with immunosuppression for acute attacks of multiple sclerosis. Neurology 39:1143, 1989.

28. Woolsey RM: Intracerebral hemorrhage (non-traumatic). In Rakel RE (editor): Conn's Current therapy, Philadelphia, 1985, WB Saunders Co.

29. Yahr MD: Parkinsonism. In Rowland LP (editor): Merrit's Textbook of neurology, ed 7, Philadelphia, 1984, Lea & Febiger.

30. Zulch KJ: Brain tumors: their biology and pathology, ed 2, New York, 1965, Springer Publishing Co Inc.

Pulmonary Disease

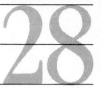

28.1 USE AND INTERPRETATION OF PULMONARY FUNCTION TESTS[22]
George T. Kiss

Indications for pulmonary function testing

1. Physiologic assessment and diagnosis
2. Monitor disease process
3. Special applications
   a. Monitor response to therapy
   b. Exercise testing
   c. Bronchial provocation
   d. Pulmonary disability
   e. Preoperative assessment

Commonly available tests

1. Tests of ventilation
   a. Static lung volume: spirometry for vital capacity parameters and closed circuit helium equilibration to determine functional residual capacity; the patient is instructed to take a maximum inhalation and then exhale completely (Fig. 28-1 illustrates a normal tracing using a bell spirometer)
   b. Dynamic lung volumes
      (1) Forced expirogram (forced vital capacity or time-volume curve) to record a maximum rapid exhalation after a maximum inhalation against time (Fig. 28-2 demonstrates a normal curve using bellows or electronic spirometer)
      (2) Flow-volume curve: to directly measure maximum exhalation and flow with a pneumotachograph or to calculate it from forced expirogram (Fig. 28-3 demonstrates the relationship between flow/volume and time/volume curves, i.e., $V = {}^{\text{volume}}/_{\text{time}}$)
   c. Arterial P_{CO_2} measurement is inversely proportional to alveolar ventilation in the absence of metabolic disturbances
   d. Radioactive xenon (inhaled) or krypton scan and washout to demonstrate and to quantitate regional alterations

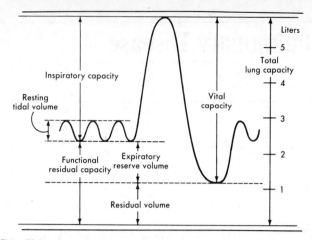

Figure 28-1
Basic spirometry. Lung volumes obtained with a bell spirometer. (From Kiss GT: Diagnosis and treatment of pulmonary disease in primary practice, Baltimore, 1984, The Williams & Wilkins Co.)

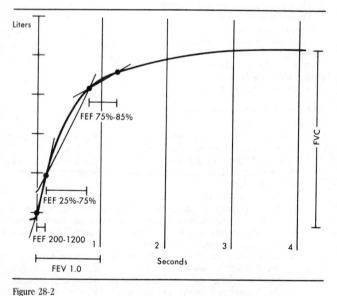

Figure 28-2
Timed vital capacity (or forced expirogram) using bellows or electronic spirometer. (From Kiss GT: Diagnosis and treatment of pulmonary disease in primary practice, Baltimore, 1984, The Williams & Wilkins Co.)

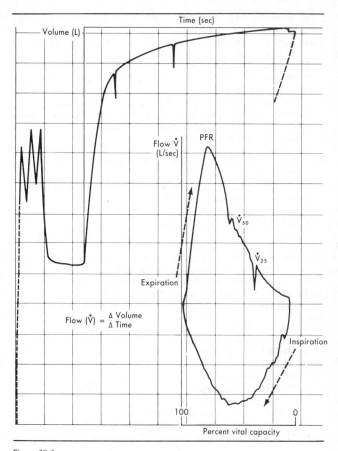

Figure 28-3
Relationship between flow-volume and time-volume curves. (From Kiss GT:
Diagnosis and treatment of pulmonary disease in primary practice, Baltimore, 1984,
The Williams & Wilkins Co.)

    e. Single-breath nitrogen washout is a useful index of uneven distribution of air
    f. Body plethysmography to measure total thoracic gas and airway resistance; total lung capacity values are higher with this method
2. Test of pulmonary mechanics
    a. Maximum voluntary ventilation (MVV): maximum air movement extrapolated to 1 min

  b. Inspiratory force: the negative force generated by a maximum inspiration against a closed airway
  c. Inspiratory pressure and compliance on ventilator patients (i.e., Δ Volume/Δ Pressure
3. Measurement of perfusion: radioactive technetium (given intravenously) or krypton lung scan to localize and to quantitate changes in pulmonary flow
4. Measurement of diffusion (CO diffusing capacity) to express transfer of gas into the blood; it is affected by ventilation, perfusion, hemoglobin level, surface area, thickness, and carbon monoxide concentration
5. Tests of oxygenation
  a. Arterial Pao_2
  b. Oxygen saturation is measured with co-oximeter (transcutaneous methods also available for a and b)
  c. Central venous Po_2 is sampled through pulmonary artery catheter
  d. Hemoglobin content
  e. Carbon monoxide (carboxyhemoglobin level)
  f. Cardiac output

Physiological assessments

Physiological assessment tests are performed according to accepted protocols and the results are expressed as percents of established normals. Therapeutic bronchodilators should be withheld if possible before testing. Fig. 28-4 compares normal obstructive and restrictive ventilatory patterns. Table 28-1 summarizes pulmonary function testing abnormalities in common disorders.

1. The presence of obstructive disorders (e.g., bronchitis, asthma) is evidenced by reduced airflows:
  a. FEV_1/FVC: % predicted
     >80 normal
     65-79 mild obstructive disease
     50-64 moderate obstructive disease
     <50 severe obstructive disease
  b. FEF 25-75: indicates small airways
  c. Peak expiratory flow rate (PEFR): reflects mostly large airways
  d. FEF 50, 25: indicate small airways (flow-volume)

Table 28-1   PFT abnormalities in common disorders

Disorder	FVC	FEV_1	FEV_1/FVC	RV	TLC	Diffusing Capacity
Asthma	↓	↓	↓	↑	N/ ↑	N
COPD	N/ ↓	↓	↓	↑	N/ ↑	N/ ↓
Kyphoscoliosis	↓	↓	N/ ↑	N/ ↓	↓	N
Interstitial fibrosis	↓	↓	N/ ↑	↓	↓	↓

KEY: ↓, Decreased; ↑, increased; N, normal; FVC, forced vital capacity; FEV_1, forced expiratory volume in 1 sec; RV, residual volume; TLC, total lung capacity

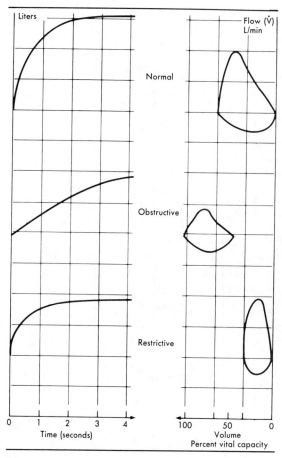

Figure 28-4
Ventilatory patterns of disease. (From Kiss GT: Diagnosis and treatment of
pulmonary disease in primary practice, Baltimore, 1984, The Williams & Wilkins
Co.)

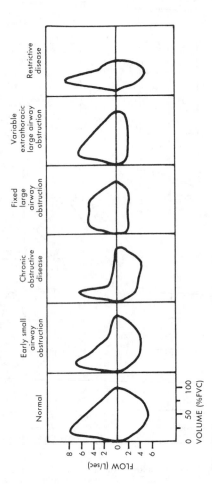

Figure 28-5
Flow-volume curves of restrictive disease and various types of obstructive diseases compared with normal curves. FVC is functional vital capacity.

e. Flow-volume tracing may also indicate extrathoracic obstruction, particularly in the inspiratory phase (Fig. 28-5 compares flow-volume curves in various disease states)

f. Patients with COPD may have a mixture of reversible and irreversible airway obstruction

  (1) Improvement in FEV_1 >15% after inhaled bronchodilator demonstrates reversibility

  (2) Negative response does not exclude reversibility, however, since patients can still have improvement in pulmonary function on long-term bronchodilator therapy

2. Increased residual volume (RV) on spirometry suggests hyperinflation (COPD, asthma); decreased RV occurs in restrictive disease (e.g., interstitial fibrosis) (Fig. 28-6 compares spirometric patterns in obstructive and restrictive disease)

3. Presence of restriction is manifested by a decrease in lung volumes, particularly VC and TLC; it occurs with neuromuscular, skeletal, pleural, and interstitial lung disorders

4. Diffusing capacity is reduced with interstitial disease, thickness of or loss of air exchange surface, and decreased ventilation or perfusion;

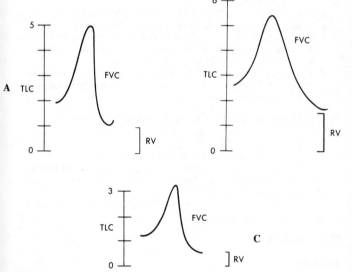

Figure 28-6
Spirometric patterns. TLC, Total lung capacity; FVC, forced vital capacity; RV, residual volume. **A,** Normal person. **B,** Patient with obstructive disease. **C,** Patient with restrictive disease. (From Kiss GT: Diagnosis and treatment of pulmonary disease in primary practice, Baltimore, 1984, The Williams & Wilkins Co.)

useful as an early sign of emphysema or predictor of oxygen desaturation or poor exercise tolerance

Special applications of pulmonary function testing

1. Monitoring treatment
   a. Asthma or bronchospasm: follow peak flow (PEFR) or FEV_1 before and after inhalation treatments
   b. Interstitial lung disease (suspected or proven): perform periodic diffusing capacity
   c. Neuromuscular disorders: follow VC or inspiratory force
2. Exercise testing: indications
   a. To elicit bronchospasm
   b. To elicit hypoxemia
3. Bronchial provocation: done with inhalation of graded methacholine doses to demonstrate susceptibility to bronchospasm
4. Disability testing to compare levels of impairment with published levels
   a. Social Security standards (reflect level of total disability)
   b. As part of comprehensive physiologic evaluation to assess degree of impairment
5. Preoperative assessment
   a. Spirometry is indicated for abdominal and thoracic surgery particularly when patient is more than 65 yr old, has a history of smoking or other lung disease, or if obese
   b. When FEV_1 <2.0 L, FEV_1/FVC <50%, and MVV <50% there is a significantly increased incidence of postoperative complications
   c. If pneumonectomy is considered at above level, residual FEV_1 can be predicted by using quantified radionucleotide perfusion scanning; a residual FEV_1 of <800 ml is usually prohibitive
   d. Postoperative prognosis can be improved, however, by cessation of smoking and an appropriate program of preoperative and perioperative respiratory treatment

Practical approach to pulmonary function testing

1. Forced expirogram/flow volume loop in asymptomatic patient
2. Proceed to full lung volumes if abnormal
3. Determine ABGs for baseline or to assess abnormality
4. Do diffusing capacity for unexplained dyspnea and for evaluation/ progress of interstitial disease; this is of little practical value in presence of severe obstructive disorder
5. Do exercise testing or bronchial provocation testing if airway disorder is suspected but not demonstrated

28.2 PNEUMONIA

Etiology

1. Bacterial
   a. *Streptococcus pneumoniae*
   b. *Haemophilus influenzae*
   c. *Legionella pneumophila*

d. *Klebsiella, Pseudomonas, E. coli*

e. *Staphylococcus aureus*

2. Atypical: usually *Mycoplasma pneumoniae;* however, may be caused by other agents (e.g., *Chlamydia psittaci,* [psittacosis], *Chlamydia trachomatis, Coxiella burnetii* [Q fever], *Chlamdyia pneumoniae* [TWAR])

3. Viral: influenza, adenovirus, CMV, respiratory syncytial virus, herpes

4. Fungal: histoplasmosis, coccidioidomycosis, cryptococcosis, *Aspergillus, Blastomyces*

5. Parasitical: *Pneumocystis carinii*

Diagnostic considerations

1. History
   a. Evaluate predisposing factors
      (1) COPD: *H. influenzae, S. pneumoniae, Legionella*
      (2) Recent seizures: aspiration pneumonia
      (3) Compromised host: *Pneumocystis carinii,* CMV, *Legionella,* gram-negative organisms, fungi, *Mycobacterium intracellulare avium* (MIA)
      (4) Alcoholism: *Klebsiella, S. pneumoniae, H. influenzae*
      (5) IV drug addict with right-sided bacterial endocarditis: *S. aureus*
   b. Distinguish between hospital-acquired vs. community-acquired pneumonia
      (1) Hospital-acquired: gram-negatives, *S. aureus*
      (2) Community-acquired: *S. pneumoniae, M. pneumoniae, H. influenzae*
   c. Consider patient's age
      (1) Infants: viral pneumonia
      (2) Young adults: *M. pneumoniae*
      (3) Adults: *S. pneumoniae*
   d. Rapidity of onset
      (1) Abrupt onset with fever, shaking chills, and copious amounts of rusty-colored sputum: *S. pneumoniae*
      (2) Insidious onset with gradual onset of fever and hacking cough with scant sputum: *M. pneumoniae*

2. Symptoms and physical exam: the presentation varies with the cause of the pneumonia and the patient's age and clinical condition
   a. A patient with *S. pneumoniae* classically presents with high fever, shaking chills, pleuritic chest pain, cough, and copious production of purulent sputum
   b. Patients with viral pneumonia usually present with generalized body aches, malaise, and dry, nonproductive cough
   c. Elderly or immunocompromised hosts may present with only minimal symptoms (e.g., low-grade fever, confusion)

3. Diagnostic methods
   a. Obtain an adequate sputum specimen for Gram stain and cultures
      (1) An expectorated sputum sample is often inadequate because of many false positives (secondary to contamination from oral flora), and many false negatives; a specimen may be considered adequate if the Gram stain shows >25 PMNs and <10 epithelial cells per low-power field

    (2) Aerosol induction with hypertonic saline (3-10%) may increase the diagnostic yield of a sputum

    (3) The use of fiberoptic bronchoscopy to obtain a sputum sample is generally reserved for critically ill patients responding poorly to initial antimicrobial therapy

  b. Chest x-ray: findings vary with the stage and type of pneumonia and the hydration of the patient

    (1) Classically, pneumococcal pneumonia presents with a segmental or lobar infiltrate, *Mycoplasma pneumoniae* shows patchy infiltrates, and viral pneumonia manifests radiographically with hazy infiltrates

    (2) Diffuse infiltrates on chest x-ray can be seen with any of the following: *Legionella* pneumonia, *M. pneumoniae,* viral pneumonia, *Pneumocystis carinii,* hypersensitivity pneumonitis, psittaccosis, Q fever, aspergillosis, aspiration pneumonia, miliary TB, and ARDS associated with pneumonia

    (3) An initial chest x-ray is also useful to rule out the presence of any complications (pneumothorax, empyema, abscesses)

  c. Additional lab evaluation

    (1) WBC with differential: a low WBC can be present with viral pneumonia or overwhelming bacterial pneumonias

    (2) Blood cultures: positive in approximately 20% of cases of pneumococcal pneumonia

    (3) Special studies

      (a) Viral titers: a fourfold increase in paired acute and convalescent sera is considered diagnostic of viral pneumonia

      (b) *Legionella* titer: a single titer of $\geq 1:256$ or a fourfold rise in indirect fluorescent antibodies to a titer of at least $1:128$ is diagnostic

      (c) *Mycoplasma pneumoniae* complement fixation titer: a single, high titer $\geq 1:32$ or a fourfold rise from acute to convalescent is diagnostic of *M. pneumoniae*

      (d) Direct immunofluorescent exam of sputum (e.g., direct fluorescent antibody [DFA] sputum evaluation for *Legionella*)

      (e) Cold agglutinins: nonspecific; positive in only about 50% of patients with *M. pneumoniae*

      (f) Counterimmunoelectrophoresis (CIE) can be performed on sputum or serum to detect bacterial antigens; coagglutination is also useful in patients partially treated with antibiotics

      (g) ABGs: useful to evaluate degree of hypoxia and need of oxygen therapy

      (h) Quellung reaction: swelling of bacterial capsule when exposed to antibody; used for diagnosis of *S. pneumoniae*

Characteristics and therapy of common pneumonias

1. *S. pneumoniae* (pneumococcal pneumonia)

  a. Most common bacterial pneumonia

  b. Predisposing factors are splenectomy, COPD, sickle cell disease, CHF, cigarette smoking, lung cancer, cerebrovascular disease, de-

mentia, institutionalization, seizure disorder, renal failure, cardio-vascular disease, and immunosuppression
c. Gram stain of sputum shows lancet-shaped gram-positive cocci
d. Treatment
    (1) IV: aqueous penicillin G 600,000 U q6h; 2 million units IV q4-6h in life-threatening infections
    (2) IM: procaine penicillin G 600,000 U q8-12h
    (3) PO: penicillin V 250-500 mg PO q6h
    (4) Erythromycin 500 mg PO/IV q6h is indicated in penicillin-allergic patients
    (5) Duration of therapy is 10-14 days

2. *H. influenzae*
    a. Common in COPD, elderly patients, and children under 6 yr of age
    b. Gram stain reveals pleomorphic, small, coccobacillary gram-negative organisms
    c. Treatment
        (1) IV
            (a) Ampicillin 1.0-1.5 g q4h in known ampicillin-susceptible strains
            (b) Cefuroxime in suspected or known ampicillin-resistant strains
            (c) Alternatives are trimethoprim/sulfamethoxazole or chloramphenicol (in patients allergic to the above antibiotics)
        (2) PO
            (a) Ampicillin 500 mg PO q6h in ampicillin-susceptible strains
            (b) Alternative antibiotics are trimethoprim/sulfomethoxazole (e.g., Bactrim-DS 1 tab bid for 7-10 days), cefaclor 250 mg tid, or cefuroxime 250 mg bid for 10 days)

3. *Mycoplasma pneumoniae* (atypical pneumonia)
    a. Generally involves young adults and children
    b. Characteristic finding on physical exam is bullous myringitis
    c. "Walking pneumonia": slow onset, nonproductive cough, myalgias, arthralgias
    d. Treatment: erythromycin 500 g PO/IV q6h
    e. Duration of therapy is 14-21 days

4. *Legionella pneumophila* pneumonia
    a. Associated with water sources, air conditioning units
    b. Sporadic cases often involve immunocompromised patients
    c. Often associated with diarrhea, bradycardia, liver abnormalities, and mentation difficulties
    d. Serological examination of the sputum for direct fluorescent antigen (DFA) is useful for rapid diagnosis
    e. Treatment: erythromycin 1 g IV q6h; in critically ill patients, addition of rifampin 600 mg PO bid is recommended; doxycycline is the drug of choice in patients allergic to erythromycin
    f. Duration of therapy is at least 2 wk

5. Aspiration pneumonia
    a. Should be suspected in alcoholics, seizure disorders, repeated vomiting, excessive sedation

   b. X-ray generally demonstrates infiltrates in the inferior segment of the right upper lobe or apical segment of the lower lobe

   c. Organisms commonly involved are *Peptostreptococcus, Fusobacterium, Bacteroides melaninogenicus,* aerobic streptococci, and mixed aerobes/anaerobes generally present in the mouth

   d. Treatment: penicillin G 2 million U IV q4-6h or clindamycin 600-900 mg IV q8h

   e. In hospitalized patients, aspiration pneumonia may be caused by more resistant organisms as a result of colonization of the oral pharynx with such organisms as *S. aureus* and gram-negatives; treatment should be directed toward them with a combination of cephalosporin and aminoglycoside (e.g., cefuroxime and gentamicin)

6. *Staphylococcus aureus* pneumonia

   a. High-risk groups are elderly patients recovering from influenza infection, narcotic abusers, and immunosuppressed patients

   b. Chest x-ray often shows a multicentric patchy appearance secondary to multiple abscess formation; pleural effusions and air fluid levels are often seen

   c. Treatment

      (1) Nafcillin 1.5-2.0 g IV q4h; alternatives are vancomycin 500 mg q6h or cephalothin 1.5-2.0 g q4h IV

      (2) Penicillin susceptible strains should be treated with penicillin G, 2 million units IV q4h

   d. Duration of therapy is at least 3 wk

7. *Klebsiella pneumoniae* and other gram-negative pneumonias[20]

   a. *Klebsiella*

      (1) Common in alcoholics

      (2) Gram stain reveals encapsulated gram-negative bacilli

      (3) Treatment: aminoglycoside plus cephalosporin (e.g., cefuroxime); antibiotic dosage must be adjusted for creatinine clearance, and levels must be carefully monitored to avoid renal impairment

   b. Other gram-negative bacilli

      (1) Common in immunosuppressed, elderly, and hospitalized patients

      (2) The risk of gram-negative nosocomial pneumonia due to retrograde colonization of the pharynx from the stomach is increased in patients with elevated gastric pH (e.g., those on H_2 blockers); sucralfate is preferable to antacids and H_2 blockers for prophylaxis of stress-ulcer bleeding in patients on respirators[12]

      (3) Treatment: amikacin and azlocillin in immunocompromised patients with suspected *Pseudomonas aeruginosa;* adequate treatment of other gram-negative pneumonias is the same as for *Klebsiella*

8. *Moraxella (Branhamella) catarrhalis*

   a. Often seen in patients with COPD or impaired immune response (secondary to glucocorticoids, neoplasms, or diabetes mellitus)

   b. Diagnosis: sputum culture

   c. Treatment: cefaclor, erythromycin, tetracycline, or combination of ampicillin and clavulanic acid (Augmentin)

Initial antibiotic therapy

1. Initial antibiotic therapy should be based on clinical, radiographic, and lab evaluation; if the clinical diagnosis is substantiated by an adequate Gram stain (e.g., lancet-shaped gram-positive cocci in a patient with suspected pneumococcal pneumonia) the choice of initial therapy is relatively simple (penicillin)

2. In otherwise healthy adult patients with community-acquired pneumonia and insidious presentation, erythromycin is the antibiotic of choice since it will adequately treat *Mycoplasma* and pneumococci

3. In immunocompromised patients with negative Gram stain, the initial antibiotic treatment should be broad spectrum but with emphasis on gram-negatives, *Legionella,* and *Staphylococcus aureus;* the following antibiotics should be considered[24]:

   a. Patients with AIDS

      (1) Trimethoprim/sulfamethoxazole or pentamidine for *Pneumocystis carinii* (see Section 25.4)

   b. Neutropenic patients

      (1) Amikacin and azlocillin for *Pseudomonas aeruginosa*

      (2) Erythromycin for *Legionella*

      (3) Nafcillin for *S. aureus*

   c. Immunocompromised, non-AIDS, non-neutropenic patients (e.g., DM, elderly, COPD)

      (1) Cefuroxime, plus

      (2) Erythromycin, plus

      (3) Aminoglycoside (if pneumonia is hospital acquired)

   NOTE: Erythromycin should be part of the initial therapy because of the high prevalence of *Legionella pneumophila* in immunocompromised hosts[7]

28.3   TUBERCULOSIS

Diagnosis[30,31]

1. Clinical manifestations: many patients are asymptomatic at the time of diagnosis; others may complain of dry, nonproductive cough, night-sweats, fever, anorexia, fatigue, dyspnea, pleuritic chest pain, and hemoptysis

2. Physical exam may reveal rales near the lung apices

3. Tuberculin test

   a. Five tuberculin units (TU) of purified protein derivative (PPD) in 0.1 ml of solution is injected intracutaneously

   b. Sensitized individuals demonstrate a dermal reaction of redness, swelling, and induration

   c. A positive reaction is defined as ≥10 mm of induration at 48 hr*

   d. Up to 25% of patients with newly diagnosed TB have a negative tuberculin skin test, particularly patients with renal failure, elderly patients, patients on steroid or immunosuppressive therapy, and patients with HIV infection, severe protein deficiency, concomitant live virus vaccination or infection (e.g., measles, polio), lymphoma, or sarcoidosis

---

*≥ 5 mm of induration is considered positive in persons with HIV infection, recent contact with TB, or fibrotic lesions on chest radiographs likely to represent old healed TB.

    e. In patients with inconclusive skin tests, sensitivity can be significantly increased by reexamining the skin test after 7 days; if results are still inconclusive, a repeat tuberculin test is advisable

4. Acid-fast stain and cultures of sputum
5. Chest x-ray
    a. Initial film may show a variety of patterns; rarely, it may be completely normal
    b. Parenchymal infiltrates most commonly involve the upper lobes (apical and posterior segments)
    c. Hilar and paratracheal adenopathy, unilateral pleural effusion, and cavitary lesions may also be present

Treatment in adults[2]

1. A 6 mo regimen is indicated in compliant patients with fully susceptible organisms
    a. Initial 2 mo
      (1) Isoniazid 5 mg/kg/day (up to 300 mg/day) PO qd, plus
      (2) Rifampin 10-20 mg/kg/day (up to 600 mg/day) PO qd, plus
      (3) Pyrazinamide 15-30 mg/kg (up to 2 g/day) PO qd
      (4) Ethambutol 15-25 mg/kg PO qd (up to 2.5 g/day) should be included in the initial 2 mo if isoniazid resistance is suspected
    b. Remaining 4 mo: isoniazid plus rifampin
2. A modified 6 mo low-dose (62 doses) regimen is also effective[5]
    a. Daily isoniazid, rifampin, pyrazinamide, and IM streptomycin (750 mg if <50 kg body weight or 1 g if >50 kg) for the initial 2 wk
    b. Isoniazid, rifampin, pyrazinamide, and streptomycin given twice weekly from wk 3 through 8
    c. Isoniazid and rifampin twice weekly from wk 9 through 26
3. Patient compliance is essential to any therapeutic regimen
4. Immunosuppressed patients (e.g., AIDS, HIV infection) should be treated for longer than 6 mo, probably for 9-12 mo[1]
5. Extrapulmonary TB is treated in the same manner as pulmonary TB

Prophylaxis[2]

1. General indications
    a. Household members and other close contacts of potentially infectious persons
    b. Newly infected persons (tuberculin skin test conversion within the past 2 yr)
    c. Persons with past tuberculosis or those with a significant tuberculin reaction and abnormal chest x-ray in whom current tuberculosis has been excluded
    d. Persons with positive PPD in the following clinical situations:
      (1) Silicosis
      (2) Diabetes mellitus
      (3) Adrenocorticosteroid therapy (long term)
      (4) Immunosuppressive therapy or diseases
      (5) AIDS or positive antibodies to HIV
      (6) Reticuloendothelial malignancies (e.g., leukemia, Hodgkin's disease)

(7) End-stage renal disease
(8) Clinical conditions associated with rapid weight loss or chronic undernutrition (e.g., post-gastrectomy, chronic malabsorption, chronic peptic ulcer disease)
(9) Tuberculin skin reactors under 35 yr of age
2. Therapy
a. Isoniazid 300 mg PO qd
b. Duration of therapy is 6-12 mo (lifetime in patients with positive PPD and silicosis)
c. Monitoring adverse effects of isoniazid in patients with a history of liver abnormalities or frequent alcohol usage and in those 35 yr of age or older; this consists of monthly symptom reviews and measurement of hepatic enzymes before starting isoniazid therapy and periodically throughout treatment; in patients younger than 35 yr a monthly symptom review is adequate
d. Possible complications of isoniazid therapy include acute hepatitis and hepatic necrosis; isoniazid should be discontinued and another drug substituted if hepatic enzymes increase to 3-5 times normal or if the patient develops signs or symptoms of hepatitis

| 28.4 | CARCINOMA OF THE LUNG

Epidemiology

1. Leading cause of cancer deaths in both men (15% of cancer deaths) and women (18% of cancer deaths)
2. Increased incidence in active or passive smokers and exposure to certain environmental (e.g., radon) and industrial agents (e.g., ionizing radiation, asbestos, nickel, uranium, vinyl chloride)

Histological classification

The World Health Organization distinguishes 12 types of pulmonary neoplasms[15]; among these the major types are squamous cell carcinoma, adenocarcinoma, small cell carcinoma, and large cell carcinoma. However, the crucial differential in the diagnosis of lung cancer is between small cell and non–small cell types, since the therapeutic approach is totally different.[34] Selected characteristics of the various histological cell types are described in Table 28-2.

Diagnosis

1. Characteristics and clinical manifestations
a. Weight loss, fatigue, fever, anorexia
b. Cough, hemoptysis, dyspnea
c. Chest, shoulder, and bone pain
d. Paraneoplastic syndromes
(1) Eaton-Lambert syndrome: myopathy characterized by increased strength and EMG amplitude with repeated effort, reversal with guanidine; this syndrome is often seen with small cell carcinoma
(2) Endocrine manifestations
(a) Ectopic ACTH, SIADH: small cell carcinoma

Table 28-2 Selected characteristics of lung carcinomas

Histological Cell Type	Percentage of Total	Frequent Location	Initial Metastases	Comments
Adenocarcinoma	33–35	Mid-lung and periphery	Lymphatics	Associated with peripheral scars
Squamous cell (epidermoid)	30–32	Central	Local invasion	Frequent cavitation and obstructive phenomena
Small-cell (oat-cell)	20–25	Central	Lymphatics	Cavitation rare Associated with deletion of short arm of chromosome 3'
Large-cell	15–20	Periphery	CNS Mediastinum	Rapid growth rate with early metastases
Bronchioloalveolar	5	Periphery	Lymphatics, hematogenous, and local invasion	No correlation with cigarette smoking Cavitation rare

        (b) Hypercalcemia secondary to PTH-like substances: squamous cell carcinoma
- (3) Neurologic: subacute cerebellar degeneration, peripheral neuropathy, cortical degeneration
- (4) Musculoskeletal: polymyositis, clubbing, hypertrophic pulmonary osteoarthropathy
- (5) Hematological/vascular: migratory thrombophlebitis, marantic thrombosis, anemia, thrombocytosis/thrombocytopenia
- (6) Cutaneous: acanthosis nigricans, dermatomyositis

e. Pleural effusion (10% of patients), recurrent pneumonias (secondary to obstruction), localized wheezing

f. Superior vena cava syndrome
- (1) Obstruction of venous return in the superior vena cava, most commonly caused by bronchogenic carcinoma; other causes are lymphomas, thyroid goiter, tuberculosis and other granulomatous diseases, pericardial constriction, syphilitic aortic aneurysms
- (2) The patient usually complains of headache, nausea, dizziness, visual changes, syncope, and respiratory distress
- (3) Physical exam reveals distention of thoracic and neck veins, edema of face and upper extremities, facial plethora, and cyanosis
- (4) Chest x-ray demonstrates a superior mediastinal mass
- (5) Treatment varies with the cause of SVC syndrome; irradiation is used when secondary to non–small cell lung carcinoma; combination chemotherapy with or without local irradiation is recommended in SVC syndrome due to small cell lung carcinoma

g. Horner's syndrome: constricted pupil, ptosis, facial anhidrosis caused by spinal cord damage between C8 and T1 secondary to a superior sulcus tumor (bronchogenic carcinoma at the extreme lung apex); a superior sulcus tumor associated with ipsilateral Horner's syndrome and shoulder pain is known as a "Pancoast tumor"

2. Cytological exam of at least three sputum specimens unless a positive cytology is obtained in the first or second specimen

3. Chest x-ray
a. The radiographic presentation often varies with the cell type; for example, squamous cell and large cell carcinoma often present as a peripheral mass, adenocarcinoma generally appears as a peripheral nodule, small cell anaplastic carcinoma can present as a perihilar mass or a peripheral nodule

b. Pleural effusion, lobar atelectasis, and mediastinal adenopathy can accompany any of the above cell types

c. Benign lesions that simulate thoracic malignancy are listed below[25]
- (1) Lobar atelectasis: pneumonia, tuberculosis, chronic inflammatory disease, allergic bronchopulmonary aspergillosis
- (2) Multiple pulmonary nodules: septic emboli, Wegener's granulomatosis, sarcoidosis, rheumatoid nodules, fungal disease, multiple pulmonary AV fistulas

       (3) Mediastinal adenopathy: sarcoidosis, lymphoma, primary tuber-
culosis, fungal disease, silicosis, pneumoconiosis, drug induced
(e.g., phenytoin, trimethadione)

       (4) Pleural effusion: CHF, pneumonia with parapneumonic effusion,
tuberculosis, viral pleuritis, ascites, pancreatitis, collagen-
vascular disease

4. Thoracentesis of pleural effusions, with cytological evaluation of the
obtained fluid (see Section 30.2)
5. CT of chest: to evaluate mediastinal and pleural extension of suspected
lung neoplasms
6. Establish tissue diagnosis of lung cancer
   a. Sputum cytology
   b. Biopsy of any suspicious lymph nodes (e.g., supraclavicular node)
   c. Flexible fiberoptic bronchoscopy: brush and biopsy specimens are
obtained from any visualized endobronchial lesions
   d. Transbronchial needle aspiration[39]: done via a special needle passed
through the bronchoscope; this technique is useful to sample mediastinal masses or paratracheal lymph nodes
   e. Transthoracic fine needle aspiration biopsy with fluoroscopic or CT
guidance to evaluate peripheral pulmonary nodules
   f. Mediastinoscopy and anterior mediastinotomy are used in suspected
tumor involvement of the mediastinum
   g. Exploratory thoracotomy is indicated in patients at high risk of having lung carcinoma (e.g., heavy smokers) who are being considered
for surgical resection to cure a pulmonary neoplasm

Screening

Routine screening of smokers with chest x-rays or sputum cytology has not
been found to alter the mortality rates from lung carcinoma and is therefore
not recommended.[13]

Staging

The most widely accepted staging system is the TNM system (tumor, node,
metastasis) recommended by the American Joint Committee on Cancer.[4]
However, in patients with small cell lung cancer, a more practical and
widely accepted staging system is the one developed by the Veterans Administration Lung Cancer Study Group (VALG).[41] This system contains
two stages:

1. Limited stage: disease confined to the regional lymph nodes and to one
hemithorax (excluding pleural surfaces)
2. Extensive stage: disease spread beyond the confines of limited stage disease

    Pretreatment staging procedures for lung cancer patients, in addition to
a complete history and physical exam, generally include the following
tests:

1. Chest x-ray (PA and lateral), ECG
2. Lab evaluation: CBC, electrolytes, platelets, calcium, phosphorus, glucose, renal and liver function studies, ABG, and skin test for tuberculosis

3. Pulmonary function studies
4. CT of chest
5. Mediastinoscopy or anterior mediastinotomy in patients being considered for possible curative lung resection
6. Biopsy of any accessible suspicious lesions
7. CT of liver and brain; radionuclide scans of bone in all patients with small cell carcinoma of the lung and patients with non–small cell lung neoplasms suspected of involving these organs
8. Bone marrow aspiration and biopsy only in patients with small cell carcinoma of the lung

Treatment

1. Non–small cell carcinoma
   a. Surgery
      (1) Surgical resection is indicated in patients with limited disease* (approximately 15-30% of newly diagnosed cases); the 5 yr survival rate is approximately 30%
      (2) Preoperative evaluation includes review of cardiac status (e.g., recent MI, major dysrhythmias) and evaluation of pulmonary function (to determine if the patient can tolerate any loss of lung tissue)
         (a) Pneumonectomy is possible if the patient has a preoperative $FEV_1 \geq 2$ L or if the MVV is >50% of predicted capacity[33]
         (b) In patients with equivocal results, a ventilation-perfusion lung scan provides information regarding the percentage of ventilation contributed by the non–tumor-bearing lung; if this value when multiplied by the FEV_1 is ≥ 1 L, the pneumonectomy is functionally tolerable[28] (e.g., if the preoperative $FEV_1 = 1.9$ and a lung scan demonstrates that the percentage of ventilation of the non–tumor-bearing lung is equal to 60%, the product of these two values [1.9×0.6] = 1.14, a value within the safe range)
   b. Treatment of unresectable non–small cell carcinoma of the lung
      (1) Radiotherapy can be used alone or in combination with chemotherapy; it is used primarily for treatment of CNS and skeletal metastases, SVC syndrome, and obstructive atelectasis; thoracic irradiation does not prolong survival in patients with locally advanced unresectable non–small cell lung cancer[18]
      (2) Chemotherapy: there are various combination regimens available (e.g., MVP [combination of mitomycin, vinblastine, and platinol]); however, the overall results are disappointing
2. Treatment of small cell bronchogenic carcinoma
   a. The main therapeutic approach consists of aggressive chemotherapy with or without irradiation; the few patients who remain free of cancer after 2 yr are at high risk for the development of second malignancies and therefore require close follow-up[18]

---

*Not involving mediastinal nodes, ribs, pleura, or distant sites.

b. Thoracic radiotherapy generally plays only a secondary role in the treatment of these patients
c. Surgical resection combined with chemotherapy (CAV, CAVP-16, VP-16 plus cisplatin) may be useful only in selected patients with limited disease

28.5 MECHANICAL VENTILATION[36,37]

Indications for mechanical ventilation

The decision to initiate mechanical ventilation is generally based on the following:

1. Clinical assessment: presence of apnea, tachypnea (>40 breaths/min), or respiratory failure that cannot be adequately corrected by any other means
2. ABGs: severe hypoxemia despite high-flow oxygen or significant CO_2 retention (e.g., Po_2 <50, Pco_2 >50)
3. Physiological parameters are of limited use since many patients with respiratory insufficiency are unable to perform PFTs and their respiratory failure mandates immediate intervention; some of the commonly accepted physiological parameters for intubation and respiratory support are
   a. Vital capacity <15 ml/kg
   b. Inspiratory force < -25 cm H_2O
   c. FEV_1 <10 ml/kg

NOTE: The clinical assessment is the most important determinant of the need for mechanical ventilation since both physiological parameters and ABGs do not distinguish between acute and chronic respiratory insufficiency (e.g., a Pco_2 >60 mm Hg and a respiratory rate >30/min) may be the "norm" for a patient with COPD, whereas the same values in a young otherwise healthy adult are indications for intubation and mechanical ventilation).

Common modes of mechanical ventilation

1. Intermittent mandatory ventilation (IMV): the patient is allowed to breathe spontaneously and the ventilator delivers a number of machine breaths at a preset rate and volume
   a. Advantages and indications
      (1) IMV is indicated in the majority of spontaneously breathing patients because it maintains respiratory muscle tone and results in less depression of cardiac output than assist/control
      (2) It is useful for weaning, because as the IMV rate is decreased the patient gradually assumes the bulk of the breathing work
   b. Disadvantages
      (1) The increased work of breathing results in increased oxygen consumption (deleterious to patients with myocardial insufficiency)
      (2) IMV is not useful in patients with depressed respiratory drive or impaired neurologic status

2. Assist/control: the patient breathes at his own rate and the ventilator senses the inspiratory effort and delivers a preset tidal volume with each patient effort; if the patient's respiratory rate decreases past a preset rate, the ventilator delivers tidal breaths at the present rate
   a. Advantages/indications: useful in patients with neuromuscular weakness, or CNS disturbances
   b. Disadvantages
      (1) Tachypnea may result in significant hypocapnia and respiratory alkalosis
      (2) Improper setting of sensitivity to the negative pressure necessary to trigger the ventilator may result in "fighting the ventilator" when the sensitivity is set too low
      (3) Increased sensitivity may result in hyperventilation; sensitivity is generally set so that an inspiratory effort of 2-3 cm will trigger ventilation
      (4) The respiratory muscle tone is not well maintained in patients on assist/control and this may result in difficulty with weaning
3. Controlled ventilation: the patient does not breathe spontaneously; the respiratory rate is determined by the physician
   a. Advantages and indications
      (1) Useful in patients who are unable to make an inspiratory effort (e.g., severe CNS dysfunction) and in patients with excessive agitation or breathing effort
      (2) Patients with excessive agitation are often sedated with morphine or benzodiazepines and paralyzed with pancuronium bromide (Pavulon); adequate sedation is necessary to eliminate awareness of paralysis
      (3) Initial pancuronium dose is 0.08 mg/kg IV in adults
      (4) Later incremental doses starting at 0.01 mg/kg may be used prn to maintain paralysis; pancuronium should be administered only by or under the supervision of experienced clinicians; a combination of neostigmine/atropine can be used to reverse the action of the pancuronium
   b. Disadvantages: paralyzed patients on controlled ventilation must be closely monitored because ventilator malfunction or disconnection is rapidly fatal

Selection of ventilator settings

1. Tidal volume (TV): 10-15 ml/kg of ideal body weight
2. Rate (number of tidal breaths delivered/minute): 8-16 depending on the desired $Paco_2$ or pH (increased rate = decreased $Paco_2$)
3. Mode: IMV, assist/control, controlled ventilation
4. Oxygen concentration (FIo_2): the initial FIo_2 should be 100% unless it is evident that a lower FIo_2 will provide adequate oxygenation
5. Obtain ABGs 15 to 30 min after initiating mechanical ventilation
6. Immediate chest x-ray is indicated after intubation to evaluate for correct placement of endotracheal tube
7. Sedation orders (e.g., morphine, diazepam) may be necessary in selected patients

8. Positive end-expiratory pressure (PEEP)
   a. The application of positive pressure may prevent the closure of edematous small airways; it is indicated when arterial oxygenation is inadequate (saturation <90%) despite an FIo_2 >50%
   b. PEEP is generally started at 5 cm of H_2O and increased by increments of 2-5 cm to maintain the Pao_2 ≥60 mm Hg
   c. The use of PEEP can result in pulmonary barotrauma and hemodynamic compromise (secondary to decreased right ventricular filling)
   d. Patients receiving PEEP should have their cardiac output frequently monitored; the measurement of mixed venous oxygen saturation is useful to evaluate the effect of PEEP on cardiac output[19]
9. Adjust the initial ventilator setting depending on results of the ABGs and clinical response
   a. Use the lowest FIo_2 necessary to maintain a Pao_2 >60 mm Hg (90% hemoglobin saturation in patients with a normal pH)
   b. Adjust minute ventilation (tidal volume × rate) to normalize the pH and the $Paco_2$
      (1) Increasing the TV or the rate will decrease $Paco_2$ and increase the pH
      (2) Do not lower the $Paco_2$ below the "norm" for that patient (e.g., some patients with COPD should be allowed to maintain their usual mildly elevated $Paco_2$ to avoid alkalosis and to provide stimulus for breathing)

Major complications of mechanical ventilation[21]

1. Pulmonary barotrauma (e.g., pneumomediastinum, pneumothorax, subcutaneous emphysema, emphysema, pneumoperitoneum): generally secondary to high levels of PEEP, excessive tidal volumes, high peak airway pressures, and coexistence of significant lung disease
2. Pulmonary thromboemboli can be prevented by vigorous leg care, TED stockings, and use of prophylactic low-dose heparin (i.e., 5000 U SQ q12h)
3. GI bleeding: prophylaxis with sucralfate suspension, 1 g qid via NG tube, is generally indicated in patients on mechanical ventilators
4. Dysrhythmias: avoid use of dysrhythmogenic drugs and prevent rapid acid-base shifts
5. Accumulation of large amount of secretions: frequent respiratory toilet is necessary in all patients on mechanical ventilators
6. Other: nosocomial infections, laryngotracheal injury, malnutrition, hypophosphatemia, oxygen toxicity, psychosis

Withdrawal of mechanical ventilatory support

1. Common criteria for ventilator weaning
   a. Improved clinical status (the patient is alert and hemodynamically stable)
   b. Adequate oxygenation (Pao_2 >60 mm Hg on 40% FIo_2)
   c. pH 7.33-7.48, with acceptable $Paco_2$
   d. Respiratory rate ≤25/min
   e. Vital capacity ≥10 ml/kg

   f. Resting minute ventilation <10 L/min, with ability to double the resting minute ventilation

   g. Maximum inspiratory pressure more negative than −20 cm H_2O

NOTE: The above criteria are only gidelines; significant variation may be present (e.g., a respiratory rate of 30 breaths/minute may be acceptable in a patient with COPD).

2. Methods of weaning

   a. Weaning via IMV

      (1) Gradually decrease the IMV as tolerated (e.g., two breaths every 3-4 hr), monitoring ABGs after each adjustment

      (2) Do not change more than one parameter at a time

      (3) When the patient is tolerating an IMV of 4-6, a trial with a T-tube can be attempted; the T-tube is attached to the endotracheal tube and delivers humidified oxygen (FIo_2 40%)

      (4) If the patient tolerates the T-tube well, extubation may be attempted

         (a) Have adequate equipment and personnel available if reintubation is necessary (start early in the day)

         (b) Suction airway and oropharynx

         (c) Deflate cuff and extubate

         (d) Administer oxygen via facemask (FIo_2 40-100%)

         (e) Auscultate the lungs for adequate air movement

         (f) Closely monitor vital signs

         (g) Obtain ABGs approximately 15 to 30 min postextubation

         (h) Reintubate if extubation is poorly tolerated

   b. Stable patients without pulmonary disease and with a good probability of quick extubation (e.g., after uncomplicated cardiac surgery) may be given a direct trial of T-tube (bypassing gradual decreases of IMV)

Failure to wean from mechanical ventilator

Failure usually results from premature attempts at weaning (e.g., patient is hemodynamically unstable). Other common reversible causes of failure to wean are

1. Hypophosphatemia and nutritional deficiency
2. Drug toxicity (e.g., excessive CNS depression from sedatives)
3. Bronchospasm
4. Excessive secretions
5. Significant acid-base disturbances
6. Hypothyroidism

 ACUTE BRONCHOSPASM

Status asthmaticus

Definition

Status asthmaticus is characterized by severe continuous bronchospasm.

Clinical manifestations[14]

1. Usually there is a history of progressively worsening dyspnea, cough, tachypnea, chest tightness, and wheezing over a period of hours to days
2. The patient is generally sitting forward, is diaphoretic, and may be unable to speak because of severe dyspnea
3. Physical exam may reveal
   a. Tachycardia and tachypnea
   b. Use of accessory respiratory muscles
   c. Pulsus paradoxus (inspiratory decline in systolic blood pressure >10 mm Hg)
   d. Wheezing; the absence of wheezing (silent chest) or decreased wheezing can indicate worsening obstruction
   e. Mental status changes; these are generally secondary to hypoxia and hypercapnia and constitute an indication for urgent intubation
   f. An important sign of impending respiratory crisis is paradoxic abdominal and diaphragmatic movement on inspiration (detected by palpation over the upper part of the abdomen in a semirecumbent position); it indicates diaphragmatic fatigue[6]; aminophylline infusion is effective in improving diaphragmatic contractility in these patients

Lab and radiographic evaluation

1. ABGs can be used in staging the severity of the asthmatic attack
   a. Mild: decreased Pa_{O_2} and Pa_{CO_2}, increased pH
   b. Moderate: decreased Pa_{O_2}, normal Pa_{CO_2}, normal pH
   c. Severe: markedly decreased Pa_{O_2}, increased Pa_{CO_2}, and decreased pH
2. CBC: leukocytosis with "left shift" may indicate coexistence of bacterial infection (e.g., pneumonia)
3. Sputum: eosinophils, Charcot-Leyden crystals; PMNs and bacteria may be found on Gram stain in patients with pneumonia
4. Chest x-ray: generally shows only evidence of thoracic hyperinflation (e.g., flattening of diaphragm, increased volume of the retrosternal airspace)

Additional evaluation

1. ECG: tachycardia and nonspecific ST-T wave changes; may also show cor pulmonale, RBBB, right axis deviation, counterclockwise rotation
2. Pulmonary function tests: FEV_1 <1 L and peak expiratory flow rate (PEFR) <80 L/min indicate severe bronchospasm

Treatment

1. Oxygen is available via nasal cannula (each L/min of flow generally adds 2% to the FI_{O_2}) or with Ventimask (24, 28, 31, 35, 40, 50 %)
   a. It is generally started at 2-4 L/min via nasal cannula or Ventimask at 40% FI_{O_2}
   b. Further adjustments are made according to the ABGs
2. Sympathomimetics: various agents and modalities are available
   a. Epinephrine (1:1000 dilution)
      (1) Dosage range is 0.3-0.5 ml SQ; may repeat after 15-20 min
      (2) Onset of action is within 15 min

      (3) Duration is less than 1-4 hr

      (4) Use with caution in patients over 40 yr or anyone with heart disease

  b. Terbutaline (Brethine)

      (1) May be given SQ 0.25 mg q6-8h

      (2) Clinically significant increase in FEV_1 occurs within 15 min and persists for 90 min to 4 hr

      (3) It generally has fewer cardiac stimulating effects than epinephrine, however, systemic vasodilatation with compensatory tachycardia can occur

  c. Metaproterenol (Alupent)

      (1) May be administered via aerosol nebulizer, bulb nebulizer, or IPPB (e.g., 0.3 ml of metaproterenol in 3 ml of saline, given via nebulizer)

      (2) Onset of action is within 5 min, duration is 3-4 hr

  d. Isoetharine (Bronkosol): 0.25-0.5 ml in 3 ml of saline via nebulizer q4h is also effective; however, its duration is less than that of metaproterenol

3. Theophylline: refer to Chapter 32 for loading and maintenance doses

4. Corticosteroids

  a. Early administration is advised, particularly in patients receiving steroids at home

  b. Patients may be started on hydrocortisone (Solu-Cortef) 2.5-4 mg/kg or methylprednisolone (Solu-Medrol) 0.5-1 mg/kg IV loading and then q6h prn; higher doses may be necessary in selected patients (particularly those receiving steroids at home); steroids given by inhalation (e.g., beclomethasone, 2 inhalations qid, maximum 20 inhalations/day) are also useful in controlling bronchospasm and tapering off oral steroids

  c. Rapid but judicious tapering of corticosteroids will eliminate serious steroid toxicity; long-term low-dose methotrexate is an effective means of reducing the systemic corticosteroid requirements of patients with severe asthma[29]

  d. The most common error regarding steroid therapy in acute bronchospasm is the use of "too little, too late"

5. Atropine analogs (e.g., ipratropium bromide, 2 inhalations qid, maximum 12 inhalations in 24 hr) may be useful in patients not responding well to beta agonists and whose bronchospasm is secondary to bronchitis; their benefit is usually limited to the initial 12-24 hr

6. IV hydration: judicious use is necessary to avoid pulmonary edema

7. IV antibiotics are indicated when there is suspicion of bacterial infection (e.g., infiltrate on chest x-ray, fever, or leukocytosis)

8. Intubation and mechanical ventilation are indicated when above measures fail to produce significant improvement

9. General anesthesia: halothane may reverse bronchospasm in a severe asthmatic who cannot be ventilated adequately by mechanical means

10. Intravenous magnesium sulfate supplementation in patients with low or borderline-low magnesium levels may improve acute bronchospasm and airflow

Exacerbation of COPD

Clinical manifestations

Patients with COPD are classically subdivided into two major groups based on their appearance:

1. "Blue bloaters" are patients with chronic bronchitis; they derive their name from the bluish tinge of their skin (secondary to chronic hypoxemia and hypercapnia) and from the frequent presence of peripheral edema (secondary to cor pulmonale); chronic cough with production of large amounts of sputum is characteristic
2. "Pink puffers" are patients with emphysema; they have a cachectic appearance but a pink skin color (adequate O_2 saturation); shortness of breath is manifested by pursed-lip breathing and use of accessory muscles for respiration

Chest x-ray

Chest x-ray usually demonstrates hyperinflation with flattened diaphragm, tenting of the diaphragm at the rib insertions and increased retrosternal air space. Decreased vascular markings and bullae may be evident in patients with emphysema.

Lab evaluation

1. CBC may reveal leukocytosis with "shift to the left"
2. Sputum may be purulent in patients with bacterial respiratory tract infections

Treatment of acute exacerbation

1. Aerosolized beta agonists (e.g., metaproterenol, isoetharine)
2. Theophylline (see Chapter 32 for dosage)
3. Inhaled parasympatholytic agents may be effective in selected patients[35]; side effects (tachycardia, urinary retention) can occur even at low dosages; ipratropium dosage is 2 inhalations qid, maximum 12 inhalations in 24 hr
4. Judicious oxygen administration
   a. Hypercapnia and further respiratory compromise may occur after high-flow oxygen therapy
   b. The use of a Venturi-type mask delivering an inspired O_2 fraction of 24-28% is preferred to nasal cannula
5. Corticosteroids (e.g., hydrocortisone, methylprednisolone) may be beneficial during acute exacerbation if bronchospasm is a significant factor; however, chronic steroid therapy should be avoided if possible
6. Antibiotics are indicated in suspected respiratory infection
   a. *H. influenzae* and *S. pneumoniae* are frequent causes of acute bronchitis
   b. Oral antibiotics of choice are ampicillin, trimethoprim/sulfamethoxazole, tetracycline, cefuroxime, or cefaclor
   c. The use of antibiotics has been shown to be beneficial in exacerbations of COPD presenting with increased dyspnea, sputum, and sputum purulence[3]

7. Iodinated glycerol (e.g., 60 mm qid) can improve cough symptoms and mucus clearance, thereby lessening the duration of acute exacerbations of chronic obstructive bronchitis[35]
8. Pulmonary toilet: careful nasotracheal suction is indicated in patients with excessive secretions and inability to expectorate them
9. Intubation and mechanical ventilation may be necessary if the above measures fail to provide satisfactory improvement

 DIFFUSE INTERSTITIAL PULMONARY DISEASE[8,9,10]

Definition

Diffuse interstitial pulmonary disease is a group of disorders involving the lung interstitium and characterized by inflammation of the alveolar structures and progressive parenchymal fibrosis.

Etiology

There are over 100 known disorders that can cause interstitial lung disease (ILD). The more common causes are
1. Occupational and environmental exposure: pneumoconiosis, asbestosis, organic dusts, gases, fumes, berylliosis, silicosis
2. Granulomatous lung disease: sarcoidosis, infections (e.g., fungal, mycobacterial)
3. Drug-induced: bleomycin, busulfan, methotrexate, chlorambucil, cyclophosphamide, BCNU (carmustine), gold salts, nitrofurantoin, amiodarone, tocainide, penicillin
4. Radiation pneumonitis
5. Connective tissue diseases: SLE, rheumatoid arthritis, dermatomyositis
6. Idiopathic pulmonary fibrosis: bronchiolitis obliterans, interstitial pneumonitis, DIP
7. Infections: viral pneumonia, *Pneumocystis*
8. Others: Wegener's granulomatosis, Goodpasture's syndrome, eosinophilic granuloma, lymphangitic carcinomatosis, chronic uremia, chronic gastric aspiration, hypersensitivity pneumonitis, lipoid pneumonia

Diagnosis

1. Clinical history: inquire about possible drug, occupational, and environmental exposure
2. Clinical manifestations and physical exam
   a. The patient generally has progressive dyspnea and nonproductive cough; other clinical manifestations vary with the underlying disease process
   b. Physical exam typically shows end-inspiratory dry rales (Velcro rales); cyanosis, clubbing, and signs of right heart failure are generally late findings
3. Chest x-ray may be normal in approximately 10% of patients; roentgenographic abnormalities usually reflect the underlying disease process and stage of the disease.
   a. Ground-glass appearance is often an early finding
   b. A coarse reticular pattern is usually a late finding

c. Additional findings on chest x-ray may include
   (1) Kerley B-lines: lymphangitic carcinomatosis, left ventricular dysfunction
   (2) Hilar and mediastinal adenopathy: sarcoidosis, pneumoconiosis
   (3) Lytic bone lesions: eosinophilic granuloma, lymphangitic carcinomatosis
d. Congestive heart failure causing interstitial changes on chest x-ray must always be ruled out
e. A differential diagnosis of interstitial x-ray pattern should include the following: pulmonary fibrosis, pulmonary edema, PCP, TB, sarcoidosis, eosinophilic granuloma, pneumoconiosis, and lymphangitic spread of carcinoma

4. Arterial blood gases provide only limited information; initial ABGs may be normal, but with progression of the disease, hypoxemia may be present
5. Pulmonary function tests: findings are generally consistent with restrictive disease (decreased VC, TLC, and diffusing capacity)
6. Bronchoscopy with bronchoalveolar lavage is useful to characterize the pulmonary inflammatory response; the effector cell population in patients with ILD consists of two major cell types:
   a. Lymphocytes (e.g., sarcoidosis, berylliosis, silicosis, hypersensitivity pneumonitis)
   b. Neutrophils (e.g., asbestosis, collagen-vascular diseases, idiopathic pulmonary fibrosis)
7. Biopsy (open lung biopsy or transbronchial biopsy) to identify the underlying disease process and exclude neoplastic involvement; transbronchial biopsy is less invasive but provides less tissue for analysis (this factor may be important in patients with irregular pulmonary involvement)
8. Gallium-67 (^{67}Ga) scanning plays a limited role in the evaluation of ILD because it is nonspecific and a negative result does not exclude disease (e.g., patients with end-stage fibrosis may have negative scan)
9. Antineutrophil cytoplasmic antibody (ANCA) is frequently positive in Wegener's

Treatment

1. Removal of offending agent (e.g., environmental exposure)
2. Treatment of infectious process with appropriate antibiotic therapy
3. Supplemental oxygen in patients with significant hypoxemia
4. Corticosteroids are beneficial in patients with sarcoidosis; in patients with interstitial lung disease caused by an inflammatory process they may suppress alveolitis; however, response to therapy is highly variable
5. Immunosuppressive therapy in selected cases (e.g., cyclophosphamide in patients with Wegener's granulomatosis)
6. Treatment of any complications (e.g., pneumothorax, pulmonary embolism)

SARCOIDOSIS

Definition

Sarcoidosis is a chronic systemic granulomatous disease of unknown cause, characterized histologically by the presence of nonspecific noncaseating granulomas.

Characteristics and clinical manifestations

1. Increased incidence in blacks, females, and patients 20-40 yr old
2. Clinical manifestations often vary with the stage of the disease and degree of organ involvement; patients may be asymptomatic, but their chest x-ray film may demonstrate findings consistent with sarcoidosis (see below)
3. Frequent presentations are:
   a. Pulmonary manifestations: dry, nonproductive cough, dyspnea, chest discomfort
   b. Constitutional symptoms: fatigue, weight loss, anorexia, malaise
   c. Visual disturbances: blurred vision, ocular discomfort, conjunctivitis, iritis, uveitis
   d. Dermatologic manifestations: erythema nodosum, macules, papules, subcutaneous nodules, hyperpigmentation
   e. Myocardial disturbances: dysrhythmias, cardiomyopathy
   f. GI disturbances: hepatomegaly
   g. Rheumatologic manifestations: arthralgias, arthritis
   h. Neurologic and other manifestations: cranial nerve palsies, diabetes insipidus, meningeal involvement, parotid enlargement

Diagnosis

1. Chest x-ray: adenopathy of the hilar and paratracheal nodes is a frequent finding; parenchymal changes may also be present, depending on the stage of the disease
2. Lab abnormalities
   a. Hypergammaglobulinemia
   b. Liver function test abnormalities
   c. Hypercalcemia, hypercalciuria (secondary to increased GI absorption, abnormal vitamin D metabolism and increased calcitriol production by sarcoid granuloma[23])
   d. Cutaneous anergy to *Trichophyton, Candida,* mumps, and tuberculin
   e. Angiotensin-converting enzyme (ACE): elevated in approximately 60% of patients with sarcoidosis; may be useful in following the course of the disease[38]
3. PFTs: may be normal or may reveal a restrictive pattern (see Section 28.1)
4. Gallium-67 scan: [67]Ga will localize in areas of granulomatous infiltrates; however, it is nonspecific; the "panda" sign is suggestive of sarcoidosis
5. Ophthalmological exam[11]: indicated in all patients with suspected sarcoidosis since ocular findings (iridocyclitis, uveitis, conjunctivitis, and keratopathy) are found in over 25% of documented cases

6. Biopsy: should be done on accessible tissues suspected of sarcoid involvement (conjunctiva, skin, lymph nodes); bronchoscopy with transbronchial biopsy is the procedure of choice in patients without another readily accessible site
7. Bronchoalveolar lavage: useful to evaluate the cellularity of the lavaged fluid
   a. Patients with sarcoidosis generally manifest lymphocytic alveolitis
   b. The levels of helper T-cell lymphocytes in bronchoalveolar lavage fluid can be used as a marker for sarcoid activity[17]
   c. Patients with high levels of T-lymphocytes (>28%) have a higher incidence of pulmonary roentgenographic and physiologic deterioration

Treatment

The majority of patients with sarcoidosis have spontaneous remission within 2 yr and do not require any treatment. Their course can be followed by periodical evaluation, chest x-rays, and PFTs. Corticosteroids should be considered in patients with severe symptoms (e.g., dyspnea, chest pain), hypercalcemia, ocular or CNS or cardiac involvement, and progressive pulmonary disease.

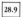

28.9 PULMONARY THROMBOEMBOLISM

Risk factors

1. Prolonged immobilization
2. Postoperative state
3. Trauma to lower extremities
4. Estrogen-containing birth control pills
5. Prior history of DVT or PE
6. Congestive heart failure
7. Pregnancy and early puerperium
8. Visceral cancer (lung, pancreas, alimentary and genitourinary tract)
9. Trauma, burns
10. Advanced age
11. Obesity
12. Hematological disease (e.g., antithrombin III deficiency, protein C deficiency, protein S deficiency, lupus anticoagulant, polycythemia vera, dysfibrinogenemia, PNH)
13. COPD, diabetes mellitus

Clinical manifestations

1. Dyspnea is the most common symptom
2. Chest pain may be nonpleuritic or pleuritic (infarction)
3. Syncope (massive PE)
4. Fever, diaphoresis
5. Hemoptysis, cough

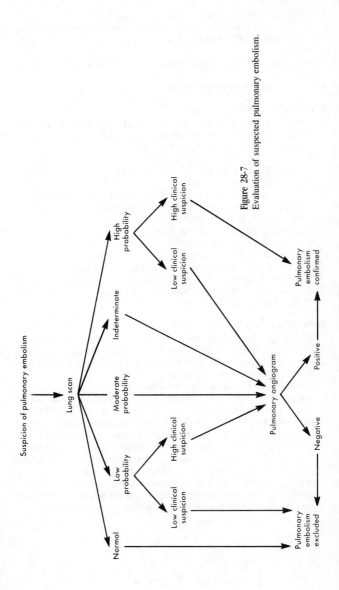

Figure 28-7
Evaluation of suspected pulmonary embolism.

Physical exam

1. Evidence of DVT may be present (see Chapter 12)
2. Cardiac exam may reveal tachycardia, increased pulmonic component of S_2, murmur of tricuspid insufficiency, right ventricular heave, right sided S_3
3. Pulmonary exam may demonstrate rales, localized wheezing, friction rub
4. Tachypnea is the most common physical finding

Diagnostic studies

1. Chest x-ray may be normal; suggestive findings include elevated diaphragm, pleural effusion, dilatation of pulmonary artery, infiltrate or consolidation, abrupt vessel cutoff
2. ECG: sinus tachycardia, $S_I Q_{III} T_{III}$ pattern, T-wave inversion in V_1-V_4, acute RBBB, new-onset atrial fibrillation; ST segment depression in lead II, right ventricular strain
3. ABGs: generally reveal decreased Pao_2 and $Paco_2$ and increased pH; normal results do not rule out pulmonary embolism
4. Lung scan and arteriography[16]
   a. A normal lung scan rules out PE
   b. A ventilation/perfusion mismatch is suggestive of PE, and a lung scan interpretation of high probability is confirmatory
   c. If the clinical suspicion of PE is high and the lung scan is interpreted as low probability, moderate probability, or indeterminate, then a pulmonary arteriogram is indicated (see Fig. 28-7); a positive arteriogram confirms the diagnosis

Treatment[26,27]

1. Thrombolytic agents (urokinase, streptokinase): provide rapid resolution of clots; this is the treatment of choice in patients with massive pulmonary embolism who are hemodynamically unstable and with no contraindications to the use of thrombolytic agents
2. Heparin by continuous infusion for at least 5 days
3. Long-term treatment: generally carried out with warfarin therapy started on day 1 or 2 and given in a dose to prolong PT 1.3-1.5 times baseline (refer to Table 12-2 for guidelines regarding antithrombotic therapy; prophylaxis of pulmonary embolism is also discussed in Chapter 12)
4. If thrombolytics and anticoagulants are contraindicated (e.g., GI bleeding, recent CNS surgery, recent trauma) or if the patient is hypotensive (secondary to massive PE) and refractory to medical therapy, acute embolectomy is indicated; in these patients and in others with recurrent PE despite adequate anticoagulant therapy, vena caval interruption is indicated by transvenous placement of a Greenfield vena caval filter[40]

References

1. Advisory committee for the elimination of tuberculosis (ACET): Tuberculosis and human immunodeficiency virus infection: recommendations, MMWR 38:236, 243, 1989.
2. American Thoracic Society: Treatment of tuberculosis and tuberculosis infection in adults and children, Am Rev Resp Dis 134, 355, 1986.
3. Anthonisen NR, et al: Antibiotic therapy in exacerbation of chronic obstructive pulmonary disease, Ann Intern Med 106:196, 1987.
4. Carr DT, Mountain CF: Staging of lung cancer, Semin Resp Med 3:154, 1982.
5. Cohn DL, Catlin BJ, et al: A 62-dose, 6-month therapy for pulmonary and extrapulmonary tuberculosis, Ann Intern Med 112:407, 1990.
6. Cohen CA, et al: Clinical manifestations of inspiratory muscle fatigue, Am J Med 73:308, 1982.
7. Cordonnier C, et al: Legionnaire's disease and hairy-cell leukemia: an unfortuitous association? Arch Intern Med 144:2373, 1984.
8. Crystal RG, et al: Interstitial lung disease of unknown cause: disorders characterized by chronic inflammation of the lower respiratory tract. I, N Engl J Med 310:154, 1984.
9. Crystal RG, et al: Interstitial lung disease of unknown cause: disorders characterized by chronic inflammation of the lower respiratory tract. II, N Engl J Med 310:235, 1984.
10. Davis WB, Crystal RG: Chronic interstitial lung disease. In Simmons DH (editor): Current pulmonology, New York, 1984, John Wiley & Sons, vol 5.
11. Dresner MS, Brecher R, Henkind P: Ophthalmology consultation in the diagnosis and treatment of sarcoidosis, Arch Intern Med 146:301, 1986.
12. Driks MR: Nosocomial pneumonia in intubated patients given sucralfate as compared with antacids or histamine type 2 blockers, N Engl J Med 317:1376, 1987.
13. Eddy DM: Screening for lung carcinoma, Ann Intern Med 111:232, 1989.
14. Edelson JD, Rebuck AS: The clinical assessment of severe asthma, Arch Intern Med 145:321, 1985.
15. Histologic typing of lung cancer, Tumor 67:253, 1981.
16. Hull RD, et al: Pulmonary angiography, ventilation lung scanning, and venography for clinically suspected pulmonary embolism with abnormal perfusion lung scan, Ann Intern Med 98:891, 1983.
17. Hunninghake GW, Crystal RG: Pulmonary sarcoidosis; a disorder mediated by excess helper T-lymphocyte activity at sites of disease activity, N Engl J Med 305:429, 1981.
18. Johnson BE, et al: Ten year survival of patients with small cell lung cancer treated with combination chemotherapy with or without irradiation, J Clin Oncol 8:396, 1990.
19. Kandel G, Aberman A: Mixed venous oxygen saturation: its role in the assessment of the critically ill patient, Arch Intern Med 143:1400, 1983.
20. Karnad A, Alvarez S: Pneumonia caused by gram-negative bacilli, Am J Med 79(suppl A):61, 1985.
21. Khan FA, Rajinder KC: Complications of acute respiratory failure, Postgrad Med 79:205, 1986.
22. Kiss GT: Diagnosis and treatment of pulmonary disease in private practice, Baltimore, 1984, The Williams & Wilkins Co.
23. Mason RS, et al: Vitamin D conversion by sarcoid lymph node homogenate, Ann Intern Med 36:938, 1984.
24. Masur H, Shelhamer J, Parrillo JE: The management of pneumonias in immunocompromised patients, JAMA 253:1769, 1985.
25. Millar WR, et al: Benign lesions which simulate thoracic malignancy, Primary Care & Cancer, p 8, September 1985.

26. Moser KM, Fedullo PF: Venous thromboembolism: three simple decisions. I, Chest 83:117, 1983.

27. Moser KM, Fedullo PF: Venous thromboembolism: three simple decisions. II, Chest 83:256, 1983.

28. Mountain CF: Biologic, physiologic, and technical determinants in surgical therapy for lung cancer. In Straus MJ (editor): Lung cancer; clinical diagnosis and treatment, New York, 1977, Grune & Stratton Inc.

29. Mullarkey MF, Lammert JK, et al: Long-term methotrexate treatment in corticosteroid-dependent asthma, Ann Intern Med 112:577, 1990.

30. National consensus conference on tuberculosis: Preventive treatment of tuberculosis, Chest 87(suppl):128S, 1985.

31. National consensus conference on tuberculosis: Standard therapy for tuberculosis, Chest 87(suppl):117S, 1985.

32. Obernauf CD, et al: Sarcoidosis and its ophthalmic manifestations, Am J Ophthalmol 86:648, 1978.

33. Olsen GN, et al: Pulmonary function evaluation of the lung resection candidate: a prospective study, Am Rev Respir Dis 111:379, 1975.

34. Patrick DM, Dales RE, et al: Severe exacerbations of COPD and asthma: incremental benefit of adding ipratropium to usual therapy, Chest 98:295, 1990.

35. Petty TL: The National Mucolytic Study: results of a randomized, double-blind, placebo-controlled study of iodinated glycerol in chronic obstructive bronchitis, Chest 97:75, 1990.

36. Popovich J Jr: The physiology of mechanical ventilation and the mechanical zoo: IPPB, PEEP, CPAP, Med Clin North Am 67:621, 1983.

37. Popovich J Jr: Mechanical ventilation: keeping all systems "go," J Respir Dis 6:69, 1985.

38. Studdy PR, Lapworth R, Bird R: Angiotensin-converting enzyme and its clinical significance, J Clin Pathol 36:938, 1983.

39. Wang KP, Terry PB: Transbronchial needle aspiration in the diagnosis and staging of bronchogenic carcinoma, Am Rev Respir Dis 127:344, 1983.

40. West JW: Pulmonary embolism, Med Clin North Am 70:877, 1986.

41. Zelen M: Keynote address on biostatistics and data retrieval, Cancer Chemother Rep 4(2);31, 1973.

Rheumatology

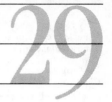

29.1 **TEMPORAL ARTERITIS AND POLYMYALGIA RHEUMATICA[1]**

Some authors consider temporal arteritis and polymyalgia rheumatica to be manifestations of the same disease, known as "giant cell arteritis."[6] Polymyalgia rheumatica occurs in 40-60% of patients with temporal arteritis while the incidence of temporal arteritis in patients with polymyalgia rheumatica varies from 15-78%.[17]

Temporal arteritis

Definition

Temporal arteritis is a systemic segmental granulomatous inflammation predominantly involving the arteries of the carotid system in patients over the age of 50. However, it can involve any large- or medium-sized arteries.

Clinical manifestations

1. Headache, often associated with marked scalp tenderness
2. Tenderness, decreased pulsation, and nodulation of the temporal arteries
3. Constitutional symptoms (fever, weight loss, anorexia, fatigue)
4. Polymyalgia syndrome (aching and stiffness of the trunk and proximal muscle groups)
5. Visual disturbances (visual loss, blurred vision, diplopia, amaurosis fugax)
6. Intermittent claudication of jaw and tongue upon mastication
7. Cough

Lab findings

1. Elevated ESR (usually >50 mm/hr by the Westergren method); however, a normal ESR does not exclude the diagnosis[7]
2. Mild to moderate normochromic normocytic anemia, elevated platelets
3. LFT abnormalities (elevation of alkaline phosphatase is most common)

Diagnosis

The clinical diagnosis requires pathologic confirmation with biopsy of at least 3 cm of the temporal artery. Overall reported sensitivity of temporal artery biopsy is 90.3%; specificity is 100%.[13] Pathological confirmation is desirable because of significant toxicity associated with subsequent long-term steroid therapy.

Therapy

1. In stable patients without significant ocular involvement, therapy is usually started with prednisone 50 mg qAM, continued for 4-6 wk until symptoms resolve; the prednisone is gradually tapered over several months; the usual length of treatment is 6 mo to 2 yr[1]
2. In very ill patients and patients with significant ocular involvement (e.g., visual loss in one eye) rapid aggressive treatment with large doses of IV methylprednisolone is indicated to provide optimum protection to the uninvolved eye and offer any chance of visual recovery of the involved eye; the optimum dose of methylprednisolone ranges from 100 mg/day to 1000 mg q12h for 5 days[22]
3. Methotrexate may be useful in patients intolerant of steroids

Polymyalgia rheumatica

Definition

Polymyalgia rheumatica (PMR) is a clinical syndrome predominantly involving individuals over the age of 50 yr and characterized by pain and stiffness involving mainly the shoulders, pelvic girdle musculature, and torso.

Clinical manifestations

1. Symmetrical polymyalgias and arthralgias involving back, shoulder, neck, and pelvic girdle muscles; duration is generally longer than 1 mo
2. Constitutional symptoms (fever, malaise, weight loss)
3. Headache in patients with coexisting temporal arteritis
4. Symptoms are worse in the morning (difficulty getting out of bed) and at nighttime
5. Muscle strength is usually within normal limits
6. Crescendo of symptoms over several weeks or months

Lab findings

The lab findings for polymyalgia rheumatica are the same as for temporal arteritis.

Diagnosis

Diagnosis is based on clinical presentation and elevated ESR, although the latter is not essential for the diagnosis. There is controversy regarding the need for temporal artery biopsy in all patients with PMR. Proponents state that because of the high incidence of temporal arteritis (with associated risk of blindness), all patients who have an elevated ESR and aching muscles should undergo a temporal artery biopsy to rule out the presence of temporal arteritis. Opponents reason that biopsy is not indicated in patients without any signs or symptoms suggestive of cranial arteritis because the diagnostic yield is too low.

Treatment

1. Abolish symptoms
   a. Low-dose corticosteroids (e.g., prednisone 10-15 mg/day) will generally produce dramatic relief of symptoms within 48 hr and confirm the diagnosis; failure to improve within 1 wk suggests other diagnoses (e.g., fibromyalgia, polymyositis, viral myalgias, hypothyroidism, depression, rheumatoid arthritis, occult neoplasm, or infection)
   b. The corticosteroid dosage is then gradually tapered over several months based on repeated clinical observation
   c. In patients with mild symptoms NSAIDs may be used instead of corticosteroids
2. Monitor closely for possible development of temporal arteritis
   a. Instruct patient to immediately report any visual or neurologic symptoms
   b. As many as one third of patients with PMR can develop temporal arteritis within 1 yr of onset of PMR[19]

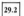 **29.2 SYSTEMIC LUPUS ERYTHEMATOSUS**

Definition

Systemic lupus erythematosus (SLE) is a chronic multisystemic disease of unknown etiology, characterized by production of autoantibodies and protean clinical manifestations.

Clinical manifestations[22,24]

SLE generally affects women (female/male ratio 7:1) in the childbearing years and may present with any of the following:
1. Common cutaneous manifestations
   a. Butterfly rash: erythematous rash over the malar eminences, generally with sparing of the nasolabial folds
   b. Discoid lupus: raised erythematous patches with subsequent edematous plaques and adherent scales
   c. Symmetrical erythematous lesions involving shoulders, chest, neck, and upper extremities
   d. Alopecia
   e. Raynaud's phenomenon
   f. Photosensitivity (particularly leg ulcerations)
   g. Nasal or oropharyngeal ulcerations
   h. Other: livedo reticularis, maculopapular eruptions, vasculitic ulcers
2. Joint disturbances: tenderness, swelling, or effusion generally involving peripheral joints; a nonerosive arthropathy of the hands occurs in 10% of patients
3. Renal disturbances: proteinuria, active renal sediment, renal insufficiency
4. Hematologic abnormalities: anemia (chronic disease, hemolysis), leukopenia, thrombotic events (secondary to lupus anticoagulant), immune thrombocytopenic purpura

5. Cardiac involvement: pericarditis, verrucous endocarditis (Libman-Sacks endocarditis), myocarditis, coronary vasculitis, conduction abnormalities, valvular thickening and dysfunction
6. Neurologic abnormalities: seizures, psychosis, depression, transverse myelitis, aseptic meningitis
7. Pulmonary involvement: pleural effusions, pleuritis, pulmonary infiltrates, vasculitis
8. GI manifestations: oral ulcers, abdominal pain, vomiting
9. Constitutional symptoms: fatigue, malaise, fever
10. Other: conjunctivitis, sicca syndrome (i.e., a manifestation of SS that can be associated with SLE)

Lab diagnosis

1. Presence of antinuclear antibody (ANA): This is a generic test used in a variety of rheumatologic disorders; distinctive profiles of ANA are associated with certain disorders; antibodies to double-strand DNA (anti-ds DNA) and to the Smith nuclear antigen (anti-Sm) are highly specific for SLE; Table 29-1 describes the ANA pattern and corresponding antibody found in various rheumatological disorders; ANA-negative SLE is very unusual; these patients generally have anti-SS-A and/or anti-SS-B antibodies
2. Drug-related lupus erythematosus (DLE)[14]

   Drugs *definitely* associated: procainamide, hydralazine, isoniazid, methyldopa, quinidine, and chlorpromazine

   Drugs *probably* associated: hydantoins, antithyroids, penicillamine, lithium, sulfasalazine, beta blockers

   Drugs *possibly* associated: estrogens, penicillin, gold salts, tetracycline, reserpine, griseofulvin, PAS

   a. Patients with DLE generally do not have CNS or renal involvement, the classical malar rash, mucosal ulcers, or alopecia
   b. Distinguishing lab characteristics in DLE are
      (1) Virtual absence of anti–ds DNA and anti-Sm
      (2) Higher frequency of antibodies to histones
      (3) Normal levels of complement
      (4) Absence of severe anemia, leukopenia, and thrombocytopenia
   c. DLE does not have the same prognostic implications as SLE since it is reversible after discontinuation of the offending agent
3. Suggested initial lab evaluation of suspected SLE
   a. Immunological evaluation: ANA, anti-DNA antibody, anti-Sm antibody
   b. Other lab tests: CBC with differential, platelet count, Coombs' test if anemia detected, 24 hr urine collection for protein if proteinuria detected, PTT and anticardiolipin antibodies in patients with thrombotic events; BUN, creatinine, urinalysis, and complement levels are also useful

Classification of SLE

The following list describes the 1982 revised criteria of the American Rheumatism Association for classification of systemic lupus erythematosus.[25] A

Table 29-1 Antinuclear antibody

ANA Pattern	Corresponding Antibody	Found in
Rim and/or homogeneous	Double strand DNA	SLE
Rim and/or homogeneous	Double and single strand DNA	SLE and other rheumatic diseases
Rim and/or homogeneous	LE cell antibody	SLE, drug-induced LE
Homogeneous	Histones	Drug-induced LE
Speckled	Sm (Smith)	SLE
Speckled	MA	SLE (severe)
Speckled	RNP	Mixed connective tissue disease
Atypical speckled	Sc1	Scleroderma
Speckled	SS-A (Ro), SS-B (La)	Sjögren's syndrome
Nucleolar	Nucleolar	Progressive systemic sclerosis

*Reproduced from Jacobs DS, et al: Laboratory test handbook with key word index, St. Louis, 1988, Mosby/Lexi-Comp.

person is said to have SLE if any four or more of the 11 criteria are present, serially or simultaneously, during an interval of observation.

1. Butterfly rash
2. Discoid rash
3. Photosensitivity
4. Oral ulcers
5. Arthritis
6. Serositis
   a. Pleuritis
   b. Pericarditis
7. Renal disorder
   a. Persistent proteinuria greater than 0.5 g/day or 3+ if quantitation not performed
   b. Cellular casts
8. Neurological disorder
   a. Seizures (in the absence of offending drugs or known metabolic derangements)
   b. Psychosis (in the absence of offending drugs)
9. Hematological disorder
   a. Hemolytic anemia with reticulocytosis
   b. Leukopenia (less than 4000/mm^3 total on two or more occasions)
   c. Lymphopenia (less than 1500/mm^3 on two or more occasions)
   d. Thrombocytopenia (less than 100,000/mm^3 in the absence of offending drugs)
10. Immunologic disorder
    a. Positive LE cell preparation

    b. Anti-DNA (presence of antibody to native DNA in abnormal titer)

    c. Anti-Sm (presence of antibody to Smith nuclear antigen)

    d. False-positive STS known to be positive for at least 6 mo and confirmed by negative TPI or FTA tests

11. Antinuclear antibody: an abnormal titer of antinuclear antibody by immunofluorescence or equivalent assay at any time and in the absence of drugs known to be associated with "drug-induced lupus" syndrome

Treatment

Therapy of SLE should be individualized, based on the severity of the disease.

1. Joint pain and mild serositis are generally well controlled with NSAIDs; antimalarials are also effective

2. Cutaneous manifestations are treated with
   a. Topical corticosteroids
   b. Antimalarials (e.g., hydroxychloroquinine [Plaquenil])
   c. Sunscreens that filter out ultraviolet B light

3. Renal disease
   a. Significant active renal disease can be treated with corticosteroids, immunosuppressants (e.g., azathioprine [Imuran]), and alkylating agents (cyclophosphamide [Cytoxan]); some studies[4] have demonstrated that IV cyclophosphamide plus low dosages of prednisone result in better preservation of renal function than high dosages of prednisone alone
   b. Use of plasmapheresis in combination with immunosuppressive agents (to prevent rebound phenomenon of antibody levels after plasmapheresis) is an experimental therapy generally reserved for rapidly progressive renal failure or life-threatening systemic vasculitis

4. CNS involvement: treatment generally consists of corticosteroid therapy; however, its efficacy is uncertain, and it is generally reserved for organic brain syndrome; anticonvulsants and antipsychotics are also indicated in selected cases; headaches are treated symptomatically

5. Hemolytic anemia: treatment of Coombs' positive hemolytic anemia consists of high doses of steroids; nonhemolytic anemia (secondary to chronic disease) does not require specific therapy

6. Thrombocytopenia
   a. Initial treatment consists of corticosteroids
   b. In patients with poor response to steroids encouraging results have been reported with the use of danazol[21] and vincristine
   c. Splenectomy generally does not cure the thrombocytopenia of SLE[12] but may be necessary as an adjunctive in managing selected cases

7. Valvular heart disease: present in 18% of patients with SLE; echocardiography can identify a subset of lesions (valvular thickening and dysfunction) other than verrucous (Libman-Sacks) endocarditis that are prone to hemodynamic deterioration[9]; the prevalence of infective endocarditis in patients with SLE is approximately 1% (similar to the prevalence after prosthetic valve surgery, but greater than that following rheumatic fever)[20]; antibiotic prophylaxis for SBE remains controversial

8. Infections are common because of compromised immune function secondary to SLE and the use of corticosteroids and cytotoxic and antimetabolite drugs; pneumococcal bacteremia is associated with high mortality

Prognosis[3,5,11,27]

1. The leading cause of death in SLE is infection (one third of all deaths); active nephritis causes approximately 18% of deaths, and CNS disease 7% of deaths; the survival rate is 75% over the first 10 yr; blacks and Hispanics generally have a worse prognosis
2. Renal histological studies and evaluation of renal function are useful in determining disease activity and predicting disease outcome (e.g., serum creatinine levels >3 mg/dl or evidence of diffuse proliferative involvement on renal biopsy are poor prognostic factors)

RHEUMATOID ARTHRITIS

Definition

Rheumatoid arthritis (RA) is a chronic systemic disorder characterized primarily by pain and inflammation in multiple joints.

Epidemiology and prognosis[28]

The incidence of RA is about 1% in the general population. The female/male ratio is approximately 3:1. Peak onset is between the ages of 20-45 yr. The course of the disease is highly variable and characterized by exacerbations and remissions. Approximately 10% of patients will have severe destructive arthritis unresponsive to any therapeutic modalities, whereas 15% of all patients experience a complete remission. Latex and ANA positivity, persistently high ESR, and presence of subcutaneous nodules are generally associated with poorer prognosis.

Clinical manifestations

The initial manifestations of RA are highly variable. In the majority of patients the onset is insidious, taking months or years to become clinically evident as a diagnosable entity. In other patients the onset is dramatic, with rapid development of severe manifestations (see below). RA can present with any of the following articular and extraarticular manifestations:

1. Articular and periarticular manifestations
   a. Morning stiffness is often the initial complaint
   b. Symmetrical polyarthritis
      (1) Joint swelling and tenderness to palpation, with significant limitation of motion of involved joints
      (2) Commonly involved joints in RA are metacarpophalangeal (MCP), metatarsophalangeal (MTP), proximal interphalangeal (PIP), wrist, knee, ankle, shoulder, and hip; however, any joint in the body can be affected
      (3) Joint deformities are generally secondary to hyperextension or flexion of the joints

      (a) Hyperextension of PIP joints and flexion of DIP joints (swan-neck deformity)

      (b) Flexion of PIP joints and extension of DIP joints (boutonniere deformity)

      (c) Carpal tunnel syndrome: numbness and pain on the palmar surface of the first three digits of the hand; it is caused by entrapment of or pressure on the median nerve as it passes in the area between the bones of the wrist and the transverse carpal ligament; tapping over the median nerve on the flexor surface of the wrist will produce a tingling sensation radiating from the wrist to the hand (positive Tinel's sign); surgical decompression is usually necessary to relieve the symptoms if NSAIDs, wrist splinting, and local corticosteroid injections are ineffective

      (d) Other: knee and ankle effusions, hoarseness secondary to cricoarytenoid arthritis, myelopathy secondary to nerve compression

2. Extraarticular manifestations

  a. Pulmonary involvement consists of one or more of the following:

    (1) Pulmonary nodules; association of rheumatoid pulmonary nodules and interstitial pneumoconiosis is known as Caplan's syndrome; pulmonary nodules are usually multiple, as opposed to the single nodules seen with lung carcinoma

    (2) Pleural effusions (exudative with low glucose concentration)

    (3) Pulmonary vasculitis

    (4) Pleuritis

  b. Ocular involvement: scleritis, episcleritis; RA is often associated with Sjögren's syndrome (characterized by dryness of eyes, mouth, and other mucous membranes secondary to lymphoplasmacytic infiltration of exocrine glands with destruction of mucus-generating glands)

  c. Vasculitis is generally seen in patients with elevated titers of rheumatoid factor (RF); it can involve any organ, and frequent manifestations are mononeuritis multiplex (e.g. foot- or wristdrop) and digital arteritis

  d. Hematological abnormalities

    (1) Normochromic normocytic/microcytic anemia (multifactorial: chronic disease, blood loss secondary to salicylates and NSAIDs)

    (2) Granulocytopenia; the presence of granulocytopenia and splenomegaly in a patient with RA is known as Felty's syndrome

    (3) Hyperviscosity, cryoglobulinemia

  e. Cardiac involvement: pericarditis, conduction defects, myocarditis, arteritis

  f. Skin: subcutaneous nodules (caused by granulomatous inflammation of surrounding arteries) may be found over the olecranon process and any bony prominences

  g. Constitutional symptoms: fever, weight loss, anorexia, malaise

h. Other: osteoporosis, myositis, compressive neuropathies, amyloidosis, mesangial glomerulonephrosis

Lab evaluation

There is no isolated lab test that can exclude or prove the diagnosis of RA. Any of the following lab abnormalities may be present:

1. Rheumatoid factor (RF): Latex positivity may be initially absent, but over the course of the disease approximately 85% of patients become latex positive; RF is not specific for RA and may be found in other conditions (e.g., osteomyelitis, infective endocarditis, liver disease)
2. ESR: generally elevated during exacerbations
3. ANA: detected in approximately 15% of patients
4. Decreased hemoglobin/hematocrit, granulocytopenia

Arthrocentesis

See Section 30.4 for procedure and interpretation of results of arthrocentesis.

Radiographic evaluation

Initially, soft tissue swelling may be the only manifestation. As the disease progresses, there is periarticular osteopenia, cortical thinning, and marginal erosion. Subluxation and joint space diminution are late findings.

Diagnosis

RA is a clinical diagnosis. The seven criteria of the American Rheumatism Association are described in Table 29-2. Existence of four or more of these criteria in a patient denotes probable RA. The major value of the criteria lies not in diagnosing the individual patient but in advancing epidemiological and clinical research.

Treatment[8]

1. Improve the patient's quality of life with
   a. Drug therapy to relieve pain and inflammation
   b. Active rehabilitation with adequate physical therapy programs
   c. Emotional support and social counseling
2. Arrest or retard the disease process with appropriate drug therapy
   a. Drug therapy of RA generally consists of a stepwise approach based on the severity of disease and clinical response
   b. There are three major categories of drugs:
      (1) Rapid acting: indicated for initial rapid relief of painful joint symptoms; examples are salicylates and other nonsteroidal antiinflammatory drugs (NSAIDs)
      (2) Disease-modifying
         (a) These agents are associated with significant toxicity
         (b) Their use is indicated in patients with severe, progressive disease
         (c) Examples are gold salts, penicillamine, and antimalarials (e.g., hydroxychloroquine)
      (3) Immunosuppressive agents (e.g., methotrexate)

Table 29-2 The 1987 revised criteria for the diagnosis of rheumatoid arthritis*

Criterion	Definition
1. Morning stiffness	Morning stiffness in and around the joints, lasting at least 1 hr before maximal improvement
2. Arthritis of three or more joint areas	At least three joint areas simultaneously have had soft tissue swelling or fluid (not bony overgrowth alone) observed by physician; 14 possible areas are right or left PIP, MCP, wrist, elbow, knee, ankle, and MTP joints
3. Arthritis of hand joints	At least one area swollen (as defined above) in a wrist, MCP, or PIP joint
4. Symmetrical arthritis	Simultaneous involvement of same joint areas (as defined in 2) on both sides of body (bilateral involvement of PIPs, MCPs, or MTPs acceptable without absolute symmetry)
5. Rheumatoid nodules	Subcutaneous nodules, over bony prominences, or extensor surfaces, or in juxtaarticular regions, observed by physician
6. Serum rheumatoid factor	Demonstration of abnormal amounts of serum rheumatoid factor by any method for which result has been positive in <5% of normal control subjects
7. Roentgenographic changes	Roentgenographic changes typical of rheumatoid arthritis on PA hand and wrist roentgenograms, which must include erosions or unequivocal bony decalcification localized in or most marked adjacent to involved joints (osteoarthritis changes alone do not qualify)

*For classification purposes, a patient shall be said to have rheumatoid arthritis if he or she has satisfied at least four of these seven criteria. Criteria 1 through 4 must have been present for at least 6 wk. Patients with two clinical diagnoses are not excluded. (Modified from Arnett FC, et al: Arthritis Rheum 31:315, 1988. Used by permission of the American Rheumatism Association.)

KEY: MCP, Metacarpophalangeal; MTP, metatarsorphalangeal; PIP, proximal interphalangeal

   c. Initial treatment of RA generally consists of high doses of salicylates (e.g., 3 to 6 g/day) or other NSAIDS
     (1) Frequent side effects of both consist of gastric irritation and GI bleeding
     (2) Patients responding poorly to a trial of NSAIDS are generally treated with gold preparations; complications of gold therapy are skin rashes, pruritus, stomatitis, leukopenia, thrombocytopenia, and proteinuria
     (3) If therapy with gold preparations is unsuccessful, the following agents may be used:
       (a) Methotrexate: possible toxicity includes bone marrow suppression, interstitial pneumonitis, GI ulceration and bleeding, and liver abnormalities
       (b) Penicillamine: can cause proteinuria, bone marrow depression, fever, and rash
       (c) Hydroxychloroquine: its use is associated with retinopathy and requires periodic ophthalmological examination
       (d) Azathioprine (Imuran): can result in bone marrow depression, nausea, vomiting, hepatitis
       (e) Sulfasalazine (Azulfidine): rash and GI disturbances may occur
   d. Systemic corticosteroids are often used for brief periods in combination with slow-remitting agents to minimize symptoms in patients with significant disease but who need to continue full-time employment for socioeconomic reasons (e.g., head of household); 100 g of methylprednisolone IV daily for 3 days often results in sustained improvement in patients with active rheumatoid arthritis[25]; low-dose steroids (e.g., 7.5 mg prednisone qd) are useful in improving the quality of life without significant toxicity when long-term steroid therapy is necessary; intraarticular steroids are frequently used as adjunctive therapy to any of the previously described agents

29.4 OSTEOARTHRITIS (DEGENERATIVE JOINT DISEASE)[16]

Definition

Osteoarthritis is a common disease of the aging process, characterized pathologically by cartilage breakdown and bone remodeling and overgrowth. It can be primary (unrelated to other conditions) or secondary to various factors (e.g., trauma, septic arthritis, inflammatory arthritis, congenital or developmental defects)

Clinical manifestations

Clinical manifestations are variable, depending on the joints involved and the stage of the disease. Onset is gradual with pain and stiffness of involved joints (generally more severe upon awakening in the morning or following a prolonged period of inactivity). Joints commonly involved are
1. Hip: the patient complains of thigh or groin pain with motion or weight-bearing
2. Knee: significant restriction of movement, bony enlargement, and crepitation (with movement) may be present

3. Cervical spine: osteophyte formation along the margins of the vertebral bodies can result in cervical pain, headache, syncope (secondary to vertebral artery compression), and paresthesias of upper extremities (secondary to nerve compression); the areas most commonly involved are C4 to C6
4. Hands: osteoarthritis generally involves the DIP, PIP, and carpometacarpal joint of the thumb; bony overgrowths (felt as hard nontender nodules) are known as Heberden's nodes for DIP joints and Bouchard's nodes for PIP joints

Lab evaluation

Generally noncontributory (normal ESR, negative ANA, absent RF, normal CBC)

Radiographic evaluation

Osteophytes may be detected on oblique views of the cervical spine in symptomatic patients; other involved joints may show thinning of joint space and subchondral bone sclerosis

Management

1. Relief of pain can be achieved with the following modalities:
   a. Medications
      (1) Acetaminophen or NSAIDs are generally used (refer to Table 33-30 for a comparison of the various NSAIDs)
      (2) Systemic corticosteroids are not indicated in osteoarthritis
      (3) Intraarticular injection of corticosteroids with local anesthetics is useful as adjunctive management of acutely inflamed joints refractory to other therapeutic modalities; frequent injections must be avoided (increased risk of steroid arthropathy)
   b. Local application of heat
   c. Periods of rest at selected times during the day
   d. Judicious exercise to maintain joint motion and muscle power; strenuous exercise or any activity which causes persistent pain should be avoided
   e. Weight reduction of painful joints with canes or crutches
   f. Surgical procedures may be necessary in patients with severe hip or knee involvement or spinal nerve compression
2. Patient education and reassurance

29.5   CRYSTAL-INDUCED ARTHRITIS

Acute gout[10,15]

Definition

Gout is a metabolic disease characterized by hyperuricemia and deposits of monosodium urate crystals in and about joints, with subsequent acute or chronic arthritis. It can be subdivided into the following phases: asymptomatic, acute gouty arthritis, interval gout, and chronic gout.

Epidemiology

Initial acute gouty arthritis occurs primarily in men aged 30-60 yr. In women it usually occurs after menopause. Attacks can be precipitated by several factors (e.g., trauma, certain foods, ethanol intake, diuretics, renal failure).

Clinical manifestations and diagnosis

1. The typical presentation is monoarticular and characterized by sudden severe pain involving the first metatarsophalangeal (MTP) joint (podagra), although the midtarsal and ankle are also frequently affected; acute asymmetric polyarthritis is uncommon
2. Physical exam reveals a warm, tender, swollen, erythematous joint; fever may be present, particularly if several joints are involved.
3. Serum uric acid level may be elevated, but it is often normal during the acute attack, later rising when the symptoms resolve
4. Aspiration and analysis of synovial fluid from the inflamed joint confirms the diagnosis; examination of the fluid with a polarized light microscope with compensator reveals monosodium urate crystals (needle-shaped, strongly negative birefringent crystals) with synovial fluid leukocytes

Treatment

1. Colchicine can be given PO or IV (see Chapter 32 for dosages)
2. Nonsteroidal antiinflammatory drugs (NSAIDs): indomethacin 50 mg q8h for 3-4 days, then gradually tapered off over approximately 1-2 wk (depending on the patient's clinical response); naproxen, sulindac, and other NSAIDS are also effective
3. Glucocorticoids (IV or IM ACTH): generally reserved for patients who cannot tolerate PO medication (e.g., postoperatively) and with contraindications to the use of IV colchicine
4. Intraarticular administration of methylprednisone or betamethasone is generally reserved for patients with monoarticular disease

Prevention of recurrences

Prevention is achieved through normalization of serum urate concentration with avoidance of foods high in purines (e.g., anchovies, sweetbreads), alcohol, aspirin, and diuretics. Uricosuric agents (e.g., probenecid) or agents to reduce uric acid synthesis (allopurinol) are used in patients with recurrent attacks despite adequate dietary restrictions. However, hypouricemic therapy should not be started for at least 2 wk after the acute attack has resolved because it may prolong the acute attack and can also precipitate new attacks by rapidly lowering the serum uric acid level. Colchicine 0.6 mg PO bid is indicated for acute gout prophylaxis before starting hypouricemic therapy. It is generally discontinued 6-8 wk following normalization of serum urate levels. Long-term colchicine therapy (0.6 mg qd-bid) may be necessary in patients with frequent gout attacks despite the use of uricosuric agents.

Table 29-3 Comparison of crystal-induced arthritides

Crystal-induced arthritis	Characteristics of Crystals (From Joint Aspiration)	Commonly Involved Joints	Comments and Therapy
Gouty arthritis	Monsodium urate crystals	First metatarsophalangeal, ankles, midfoot	See p. 551
Calcium pyrophosphate deposition disease (pseudogout)	Calcium pyrophosphate dihydrate crystals Rhomboid or polymorphic shaped, weakly positive, birefringent crystals	Knees, wrists	X-rays of involved joint may reveal linear calcifications (chondrocalcinosis) on articular cartilage Possible associated conditions must be ruled out: hyperparathyroidism, hypothyroidism, hemochromatosis, hypomagnesemia Therapy: NSAIDs, joint immobilization, intraarticular steroids

Hydroxyapatite arthropathy	Calcium hydroxyapatite crystals Crystals form nonbirefringent clumps with synovial fluid when placed on slide Diagnosis often requires electron microscopy because of small size of the crystals	Knees, hips, shoulders	Usually affects younger patients than the other crystal-induced arthritides Therapy: NSAIDs, joint immobilization, intraarticular steroids
Calcium oxalate–induced arthritis	Calcium oxalate crystals Bipyramidal shaped, positive birefringent crystals	DIP, PIP joints of hands	Often seen in dialysis patients taking large doses of ascorbic acid (metabolized to oxalate) Therapy: NSAIDs, joint immobilization, intraarticular steroids

Table 29-4 Comparison of seronegative spondyloarthropathies[2]

Spondyloarthropathy	Ankylosing Spondylitis	Reiter's Syndrome	Psoriatic Arthritis	Arthritis Associated with GI Disease
Characteristics and presentation	• Insidious onset of constant back pain lasting longer than 3 mo in patient under 40 yr of age • Pain and stiffness are improved by exercise; patients often walk around at night to gain relief from nocturnal back pain • Associated with anterior uveitis (25%), aortitis (5%)	• Arthritis usually follows episode of urethritis • Eye involvement: bilateral conjunctivitis, uveitis, keratitis, retinitis • Dermatitis: usually painless mucocutaneous lesions on glans penis and mouth, hyperkeratotic lesions on palms and soles (keratoderma blenorrhagicum)	• Arthritis usually involves DIP joints often resulting in "sausage" digits • Skin lesions usually precede arthritis • Nail changes (pitting) often accompany psoriatic arthritis	Occurs with Whipple's disease (up to 90% of patients) Crohn's disease (20%) Following intestinal bypass (15%) Ulcerative colitis (10%) Remission of underlying disorder usually results in complete remission of the arthritis May be associated with erythema nodosum, pyoderma gangrenosum, anterior uveitis
Association with HLA-B27	Strong association	Strong association	No significant association	No significant association except in patients with IBD and sacroiliitis

Characteristic radiographic patterns of spine	Radiographs of spine initially show straightening of lumbar part of spine; in advanced disease, diffuse syndesmophyte formation may result in fusion of entire spine (bamboo spine)	Unlike ankylosing spondylitis, distribution of syndesmophytes is asymmetrical and nonmarginal	Similar to Reiter's syndrome	Radiographic evaluation may be normal or may reveal sacroiliitis
Peripheral arthritis	• Oligoarticular • Hips, shoulders	• Oligoarticular • Asymmetric • Lower extremities	• DIP joints • Usually asymmetrical and oligoarticular but can be variable	• Large joints (knees, ankles) • Symmetrical
Therapy	NSAIDs Physical therapy	IV penicillin Joint immobilization NSAIDs Topical corticosteroids for conjunctivitis Long-term tetracycline for persistent urethritis	• Treat skin disease • NSAIDs • Methotrexate • Gold therapy	Treat underlying disorder Sulfasalazine (Azulfidine) for sacroiliitis associated with IBD

Joint diseases caused by other chemical species of crystals

Other joint disorders resulting from the accumulation of chemical crystals are described in Table 29-3.

29.6   SPONDYLOARTHROPATHIES[2]

Spondyloarthropathies are defined as seronegative arthritis syndromes characterized clinically by back pain, extraarticular disorders, and peripheral arthritis. The principal differences among the seronegative spondyloarthropathies are summarized in Table 29-4.

References

1. Allen NB, Studenski SA: Polymyalgia rheumatica and temporal arteritis, Med Clin North Am 70:369, 1986.
2. Arnett FC: Seronegative polyarthritis. In Cohen AS, Bennett JC (editors): Rheumatology and immunology, ed 2, New York, 1986, Grune & Stratton Inc, p 223.
3. Austin HA, et al: Prognostic factors in lupus nephritis: contribution of renal histologic data, Am J Med 75:382, 1983.
4. Austin HA, et al: Therapy of lupus nephritis: controlled trial of prednisone and cytotoxic drugs, N Engl J Med 314:614, 1986.
5. Ballou SP, Kushner I: Lupus patients who lack detectable anti-DNA: clinical features and survival, Arthritis Rheum 25:1126, 1982.
6. Bengtsson BA, Malmvall BE: The epidemiology of giant cell arteritis including temporal arteritis and polymyalgia rheumatica: incidence of different clinical presentations and eye complications, Arthritis Rheum 24:899, 1981.
7. Biller J, et al: Temporal arteritis associated with normal sedimentation rate, JAMA 247:486, 1982.
8. Dugowson CE, Gilliland BC: Management of rheumatoid arthritis, DM 32(1):1, 1986.
9. Galve EG, Candell-Riera J, et al: Prevalence, morphologic types, and evaluation of cardiac valvular disease in systemic lupus erythematosus, N Engl J Med 319:817, 1988.
10. German DC, Holmes EW: Hyperuricemia and gout, Med Clin North Am 70:419, 1986.
11. Ginzler EM, et al: A multicenter study of outcome in systemic lupus erythematosus: entry variables as predictors of prognosis, Arthritis Rheum 25:601, 1982.
12. Hall S, et al: Splenectomy does not cure the thrombocytopenia of systemic lupus erythematosus, Ann Intern Med 102:325, 1985.
13. Hedges TR III, Gieger GL, Albert DM: The clinical value of negative temporal artery biopsy specimens, Arch Ophthalmol 101:1251, 1983.
14. Hess E: Drug-related lupus, N Engl J Med 318:1460, 1988.
15. Holmes EW: Clinical gout and the pathogenesis of hyperuricemia. In McCarthy DJ (editor): Arthritis and allied conditions, ed 10, Philadelphia, 1985, Lea & Febiger.
16. Howell DS, Pita JC, Woessner JF Jr: Discussion: Which comes first—crystals, necrosis, or inflammation? J Rheumatol 10(suppl 9):59, 1983.
17. Hunder GG, Allen GL: Giant cell arteritis: a review, Bull Rheum Dis 29:980, 1978-1979.
18. Huskisson EC: The drug treatment of osteoarthritis, Scand J Rheumatol 43(suppl): 57, 1982.
19. Jones JG, Hazelman BL: Prognosis and management of polymyalgia rheumatica, Ann Rheum Dis 40:1 1981.

20. Krane SM, Simon LS: Rheumatoid arthritis: clinical features and pathogenetic mechanisms, Med Clin North Am 70:263, 1986.
21. Marino C, Cook P: Danazol for lupus thrombocytopenia, Arch Intern Med 145:2251, 1985.
22. Pisetsky DS: Systemic lupus erythematosus, Med Clin North Am 70:337, 1986.
23. Rosenfield SI, et al: Treatment of temporal arteritis with ocular involvement, Am J Med 80:143, 1986.
24. Rothfield NF: Systemic lupus erythematosus: clinical aspects and treatment. In McCarthy DJ (editor): Arthritis and allied conditions, Philadelphia, 1985, Lea & Febiger.
25. Tan EM, et al: The 1982 revised criteria for the classification of systemic lupus erythematosus, Arthritis Rheum 25:1271, 1982.
26. The viral etiology of rheumatoid arthritis, Lancet 1:772, 1984.
27. Wasicek CCA, Reichlin M: Clinical and serological differences between systemic lupus erythematosus patients with antibodies to Ro versus patients with antibodies to Ro and La, J Clin Invest 69:835, 1982.
28. Zwaifler NS: Rheumatoid arthritis: a clinical perspective. In Lawrence RC, Shulman LE (editors): Current topics in rheumatology: epidemiology of the rheumatic diseases, Brookfield Vt, 1984, Gower Publishing Co.

Procedures and Interpretation of Results

LUMBAR PUNCTURE

Indications

1. Suspected meningitis
2. Suspected encephalitis
3. Diagnosis of meningeal carcinomatosis and meningeal leukemia
4. Diagnosis of tertiary syphilis
5. Follow-up of therapy for meningitis (selected cases)
6. Evaluation for Guillain-Barré syndrome
7. Evaluation for multiple sclerosis
8. Staging of lymphomas
9. Evaluation of dementia (in selected cases)
10. Treatment of pseudotumor cerebri
11. Suspected subarachnoid hemorrhage (only after normal head CT scan)
12. Introduction of drugs, anesthetics, or radiographic media in the CNS

Contraindications

1. Infection at the site of lumbar puncture
2. Increased intracranial pressure
3. Severe hemorrhagic diathesis
4. Presence of a CNS mass lesion
5. Suspected venous sinus occlusion

Procedure[2,3,4,14]

1. Perform a careful ophthalmoscopic exam; if increased intracranial pressure and/or a CNS space occupying lesion is suspected, CT scan of the head should be done before LP
2. Place the patient in a lateral decubitus position with spine flexed (draw shoulders forward and bring thighs toward the abdomen, Fig. 30-1)
3. Identify the L4-5 interspace (imaginary line connecting the iliac crests)
4. Clean area with povidone-iodine solution
5. Anesthetize skin and subcutaneous tissues with 1-2% lidocaine
6. Gently introduce the spinal needle (with bevel turned upward) in the L4-5 interspace in a horizontal direction and with a slight cephalad inclination (Fig. 30-2)

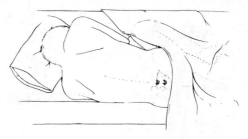

Figure 30-1
Lateral decubitus position. (From Suratt PM, Gibson RS [editors]: Manual of medical procedures, St Louis, 1982, The CV Mosby Co.)

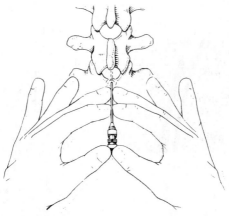

Figure 30-2
Insert spinal needle into subcutaneous tissue and slowly advance needle into subarachnoid space. (From Suratt PM, Gibson RS [editors]: Manual of medical procedures, St Louis, 1982, The CV Mosby Co.)

7. Measure opening pressure (normal is 100-200 mm Hg)
   a. If the pressure is elevated, instruct the patient to relax and ensure that there is no abdominal compression or breath holding (straining and pressure on the abdominal wall will increase the CSF pressure) (Fig. 30-3)
   b. If the pressure is markedly elevated, remove only 5 ml of spinal fluid and remove the spinal needle immediately

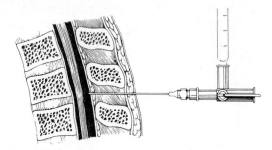

Figure 30-3
Measure opening pressure. Note position of stopcock. (From Suratt PM, Gibson RS [editors]: Manual of medical procedures, St Louis, 1982, The CV Mosby Co.)

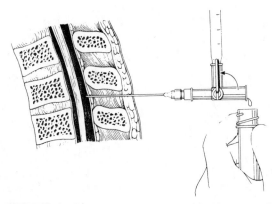

Figure 30-4
Collect cerebrospinal fluid. (From Suratt PM, Gibson RS [editors]: Manual of medical procedures, St Louis, 1982, The CV Mosby Co.)

8. Collect 5-10 ml of spinal fluid in four collection tubes (2 ml/tube) (Fig. 30-4)
9. Measure closing pressure, then remove manometer and stopcock, and replace stylet before removing the spinal needle; apply pressure to the puncture site with sterile gauze for a few minutes
10. Instruct the patient to remain in a horizontal position for approximately 4 hours to minimize post–lumbar puncture headache (caused by CSF fluid leakage through the puncture site)

11. Process the CSF fluid
    a. Tube 1: protein, glucose
    b. Tube 2: Gram stain of the centrifuged specimen
    c. Tube 3: save the fluid until further notice
    d. Tube 4: cell count (total and differential)
12. Consider additional tests (if indicated)
    a. Bacterial cultures in suspected bacterial meningitis
    b. Assay for cryptococcal antigen in immunocompromised patients
    c. Countercurrent immunoelectrophoresis (CIE): to detect specific polysaccharide bacterial antigens *(N. meningitidis, H. influenzae, S. pneumoniae)* in the CSF of patients with inconclusive Gram staining (e.g., patients with partially treated meningitis)
    d. Oligoclonal banding and assay for myelin basic protein are useful to diagnose multiple sclerosis
    e. VDRL, AFB stain, Wright stain of sediment, India ink preparation, Lyme titer antibody, fungal or viral cultures, and cytologic exam should not be routinely ordered, but only when specifically indicated

Interpretation of results[5]

1. Appearance of the fluid
   a. Clear: normal
   b. Yellow color (xanthochromia) in the supernatant of centrifuged CSF within 1 hr or less after collection is usually the result of previous bleeding (subarachnoid hemorrhage); it may also be caused by increased CSF protein, melanin from meningeal melosarcomas, or carotenoids
   c. Pinkish color is usually the result of a bloody tap; the color generally clears progressing from tubes 1 to 4 (the supernatant is usually crystal clear in traumatic taps)
   d. Turbidity usually indicates the presence of leukocytes (bleeding introduces approximately 1 WBC/500 RBC into the CSF)
2. CSF pressure: elevated pressure can be seen with meningitis, meningoencephalitis, pseudotumor cerebri, mass lesions, and intracerebral bleeding
3. Cell count: in the adult, the CSF is normally free of cells (although up to 5 mononuclear cells/mm^3 is considered normal); the presence of granulocytes is never normal
   a. Neutrophils: seen in bacterial meningitis, early viral meningoencephalitis and early TB meningitis
   b. Increased lymphocytes: TB meningitis, viral meningoencephalitis, syphilitic meningoencephalitis, fungal meningitis
4. Protein: serum proteins are generally too large to cross the normal blood/CSF barrier; however, increased CSF protein is seen with meningeal inflammation, traumatic tap, increased CNS synthesis, tissue degeneration, obstruction to CSF circulation, and Guillain-Barré syndrome
5. Glucose
   a. Decreased glucose is seen with bacterial meningitis, TB meningitis, fungal meningitis, subarachnoid hemorrhage, and some cases of viral meningitis

Table 30-1 CSF abnormalities in various CNS conditions

	Appearance	Glucose (mg/dl)	Protein (mg/dl)	Cell Count (cells/mm^3) and Cell Type	Pressure (mm Hg)
Normal	Clear	50-80	20-45	<6 Lymphocytes	100-200
Acute bacterial meningitis	Cloudy	↓/↓*	↑	↑↑ PMN†	↑/↑
Aseptic (viral) meningitis	Clear/cloudy	N	↑	↑, Usually mononuclear cells May be PMN in early stages	N/↑
Hemorrhage	Bloody/xanthochromic	N/↓	↑	↑↑ RBC	↑/↑
Neoplasm	Clear/xanthochromic	N/↓	N/↑	N/↑ Lymphocytes	↑/↑
Tuberculous meningitis	Cloudy	↓	↑	↑ PMN (early) Lymphocytes (later)	↑/↑
Fungal meningitis	Clear/cloudy	↓	↑	↑ Monocytes	↑/↑
Neurosyphilis	Clear/cloudy	N	↑	↑ Monocytes	N/↑
Guillain-Barré syndrome	Clear/cloudy	N	↑	N/↑ Lymphocytes	N

*↑, Increased; ↑↑, markedly increased; ↓, decreased; ↓↓, markedly decreased; N, normal.
†PMN, polymorphonucleocytes; RBC, red blood cells.

b. A mild increase in CSF glucose can be seen in patients with very elevated serum glucose levels

NOTE: Table 30-1 describes CSF abnormalities found in various CNS conditions.

30.2 THORACENTESIS[9]

Major indications

1. Presence of any pleural effusion of unknown cause
2. Relief of dyspnea caused by large pleural effusion

Contraindications

1. Clotting abnormalities
2. Thrombocytopenia
3. Uncooperative patient, or patient with severe cough or hiccups

Localization of pleural effusion

1. Physical exam: dullness to percussion
2. Chest x-ray: posteroanterior view is usually sufficient in identifying the fluid collection, but in case of equivocal effusions, a lateral decubitus chest x-ray can demonstrate layering out of the pleural fluid
3. Fluoroscopy or ultrasound[11]: useful before thoracentesis if the fluid collection is
   a. <10 mm thick
   b. Not freely moveable on the lateral decubitus x-ray view

Procedure[14]

1. Position patient in a sitting position with arms and head resting supported on a bedside adjustable table (Fig. 30-5)
2. Identify the area of effusion by gentle percussion
3. Clean the area with povidone-iodine solution, and maintain strict aseptic technique

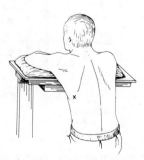

Figure 30-5

Patient position for thoracentesis. (From Suratt PM, Gibson RS [editors]: Manual of medical procedures, St Louis, 1982, The CV Mosby Co.)

4. Insert the needle in the posterior chest (approximately 5-10 cm lateral to the spine) in an interspace below the point of dullness to percussion
5. Anesthetize the skin and subcutaneous tissues with 1-2% lidocaine
6. Make sure that the needle is positioned and advanced above the superior margin of the rib (the intercostal nerve and the blood supply are located near the inferior margin)
7. Gently advance a 20-gauge needle; anesthetize the pleura and gently aspirate until pleural fluid is noted in the syringe, then remove the needle and note the depth of insertion needed for the thoracentesis needle
8. In the previous puncture site, insert a 17-gauge needle (flat bevel) attached to a 30 ml syringe via a three-way stopcock connected to a drainage tube (Fig. 30-6)
9. Slowly advance the needle (above the superior margin of the rib), and gently aspirate while advancing
10. When pleural fluid is noted, place a snap-on clip or a hemostat on the needle to prevent it from inadvertently advancing forward
11. Remove the necessary amount of pleural fluid (usually 100 ml for diagnostic studies), but do not remove more than 1500 ml of fluid at any one time because of increased risk of pulmonary edema or hypotension[6] (pneumothorax from needle laceration of the visceral pleura is also much more likely to occur if an effusion is completely drained[7])
12. Gently remove the needle
13. Obtain serum LDH, albumin, glucose levels, and total protein level
14. Process the pleural fluid; the *initial* lab studies should be aimed only at distinguishing an exudate from a transudate
    a. Tube 1: protein, LDH, albumin

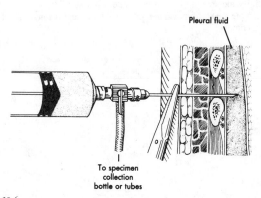

Figure 30-6
Fluid removal through thoracentesis needle and a three-way stopcock. (From Suratt PM, Gibson RS [editors]: Manual of medical procedures, St Louis, 1982, The CV Mosby Co.)

Table 30-2   Evaluation of pleural and peritoneal effusions

Test	Exudate (IU/dl)	Transudate (IU/dl)
Fluid LDH	>200	<200
Fluid protein	>3 g	<3 g
Fluid/serum LDH ratio	>0.6	<0.6
Fluid/serum protein ratio	>0.5	<0.5
Specific gravity	>1.016	<1.016

   b. Tubes 2, 3, 4: save the fluid until further notice

   NOTE: Do not order further tests until the presence of an exudate is confirmed on the basis of protein and LDH determinations[8] (Table 30-2), however, if the results of protein and LDH determinations cannot be obtained within a reasonable time (resulting in unnecessary delay), additional lab tests should be ordered at the time of thoracentesis

15. A serum/effusion albumin gradient of ≤1.2 g/dl is indicative of exudative effusions, especially in CHF patients treated with diuretics

16. Note the appearance of the fluid:
   a. A grossly hemorrhagic effusion can be secondary to a traumatic tap or neoplasm
   b. A milky appearance indicates either
     (1) Chylous effusion—due to trauma or tumor invasion of the thoracic duct; lipoprotein electrophoresis of the effusion reveals chylomicrons and triglyceride levels >115 mg/dl
     (2) Pseudochylous effusion—often seen with chronic inflammation of the pleural space (e.g., TB, connective tissue diseases)

Evaluation of results

1. For differential diagnosis of pleural effusions refer to Chapter 6
2. If transudate, consider CHF, cirrhosis, chronic renal failure, and other hypoproteinemic states and perform direct subsequent work-up accordingly
3. If exudate, consider ordering these tests on the pleural fluid:
   a. Cytological exam for malignant cells (for suspected neoplasm)
   b. Gram stain, cultures (aerobic and anaerobic), and sensitivities (for suspected infectious process)
   c. AFB stain and cultures (for suspected TB)
   d. pH: a value <7.0 suggests parapneumonic effusion[11] or empyema; a pleural fluid pH must be drawn anaerobically and iced immediately; the syringe should be prerinsed with 0.2 ml of 1:1000 heparin
   e. Glucose: a low glucose level suggests parapneumonic effusions and rheumatoid arthritis
   f. Amylase: a high amylase level suggests pancreatitis or ruptured esophagus

Complications of thoracentesis[4]

1. Pneumothorax
2. Hemorrhage
3. Vasovagal episode
4. Infection
5. Unilateral pulmonary edema
6. Puncture of liver or spleen
7. Subcutaneous emphysema
8. Air embolism

30.3   PARACENTESIS

Indications

1. Ascites of undetermined etiology
2. Evaluation for possible peritonitis
3. Relief of abdominal pain and discomfort caused by tense ascites
4. Relief of dyspnea caused by elevated diaphragm (from ascites)
5. Evaluation of possible intraabdominal hemorrhage in a patient with blunt abdominal trauma
6. Institution of peritoneal dialysis

Contraindications

1. Bleeding disorders
2. Bowel distention
3. Infection or surgical scars at the site of needle entry

Procedure[4,14]

1. Have patient empty the bladder (insertion of a Foley catheter is not recommended but may be necessary in certain patients)
2. To identify the site of paracentesis, first locate the rectus muscle; a good site is approximately 2-3 cm lateral to the rectus muscle border in the lower abdominal quadrants (Fig. 30-7). Avoid the following:

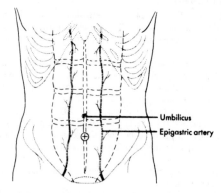

Figure 30-7
Anatomic landmarks for paracentesis. (From Suratt PM, Gibson RS [editors]: Manual of medical procedures, St Louis, 1982, The CV Mosby Co.)

   a. Rectus muscles (increased risk of hemorrhage from epigastric vessels)

   b. Surgical scars (increased risk of perforation caused by adhesion of bowel to the wall of the peritoneum)

   c. Areas of skin infection (increased risk of intraperitoneal infection)

   NOTE: An alternate site is on the linea alba 3-4 cm below the umbilicus

3. Cleanse the area with povidone-iodine and drape the abdomen
4. Anesthetize the puncture site with 1-2% lidocaine
5. Cautiously insert the needle (attached to a syringe) perpendicular to the skin; a small pop is felt as the needle advances through the anterior and posterior muscular fascia, and entrance into the peritoneal cavity is evidenced as a sudden "give" (use caution to avoid the sudden thrust forward of the needle)
6. Remove the necessary amount of fluid (generally not more than 1 L, particularly in cirrhotic patients)
7. If diagnostic paracentesis, process the fluid as follows:

   a. Tube 1: LDH, glucose

   b. Tube 2: protein, specific gravity, albumin

   c. Tube 3: cell count and differential

   d. Tube 4: save until further notice

8. Draw serum LDH, protein, albumin
9. Gram stain, AFB stain, bacterial and fungal cultures, amylase, and triglycerides should be ordered only when indicated
10. If malignant ascites is suspected, consider a carcinoembryonic antigen (CEA) level on the paracentesis fluid and cytological evaluation
11. In suspected spontaneous bacterial peritonitis (SBP) the incidence of positive cultures can be increased by injecting 10 to 20 ml of ascitic fluid into blood culture bottles[12]

Interpretation of results[1]

1. Peritoneal effusion can be classified as exudative or transudative based on its characteristics (Table 30-2)
2. For the differential diagnosis of ascites refer to Chapter 6
3. Table 30-3 describes the characteristics of ascitic fluid in various conditions
4. An ascitic fluid PMN count of >500/μl indicates spontaneous bacterial peritonitis (see Section 25.13)
5. A blood–ascitic fluid albumin gradient of less than 1.1 g/dl indicates malignant ascites

Complications

1. Persistent leakage of ascitic fluid
2. Hypotension and shock
3. Bleeding
4. Perforated bowel
5. Abscess formation in area of puncture site
6. Peritonitis

Table 30-3 Characteristics of ascitic fluid in various conditions[2-6]

Etiology	Appearance	Total Protein (g/dl)	LDH (IU)	Specific Gravity	Glucose (mg/dl)	WBC/mm³	RBC/mm³	Amylase
Neoplasm	Bloody Clear Chylous	>2.0	>200	Variable	<60	↑*	↑↑	
Cirrhosis	Straw-colored	<2.5	<200	<1.016	<60	→	→	
Nephrosis	Straw-colored	<2.5	<200	<1.016	>60	→	→	
CHF	Straw-colored	<2.5	<200	<1.016	>60	→	→	
Pyogenic	Turbid	>2.5	>200	>1.016	>60	↑ PMN†	→	
Pancreatic	Clear Hemorrhagic Turbid Chylous	>2.5	>200	Variable	>60	Variable	Variable	↑↑

* ↑, High; ↑↑, markedly high; ↓, low.
† PMN, Polymorphonuclear leukocytes.

30.4 ARTHROCENTESIS

Indications

1. Presence of effusion of unexplained etiology
2. Steroid injection
3. Decompression of a hemorrhagic effusion in traumatized joints
4. Evaluation of antibiotic response in patients with infectious arthritis
5. Removal of purulent fluid in distended infected joints

Contraindication

1. Infection at the arthrocentesis site

Procedure[14]

1. Palpate the joint and identify the extensor surface (vessels and nerves are less commonly found here)
2. With firm pressure, use a ballpoint pen that has the writing portion retracted to mark the specific area of the joint to be aspirated
3. Clean the skin with an antiseptic solution
4. Use a 25-gauge needle to infiltrate the skin with 1-2% lidocaine
5. Gently insert an 18- or 20-gauge needle connected to a 20-30 ml syringe; a slight "pop" may be felt as the needle penetrates through the capsule (Fig. 30-8 shows arthrocentesis of knee joint)
6. Apply gentle suction to the syringe to aspirate the fluid
7. Gently remove the needle and apply slight pressure to the puncture site
8. Process the aspirated synovial fluid:
   a. Tube 1 (no heparin): viscosity, mucin clot

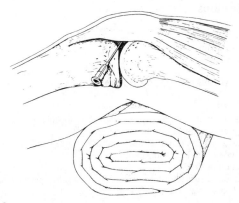

Figure 30-8
Arthrocentesis of knee joint, anteromedial approach. Flex knee and insert needle approximately 1 cm below patella. (From Suratt PM, Gibson RS [editors]: Manual of medical procedures, St Louis, 1982, The CV Mosby Co.)

b. Tube 2 (containing heparin): glucose
c. Tube 3 (containing heparin): Gram stain, culture and sensitivity, cytology, cell count and differential
d. Glass slide: place a drop of fluid and examine under polarized light
e. Plate with Thayer-Martin medium: used in cases of suspected gonococcal arthritis; Lyme titer, cultures for anaerobes, *Mycobacterium tuberculosis,* and fungi should be ordered only when clearly indicated

9. Draw serum glucose

Interpretation of results[4,5,13]

1. Color: normally it is clear or pale yellow; cloudiness indicates inflammatory process or presence of crystals, cell debris, fibrin, or triglycerides
2. Viscosity: normally it has a high viscosity because of hyaluronate; when fluid is placed on a slide it can be stretched to a string >2 cm in length before separating (low viscosity indicates breakdown of hyaluronate [lysosomal enzymes from leukocytes] or the presence of edema fluid)
3. Mucin clot: add 1 ml of fluid to 5 ml of a 5% acetic acid solution and allow 1 minute for the clot to form; a firm clot (does not fragment on shaking) is normal and indicates the presence of large molecules of hyaluronic acid (this test is nonspecific and infrequently done)
4. Glucose: normally it approximately equals serum glucose, a difference of more than 40 mg/dl is suggestive of infection
5. Microscopic examination for crystals (also refer to Section 29.5)
   a. Gout: monosodium urate crystals (MSU)
   b. Pseudogout: calcium pyrophosphate dihydrate crystals (CPPD)

NOTE: Synovial fluid is classified into three major groups based on its characteristics (Table 30-4)

Complications

1. Infection
2. Hemorrhage
3. Tendon rupture
4. Nerve palsies

30.5 BONE MARROW EXAMINATION

Indications[10,14]

1. Evaluation of anemia, leukopenia, thrombocytopenia, pancytopenia
2. Staging of lymphoma or solid tumors
3. Diagnosis and evaluation of treatment of dysproteinemias, leukemias
4. Evaluation of iron metabolism
5. Evaluation of FUO
6. Evaluation of suspected tuberculosis or of fungal or parasitic infections
7. Unexplained splenomegaly

Contraindications

1. Skin infection, osteomyelitis, or previous radiation therapy in the area of proposed aspiration or biopsy

Table 30-4 Classification and interpretation of synovial fluid analysis[4,5,13]

Group	Diseases	Appearance	Viscosity	Mucin Clot	WBC/mm³	% PMN*	Glucose (mg/dl) (Blood-Synovial Fluid)
Normal	—	Clear	↑↑	Firm	<200	<25	<10
I (noninflammatory)	Osteoarthritis, aseptic necrosis, traumatic arthritis, erythema nodosum, osteochondritis dissecans	Clear, yellow (may be xanthochromic if traumatic arthritis)	↑	Firm	↑ Up to 10,000	<25	<10
II (inflammatory)	Crystal-induced arthritis, rheumatoid arthritis, Reiter's syndrome, collagen vascular disease, psoriatic arthritis, serum sickness, rheumatic fever	Clear, yellow Turbid	↓	Friable	↑↑ Up to 100,000	40-90	<40
III (septic)	Bacterial (staphylococcal, gonococcal, TB)	Turbid	↓/↑	Friable	↑↑↑ Up to 5,000,000	40-100	20-100

*PMN, polymorphonuclear leukocytes.

↑↑, Elevated; ↑↑, markedly high; ↓, decreased. Note that there is considerable overlap in the numbers listed above.

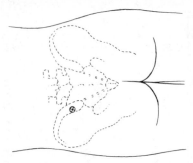

Figure 30-9
Posterior iliac crest anatomy. (From Suratt PM, Gibson RS [editors]: Manual of medical procedures, St Louis, 1982, The CV Mosby Co.)

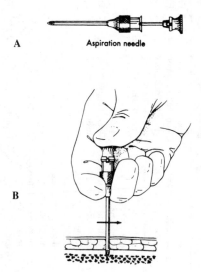

Figure 30-10
A, Bone marrow aspiration needle. B, Insert the needle with the stylet in place. (From Suratt PM, Gibson RS [editors]: Manual of medical procedure, St Louis, 1982, The CV Mosby Co.)

2. Uncooperative patient
3. Severe hemorrhagic diathesis (except for thrombocytopenia)

Procedure[10,14]

1. The preferred site is the posterior iliac crest; other sites are the sternum, anterior iliac crest, and greater femoral trochanter
2. Position the patient prone or lateral decubitus (Fig. 30-9)
3. Examine the site for evidence of infection, mark the area site by making an indentation in the skin with a coin or the end of a ballpoint pen (writing tip retracted)
4. Cleanse the area with povidone-iodine solution and drape a sterile field
5. Anesthetize the skin and subcutaneous tissues with 1-2% lidocaine using a 23-gauge needle; then with a 21-gauge needle, anesthetize the periosteum
6. Make a small (3 mm) skin incision with a scalpel blade at the site of insertion of the aspiration needle (to facilitate its entry)
7. Hold the bone marrow needle (with stylet in place, Fig. 30-10) perpendicular to the skin and gently advance it to the periosteum
8. Use a steady twisting motion to penetrate periosteum and the cortical bone; a "give" is felt upon entering the marrow cavity
9. Remove the stylet, attach a 2 ml syringe to the needle, and warn patient that the aspiration will cause a brief period of pain
10. Aspirate 0.2-0.4 ml of marrow contents, remove the syringe, reinsert the stylet, and place a drop of aspirate on each of 4 to 6 slides; prepare the slides as shown in Fig. 30-11; the presence of grossly visible bone spicules indicates a suitable specimen
11. Remove the needle (with stylet in place) using a twisting motion and apply a pressure dressing to the site until the bleeding stops
12. If biopsy is necessary, prepare the Jamshidi needle (Fig. 30-12) and advance it into the cortical bone with a steady rotating movement until it is firmly lodged; then remove the stylet and with a rotating motion advance the needle another 5-15 mm (Fig. 30-13)
13. Redirect the needle tip and rotate it 360 degrees to break off the biopsy specimen
14. Remove the needle with a twisting motion and apply a sterile pressure dressing to the site until the bleeding stops
15. Remove the specimen from the needle by inserting the obturator into the distal end of the needle (Fig. 30-14)

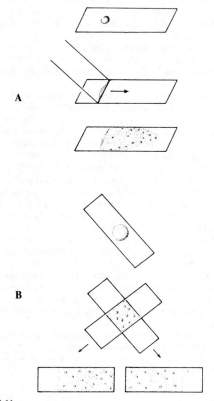

Figure 30-11
Slide preparation. (From Suratt PM, Gibson RS [editors]: Manual of medical procedures, St Louis, 1982, The CV Mosby Co.)

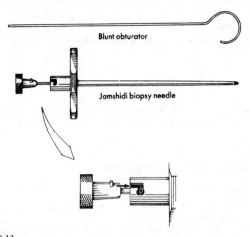

Blunt obturator

Jamshidi biopsy needle

Figure 30-12
Preparation of the biopsy needle. (From Suratt PM, Gibson RS [editors]: Manual of medical procedures, St Louis, 1982, The CV Mosby Co.)

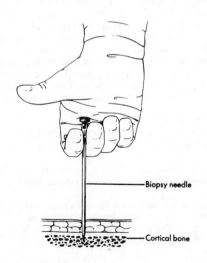

Biopsy needle

Cortical bone

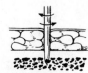

Figure 30-13
Insert the needle through the incision, penetrating cortical bone with a steady rotating movement. (From Suratt PM, Gibson RS [editors]: Manual of medical procedures, St Louis, 1982, The CV Mosby Co.)

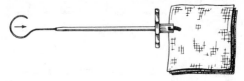

Figure 30-14
Remove the specimen from the biopsy needle. (From Suratt PM, Gibson RS [editors]: Manual of medical procedures, St Louis, 1982, The CV Mosby Co.)

30.6   RADIAL ARTERY CANNULATION

Major indications

1. Monitoring of blood pressure during use of potent vasoactive agents (e.g., nitroprusside, dopamine)
2. Monitoring of blood pressure in critically ill hypotensive patients (e.g., shock) or during major surgery (e.g., cardiovascular)
3. Frequent arterial blood gas analysis or other blood tests in patients with limited vascular access

Procedure[14]

1. Evaluate patency of the ulnar artery with the Allen test (Fig. 30-15): simultaneously compressing the radial and ulnar arteries, have the patient clench and elevate the fist to let blood drain from the hand; keep pressure on both arteries until the hand blanches; then have the patient open the hand while pressure is maintained on both arteries; release the ulnar artery and observe the hand for blushing; the presence of blushing and return of normal color to the hand indicate patency of the ulnar artery and adequate blood supply if radial occlusion occurs with the catheter
2. Hyperextend the hand over a wrist roll and immobilize it and the lower arm (Fig. 30-16)
3. Sterile drape and clean the area with povidone-iodine solution
4. Anesthetize the skin and then insert the angiocatheter through the skin at a 30-45 degree angle, advancing it parallel to the artery; gently cannulate the artery (Fig. 30-17)
5. Detach the syringe and connect the catheter to the pressure tubing and functioning irrigation system; an arterial pressure tracing indicates intraarterial positioning
6. Secure the catheter line to the skin with a silk ligature and apply sterile dressing and adhesive tape to prevent accidental disconnection
7. Remove the wrist from its hyperextended position and splint the dorsal aspect to prevent accidental disconnection

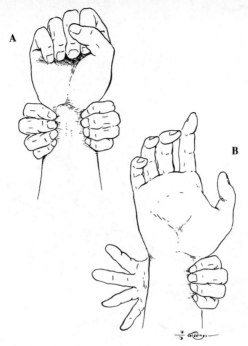

Figure 30-15
Allen test for ulnar artery patency. (From Van Way CW, Buerk CA: Surgical skills in patient care, St Louis, 1978, The CV Mosby Co.)

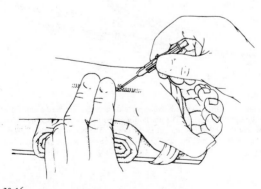

Figure 30-16
Hyperextend the hand over a wrist roll; immobilize the hand and lower arm. (From Suratt PM, Gibson RS [editors]: Manual of medical procedures, St Louis, 1982, The CV Mosby Co.)

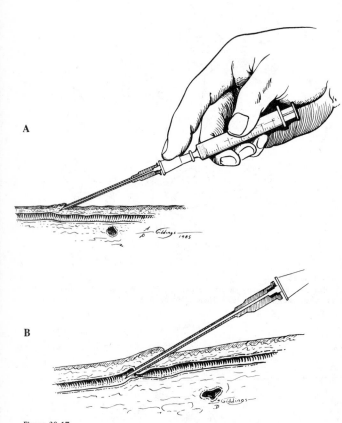

Figure 30-17
Cannulation of an artery with an over-needle device. **A,** The needle and catheter are inserted through the skin. **B,** The needle tip enters the artery. Blood can be aspirated, but the catheter is not yet in the artery. The barrel is gently lowered, raising the needle tip, and the needle is advanced farther so the catheter can enter the artery.

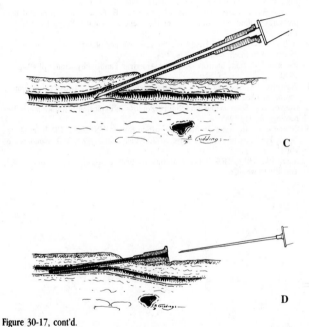

Figure 30-17, cont'd.
C. After the needle is in the artery, the catheter is threaded over it. **D,** The needle is then withdrwan, leaving the catheter in place. (From Van Way CW, Buerk CA: Surgical skills in patient care, St Louis, 1978, The CV Mosby Co.)

References

1. Albillos A, et al: Ascitic fluid polymorphonuclear cell count and serum to ascites albumin gradient in the diagnosis of bacterial peritonitis, Gastroenterology 98:134, 1990.
2. Bauer JD: Clinical laboratory methods, ed 9, St Louis, 1982, The CV Mosby Co.
3. Bennington JL: Saunders' dictionary and encyclopedia of laboratory medicine and technology, Philadelphia, 1984, WB Saunders Co.
4. Eknoyan G: Medical procedures manual, Chicago, 1982, Year Book Medical Publishers Inc.
5. Henry JB, Todd SD: Clinical diagnosis and management by laboratory methods, Philadelphia, 1984, WB Saunders Co.
6. Light RW: Management of parapneumonic effusions, Arch Intern Med 141:1339, 1981.
7. Light RW: Pleural diseases, Philadelphia, 1983, Lea & Febiger.
8. Light RW, Jenkinson SG, Mihn VD, George RB: Observation on pleural fluid pressures as fluid is withdrawn during thoracentesis, Am Rev Respir Dis 121:799, 1980.
9. Hall WJ, Mayewski RJ: Diagnostic thoracentesis and pleural biopsy in pleural effusions, Ann Intern Med 103:798, 1985.
10. Paulman PM: Bone marrow sampling, American Family Physician, vol 40, p 85, 1990.
11. Peterman TA, Speicher CE: Evaluating pleural effusions: a two-stage laboratory approach, JAMA 252:1051, 1984.
12. Runyon BA: Spontaneous bacterial peritonitis: an explosion of information, Hepatology 8:171, 1988.
13. Schumacher HR: Synovial fluid analysis. In Kelley WN, Harris ED Jr, et al (editors): Textbook of rheumatology, ed 2, Philadelphia, 1985, WB Saunders Co, vol 1.
14. Suratt PM, Gibson RS (editors): Manual of medical procedures, St Louis, 1982, The CV Mosby Co.

Laboratory Values and Interpretation of Results

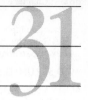

This chapter covers over 150 of the most common laboratory tests. Each test is approached with the following format:

1. Laboratory test
2. Normal range in adult patients
3. Common abnormalities, such as positive test, increased or decreased value
4. Causes of abnormal result

The normal ranges may differ slightly, depending on the laboratory. The reader should be aware of the "normal range" of the particular laboratory performing the test. Every attempt has been made to present current laboratory test data with emphasis on practical considerations. Normal values are given using the present (traditional) reference interval, followed by the Système Internationale (SI) reference interval, the conversion factor (CF), and the suggested minimum increment (SMI). For example,

Test	Present reference interval	SI reference interval	CF	SMI
Fasting glucose	70-110 mg/dl	3.6-6.1 mmol/L	0.05551	0.1 mmol/L

ACETONE (serum or plasma)

Normal:
  Negative
Elevated in:
  DKA, starvation, isopropanol ingestion

ACE LEVEL; *see* ANGIOTENSIN CONVERTING ENZYME

ACID PHOSPHATASE (serum)

Normal range:
  0-5.5 U/L (0-90 nkat/L) [CF: 16.67, SMI: 2 nkat/L]
Elevated in:
  Carcinoma of prostate, other neoplasms (breast, bone), Paget's disease, osteogenesis imperfecta, malignant invasion of bone, Gaucher's dis-

ease, multiple myeloma, myeloproliferative disorders, benign prostatic hypertrophy, prostatic palpation or surgery, hyperparathyroidism, liver disease, chronic renal failure

ACID SERUM TEST; *see* HAM TEST

ACTIVATED PARTIAL THROMBOPLASTIN TIME (APTT, aPTT); *see* PARTIAL THROMBOPLASTIN TIME

ALANINE AMINOTRANSFERASE (ALT, SGPT)
Normal range:
   0-35 U/L (0.058 μkat/L) [CF: 0.02 μkat/L]
Elevated in:
   Liver disease (hepatitis, cirrhosis, Reye's syndrome), hepatic congestion, infectious mononucleosis, MI, myocarditis, severe muscle trauma, dermatomyositis/polymyositis, muscular dystrophy, drugs (antibiotics, narcotics, antihypertensive agents, heparin, labetalol, lovastatin, NSAIDs, amiodarone, chlorpromazine, phenytoin), malignancy, renal and pulmonary infarction, convulsions, eclampsia, shock liver

ALBUMIN (serum)
Normal range:
   4-6 g/dl (40-60 g/L) [CF: 10, SMI: 1 g/L]
Elevated in:
   Dehydration
Decreased in:
   Liver disease, nephrotic syndrome, poor nutritional status, rapid IV hydration, protein-losing enteropathies (inflammatory bowel disease), severe burns, neoplasia, chronic inflammatory diseases, pregnancy, oral contraceptives, prolonged immobilization

ALDOLASE (serum)
Normal range:
   0-6 U/L (0-100 nkat/L) [CF: 16.67, SMI: 20 nkat/L]
Elevated in:
   Muscular dystrophy, rhabdomyolysis, dermatomyositis/polymyositis, trichinosis, acute hepatitis and other liver diseases, MI, prostatic carcinoma, hemorrhagic pancreatitis, gangrene, delirium tremens
Decreased in:
   Loss of muscle mass, late stages of muscular dystrophy

ALKALINE PHOSPHATASE (serum)
Normal range:
   30-120 U/L (0.5-2 μkat/L) [CF: 0.01667, SMI: 0.1 μkat/L]
Elevated in:
   Biliary obstruction, cirrhosis (particularly primary biliary cirrhosis), liver disease (hepatitis, infiltrative liver diseases, fatty metamorphosis), Paget's disease of bone, osteitis deformans, rickets, osteomalacia, hypervitaminosis D, hyperparathyroidism, hyperthyroidism, ulcerative colitis, bowel perforation, bone metastases, healing fractures, bone neoplasms, acromegaly, infectious mononucleosis, CMV infections,

sepsis, pulmonary infarction, CHF, hypernephroma, leukemia, myelofibrosis, multiple myeloma, drugs (estrogens, albumin, erythromycin and other antibiotics, cholestasis-producing drugs [phenothiazines])

Decreased in:
Hypothyroidism, pernicious anemia, hypophosphatemia, hypervitaminosis D, malnutrition

ALPHA-1-FETOPROTEIN (serum); *see* α-1 FETOPROTEIN

ALT; *see* ALANINE AMINOTRANSFERASE

AMMONIA (serum)

Normal range:
10-80 μg/dl (5-50 μmol/L) [CF: 0.5872, SMI: 5 μmol/L]
Elevated in:
Hepatic failure, hepatic encephalopathy, Reye's syndrome, portacaval shunt, drugs (diuretics, polymyxin B, methicillin)

Decreased in:
Drugs (neomycin, lactulose, tetracycline), renal failure

AMYLASE (serum)

Normal range:
0-130 U/L (0-2.17 μkat/L) [CF: 0.01667, SMI: 0.01 μkat/L]
Elevated in:
Acute pancreatitis, pancreatic neoplasm, abscess, pseudocyst, ascites, macroamylasemia, perforated peptic ulcer, intestinal obstruction, intestinal infarction, acute cholecystitis, appendicitis, ruptured ectopic pregnancy, salivary gland inflammation, peritonitis, burns, diabetic ketoacidosis, renal insufficiency, drugs (morphine), carcinomatosis of lung, esophagus, ovary, acute ethanol ingestion

Decreased in:
Advanced chronic pancreatitis, hepatic necrosis

AMYLASE, URINE; *see* URINE AMYLASE

ANA; *see* ANTINUCLEAR ANTIBODY

ANGIOTENSIN CONVERTING ENZYME (ACE level)

Normal range:
<40 nmol/ml/min (<670 nkat/L) [CF: 16.67, SMI: 10 nkat/L]
Elevated in:
Sarcoidosis, primary biliary cirrhosis, alcoholic liver disease, hyperthyroidism, hyperparathyroidism, diabetes mellitus, amyloidosis, multiple myeloma, lung disease (asbestosis, silicosis, berylliosis, allergic alveolitis, coccidioidomycosis), Gaucher's disease, leprosy

ANION GAP

Normal range:
8-16 mEq/L
Elevated in:
Lactic acidosis

Ketoacidosis (DKA, alcoholic starvation)
Uremia (chronic renal failure)
Ingestion of toxins (paraldehyde, methanol, salicylates, ethylene glycol)
Decreased in:
Hypoalbuminemia, severe hypermagnesemia, IgG myeloma, lithium tox-
icity, lab error (falsely decreased sodium or overestimation of bicar-
bonate or chloride)

ANTICOAGULANT; *see* CIRCULATING ANTICOAGULANT

ANTI-DNA
Normal range:
Absent
Present in:
SLE, chronic active hepatitis, infectious mononucleosis, biliary cirrhosis

ANTIGLOMERULAR BASEMENT ANTIBODY; *see* GLOMERULAR BASEMENT MEMBRANE ANTIBODY

ANTIMITOCHONDRIAL ANTIBODY
Normal range:
<1:20 titer
Elevated in:
Primary biliary cirrhosis (85-95%), chronic active hepatitis (25%-30%),
cryptogenic cirrhosis (25-30%)

ANTINUCLEAR ANTIBODY (ANA)
Normal range:
<1:20 titer
Positive test:
SLE (more significant if titer >1:160), drugs (phenytoin, ethosuximide,
primidone, methyldopa, hydralazine, carbamazepine, penicillin, procainamide, chlorpromazine, griseofulvin, thiazides), chronic active
hepatitis, age over 60 yr (particularly age over 80), rheumatoid arthritis, scleroderma, mixed connective tissue disease, necrotizing vasculitis, Sjögren's syndrome (SS), tuberculosis, pulmonary interstitial fibrosis
NOTE: Refer to Section 29.2 for further information.

ANTI-RNP ANTIBODY; *see* EXTRACTABLE NUCLEAR ANTIGEN

ANTI-Sm (anti-Smith) ANTIBODY; *see* EXTRACTABLE NUCLEAR ANTIGEN

ANTI–SMOOTH MUSCLE ANTIBODY; *see* SMOOTH MUSCLE ANTIBODY

ANTI–STREPTOLYSIN O TITER (STREPTOZYME, ASLO titer)
Normal range for adults:
<160 Todd units
Elevated in:
Streptococcal upper airway infection, acute rheumatic fever, acute glom-
erulonephritis, increased levels of β-lipoprotein

NOTE: A fourfold increase in titer between acute and convalescent specimens is diagnostic of streptococcal upper airway infection regardless of the initial titer.

ANTITHROMBIN III

Normal range:
   81-120% of normal activity; 17-30 mg/dl
Decreased in:
   Hereditary deficiency of antithrombin III, DIC, pulmonary embolism, cirrhosis, thrombolytic therapy, chronic liver failure, post-surgery, third trimester of pregnancy, oral contraceptives, nephrotic syndrome, IV heparin >3 days, sepsis
Elevated in:
   Warfarin drugs, post-MI

ARTERIAL BLOOD GASES

Normal range:
   Po_2: 75-100 mm Hg
   Pco_2: 35-45 mm Hg
   HCO_3^-: 24-28 mEq/L
   pH: 7.35-7.45
Abnormal values:
   Refer to Chapter 19

ASLO TITER; *see* ANTI–STREPTOLYSIN O TITER

ASPARTATE AMINOTRANSFERASE (AST, SGOT)

Normal range:
   0-35 U/L (0-0.58 µkat/L) [CF: 0.01667, SMI: 0.01 µkat/L]
Elevated in:
   Liver disease (hepatitis, cirrhosis, Reye's syndrome), hepatic congestion, infectious mononucleosis, MI, myocarditis, severe muscle trauma, dermatomyositis/polymyositis, muscular dystrophy, drugs (antibiotics, narcotics, antihypertensive agents, heparin, labetalol, lovastatin, NSAIDs, phenytoin, amiodarone, chlorpromazine), malignancy, renal and pulmonary infarction, convulsions, eclampsia

BASOPHIL COUNT

Normal range:
   0.4-1% of total WBC; 40-100 mm^3
Elevated in:
   Leukemia, inflammatory processes, polycythemia vera, Hodgkin's lymphoma, hemolytic anemia, after splenectomy, myeloid metaplasia
Decreased in:
   Stress, hypersensitivity reaction, steroids, pregnancy, hyperthyroidism

BILE, URINE; *see* URINE BILE

BILIRUBIN, DIRECT (conjugated bilirubin)

Normal range:
   0-0.2 mg/dl (0-4 µmol/L) [CF: 17.10, SMI: 2 µmol/L]

Elevated in:
   Hepatocellular disease, biliary obstruction, drug-induced cholestasis, hereditary disorders (Dubin-Johnson syndrome, Rotor's syndrome)

BILIRUBIN, INDIRECT (unconjugated bilirubin)

Normal range:
   0-1.0 mg/dl (2-18 μmol/L) [CF: 17.10, SMI: 2 μmol/L]
Elevated in:
   Hemolysis, liver disease (hepatitis, cirrhosis, neoplasm), hepatic congestion secondary to congestive heart failure, hereditary disorders (Gilbert's disease, Crigler-Najjar syndrome)

BILIRUBIN, TOTAL

Normal range:
   0-1.0 mg/dl (2-18 μmol/L) [CF: 17.10, SMI: 2 μmol/L]
Elevated in:
   Liver disease (hepatitis, cirrhosis, cholangitis, neoplasm, biliary obstruction, infectious mononucleosis), hereditary disorders (Gilbert's disease, Dubin-Johnson syndrome), drugs (steroids, diphenylhydantoin, phenothiazines, penicillin, erythromycin, clindamycin, captopril, amphotericin B, sulfonamides, azathioprine, isoniazid, 5-aminosalicylic acid, allopurinol, methyldopa, indomethacin, halothane, oral contraceptives, procainamide, tolbutamide, labetalol), hemolysis, pulmonary embolism or infarct, hepatic congestion secondary to CHF

BILIRUBIN, URINE; *see* URINE BILE

BLEEDING TIME (modified Ivy method)

Normal range:
   2 to 9½ min
Elevated in:
   Thrombocytopenia, capillary wall abnormalities, platelet abnormalities (Bernard-Soulier, Glanzmann's), drugs (aspirin, warfarin, antiinflammatory medications, streptokinase, urokinase, dextran, β lactam antibiotics, moxalactam), DIC, cirrhosis, uremia, myeloproliferative disorders, Von Willebrand's

BUN; *see* UREA NITROGEN

C3; *see* COMPLEMENT C3

C4; *see* COMPLEMENT C4

CALCITONIN (serum)

Normal range:
   <100 pg/ml (<100 ng/L) [CF: 1, SMI: 10 ng/L]
Elevated in:
   Medullary carcinoma of the thyroid (particularly if level >1500 pg/ml), carcinoma of the breast, APUDomas, carcinoids, renal failure, thyroiditis

CALCIUM (serum)

Normal range:
8.8-10.3 mg/dl (2.2-2.58 mmol/L) [CF: 0.2495, SMI: 0.02 mmol/L]
Abnormal values:
Refer to Section 22.8

CALCIUM, URINE; *see* URINE CALCIUM

CARBON MONOXIDE; *see* CARBOXYHEMOGLOBIN

CARBOXYHEMOGLOBIN

Normal range:
Saturation of hemoglobin <2%, smokers <9% (coma: 50%; death: 80%)
Elevated in:
Smoking, exposure to smoking, exposure to automobile exhaust fumes, malfunctioning gas-burning appliances

CARCINOEMBRYONIC ANTIGEN (CEA)

Normal range:
Nonsmokers: 0-2.5 ng/ml (0-2.5 μg/L) [CF: 1, SMI: 0.1 μg/L]
Smokers: 0-5 ng/ml (0-5 μg/L) [CF: 1, SMI: 0.1 μg/L]
Elevated in:
Colorectal carcinomas, pancreatic carcinomas, and metastatic disease usually produce higher elevations (>20 ng/ml)
Carcinomas of the esophagus, stomach, small intestine, liver, breast, ovary, lung and thyroid usually produce lesser elevations
Benign conditions (smoking, inflammatory bowel disease, hypothyroidism, cirrhosis, pancreatitis, infections) usually produce levels <10 ng/ml

CAROTENE (serum)

Normal range:
50-250 μg/dl (0.9-4.6 μmol/L) [CF: 0.01863, SMI: 0.1 μmol/L]
Elevated in:
Carotenemia, chronic nephritis, diabetes mellitus, hypothyroidism, nephrotic syndrome
Decreased in:
Fat malabsorption, steatorrhea, pancreatic insufficiency, lack of carotenoids in diet

CATECHOLAMINES, URINE; *see* URINE CATECHOLAMINES

CBC; *see* COMPLETE BLOOD COUNT

CEA; *see* CARCINOEMBRYONIC ANTIGEN

CEREBROSPINAL FLUID (CSF)

Normal range:
Appearance: clear
Glucose: 40-70 mg/dl (2.2-3.9 mmol/L) [CF: 0.055, SMI: 0.1 mmol]
Protein: 20-45 mg/dl (0.20-0.45 g/L) [CF: 0.01, SMI: 0.1 g/L]
Chloride: 116-122 mEq/L (116-122 mmol/L) [CF: 1, SMI: 1 mmol/L]

Pressure: 100-200 mm H_2O

Cell count (cells/mm^3) and cell type: <6 lymphocytes, no polymorpho-
nucleotes

Refer to Section 30.1 for interpretation of abnormalities

CERULOPLASMIN (serum)

Normal range:

20-35 mg/dl (200-350 mg/L) [CF: 10, SMI: 10 mg/L]

Elevated in:

Pregnancy, estrogens, oral contraceptives, neoplastic diseases (leukemias, Hodgkin's lymphoma, carcinomas), inflammatory states, SLE,
primary biliary cirrhosis, rheumatoid arthritis

Decreased in:

Wilson's disease (values often <10 mg/dl), nephrotic syndrome, advanced liver disease, malabsorption, total parenteral nutrition, Menkes' syndrome

CHLORIDE (serum)

Normal range:

95-105 mEq/L (95-105 mmol/L) [CF: 1, SMI: 1 mmol/L]

Elevated in:

Dehydration, excessive infusion of normal saline

Hyperparathyroidism, renal tubular disease, metabolic acidosis, prolonged diarrhea

Drugs (ammonium chloride administration, acetazolamide, boric acid,
triamterene)

Decreased in:

CHF, SIADH, Addison's disease, vomiting, gastric suction, salt-losing
nephritis, continuous infusion of D$_5$W, thiazide diuretic administration, diaphoresis, diarrhea, burns

CHLORIDE, URINE; *see* URINE CHLORIDE

CHOLESTEROL, TOTAL

Normal range:

Varies with age (see Chapter 9)

Generally <200 mg/dl (<5.20 mmol/L) [CF: 0.02586, SMI: 0.05 mmol/
L]

Elevated in:

Primary hypercholesterolemia, biliary obstruction, diabetes mellitus,
nephrotic syndrome, hypothyroidism, primary biliary cirrhosis, high
cholesterol diet, third trimester of pregnancy, MI, drugs (steroids,
phenothiazines, oral contraceptives)

Decreased in:

Starvation, malabsorption, sideroblastic anemia, thalassemia, abetalipoproteinemia, hyperthyroidism, Cushing's syndrome, hepatic failure,
multiple myeloma, polycythemia vera, chronic myelocytic leukemia,
myeloid metaplasia, Waldenstrom's macroglobulinemia, myelofibrosis

CHOLESTEROL, LOW DENSITY LIPOPROTEIN; *see* LOW DENSITY
LIPOPROTEIN CHOLESTEROL

CHOLESTEROL, HIGH DENSITY LIPOPROTEIN; *see* HIGH DENSITY LIPOPROTEIN CHOLESTEROL

CIRCULATING ANTICOAGULANT (lupus anticoagulant)

Normal:
Negative
Detected in:
SLE, drug-induced lupus, long-term phenothiazine therapy, multiple myeloma, ulcerative colitis, rheumatoid arthritis, postpartum, hemophilia, neoplasms, chronic inflammatory states

CK; *see* CREATINE KINASE

CO; *see* CARBOXYHEMOGLOBIN

COAGULATION FACTORS

Factor reference ranges:
V: >10%
VII: >10%
VIII: 50-170%
IX: 60-136%
X: >10%
XI: 50-150%
XII: >30%

COLD AGGLUTININS TITER

Normal range:
<1:32
Elevated in:
Primary atypical pneumonia (mycoplasma pneumonia), infectious mononucleosis, CMV infection
Other: hepatic cirrhosis, acquired hemolytic anemia, frostbite, multiple myeloma, lymphoma, malaria

COMPLEMENT (C3, C4)

Normal range:
C3 70-160 mg/dl (0.7-1.6 g/L) [CF: 0.01, SMI: 0.1 g/L]
C4 20-40 mg/dl (0.2-0.4 g/L) [CF: 0.01, SMI: 0.1 g/L]
Abnormal values:
Refer to Tables 31-1, 31-2

COMPLETE BLOOD COUNT
WBC 3200-9800 mm^3 (3.2-9.8 10^9/L) [CF: 0.001, SMI: 0.1 × 10^9/L]
RBC
  Male: 4.3-5.9 10^6/mm^3 (4.3-5.9 10^{12}/L) [CF: 1, SMI: 0.1 × 10^{12}/L]
  Female: 3.5-5 10^6/mm^3 (3.5-5 10^{12}/L) [CF: 1, SMI: 0.1 × 10^{12}/L]
Hemoglobin
  Male: 13.6-17.7 g/dl (136-172 g/L) [CF: 10, SMI: 1 g/L]
  Female: 12-15 g/dl (120-150 g/L) [CF: 10, SMI: 1 g/L]

Table 31-1 Summary of complement deficiencies in humans and their association with repeated infection and/or collagen disease

Deficient Component	Patients	Disease/Symptoms
C1r	4	SLE (1), renal disease (1), repeated infections (1)
C1s	2	SLE (2)
C4	3	SLE (3)
C2	23	LE (7), vasculitis (3), MPGN (1), dermatomyositis (1)
C3	4	Repeated infections (3), fever/rash/arthralgias (1)
C5	3	SLE (1), gonococcal disease
C6	5	Relapsing meningococcal meningitis (4), gonococcal disease (1)
C7	5	Raynaud's disease (1), chronic renal disease (1), gonococcal disease (2), SLE (1)
C8	3	SLE (1), gonococcal disease (1)

Adapted with permission from Sonnenwirth AC, Jarrett L (editors): Gradwohl's Clinical laboratory methods and diagnosis, ed 8, St Louis, 1980, The CV Mosby Co, p 1233.

Table 31-2 General guide to the evaluation of C4 and C3 protein levels in the presence of decreased hemolytic complement activity

	Normal C4	Decreased C4
Normal C3	Alterations in vitro (eg, improper specimen handling) Coagulation-associated complement consumption Inborn errors (other than C4 or C3)	Immune complex disease Hypergammaglobulinemic states Cryoglobulinemia Hereditary angioedema Inborn C4 deficiency
Decreased C3	Acute glomerulonephritis Membranoproliferative glomerulonephritis Immune complex disease Active SLE Inborn C3 deficiency	Active SLE Serum sickness Chronic active hepatitis Subacute bacterial endocarditis Immune complex disease

Adapted with permission from Sonnenwirth AC, Jarrett L (editors): Gradwohl's Clinical laboratory methods and diagnosis, ed 8, St Louis, 1980, The CV Mosby Co, p 1233.

Hematocrit
  Male: 39-49% (0.39-0.49) [CF: 0.01, SMI: 0.01]
  Female: 33-43% (0.33-0.43) [CF: 0.01, SMI: 0.01]
MCV: 76-100 μm^3 (76-100 fL) [CF: 1, SMI: 1 fL]
MCH: 27-33 pg (27-33 pg) [CF: 1, SMI: 1 pg]
MCHC: 33-37 g/dl (330-370 g/L) [CF: 10, SMI: 10 g/L]
RDW: 11.5-14.5%
Platelet count: 130-400 × $10^3/mm^3$ (130-400 × 10^9/L) [CF: 1, SMI: 5 × 10^9/L]
Differential:
  2-6 stabs (bands, early mature neutrophils)
  60-70 segs (mature neutrophils)
  1-4 eosinophils
  0-1 basophils
  2-8 monocytes
  25-40 lymphocytes

CONJUGATED BILIRUBIN; *see* BILIRUBIN, DIRECT

COOMBS, DIRECT

Normal:
  Negative
Positive:
  Autoimmune hemolytic anemia, erythroblastosis fetalis, transfusion reactions, drugs (α-methyldopa, penicillins, tetracycline, sulfonamides, levodopa, cephalosporins, quinidine, insulin)
False positive:
  May be seen with cold agglutinins

COOMBS, INDIRECT

Normal:
  Negative
Positive:
  Acquired hemolytic anemia, incompatible cross-matched blood, anti-Rh antibodies, drugs (methyldopa, mefenamic acid, levodopa)

COPPER (serum)

Normal range:
  70-140 μg/dl (11-22 μmol/L) [CF: 0.1574, SMI: 0.2 μmol/L]
Decreased in:
  Wilson's disease, Menkes' syndrome, malabsorption, malnutrition, nephrosis, TPN

COPPER, URINE; *see* URINE COPPER

CORTISOL (plasma)

Normal range:
  Varies with time of collection (circadian variation):
    8 AM: 4-19 μg/dl (110-520 nmol/L) [CF: 27.59, SMI: 10 nmol/L]
    4 PM: 2-15 μg/dl (50-410 nmol/L) [CF: 27.59, SMI: 10 nmol/L]

Elevated in:
   Ectopic ACTH production (i.e., oat cell carcinoma of lung), loss of normal diurnal variation, pregnancy, chronic renal failure
   Iatrogenic, stress, adrenal or pituitary hyperplasia or adenomas
Decreased in:
   Primary adrenocortical insufficiency, anterior pituitary hypofunction, secondary adrenocortical insufficiency, adrenogenital syndromes

CPK; *see* CREATINE KINASE

C-REACTIVE PROTEIN

Normal range:
   6.8-820 µg/dl (68-8200 µg/L) [CF: 10, SMI: 10 µg/L]
Elevated in:
   Rheumatoid arthritis, rheumatic fever, inflammatory bowel disease, bacterial infections, MI, oral contraceptives, third trimester of pregnancy (acute phase reactant), inflammatory and neoplastic diseases

CREATINE KINASE (CK, CPK)

Normal range:
   0-130 U/L (0-2.16 µkat/L) [CF: 0.01667, SMI: 0.01 µkat/L]
Elevated in:
   MI, myocarditis, rhabdomyolysis, myositis, crush injury/trauma, polymyositis, dermatomyositis, vigorous exercise, muscular dystrophy, myxedema, seizures, malignant hyperthermia syndrome, IM injections, CVA, pulmonary embolism and infarction, acute dissection of aorta
Decreased in:
   Steroids, decreased muscle mass, connective tissue disorders, alcoholic liver disease, metastatic neoplasms

CREATINE KINASE ISOENZYMES

CK-MB
   Elevated in: MI, myocarditis, pericarditis, muscular dystrophy, cardiac defibrillation, cardiac surgery, extensive rhabdomyolysis, strenuous exercise (marathon runners), mixed connective tissue disease, cardiomyopathy, hypothermia
CK-MM
   Elevated in: crush injury, seizures, malignant hyperthermia syndrome, rhabdomyolysis, myositis, polymyositis, dermatomyositis, vigorous exercise, muscular dystrophy, IM injections, acute dissection of aorta
CK-BB
   Elevated in: CVA, subarachnoid hemorrhage, neoplasms (prostate, GI tract, brain, ovary, breast, lung), severe shock, bowel infarction, hypothermia

CREATININE (serum)

Normal range:
   0.6-1.2 mg/dl (50-110 µmol/L) [CF: 88.4, SMI: 10 µmol/L]

Elevated in:
  Renal insufficiency (acute and chronic), decreased renal perfusion (hypotension, dehydration, CHF), urinary tract infection, rhabdomyolysis, ketonemia
  Drugs (antibiotics [aminoglycosides, cephalosporins], hydantoin, diuretics, methyldopa)
Falsely elevated in:
  DKA, administration of some cephalosporins (e.g., cefoxitin, cephalothin)
Decreased in:
  Decreased muscle mass (including amputees and older persons), pregnancy, prolonged debilitation

CREATININE CLEARANCE

Normal range:
  75-124 ml/min (1.24-2.08 ml/sec) [CF: 0.01667, SMI: 0.02 ml/sec]
Elevated in:
  Pregnancy, exercise
Decreased in:
  Renal insufficiency, drugs (cimetidine, procainamide, antibiotics, quinidine)

CREATININE, URINE; *see* URINE CREATININE

CRYOGLOBULINS (serum)

Normal range:
  Not detectable
Present in:
  Collagen-vascular diseases, CLL, hemolytic anemias, multiple myeloma, Waldenstrom's macroglobulinemia, chronic active hepatitis, Hodgkin's disease

CSF; *see* CEREBROSPINAL FLUID

ELECTROLYTES, URINE; *see* URINE ELECTROLYTES

ELECTROPHORESIS, HEMOGLOBIN; *see* HEMOGLOBIN ELECTROPHORESIS

ELECTROPHORESIS, PROTEIN; *see* PROTEIN ELECTROPHORESIS

ENA-COMPLEX; *see* EXTRACTABLE NUCLEAR ANTIGEN

EOSINOPHIL COUNT

Normal range:
  1-4% eosinophils (0-440/mm^3)
Elevated in:
  Allergy, parasitic infestations (trichinosis, aspergillosis, hydatidosis), angioneurotic edema, drug reactions, warfarin sensitivity, collagen-vascular diseases, acute hypereosinophilic syndrome, eosinophilic nonallergic rhinitis, myeloproliferative disorders, Hodgkin's lymphoma, radiation therapy, NHL, L-tryptophan ingestion

ERYTHROCYTE SEDIMENTATION RATE (Westergren)

Normal range:
Male: 0-15 mm/hr
Female: 0-20 mm/hr

Elevated in:
Collagen-vascular diseases, infections, MI, neoplasms, inflammatory states (acute phase reactant)

EXTRACTABLE NUCLEAR ANTIGEN (ENA complex, anti-RNP antibody, anti-Sm, anti-Smith)

Normal:
Negative

Present in:
SLE, rheumatoid arthritis, Sjögren's syndrome, MCTD

FDP; *see* FIBRIN DEGRADATION PRODUCT

FECAL FAT, QUANTITATIVE (72 hr collection)

Normal range:
2-6 g/24 hr (7-21 mmol/dl) [CF: 3.515, SMI: 1 mmol/dl]

Elevated in:
Malabsorption syndrome (refer to Section 23.5)

FERRITIN (serum)

Normal range:
18-300 ng/ml (18-300 μg/L) [CF: 1, SMI: 10 μg/L]

Elevated in:
Hyperthyroidism, inflammatory states, liver disease (ferritin elevated from necrotic hepatocytes), neoplasms (neuroblastomas, lymphomas, leukemia, breast carcinoma), iron replacement therapy, hemochromatosis

Decreased in:
Iron deficiency anemia

α-1 FETOPROTEIN

Normal range:
0-20 ng/ml (0-20 μg/L) [CF: 1, SMI: 1 μg/L]

Elevated in:
Hepatocellular carcinoma (usually values >1000 ng/ml), germinal neoplasms (testis, ovary, mediastinum, retroperitoneum), liver disease (alcoholic cirrhosis, acute hepatitis, chronic active hepatitis), fetal anencephaly, spina bifida

FIBRIN DEGRADATION PRODUCT (FDP)

Normal range:
<10 μg/ml

Elevated in:
DIC, primary fibrinolysis, pulmonary embolism, severe liver disease
NOTE: The presence of rheumatoid factor may cause falsely elevated FDP

FIBRINOGEN

Normal range:

200-400 mg/dl (2-4 g/L) [CF: 0.01, SMI: 0.1 g/L]

Elevated in:

Tissue inflammation/damage (acute-phase protein reactant), oral contraceptives, pregnancy, acute infection, MI

Decreased in:

DIC, hereditary afibrinogenemia, liver disease, primary or secondary fibrinolysis, cachexia

FLUORESCENT TREPONEMAL ANTIBODY; *see* FTA-ABS

FOLATE (FOLIC ACID)

Normal range:

Plasma: 2-10 ng/ml (4-22 nmol/L) [CF: 2.266, SMI: 2 nmol/L]

RBC: 140-960 ng/ml (550-2200 nmol/L) [CF: 2.266, SMI: 10 nmol/L]

Decreased in:

Folic acid deficiency (inadequate intake, malabsorption), alcoholism, drugs (methotrexate, trimethoprim, phenytoin, oral contraceptives, azulfadine), vitamin B_{12} deficiency (defective red cell folate absorption)

FREE T_4; *see* T_4, FREE

FREE THYROXINE INDEX

Normal range:

1.1-4.3

Refer to Section 22.7 for interpretation of abnormal values

FTA-ABS (serum)

Normal:

Nonreactive

Reactive in:

Syphilis, other treponemal diseases (yaws, pinta, bejel)

GAMMA-GLUTAMYL TRANSFERASE (GGT); *see* γ-GLUTAMYL TRANSFERASE

GASTRIN (serum)

Normal range:

0-180 pg/ml (0-180 ng/L) [CF: 1, SMI: 10 ng/L]

Elevated in:

Zollinger-Ellison syndrome (gastrinoma), pernicious anemia, hyperparathyroidism, retained gastric antrum, chronic renal failure, gastric ulcer, chronic atrophic gastritis, pyloric obstruction, malignant neoplasms of the stomach, H_2 blockers, omeprazole

GLOMERULAR BASEMENT MEMBRANE ANTIBODY

Normal:

Negative

Present in:

Goodpasture's syndrome

GLUCOSE, FASTING

Normal range:
70-110 mg/dl (3.9-6.1 mmol/L) [CF: 0.05551, SMI: 0.1 mmol/L]
Elevated in:
Diabetes mellitus, stress, infections, MI, CVA, Cushing's syndrome, acromegaly, acute pancreatitis, glucagonoma, hemochromatosis, drugs (glucocorticoids, diuretics [thiazides, loop diuretics]), glucose intolerance
Decreased:
See Section 22.4

GLUCOSE, POSTPRANDIAL

Normal range:
<140 mg/dl (<7.8 mmol/L) [CF: 0.05551, SMI: 0.1 mmol/L]
Elevated in:
Diabetes mellitus, glucose intolerance
Decreased in:
Post-gastrointestinal resection, reactive hypoglycemia, hereditary fructose intolerance, galactosemia, leucine sensitivity

GLUCOSE TOLERANCE TEST

Normal values above fasting:
30 min: 30-60 mg/dl (1.65-3.3 mmol/L) [CF: 0.05551, SMI: 0.1 mmol/L]
60 min: 20-50 mg/dl (1.1-2.75 mmol/L) [CF: 0.05551, SMI: 0.1 mmol/L]
120 min: 5-15 mg/dl (0.28-0.83 mmol/L) [CF: 0.05551, SMI: 0.1 mmol/L]
180 min: fasting level or below
Elevated in:
Glucose intolerance, diabetes mellitus, Cushing's syndrome, acromegaly, pheochromocytoma

GLUCOSE-6-PHOSPHATE DEHYDROGENASE SCREEN (blood)

Normal:
G_6PD enzyme activity is detected
Abnormal:
If a deficiency is detected, quantitation of G_6PD is necessary; a G_6PD screen may be falsely interpreted as "normal" after an episode of hemolysis because most G_6PD deficient cells have been destroyed.

γ-GLUTAMYL TRANSFERASE (GGT)

Normal range:
0-30 U/L (0.050 μkat/L) [CF: 0.01667, SMI: 0.01 μkat/L]
Elevated in:
Chronic alcoholic liver disease, neoplasms (hepatoma, metastatic disease to the liver, carcinoma of the pancreas), SLE, CHF, trauma, nephrotic syndrome, sepsis, cholestasis, drugs (phenytoin, barbiturates)

GLYCATED (GLYCOSYLATED) HEMOGLOBIN (HbA$_{1c}$)

Normal range:
  4.0-6.7%
Elevated in:
  Uncontrolled diabetes mellitus (glycated hemoglobin levels reflect the level of glucose control over the preceding 120 days)
Decreased in:
  Hemolytic anemias, decreased RBC survival, pregnancy, chronic blood loss, chronic renal failure, insulinoma

HAM TEST (acid serum test)

Normal:
  Negative
Positive in:
  Paroxysmal nocturnal hemoglobinuria (PNH)
False positive in:
  Hereditary or acquired spherocytosis, recent transfusion with aged RBC, aplastic anemia, myeloproliferative syndromes, leukemia, hereditary dyserythropoietic anemia type II (HEMPAS)

HAPTOGLOBIN (serum)

Normal range:
  50-220 mg/dl (0.50-2.2 g/L) [CF: 0.01, SMI: 0.01 g/L]
Elevated in:
  Inflammation (acute phase reactant), collagen-vascular diseases, infections (acute phase reactant), drugs (androgens)
Decreased in:
  Hemolysis (intravascular > extravascular), megaloblastic anemia, severe liver disease, large tissue hematomas, infectious mononucleosis, drugs (oral contraceptives)

HDL; *see* HIGH DENSITY LIPOPROTEIN CHOLESTEROL

HEMATOCRIT

Normal range:
  Male: 39-49% (0.39-0.49) [CF: 0.01, SMI: 0.01]
  Female: 33-43% (0.33-0.43) [CF: 0.01, SMI: 0.01]
Elevated in:
  Polycythemia vera, smoking, COPD, high altitudes, dehydration, hypovolemia
Decreased in:
  Blood loss (GI, GU), anemia (refer to Sections 24.1-24.3), pregnancy

HEMOGLOBIN

Normal range:
  Male: 13.6-17.7 g/dl (136-172 g/L) [CF: 10, SMI: 1 g/L]
  Female: 12.0-15.0 g/dl (120-150 g/L) [CF: 10, SMI: 1 g/L]

Elevated in:
   Hemoconcentration, dehydration, polycythemia vera, COPD, high altitudes, false elevations (hyperlipemic plasma, WBC >50,000 mm³), stress

Decreased in:
   Hemorrhage (GI, GU), anemia (refer to Sections 24.1-24.3)

HEMOGLOBIN ELECTROPHORESIS

Normal range:
   Hb A_1: 95-98%
   Hb A_2: 1.5-3.5%
   Hb F: <2%
   Hb C: absent
   Hb S: absent

HEMOGLOBIN, GLYCATED; *see* GLYCATED HEMOGLOBIN

HEMOGLOBIN, GLYCOSYLATED; *see* GLYCATED HEMOGLOBIN

HEMOGLOBIN, URINE; *see* URINE HEMOGLOBIN

HEMOSIDERIN, URINE; *see* URINE HEMOSIDERIN

HEPATITIS A ANTIBODY

Normal:
   Negative
Present in:
   Viral hepatitis A; can be IgM or IgG (if IgM, acute hepatitis A; if IgG, previous infection with hepatitis A)

HEPATITIS B SURFACE ANTIGEN (HB$_s$Ag)

Normal:
   Not detected
Detected in:
   Acute viral hepatitis Type B, chronic hepatitis B

HIGH DENSITY LIPOPROTEIN (HDL) CHOLESTEROL

Normal range:
   Male: 30-70 mg/dl (0.8-1.8 mmol/L) [CF: 0.02586, SMI: 0.05 mmol/L]
   Female: 30-90 mg/dl (0.8-2.35 mmol/L) [CF: 0.02586, SMI: 0.05 mmol/L]
Increased:
   Use of gemfibrozil, nicotinic acid, estrogens, regular aerobic exercise, small (1 oz) daily alcohol intake
Decreased:
   Deficiency of apoproteins, liver disease, probucol ingestion, Tangier disease

NOTE: A cholesterol/HDL ratio >4.5 is associated with ↑ risk of coronary artery disease.

HLA ANTIGENS

Associated disorders:
   See Table 31-3

Table 31-3 HLA antigens associated with specific diseases

Antigen	Condition
HLA-B27	Ankylosing spondylitis
	Reiter's syndrome
	Psoriatic arthritis
HLA-A10, B18, Dw2	C2 deficiency
HLA-A2, B40, Cw3	C4 deficiency
HLA-B7, Dw2	Multiple sclerosis
HLA-A3	Hemochromatosis
HLA-B8, Dw3	Celiac disease
HLA-B8, Dw3	Dermatitis herpetiforis
HLA-B8	Myasthenia gravis
HLA-B8	Chronic active hepatitis in children
HLA-Drw4	Active chronic hepatitis in adults
HLA-B13, Bw17	Psoriasis

From Cerra FB: Manual of critical care, St Louis, 1987, The CV Mosby Co.

5-HYDROXYINDOLE-ACETIC ACID, URINE; *see* URINE 5-HYDROXYINDOLE–ACETIC ACID

IMMUNE COMPLEX ASSAY

Normal:
    Negative
Detected in:
    Collagen-vascular disorders, glomerulonephritis, neoplastic diseases, malaria, primary biliary cirrhosis, chronic acute hepatitis, bacterial endocarditis, vasculitis

IMMUNOGLOBULINS

Normal range:
    IgA: 50-350 mg/dl (0.5-3.5 g/L) [CF: 0.01, SMI: 0.01 g/L]
    IgD: <6 mg/dl (<60 mg/L) [CF: 0.01, SMI: 0.01 g/L]
    IgE: <25 μg/dl (<0.00025 g/L) [CF: 0.01, SMI: 0.01 g/L]
    IgG: 800-1500 mg/dl (8-15 g/L) [CF: 0.01, SMI: 0.01 g/L]
    IgM: 45-150 mg/dl (0.45-1.5 g/L) [CF: 0.01, SMI: 0.01 g/L]
Elevated in:
    IgA: lymphoproliferative disorders, Berger's nephropathy, chronic infections, autoimmune disorders, liver disease
    IgE: allergic disorders, parasitic infections, immunological disorders, IgE myeloma
    IgG: chronic granulomatous infections, infectious diseases, inflammation, myeloma, liver disease
    IgM: primary biliary cirrhosis, infectious diseases (brucellosis, malaria), Waldenstrom's macroglobulinemia, liver disease

Decreased in:
IgA: nephrotic syndrome, protein-losing enteropathy, congenital deficiency, lymphocytic leukemia, ataxia-telengiectasia, chronic sinopulmonary disease
IgE: hypogammaglobulinemia, neoplasm (breast, bronchial, cervical), ataxia-telengiectasia
IgG: congenital or acquired deficiency, lymphocytic leukemia, phenytoin, methylprednisolone, nephrotic syndrome, protein-losing enteropathy
IgM: congenital deficiency, lymphocytic leukemia, nephrotic syndrome

IRON-BINDING CAPACITY (TIBC)

Normal range:
250-460 µg/dl (45-82 µmol/L) [CF: 0.1791, SMI: 1 µmol/L]
Elevated in:
Iron deficiency anemia, pregnancy, polycythemia
Decreased in:
Anemia of chronic disease, hemochromatosis, chronic liver disease, hemolytic anemias, malnutrition (protein depletion)

LACTATE (blood)

Normal range:
0.5-2 mEq/L (0.5-2 mmol/L) [CF: 1, SMI: 0.1 mmol/L]
Elevated:
See Chapter 19

LACTATE DEHYDROGENASE (LDH)

Normal range:
50-150 U/L (0.82-2.66 µkat/L) [CF: 0.01667, SMI: 0.02 µkat/L]
Elevated in:
Infarction of myocardium, lung, kidney
Diseases of cardiopulmonary system, liver, collagen, CNS
Hemolytic anemias, megaloblastic anemias, transfusions, seizures, muscle trauma, muscular dystrophy, acute pancreatitis, hypotension, shock, infectious mononucleosis, inflammation, neoplasia, intestinal obstruction, hypothyroidism

LACTATE DEHYDROGENASE ISOENZYMES

Normal range:
LDH_1: 22-36% (cardiac, RBC) (0.22-0.36) [CF: 0.01, SMI: 0.01]
LDH_2: 35-46% (cardiac, RBC) (0.35-0.46)
LDH_3: 13-26% (pulmonary) (0.15-0.26)
LDH_4: 3-10% (striated muscle, liver) (0.03-0.1)
LDH_5: 2-9% (striated muscle, liver) (0.02-0.09)
Normal ratios:
$LDH_1 < LDH_2$
$LDH_5 < LDH_4$
Abnormal values:
$LDH_1 > LDH_2$: MI (can also be seen with hemolytic anemias, pernicious anemia, folate deficiency, renal infarct)

$LDH_5 > LDH_4$: liver disease (cirrhosis, hepatitis, hepatic congestion)

LAP SCORE; *see* LEUKOCYTE ALKALINE PHOSPHATASE

LDH; *see* LACTATE DEHYDROGENASE

LDL; *see* LOW DENSITY LIPOPROTEIN CHOLESTEROL

LEGIONELLA TITER

Normal:
Negative
Positive in:
Legionnaire's disease (presumptive: $\geq 1:256$ titer; definitive: fourfold titer increase to $\geq 1:128$)

LEUKOCYTE ALKALINE PHOSPHATASE

Normal range:
13-100 (33-188 U)
Elevated in:
Leukemoid reactions, neutrophilia secondary to infections (except in sickle cell crisis—no significant increase in LAP score), Hodgkin's disease, polycythemia vera, hairy cell leukemia, aplastic anemia, Down's syndrome, myelofibrosis
Decreased in:
Acute and chronic granulocytic leukemia, thrombocytopenic purpura, paroxysmal nocturnal hemoglobinuria (PNH), hypophosphatemia, collagen disorders

LEUKOCYTE COUNT; *see* COMPLETE BLOOD COUNT

LIPASE

Normal range:
0-160 U/L (0-2.66 μkat/L) [CF: 0.01667, SMI: 0.02 μkat/L]
Elevated in:
Acute pancreatitis, perforated peptic ulcer, carcinoma of pancreas (early stage), pancreatic duct obstruction

LIPOPROTEIN CHOLESTEROL, LOW DENSITY; *see* LOW DENSITY LIPOPROTEIN CHOLESTEROL

LIPOPROTEIN CHOLESTEROL, HIGH DENSITY; *see* HIGH DENSITY LIPOPROTEIN CHOLESTEROL

LOW DENSITY LIPOPROTEIN (LDL) CHOLESTEROL

Normal range:
50-190 mg/dl (1.30-4.90 mmol/L) [CF: 0.02586, SMI: 0.05 mmol/L]
Elevated in:
Primary hyperlipoproteinemia, diet high in saturated fats, acute MI, hypothyroidism, primary biliary cirrhosis, nephrosis, diabetes mellitus
Decreased in:
Abetalipoproteinemia, advanced liver disease, malabsorption, malnutrition

LUPUS ANTICOAGULANT; *see* CIRCULATING ANTICOAGULANT

LYMPHOCYTES

Normal range:
15-40%: total lymphocyte count 800-2600/mm^3
total T lymphs 800-2200/mm^3
CD2 65-85% lymphs
helper-inducer T (T4) >400/mm^3
CD4 45-75% of T
suppressor-cytotoxic T 250-750/mm^3
T8 (CD8) 18-40% of T
helper/suppressor ratio >0.9

Elevated in:
Chronic infections, infectious mononucleosis and other viral infections, CLL, Hodgkin's disease, ulcerative colitis, hypoadrenalism, ITP

Decreased in:
AIDS, ARC, bone marrow suppression from chemotherapeutic agents or chemotherapy, aplastic anemia, neoplasms, steroids, adrenocortical hyperfunction, neurologic disorders (multiple sclerosis, myasthenia gravis, Guillain-Barré syndrome)

MAGNESIUM (serum)

Normal range:
1.8-3.0 mg/dl (0.80-1.20 mmol/L) [CF: 0.4114, SMI: 0.02 mmol/L]
For interpretation of abnormal values refer to Section 26.4

MEAN CORPUSCULAR VOLUME (MCV)

Normal range:
76-100 μm^3 (76-100 fL) [CF: 1, SMI: 1 fL]

Elevated in:
Vitamin B$_{12}$ deficiency, folic acid deficiency, liver disease, alcohol abuse, reticulocytosis, hypothyroidism, marrow aplasia, myelofibrosis

Decreased in:
Iron deficiency, thalassemia syndrome and other hemoglobinopathies, anemia of chronic disease, sideroblastic anemia, chronic renal failure, lead poisoning

METANEPHRINES, URINE; *see* URINE METANEPHRINES

MONOCYTE COUNT

Normal range:
2-8%

Elevated in:
Viral diseases, parasites, infections, neoplasms, inflammatory bowel disease, monocytic leukemia, lymphomas, myeloma, sarcoidosis

Decreased in:
Aplastic anemia, lymphocytic leukemia, glucocorticoid administration

MYOGLOBIN, URINE; *see* URINE MYOGLOBIN

NEUTROPHIL COUNT

Normal range:
  50-70%
  Subsets
    stabs (bands, early mature neutrophils): 2-6%
    segs (mature neutrophils): 60-70%
Elevated in:
  Acute bacterial infections, acute MI, stress, neoplasms, myelocytic leukemia
Decreased in:
  Viral infections, aplastic anemias, immunosuppressive drugs, radiation therapy to bone marrow, agranulocytosis, drugs (antibiotics, antithyroidals), lymphocytic and monocytic leukemias

5' NUCLEOTIDASE

Normal range:
  2-16 IU/L (3-27 × 10^{-8}kat/L) [CF: 1.67 × 10^{-8}, SMI: 1 × 10^{-8}kat/L]
Elevated in:
  Biliary obstruction, metastatic neoplasms to liver, primary biliary cirrhosis

OSMOLALITY, SERUM

Normal range:
  280-300 mOsm/kg (280-300 mmol/kg) [CF: 1, SMI: 1 mmol/kg]
  It can also be estimated by the following formula:

$$2([Na] + [K]) + \frac{Glucose}{18} + \frac{BUN}{2.8}$$

Elevated in:
  Dehydration, hypernatremia, diabetes insipidus, uremia, hyperglycemia, mannitol therapy, ingestion of toxins (ethylene glycol, methanol, ethanol)
Decreased in:
  SIADH, hyponatremia, overhydration

OSMOLALITY, URINE; *see* URINE OSMOLALITY

PARTIAL THROMBOPLASTIN TIME (PTT), ACTIVATED PARTIAL THROMBOPLASTIN TIME (APTT)

Normal range:
  25-41 sec
Elevated in:
  Heparin therapy, coagulation factor deficiency (I, II, V, VIII, IX, X, XI, XII), liver disease, vitamin K deficiency, DIC, circulating anticoagulant, warfarin therapy, specific factor inhibition (PCN reaction, rheumatoid arthritis), thrombolytic therapy
  NOTE: Useful to evaluate the intrinsic coagulation system.

pH, BLOOD
Normal values:
  Arterial: 7.35-7.45
  Venous: 7.32-7.42
For abnormal values refer to Chapter 19

pH, URINE; *see* URINE pH

PHOSPHATASE, ACID; *see* ACID PHOSPHATASE

PHOSPHATASE, ALKALINE; *see* ALKALINE PHOSPHATASE

PHOSPHORUS (serum)
Normal range:
  2.5-5 mg/dl (0.8-1.6 mmol/L) [CF: 0.3229, SMI: 0.05 mmol/L]
Elevated in:
  Renal failure, dehydration, Addison's disease, myelogenous leukemia, hypervitaminosis D, hypoparathyroidism, pseudohypoparathyroidism, bone metastases, sarcoidosis, milk-alkali syndrome, immobilization, magnesium deficiency, transfusions, hemolysis
Decreased in:
  Starvation (e.g., alcoholics), DKA, TPN, continuous IV dextrose administration, vitamin D deficiency, hyperparathyroidism, pseudohyperparathyroidism, antacids containing aluminum hydroxide, insulin administration, nasogastric suctioning, vomiting, diuretics, steroids, gram-negative septicemia

PLATELET COUNT
Normal range:
  130-400 × 10³/mm³ (130-400 × 10⁹/L) [CF: 1, SMI: 5 × 10⁹/L]
Elevated in:
  Neoplasms (GI tract), CML, polycythemia vera, myelofibrosis with myeloid metaplasia, infections, after splenectomy, postpartum, after hemorrhage, hemophilia, iron deficiency, pancreatitis, cirrhosis
Decreased:
  See Section 24.11

POTASSIUM (serum)
Normal range:
  3.5-5 mEq/L (3.5-5 mmol/L) [CF: 1, SMI: 0.1 mmol/L]
For interpretation of abnormal values refer to Section 26.3

POTASSIUM, URINE; *see* URINE POTASSIUM

PROLACTIN
Normal range:
  <20 ng/ml (<20 μg/L) [CF: 1, SMI: 1 μg/L]
Elevated in:
  Prolactinomas (level >200 highly suggestive), drugs (phenothiazines, cimetidine, tricyclic antidepressants, metoclopramide, estrogens, antihypertensives [methyldopa], verapamil, haloperidol), postpartum, stress, hypoglycemia, hypothyroidism

PROTEIN (serum)

Normal range:

6-8 g/dl (60-80 g/L) [CF: 10, SMI: 1 g/L]

Elevated in:

Dehydration, multiple myeloma, Waldenstrom's macroglobulinemia, sarcoidosis, collagen-vascular diseases

Decreased in:

Malnutrition, low-protein diet, overhydration, malabsorption, pregnancy, severe burns, neoplasms, chronic diseases, cirrhosis, nephrosis

PROTEIN ELECTROPHORESIS (serum)

Normal range:

Albumin: 60-75% (0.6-0.75) [CF: 0.01, SMI: 0.01]

α-1: 1.7-5% (0.02-0.05)

α-2: 6.7-12.5% (0.07-0.13)

β: 8.3-16.3% (0.08-0.16)

γ: 10.7-20% (0.11-0.2)

Albumin: 3.6-5.2 g/dl (36-52 g/L) [CF: 0.01, SMI: 1 g/L]

α-1: 0.1-0.4 g/dl (1-4 g/L)

α-2: 0.4-1 g/dl (4-10 g/L)

β: 0.5-1.2 g/dl (5-12 g/L)

γ: 0.6-1.6 g/dl (6-16 g/L)

Elevated: .

Albumin: dehydration

α-1: neoplastic diseases, inflammation

α-2: neoplasms, inflammation, infection, nephrotic syndrome

β: hypothyroidism, biliary cirrhosis, diabetes mellitus

γ: *see* IMMUNOGLOBULINS

Decreased:

Albumin: malnutrition, chronic liver disease, malabsorption, nephrotic syndrome, burns, SLE

α-1: emphysema (α-1 antitrypsin deficiency), nephrosis

α-2: hemolytic anemias (decreased haptoglobin), severe hepatocellular damage

β: hypocholesterolemia, nephrosis

γ: *see* IMMUNOGLOBULINS

PROTHROMBIN TIME (PT)

Normal range:

10-12 sec

Elevated in:

Liver disease, oral anticoagulants (Warfarin), heparin, factor deficiency (I, II, V, VII, X), DIC, vitamin K deficiency, afibrinogenemia, dysfibrinogenemia, drugs (salicylate, chloral hydrate, diphenylhydantoin, estrogens, antacids, phenylbutazone, quinidine, antibiotics, allopurinol, anabolic steroids)

Decreased in:

Vitamin K supplementation, thrombophlebitis, drugs (gluthetimide, estrogens, griseofulvin, diphenhydramine)

PROTOPORPHYRIN (free erythrocyte)

Normal range:
16-36 µg/dl of RBC (0.28-0.64 µmol/L) [CF: 0.0177, SMI: 0.02 µmol/L]

Elevated in:
iron deficiency, lead poisoning, sideroblastic anemias, anemia of chronic disease, hemolytic anemias, erythropoietic protoporphyria

PT; *see* PROTHROMBIN TIME

PTT; *see* PARTIAL THROMBOPLASTIN TIME

RDW; *see* RED BLOOD CELL DISTRIBUTION WIDTH

RED BLOOD CELL COUNT

Normal range:
Male: 4.3-5.9 × 10^6/mm^3 (4.3-5.9 × 10^{12}/L) [CF: 1, SMI: 0.1 × 10^{12}/L]

Female: 3.5-5 × 10^6/mm^3 (3.5-5 × 10^{12}/L) [CF: 1, SMI: 0.1 × 10^{12}/L]

Elevated in:
Polycythemia vera, smokers, high altitude, cardiovascular disease, renal cell carcinoma and other erythropoietin-producing neoplasms, stress, hemoconcentration/dehydration

Decreased in:
Anemias, hemolysis, chronic renal failure, hemorrhage, failure of marrow production

RED BLOOD CELL DISTRIBUTION WIDTH (RDW)
Measures variability of red cell size (anisocytosis)

Normal range:
11.5-14.5

Normal RDW and:
Elevated MCV: aplastic anemia, preleukemia
Normal MCV: normal, anemia of chronic disease, acute blood loss or hemolysis, CLL, CML, nonanemic enzymopathy or hemoglobinopathy
Decreased MCV: anemia of chronic disease, heterozygous thalassemia

Elevated RDW and:
Elevated MCV: vitamin B_{12} deficiency, folate deficiency, immune hemolytic anemia, cold agglutinins, CLL with high count, liver disease
Normal MCV: early iron deficiency, early vitamin B_{12} deficiency, early folate deficiency, anemic globinopathy
Decreased MCV: iron deficiency, RBC fragmentation, Hb H, thalassemia intermedia

RED BLOOD CELL FOLATE; *see* FOLATE, RBC

RED BLOOD CELL MASS (VOLUME)

Normal range:
Male: 20-36 ml/kg of BW (1.15-1.21 L/m^2 BSA)
Female: 19-31 ml/kg of BW (0.95-1.00 L/m^2 BSA)

Elevated in:

Polycythemia vera, hypoxia (smokers, high altitude, cardiovascular disease), hemoglobinopathies with high O_2 affinity, erythropoietin-producing tumors (renal cell carcinoma)

Decreased in:

Hemorrhage, chronic disease, failure of marrow production, anemias, hemolysis

RETICULOCYTE COUNT

Normal range:

0.5-1.5%

Elevated in:

Hemolytic anemia (sickle cell crisis, thalassemia major, autoimmune hemolysis, hemorrhage, postanemia therapy (folic acid, ferrous sulfate, vitamin B_{12})

Decreased in:

Aplastic anemia, marrow suppression (sepsis, chemotherapeutic agents, radiation), hepatic cirrhosis, blood transfusion, anemias of disordered maturation (iron deficiency anemia, megaloblastic anemia, sideroblastic anemia, anemia of chronic disease)

RHEUMATOID FACTOR

Normal:

Negative

Present in titer >1:20:

Rheumatoid arthritis, SLE, chronic inflammatory processes, old age, infections, liver disease

RNP; *see* EXTRACTABLE NUCLEAR ANTIGEN

SEDIMENTATION RATE; *see* ERYTHROCYTE SEDIMENTATION RATE

SGOT; *see* ASPARTATE AMINOTRANSFERASE

SGPT; *see* ALANINE AMINOTRANSFERASE

SHILLING TEST; *see* Fig. 24-1

SMOOTH MUSCLE ANTIBODY

Normal:

Negative

Present in:

Chronic active hepatitis ($\geq 1:80$), primary biliary cirrhosis ($\leq 1:80$), infectious mononucleosis

SODIUM (serum)

Normal range:

135-147 mEq/L (135-147 mmol/L) [CF: 1, SMI: 1 mmol/L]

For interpretation of abnormal values refer to Section 26.2)

STREPTOZIME; *see* ANTI-STREPTOLYSIN O TITER

SUCROSE HEMOLYSIS TEST (sugar water test)

Normal:
  Absence of hemolysis
Positive in:
  Paroxysmal nocturnal hemoglobinuria (PNH)
  False positive: autoimmune hemolytic anemia, megaloblastic anemias
  False negative: may occur with use of heparin or EDTA

T_3 (TRIIODOTHYRONINE)

Normal range:
  75-220 ng/dl (1.2-3.4 nmol/L) [CF: 0.01536, SMI: 0.1 nmol/L]
Abnormal values:
  Refer to Section 22.7

T_3 RESIN UPTAKE (T_3RU)

Normal range:
  25-35% (0.25-0.35) [CF: 0.01, SMI: 0.01]
Abnormal values:
  Refer to Section 22.7

T_4, FREE (free thyroxine)

Normal range:
  0.8-2.8 ng/dl (10-36 pmol/L) [CF: 12.87, SMI: 1 pmol/L]
Abnormal values:
  Refer to Section 22.7

THROMBIN TIME (TT)

Normal range:
  11.3-18.5 sec
Elevated in:
  Thrombolytic and heparin therapy, DIC, hypofibrinogenemia, dysfibrin-
    ogenemia

THYROID STIMULATING HORMONE (TSH)

Normal range:
  2-11.0 μU/ml (2-11 mU/L) [CF: 1, SMI: 1 mU/L]
Elevated in:
  Hypothyroidism, drugs (haloperidol, chlorpromazine, metoclopramide,
    domperidone), TSH antibodies, pituitary resistance to thyroid hor-
    mone
Decreased in:
  Hyperthyroidism, acute medical illness, drugs (dopamine, corticoster-
    oids, bromocriptine, levodopa, pyridoxine), hyponatremia, malnutri-
    tion

THYROXINE (T_4)

Normal range:
  4-11 μg/dl (51-142 nmol/L) [CF: 12.87, SMI: 1 nmol/L]
Abnormal values:
  Refer to Section 22.7

TIBC; *see* IRON BINDING CAPACITY

TRANSFERRIN
Normal range:
   170-370 mg/dl (1.7-3.7 g/L) [CF: 0.01, SMI: 0.01 g/L]
Elevated in:
   Iron deficiency anemia, oral contraceptive administration, viral hepatitis
Decreased in:
   Nephrotic syndrome, liver disease, hereditary deficiency, protein malnu-
      trition, neoplasms, chronic inflammatory states, chronic illness,
      thalassemia

TRIGLYCERIDES
Normal range:
   <160 mg/dl (<1.80 mmol/L) [CF: 0.01129, SMI: 0.02 mmol/L]
Elevated in:
   Hyperlipoproteinemias (Types I, IIb, III, IV, V), hypothyroidism, preg-
      nancy, estrogens, acute MI, pancreatitis, alcohol intake, nephrotic
      syndrome, diabetes mellitus, glycogen storage disease
Decreased in:
   Malnutrition, congenital abetalipoproteinemias, drugs (e.g., gemfibrozil,
      nicotinic acid, clofibrate)

TRIIODOTHYRONINE; *see* T_3

TSH; *see* THYROID STIMULATING HORMONE

TT; *see* THROMBIN TIME

UNCONJUGATED BILIRUBIN; *see* BILIRUBIN, INDIRECT

UREA NITROGEN
Normal range:
   8-18 mg/dl (3-6.5 mmol/L) [CF: 0.357, SMI: 0.5 mmol/L]
Elevated in:
   Drugs (aminoglycosides and other antibiotics, diuretics, lithium, corti-
      costeroids), dehydration, gastrointestinal bleeding, decreased renal
      blood flow (shock, CHF, MI), renal disease (glomerulonephritis,
      pyelonephritis, diabetic nephropathy), urinary tract obstruction (pros-
      tatic hypertrophy)
Decreased in:
   Liver disease, malnutrition, third trimester of pregnancy, overhydration

URIC ACID (serum)
Normal range:
   2-7 mg/dl (120-420 μmol/L) [CF: 59.48, SMI: 10 μmol/L]
Elevated in:
   Renal failure, gout, excessive cell lysis (chemotherapeutic agents, radia-
      tion therapy, leukemia, lymphoma, hemolytic anemia), hereditary en-
      zyme deficiency (hypoxanthine-guanine-phosphoribosyl transferase),
      acidosis, myeloproliferative disorders, diet high in purines or protein,
      drugs (diuretics, low doses of ASA, ethambutol, nicotinic acid), lead

poisoning, hypothyroidism, Addison's disease, nephrogenic diabetes insipidus, active psoriasis, polycystic kidneys

Decreased in:

Drugs (allopurinol, high doses of ASA, probenecid, warfarin, corticosteroid), deficiency of xanthine oxidase, SIADH, renal tubular deficits (Fanconi's syndrome), alcoholism, liver disease, diet deficient in protein or purines, Wilson's disease, hemochromatosis

URINALYSIS

Normal range:

Color: light straw	Protein: absent
Appearance: clear	Ketones: absent
pH: 4.5-8 (average, 6)	Glucose: absent
Specific gravity: 1.005-1.030	Occult blood: absent

Microscopic exam:
RBC: 0-5 (high-power field)
WBC: 0-5 (high-power field)
Bacteria (spun specimen): absent
Casts: 0-4 hyaline (low-power field)

URINE AMYLASE

Normal range:

35-260 U Somogyi/hr (6.5-48.1 U/hr) [CF: 0.185, SMI: 1 U/hr]

Elevated in:

Pancreatitis, carcinoma of the pancreas

URINE BILE

Normal:

Absent

Abnormal:

Urine bilirubin:

Hepatitis (viral, toxic, drug-induced), biliary obstruction

Urine urobilinogen:

Hepatitis (viral, toxic, drug-induced), hemolytic jaundice, liver cell dysfunction (cirrhosis, infection, metastases)

URINE CALCIUM

Normal range:

<250 mg/24 hr (<6.2 mmol/dl) [CF: 0.02495, SMI: 0.1 mmol/dl]

Elevated in:

Primary hyperparathyroidism, hypervitaminosis D, bone metastases, multiple myeloma, increased calcium intake, steroids, prolonged immobilization, sarcoidosis, Paget's disease, idiopathic hypercalciuria, renal tubular acidosis

Decreased in:

Hypoparathyroidism, pseudohypoparathyroidism, vitamin D deficiency, vitamin D−resistant rickets, diet low in calcium, drugs (thiazide diuretics, oral contraceptives), familial hypocalciuric hypercalcemia, renal osteodystrophy

URINE CATECHOLAMINES

Normal range:

Norepinephrine: <100 µg/24 hr (<590 nmol/day) [CF: 5.911, SMI: 10 nmol/day]

Epinephrine: <10 µg/24 hr (55 nmol/day) [CF: 5.458, SMI: 5 nmol/day]

Elevated in:

Pheochromocytoma, neuroblastoma, severe stress

URINE CHLORIDE

Normal range:

110-250 mEq/day (110-250 mmol/day) [CF: 1, SMI: 1 mmol/day]

Elevated in:

Corticosteroids, Bartter's syndrome

Decreased in:

Chloride depletion (vomiting, diuretics), colonic villous adenoma

URINE COPPER

Normal range:

<40 µg/24 hr (<0.6 µmol/day) [CF: 0.01574, SMI: 0.2 µmol/day]

URINE CORTISOL, FREE

Normal range:

10-110 µg/24 hr (30-300 nmol/day) [CF: 2.759, SMI: 10 nmol/day]

Elevated:

Refer to CORTISOL (serum)

URINE CREATININE (24 hr)

Normal range:

Male: 0.8-1.8 g/day (7-16 mmol/day) [CF: 8.840, SMI: 0.1 mmol/day]

Female: 0.6-1.6 g/day (5.3-14 mmol/day)

NOTE: Useful test as an indicator of completeness of 24 hr urine collection.

URINE GLUCOSE (qualitative)

Normal:

Absent

Present in:

Diabetes mellitus, renal glycosuria (decreased renal threshold for glucose), glucose intolerance

URINE HEMOGLOBIN, FREE

Normal:

Absent

Present in:

Hemolysis (with saturation of serum haptoglobin binding capacity and renal threshold for tubular absorption of hemoglobin)

URINE HEMOSIDERIN

Normal:

Absent

Present in:
Paroxysmal nocturnal hemoglobinuria (PNH), chronic hemolytic anemia, hemochromatosis

URINE 5-HYDROXYINDOLE – ACETIC ACID (URINE 5-HIAA)

Normal range:
2-8 mg/24 hr (10-40 μmol/day) [CF: 5.23, SMI: 5 μmol/day]
Elevated in:
Carcinoid tumors, after ingestion of certain foods (bananas, plums, tomatoes, avocados, pineapples, eggplant, walnuts), drugs (MAO inhibitors, phenacetin, methyldopa, glycerol guaiacolate, acetaminophen, salicylates, phenothiazines, imipramine, methocarbamol, reserpine, metamphetamine)

URINE INDICAN

Normal:
Absent
Present in:
Malabsorption secondary to intestinal bacterial overgrowth

URINE KETONES (semiquantitative)

Normal:
Absent
Present in:
DKA, alcoholic ketoacidosis, starvation, isopropanol ingestion

URINE METANEPHRINES

Normal range:
0-2.0 mg/24 hr (0-11.0 μmol/day) [CF: 5.458, SMI: 0.5 μmol/day]
Elevated in:
Pheochromocytoma, neuroblastoma, drugs (caffeine, phenothiazines, MAO inhibitors), stress

URINE MYOGLOBIN

Normal:
Absent
Present in:
Severe trauma, hyperthermia, polymyositis/dermatomyositis, carbon monoxide poisoning

URINE NITRITE

Normal:
Absent
Present in:
Urinary tract infections

URINE OCCULT BLOOD

Normal:
Negative

Positive in:
   Trauma to urinary tract, renal disease (glomerulonephritis, pyelonephritis), renal or ureteral calculi, bladder lesions (carcinoma, cystitis), prostatitis, prostatic carcinoma, menstrual contamination, hematopoietic disorders (hemophilia, thrombocytopenia), anticoagulants, ASA

URINE OSMOLALITY
Normal range:
   50-1200 mOsm/kg (50-1200 mmol/kg) [CF: 1, SMI: 1 mmol/kg]
Elevated in:
   SIADH, dehydration, glycosuria, adrenal insufficiency, high-protein diet
Decreased in:
   Diabetes insipidus, excessive water intake, IV hydration with D_5W, acute renal insufficiency, glomerulonephritis

URINE pH
Normal range:
   4.6-8 (average 6)
Elevated in:
   Bacteriuria, vegetarian diet, renal failure with inability to form ammonia, drugs (antibiotics, sodium bicarbonate, acetazolamide)
Decreased in:
   Acidosis (metabolic, respiratory), drugs (ammonium chloride, methenamine mandelate), diabetes mellitus, starvation, diarrhea

URINE POTASSIUM
Normal range:
   25-100 mEq/24 hr (25-100 mmol/day) [CF: 1, SMI: 1 mmol/day]
Elevated in:
   Aldosteronism (primary, secondary), glucocorticoids, alkalosis, renal tubular acidosis, excessive dietary potassium intake
Decreased in:
   Acute renal failure, potassium-sparing diuretics, diarrhea, hypokalemia

URINE PROTEIN (quantitative)
Normal range:
   <150 mg/24 hr (<0.15 g/day) [CF: 0.001, SMI: 0.01 g/day]
Elevated in:
   Renal disease (glomerular, tubular, interstitial), CHF, hypertension, neoplasms of renal pelvis and bladder, multiple myeloma, Waldenstrom's macroglobulinemia

URINE SODIUM (quantitative)
Normal range:
   40-220 mEq/day (40-220 mmol/day) [CF: 1, SMI: 1 mmol/day]
Elevated in:
   Diuretic administration, high sodium intake, salt-losing nephritis, acute tubular necrosis, vomiting, Addison's disease, SIADH, hypothyroidism, CHF, hepatic failure

URINE SPECIFIC GRAVITY

Normal range:
1.005-1.03

Elevated in:
Dehydration, excessive fluid losses (vomiting, diarrhea, fever), x-ray contrast media, diabetes mellitus, CHF, SIADH, adrenal insufficiency, decreased fluid intake

Decreased in:
Diabetes insipidus, renal disease (glomerulonephritis, pyelonephritis), excessive fluid intake or IV hydration

URINE VANILLYLMANDELIC ACID (VMA)

Normal range:
<6.8 mg/24 hr (<35 μmol/day) [CF: 5.046, SMI: 1 μmol/day]

Elevated in:
Pheochromocytoma, neuroblastoma, ganglioblastoma, drugs (isoproterenol, methocarbamol, levodopa, sulfonamides, chlorpromazine), severe stress, after ingestion of bananas, chocolate, vanilla, tea, coffee

Decreased in:
Drugs (MAO inhibitors, reserpine, guanethidine, methyldopa)

VDRL

Normal range:
Negative

Positive test:
Syphilis, other treponemal diseases (yaws, pinta, bejel)

NOTE: A false-positive test may be seen in patients with SLE and other autoimmune diseases, infectious mononucleosis, atypical pneumonia, malaria, leprosy.

VISCOSITY

Normal range:
1.4-1.8 relative to water (1.10-1.22 centipoise)

Elevated in:
Monoclonal gammopathies (Waldenstrom's macroglobulinemia, multiple myeloma), hyperfibrinogenemia, SLE, rheumatoid arthritis, polycythemia, leukemia

WESTERGREN; *see* ERYTHROCYTE SEDIMENTATION RATE

D-XYLOSE ABSORPTION

Normal range:
21-31% excreted in 5 hr (0.21-0.31) [CF: 0.01, SMI: 0.01]

Decreased in:
Malabsorption syndrome (refer to Section 23.5)

Medications

This section provides essential and concise information on more than 150 commonly prescribed medications.[2-6] For the reader's convenience, the common synonyms are cross-indexed to the generic names. Each drug is listed by its principal generic name and is approached with the following format:

1. Generic name (common synonyms)
2. Preparations
3. Adult dosage
4. Indications
5. Action
6. Contraindications and precautions

Hypersensitivity or allergic reaction to a medication or any of its components is a definite contraindication to its use. When prescribing multiple medications for the same patient, all the possible drug interactions must be carefully considered.

Every attempt has been made to cover the most important aspects of each drug and to keep medication dosages in conformity with the latest practices of the general medical community. However, it is *strongly recommended that the reader become completely familiar with the manufacturer's product information before prescribing any of these medications*. This is particularly important when prescribing for patients with renal or hepatic impairment and for elderly or debilitated patients. THE USE OF ANY DRUG IN WOMEN WHO ARE PREGNANT OR OF CHILDBEARING AGE REQUIRES THAT THE ANTICIPATED BENEFIT BE WEIGHED AGAINST THE POSSIBLE HAZARD. PLEASE NOTE THAT THIS SECTION DOES NOT LIST PREGNANCY AS A CONTRAINDICATION TO THE USE OF ANY OF THESE MEDICATIONS. *REFER TO THE MANUFACTURER'S PRODUCT INFORMATION FOR POSSIBLE WARNINGS. CONTRAINDICATIONS, OR ADVERSE REACTIONS BEFORE PRESCRIBING ANY OF THESE MEDICATIONS FOR PREGNANT WOMEN.*

Fig. 32-1 shows the composition of a prescription order.

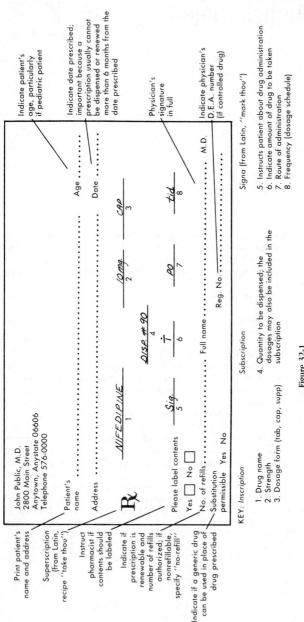

Figure 32-1
Composition of a prescription order.

Print patient's name and address

Superscription (from Latin, recipe "take thou")

Instruct pharmacist if contents should be labeled

Indicate if prescription is renewable and number of refills authorized; if nonrefillable, specify "no-refill"

Indicate if a generic drug can be used in place of drug prescribed

Indicate patient's age, particularly if pediatric patient

Indicate date prescribed; important because a prescription usually cannot be dispensed or renewed more than 6 months from the date prescribed

Physician's signature in full

Indicate physician's D.E.A. number (if controlled drug)

John Public, M.D.
2800 Main Street
Anytown, Anystate 06606
Telephone 576-0000

Patient's name ....

Address ....

℞

NIFEDIPINE
1

10 mg.
2

CAP
3

Disp. # 90
4

Sig.
5

T̄
6

po
7

tid
8

Age ....

Date ....

Please label contents ....

Yes ☐   No ☐

No. of refills ....

Substitution permissible   Yes   No

Full name .... M.D.

Reg. No. ....

KEY: *Inscription*

1. Drug name
2. Strength
3. Dosage form (tab, cap, supp)

Subscription

4. Quantity to be dispensed; the dosages may also be included in the subscription

Signa (from Latin, "mark thou")

5. Instructs patient about drug administration
6. Indicate amount of drug to be taken
7. Route of administration
8. Frequency (dosage schedule)

ACETAZOLAMIDE (Diamox)

Preparations: *tab* 125, 250 mg; *inj* 500 mg; *cap* 500 mg (Diamox Sequels)
Adult dosage
1. Glaucoma: 250 mg-1 g/24 hr, in divided doses for amounts >250 mg
2. Drug-induced edema: 250-375 mg qod
3. Edema from CHF: 250-375 mg (5 mg/kg) qd or qod
4. Epilepsy: 8-30 mg/kg in divided doses

Indications: Adjunctive treatment of
1. Chronic single glaucoma, secondary glaucoma, preoperatively in acute angle-closure glaucoma (Diamox sequels, Diamox)
2. Edema (drug-induced or from CHF) (Diamox)
3. Centrencephalic epilepsies (Diamox)

Action: Carbonic anhydrase inhibitor
Contraindications and precautions: Marked hepatic or renal disease, hyperchloremic acidosis, hyponatremia, hypokalemia, chronic noncongestive angle-closure glaucoma, adrenal failure

ACHROMYCIN; *see* TETRACYCLINE

ACYCLOVIR (Zovirax)

Preparations: *cap* 200 mg; *oint* 5%, 15 g tube; *inj* 500 mg acyclovir/10 ml vial; *susp* 200 mg/5 ml (473 ml bottles)
Adult dosage
1. Initial genital herpes: 200 mg PO q4h while awake (5 caps/day) × 10 da
2. Chronic suppressive therapy for recurrent disease: 400 mg PO bid for up to 12 mo
3. Intermittent therapy: 200 mg q4h 5 times daily × 5 days; therapy should be initiated at the earliest sign or symptom of recurrence
4. Apply ointment to affected areas 6 times/day × 7 days; not for use in the eye
5. Herpes simplex infections in the immunocompromised patient: 5 mg/kg IV infused slowly over 1 hr q8h (15 mg/kg/day) × 7 days
6. Severe initial clinical episodes of genital herpes: same as above, except × 5 days
7. Acute treatment of herpes zoster: 800 mg PO q4h, 5 times daily × 7-10 days

Indications: See above
Action: Antiviral nucleoside analog; competes for DNA polymerase
Contraindications and precautions: Hypersensitivity to any of its components; decrease the dosage in patients with creatinine clearance < 50 ml/min

ADALAT; *see* NIFEDIPINE

ADENOCARD; *see* ADENOSINE

ADENOSINE (Adenocard)

Preparations: *inj* 3 mg/ml (2 ml vial)
Adult dosage: Initially 6 mg by rapid IV bolus; if not effective, in 1-2 min, 12 mg by IV bolus; may repeat
Indications: Paroxysmal supraventricular tachycardia, including that associated with WPW syndrome
Contraindications and precautions
1. Second- or third-degree AV block, sick sinus syndrome (unless paced), atrial flutter, atrial fibrillation, ventricular tachycardia
2. Use lower doses in patients receiving dypyridamole

ADRENALIN; *see* EPINEPHRINE

ALBUMIN

Preparations
  5% solution 50, 250, 500, 1000 ml bottles containing respectively 2.5, 12.5, 25, 50 g of albumin
  25% solution (salt-poor albumin) 20, 50, 100 ml vials containing respectively 5, 12.5, 25 g of albumin
Adult dosage
1. 5% solution: For patients in shock with acute plasma volume depletion
2. 25% solution: For albumin replacement in patients with hypoproteinemia

ALBUTEROL (Ventolin, Proventil)

Preparations
  Inhaler 17 g canister, 0.09 mg/metered dose; *syrup* 2 mg/5 ml, bottles of 16 fl oz; *tab* 2, 4 mg
Adult dosage
1. Inhaler: 2 inhalations q4-6h
2. Syrup: Initially 2 mg (1 tsp) to 4 mg (2 tsp) tid-qid
3. Tab: Initially 2-4 mg tid-qid
Indications: Relief of bronchospasm in patients with reversible obstructive airway disease and for prevention of exercise-induced bronchospasm
Action: Sympathomimetic bronchodilator
Contraindications and precautions
1. Hypersensitivity to any of its components
2. Use with caution in patients with cardiovascular disorders, hyperthyroidism, diabetes mellitus, hypertension, coronary insufficiency
3. Avoid concomitant use of MAO inhibitors, tricyclic antidepressants, and other sympathomimetic aerosol bronchodilators or epinephrine

ALDACTONE; *see* SPIRONOLACTONE

ALDOMET; *see* METHYLDOPA

ALLOPURINOL (Zyloprim)

Preparations: *tab* 100, 300 mg
Adult dosage
1. Initially 100 mg/day; increase by 100 mg at weekly intervals until a serum uric acid of ≤6 mg/dl is attained or a total dose of 800 mg/day
2. Maintenance (average dosages)
   a. Mild gout: 200-300 mg/day
   b. Severe gout: 400-600 mg/day in divided doses
3. A prophylactic dose of colchicine (0.5 mg bid) is recommended by some to prevent an increase in attacks of gout when allopurinol therapy is initiated
4. Secondary hyperuricemia associated with therapy of malignancies: 600-800 mg/day in divided doses for 3 days
   NOTE: Reduce the dosage in patients with renal insufficiency and those receiving mercaptopurine or azathioprine.

Indications: Gout, hyperuricemia associated with treatment of malignancies, management of patients with recurrent calcium oxalate calculi whose daily uric acid excretion is >800 mg/day (male patients) and >750 mg/day (female patients)
Action: Xanthine oxidase inhibitor; it decreases both serum and urine uric acid levels
Contraindications and precautions
1. Allopurinol hypersensitivity
2. Use with caution in patients with renal insufficiency (decrease dosage) and in patients receiving dicumarol (prolonged prothrombin time), thiazide diuretics (increased allopurinol toxicity), ampicillin or amoxicillin (increased frequency of skin rash), chlorpropamide (increased risk of hypoglycemia), cyclophosphamide, and other cytotoxic agents (possible enhancement of bone marrow suppression)

ALPRAZOLAM (Xanax)

Preparations: *tab* 0.25, 0.5, 1 mg
Adult dosage
1. Initially 0.25-0.5 mg tid
2. Maximum daily dose is 4 mg
3. Use 0.25 mg bid or tid in elderly or debilitated patients

Indications: Management of anxiety disorders and anxiety associated with depression
Action: Benzodiazepine; exact mechanism of action is unknown
Contraindications and precautions: Hypersensitivity to benzodiazepines, acute narrow-angle glaucoma, use during activities requiring complete mental alertness, concomitant use of ethanol and other CNS depressants

ALUPENT; *see* METAPROTERENOL

AMANTADINE (Symmetrel)

Preparations: *cap* 100 mg; *syrup* 10 mg/ml (16 fl oz)
Adult dosage
1. Drug-induced extrapyramidal reactions: 100 mg bid
2. Parkinsonism: 100 mg/day initially, may increase gradually to maximum of 400 mg/day in divided doses
3. Prophylaxis and treatment of Influenza A: 200 mg/day
   NOTE: Decrease the dosage in renal insufficiency, CHF, peripheral edema, or orthostatic hypotension.
   NOTE: A parkinsonian crisis may be caused by abrupt discontinuation of the drug.

Indications: Parkinsonism, drug-induced extrapyramidal reactions, prophylaxis and treatment of Influenza A
Action: Antiviral agent with ability to release dopamine
Contraindications and precautions
1. Hypersensitivity to the drug, lactation
2. Use with caution in patients with history of seizures (increased risk of seizure activity), CHF, peripheral edema, liver disease, recurrent eczematous rash, psychosis or psychoneurosis not controlled by chemotherapeutic agents
3. Decrease the dosage in elderly patients and in those with diminished renal function

AMIKACIN SULFATE (Amikin)

Preparations: *inj* 100 mg/2 ml vial, 500 mg/2 ml vial, 1 g/4 vial
Adult dosage
1. Loading dose: 5-7.5 mg/kg
2. Maintenance dose: 5 mg/kg q8h or 7.5 mg/kg q12h; do not exceed 1.5 g/day total dose; 24 hr following initiation of therapy, obtain a serum peak level 30 min after IV administration of the drug (1 hr after IM administration) and a trough level just prior to the next dose; therapeutic *peak* concentration is 15-30 μg/ml, *trough* 5-10 μg/ml; serum creatinine should be monitored qd-qod while the patient is receiving amikacin; modify maintenance doses based on the calculated CCr (see Appendix IV); Table 32-1 shows suggested reductions in maintenance dose based on the CCr

Indications: Infections caused by susceptible bacterial organisms

Table 32-1 Adjustment of amikacin dosages based on creatinine clearance

CCr	Maintenance Dose Relative to Loading Dose (%)
70	88 q12h
50	79 q12h
25	57 q12h
10	56 q24h

KEY: CCr, Creatinine clearance

Action: Bacterial aminoglycoside; it attaches to the 30S and 50S ribosomal subunits

Contraindications and precautions
1. Hypersensitivity to amikacin
2. Avoid concurrent use of diuretics and concurrent and sequential use of neurotoxins and nephrotoxins because of potential added toxicity.

AMIKIN; *see* AMIKACIN SULFATE

AMINOPHYLLINE; *see* THEOPHYLLINE

AMITRIPTYLINE (Elavil)

Preparations: *tab* 10, 25, 50, 75, 100, 150 mg; *inj* 10 mg/ml (10 ml vial)

Adult dosage
1. Initially 50-75 mg PO/day in divided doses or given as a single dose qhs; may increase by 25 mg prn to a total of 150 mg/day
2. Usual maintenance dosage is 50-100 mg/day
3. IM Dosage is 20-30 mg qid

NOTE: Use lower dosages in elderly and adolescent patients.

Indications: Relief of symptoms of depression

Action: Antidepressant with sedative effects; it interferes with reuptake of norepinephrine and serotonin

Contraindications and precautions
1. Hypersensitivity to amitryptiline
2. Concomitant use of MAO inhibitors or disulfiram; use during acute recovery phase of MI; concomitant use of ethanol or other CNS depressants
3. Use with caution in patients with a history of seizures, urinary retention, angle-closure glaucoma, increased intraocular pressure, cardiovascular disorders, hyperthyroidism
4. Avoid concomitant use of ethchlorvynol, cimetidine, anticholinergic agents, sympathomimetic drugs, electroshock therapy
5. Use with caution in patients with suicidal tendencies

AMOXICILLIN (Amoxil)

Preparations: *cap* 250, 500 mg; *susp* 125, 250 mg/5 ml (80, 100, 150, 200 ml)

Adult dosage
1. Infections of the lower respiratory tract: 500 mg q8h
2. Infections of ear, nose, throat, GU, skin, soft tissues: 250 mg q8h
3. Acute uncomplicated gonorrhea*: 3 g PO (single dose) plus probenicid 1 g PO (single dose) and tetracycline 500 mg PO qid for 7 days

Indications: Infections caused by susceptible bacterial organisms

Action: Semisynthetic broad-spectrum penicillin; it inhibits biosynthesis of cell wall mucopeptide

Contraindications and precautions: Hypersensitivity to penicillins

*Useful only for documented sensitive strains.

AMOXICILLIN/POTASSIUM CLAVULANATE (Augmentin)

Preparations: *tab* 250, 500 g; *chewable tab* 125, 250 mg; *oral susp* 125, 250 mg/5 ml (75, 150 ml)
Adult dosage: 250-500 mg q8h
Indications: Infections caused by susceptible bacterial organisms
Action: Same as for amoxicillin; the addition of clavulinic acid provides protection against β-lactamase producing strains of *Staphylococcus aureus*
Contraindications and precautions: Allergy to penicillins

AMOXIL; *see* AMOXICILLIN

AMPHOTERICIN B (Fungizone)

Preparations: *cream* 30 mg/g, 20 g tube; *lotion* 30 mg/ml, 30 ml bottle; *ointment* 30 mg/g, 20 g tube; *inj* 5 mg/ml (after reconstitution) (10 ml vial)
Adult dosage
  1. Cream/lotion/ointment: Apply to candidal lesions bid or qid
  2. IV: Initially 0.25 mg/kg in a concentration of 0.1 mg/ml infused slowly over 6 hr; total daily dosage should not exceed 1.5 mg/kg
Indications
  1. Cream/lotion/ointment: cutaneous and mucocutaneous mycotic infections caused by *Candida* sp
  2. IV: progressive, potentially fatal fungal infections
Action: It binds to sterols in the fungal cytoplasmic membrane; it increases membrane permeability with resultant leakage of molecules
Contraindications and precautions
  1. Hypersensitivity to any of its components
  2. Caution when using nephrotoxic antibiotics or antineoplastic agents concomitantly
  3. Avoid concomitant use of corticosteroids (unless necessary to control drug reactions)
  4. Perform frequent renal and hepatic function tests; discontinue therapy if BUN >40 mg/dl, creatinine >3 mg/dl, or if LFT abnormalities are noted; monitor serum potassium

AMPICILLIN

Preparations: *cap* 250, 500 mg; *susp* 125, 250, 500 mg/5 ml (80, 100, 150, 200 ml) *inj* 125, 250, 500 mg, 1 g, 2 g vials
Adult dosage
  1. Infections of the respiratory tract and soft tissues
     a. PO: 250-500 mg q6h
     b. IM/IV: 500 mg-1g q6h
  2. Infections of the GI or GU tracts
     a. PO: 500 mg q6h
     b. IM/IV: 500 mg-1g q6h
  3. Urethritis caused by ampicillin-sensitive *Neisseria gonorrhoeae*
     PO: 3.5 g with 1 g of probenecid administered simultaneously followed by tetracycline 500 mg PO qid for 7 days
  4. Bacterial meningitis or septicemia: 150-200 mg/kg/day IV in equally divided doses q3-4h

Indications: Infections caused by susceptible bacterial organisms
Action: Semisynthetic penicillin; it inhibits cell wall synthesis
Contraindications and precautions: Penicillin hypersensitivity

AMYL NITRATE

Preparations: *ampul* 0.3 ml
Indications: Identification of cardiac murmurs
1. Increased murmur: AS, IHSS, PS, MS, TS, TR
2. Decreased murmur: MR, VSD, Austin-Flint murmur
Action: Vasodilating agent

ANAPROX; *see* NAPROXEN

ANCEF; *see* CEFAZOLIN

ANTIVERT; *see* MECLIZINE

APRESOLINE; *see* HYDRALAZINE

ATARAX; *see* HYDROXYZINE

ATENOLOL (Tenormin)

Preparations: *tab* 50, 100 mg; *inj* 5 mg/10 ml
Adult dosage: Initially 50 mg PO qd, may increase to 100 mg qd if no significant effect is noted after 2 wk; for dosage in acute MI, refer to Table 20-4
Indications: Hypertension, angina pectoris, acute MI
Action: β-1 (cardioselective) adrenergic receptor blocking agent
Contraindications and precautions
1. Bradycardia, second- or third-degree heart block, CHF, cardiogenic shock
2. Use with caution in patients with bronchospastic disease; if dosages greater than 50 mg/day are needed, divide to achieve lower peak blood levels
3. β blockage may mask tachycardia associated with hypoglycemia and thyrotoxicosis
4. Use with caution in patients with impaired renal function and those receiving catecholamine-depleting drugs
5. Abrupt cessation of atenolol therapy in patients with CAD can result in exacerbation of angina

ATIVAN; *see* LORAZEPAM

ATROPINE

Preparations: *inj* 0.3, 0.4, 0.5, 0.6, 1.0, 1.3 mg; *tab* 0.4 mg
Adult dosage
1. Bradycardia: 600 μg to 1 mg q5min prn to maximum total dose of 2 mg

2. Preanesthesia: 400-600 μg SQ/IM/IV 1 hr before induction
3. Anticholinesterase poisoning: 2-3 mg parenterally; repeat until signs of atropine toxicity appear

Indications: Bradycardia, asystole, preanesthesia, anticholinesterase poisoning

Action: Anticholinergic agent

Contraindications and precautions: Acute glaucoma, GI obstruction, obstructive uropathy, prostatism

ATROVENT; *see* IPRATROPIUM BROMIDE

AUGMENTIN; *see* AMOXICILLIN/POTASSIUM CLAVULANATE

AXSAIN; *see* CAPSAICIN

AZACTAM; *see* AZTREONAM

AZT; *see* ZIDOVUDINE

AZTREONAM (Azactam)

Preparations: *inj* 500 mg (1, 2 g vial)

Adult dosage: Sepsis, 1-2 g IV q8h; decrease in patients with renal impairment

Indications: Treatment of aerobic gram-negative bacterial infections

Action: Monobactam antibiotic; bactericidal through the inhibition of bacterial cell wall synthesis

Contraindications and precautions: In patients with impaired hepatic or renal function, appropriate monitoring and dosage adjustment are recommended during therapy

AZULFADINE; *see* SULFASALAZINE

BACTRIM; *see* TRIMETHOPRIM AND SULFAMETHOXAZOLE

BENADRYL; *see* DIPHENHYDRAMINE

BENEMID; *see* PROBENECID

BENZTROPINE MESYLATE (Cogentin)

Preparations: *tab* 0.5, 1, 2 mg; *inj* (IM/IV) 2 ml ampule (1 mg/ml)

Adult dosage
1. Postencephalitic and idiopathic parkinsonism: 1-2 mg/day to maximum of 6 mg/day in two divided doses; initiate at low dosage and then increase by 0.5 mg increments at 6-day intervals
2. Drug-induced extrapyramidal symptoms: 1-4 mg qd

Indications: Control of extrapyramidal disorders caused by neuroleptic drugs and as an adjunct in the therapy of parkinsonism

Action: Competitive antagonist of acetylcholine; antihistaminic

Contraindications and precautions
1. Narrow-angle glaucoma
2. Use with caution in patients with prostatic hypertrophy, hypertension. GI or GU obstructive disease, hot climate (can cause anhidrosis)

BICILLIN; *see* PENICILLIN G BENZATHINE

BRETHINE; *see* TERBUTALINE

BRETHAIRE; *see* TERBUTALINE

BRETYLIUM TOSYLATE (Bretylol)

Preparations: *inj* 50 mg/ml
Adult dosage: 5-10 mg/kg IV over 5-10 min with additional doses of 10 mg/kg prn to maximum of 40 mg/kg total; maintenance IV infusion is 1-2 mg/min
   NOTE: Reduce the dosage in patients with impaired renal function.
Indications
1. Prophylaxis and therapy of ventricular fibrillation
2. Life-threatening ventricular dysrhythmias that have failed to respond to adequate doses of a first-line antidysrhythmic agent
Action: Suppression of ventricular dysrhythmias; the precise mechanism of action has not been clearly defined
Contraindications and precautions
1. Suspected digitalis-induced ventricular dysrhythmias
2. Use with caution in patients with fixed cardiac output (severe aortic stenosis or severe pulmonary hypertension)

BRETYLOL; *see* BRETYLIUM TOSYLATE

BREVIBLOC; *see* ESMOLOL

BROMOCRIPTINE MESYLATE (Parlodel)

Preparations: *tab* 2.5 mg; *cap* 5 mg
Adult dosage
1. Parkinsonism: initial dose is 1.25 mg (half of a 2.5 mg tab) bid
2. Female infertility: initial dose is 2.5 mg bid or tid
3. Prevention of physiological lactation: 2.5 mg bid × 14 days; do not start treatment sooner than 4 hr after delivery
4. Amenorrhea/galactorrhea: 2.5 mg qd × 1 wk then increase to bid; maximum duration of therapy is 6 mo
5. Acromegaly: 1-25-2.5 mg qhs for initial 3 days; increase by 1.25-2.5 mg prn every 3-7 days
Indications: Parkinsonism, prevention of physiological lactation, amenorrhea/galactorrhea, female infertility associated with hyperprolactinemia (in absence of demonstrable pituitary tumor), acromegaly
Action: Dopamine receptor agonist; it inhibits prolactin secretion

Contraindications and precautions
1. Sensitivity to ergot alkaloids
2. Use with caution in patients with renal and hepatic disease
3. Avoid use of phenothiazines during bromocriptine therapy
4. Evaluate the sella turcica in patients with amenorrhea/galactorrhea and infertility to rule out pituitary tumors before starting therapy with bromocriptine

BRONKOSOL; *see* ISOETHARINE

BUSPAR; *see* BUSPIRONE

BUSPIRONE (Buspar)

Preparations: *tab* 5, 10 mg
Adult dosage: Initial dosage is 5 mg PO tid, may increase by 5 mg/day q3d prn; optimal daily dose is 20-30 mg; maximum daily dose is 60 mg
Indications: Management of anxiety disorders
Action: Anxiolytic; its mechanism of action is unknown
Contraindications and precautions: Avoid concurrent use of other CNS agents; concomitant use of MAO inhibitors may be hazardous (elevation of blood pressure)

CALAN; *see* VERAPAMIL

CALCIMAR; *see* CALCITONIN SALMON

CALCITONIN SALMON (Calcimar)*

Preparations: *inj* 2 ml vial (200 IU/ml)
Adult dosage
1. Paget's disease: 100 IU/day SQ/IM initially; 50 IU qd or qod maintenance
2. Hypercalcemia: 4 IU/kg q12h SQ/IM initially; may increase dosage to 8 IU/kg q12h SQ/IM after 24-48 hr if response is unsatisfactory; if response is still unsatisfactory, may increase dosage again, to 8 IU/kg SQ/IM q6h after 2 more days
3. Postmenopausal osteoporosis: 100 IU/day SQ/IM
Indications: Symptomatic Paget's disease of bone, hypercalcemia, postmenopausal osteoporosis (in addition to supplemental calcium, adequate vitamin D intake, and adequate diet)
Action: Synthetic polypeptide with the same amino acid sequence as salmon calcitonin; it acts primarily on bone to inhibit the ongoing bone resorptive process
Contraindications and precautions
1. Clinical allergy to synthetic salmon calcitonin
2. Periodical examination of urine sediment is recommended for patients on chronic therapy

---

*For skin testing to assess allergic susceptibility: Prepare a 1 IU per 0.1 ml dilution with NS and inject intracutaneously into the forearm.

CALCITRIOL (Rocaltrol)

Preparations: *cap* 0.25, 0.5 μg
Adult dosage
  1. Dialysis patients: initial dosage is 0.25 μg/day; may increase by 0.25 μg/day at 4-8 wk intervals if a satisfactory response is not obtained
  2. Hypoparathyroidism: initial dosage is 0.25 μg/day given in AM; may increase by 0.25 μg/day at 2-4 wk intervals

Indications: Hypocalcemia secondary to chronic renal dialysis, postsurgical and idiopathic hypoparathyroidism, pseudohypoparathyroidism

Action: Synthetic vitamin D analog; it is the most potent metabolite of vitamin D available

Contraindications and precautions
  1. Hypercalcemia, evidence of vitamin D toxicity
  2. Monitor serum calcium level frequently, particularly during titration period
  3. Use with caution in patients on digitalis (hypercalcemia may precipitate cardiac dysrhythmias in these persons)
  4. In patients with normal renal function, maintain adequate fluid intake

CALCIUM CARBONATE (Os-Cal)

Preparations: *tab*
  1. Os-Cal 250 = 625 mg calcium carbonate (each tab contains 250 mg of elemental calcium and 125 USP units of vitamin D)
  2. Os-Cal 500 = 1250 mg calcium carbonate (each tab contains 500 mg of elemental calcium)
  3. Os-Cal Forte = 250 mg elemental calcium plus vitamins and minerals

Adult dosage: 1 tab tid
Indications: Calcium replacement therapy
Contraindications and precautions: Hypercalcemia, vitamin D intoxication

CAPOTEN; *see* CAPTOPRIL

CAPTOPRIL (Capoten)

Preparations: *tab* 12.5, 25, 50, 100 mg
Adult dosage
  1. Hypertension: 25 mg PO, bid-tid initially; maximum dosage is 150 mg tid
  2. Heart failure: 6.25-12.5 mg tid initially; maximum daily dose is 450 mg
  3. Decrease dosage in patients with renal insufficiency

Indications: Hypertension; heart failure not adequately controlled with diuretics and digitalis
Action: ACE inhibitor

Contraindications and precautions
1. Bilateral or unilateral renal artery stenosis
2. Use with caution in patients with renal impairment and collagen-vascular disease
3. A CBC and urinalysis should be done before initiation of therapy with captopril

CAPSAICIN (Axsain, Zostrix)

Preparations: *cream* (Axsain) 0.075%, 2 oz tube; (Zostrix) 0.025%, 45 g tube
Adult dosage: Apply to affected area tid-qid
Indications: Painful diabetic neuropathy and postsurgical pain (Axsain); postherpetic neuralgia (Zostrix)
Action: Capsaicin removes substance P from the nerve endings, impairing the transmission of pain impulses to the brain
Contraindications and precautions: Avoid the eyes; wash hands immediately after application; do not use on broken or irritated skin

CARAFATE; *see* SUCRALFATE

CARDIOQUIN; *see* QUINIDINE

CARDIZEM; *see* DILTIAZEM

CATAPRES; *see* CLONIDINE

CECLOR; *see* CEFACLOR

CEFACLOR (Ceclor)

Preparations: *oral susp* 125, 250 mg/5 ml; *cap* 250, 500 mg
Adult dosage: Usual dosage is 250 mg PO q8h; may double in severe infections
Indications: Infections caused by susceptible bacterial strains
Actions: Semisynthetic cephalosporin; its bactericidal action results from inhibition of cell wall synthesis
Contraindications and precautions
1. Known allergy to cephalosporins
2. Administer with caution in patients with a history of allergy to penicillin

CEFAZOLIN (Ancef, Kefzol)

Preparations: *inj* 250 mg, 500 mg, 1 g vials
Adult dosage
1. Treatment of infections: 250 mg-2 g q8h IV/IM
2. Surgical prophylaxis; 1 g IM/IV 30-60 min before surgery and 500 mg-1 g q6-8h × 24 hr
NOTE: Decrease the dosage in patients with impaired renal function.

Indications: Infections caused by susceptible bacterial strains and for surgical prophylaxis
Action: Semisynthetic cephalosporin
Contraindications and precautions
1. Use with caution in patients allergic to penicillin
2. Do not use in patients allergic to cephalosporins

CEFOTAN; *see* CEFOTETAN

CEFOTETAN (Cefotan)

Preparations: *inj* 1, 2 g vials
Adult dosage: Sepsis, 1-3 g IV/IM q12h; decrease the dosage in patients with impaired renal function
Indications: Serious intraabdominal and gynecological infections, prophylaxis for postoperative infection following GI, obstetrical, and gynecological surgical procedures
Action: Semisynthetic cephalosporin; its bactericidal action results from the inhibition of cell wall synthesis
Contraindications and precautions: Hypersensitivity to cephalosporins. Use with caution in patients allergic to penicillin

CEFOXITIN (Mefoxin)

Preparations: *inj* 1, 2 g vials
Adult dosage
1. Treatment of infections: 1-2 g q6-8h IV to maximum of 12 g/day (2 g q4h)
2. Surgical prophylaxis: 2 g IV/IM 30 min before surgery, then 2 g q6h for 24 hr (72 hr for prosthetic arthroplasty)
NOTE: Decrease the dosage in patients with impaired renal function.
Indications: Infections caused by susceptible organisms; surgical prophylaxis
Action: Semisynthetic cephalosporin; its bactericidal action results from the inhibition of cell wall synthesis
Contraindications and precautions: Hypersensitivity to cephalosporins: use with caution in patients allergic to penicillin

CEFTAZIDIME (Fortaz)

Preparations: *inj* 0.5, 1, 2 g vials
Adult dosage
1. Uncomplicated UTI: 250 mg IV/IM q12h
2. Complicated UTI: 500 mg-1g IV/IM q8-12h
3. Uncomplicated pneumonia and mild skin infections: 500 mg-1 g q8h
4. Bone and joint infections: 2 g IV q12h
5. Meningitis, serious gynecological and intraabdominal infections, and severe life-threatening infections: 2 g IV q8h
6. Pseudomonal lung infections in patients with cystic fibrosis: 30-50 mg/kg IV q8h, up to 6 g/day
7. Usual recommended dosage: 1 g IV/IM q8-12h
NOTE: Decrease the dosage in patients with impaired renal function.

Indications: Infections caused by susceptible bacterial strains; useful in infections caused by *Pseudomonas* strains
Action: Semisynthetic cephalosporin; its bactericidal action results from the inhibition of cell wall synthesis
Contraindications and precautions: Hypersensitivity to cephalosporins; use with caution in patients allergic to penicillin

CEFTIN; *see* CEFUROXIME

CEFUROXIME (Ceftin, Zinacef)

Preparations: *tab* (Ceftin) 250, 500 mg; *inj* (Zinacef) 750 mg, 1.5 g vials
Adult dosage: PO 250-500 mg bid; IV/IM 750 mg-1.5 g q6-8h depending on severity of the infection
NOTE: Decrease the dosage in patients with renal impairment.
Indications: Infections caused by susceptible bacterial organisms
Action: Semisynthetic cephalosporin; its bactericidal action results from inhibition of cell wall synthesis
Contraindications and precautions: Hypersensitivity to cephalosporins; use with caution in patients allergic to penicillin

CEPHALEXIN (Keflex)

Preparations: *cap* 250, 500 mg; *susp* 125, 250 mg/5 ml; *tab* 1 g
Adult dosage: 250 mg-1 g q6h depending on severity of infection
NOTE: Decrease the dosage in patients with renal impairment.
Indications: Infections caused by susceptible bacterial organisms
Action: Semisynthetic cephalosporin; its bactericidal action results from inhibition of cell wall synthesis
Contraindications and precautions: Hypersensitivity to cephalosporins; use with caution in patients allergic to penicillin

CEPHALOTHIN (Keflin)

Preparations: *inj* 1, 2, 4 g vials
Adult dosage: 500 mg-1 g IV/IM q4-6h depending on severity of infection
NOTE: Decrease the dosage in patients with impaired renal function.
Indications: Infections caused by susceptible bacterial organisms
Action: Semisynthetic cephalosporin; its bactericidal action results from inhibition of cell wall synthesis
Contraindications and precautions: Hypersensitivity to cephalosporins; use with caution in patients allergic to penicillin

CEPHULAC; *see* LACTULOSE

CHARCOAL, ACTIVATED

Preparations: *bottles* containing 30 g of activated charcoal, USP, suspended in 4 oz of water
Adult dosage: 30-120 g; usually followed by a cathartic to hasten the elimination of charcoal-absorbed drugs
Indications: Drug overdose or poisoning

CHLORDIAZEPOXIDE (Librium)

Preparations: *cap* 5, 10, 25 mg; *tab* 5, 10, 25 mg; *inj* 100 mg/5 ml amp
Adult dosage
1. Relief of mild and moderate anxiety disorders: PO 5-10 mg tid-qid
2. Relief of severe anxiety disorders: PO 20-25 mg tid-qid; IM/IV: 50-100 mg initially, then 25-50 mg tid-qid prn
3. Withdrawal symptoms of acute alcoholism: 50-100 mg IM/IV initially, repeat in 2-4 hr if necessary (up to 300 mg/day)
4. Preoperative apprehension and anxiety: IM 50-100 mg 1 hr before surgery

NOTE: Decrease the dosage in elderly or debilitated patients.
NOTE: An IV injection should be given slowly over 1 min.
Indications: Management of anxiety disorders, short-term relief of symptoms of anxiety, withdrawal symptoms of acute alcoholism, preoperative apprehension and anxiety
Action: Benzodiazepine; exact mechanism of action is unknown, but it is believed to act on the limbic system of the brain
Contraindications and precautions
1. Do not use concomitantly with ethanol or other CNS depressants
2. Abrupt discontinuation can result in withdrawal symptoms
3. Do not use in patients in shock or comatose states
4. Use with caution in patients with renal or hepatic impairment, patients with a history of porphyria (possible exacerbation of symptoms)
5. Concomitant use of other psychotropic agents is not recommended

CHLORPROMAZINE (Thorazine)

Preparations: *tab* 10, 25, 50, 100, 200 mg; *syrup* 10 mg/5 ml; *inj* 25 mg/ml; *supp* 25, 100 mg; *SR cap* 30, 75, 150, 200, 300 mg; *conc* 30 mg/ml (120 ml), 100 mg/ml (60, 240 ml)
Adult dosage
1. Excessive anxiety, tension, and agitation: 10-25 mg PO tid (in severe cases may increase dosage by 20-50 mg semiweekly until patient becomes calm and cooperative)
2. Prompt control of severe symptoms: 25 mg IM (if necessary repeat in 1 hr; subsequent doses should be oral, 25 mg to 50 mg tid)
3. Nausea and vomiting: 10-25 mg PO q4-6h prn; 25 mg IM, if no hypotension occurs; give 25-50 mg IM q3-4h prn until the vomiting stops, then switch to PO dosage; 100 mg supp PR q6-8h
4. Intractable hiccups: 25-50 mg PO tid or qid; if symptoms persist, give 25-50 mg IM
Indications: Management of manifestations of psychotic disorders, control of nausea and vomiting, relief of intractable hiccups
Action: Phenothiazine neuroleptic; the principal pharmacologic actions are psychotropic but it also exerts sedative and antiemetic activity
Contraindications and precautions
1. Comatose states, presence of large amounts of CNS depressants, bone marrow depression, Reye's syndrome, hypersensitivity to phenothiazines

2. Use with caution in patients with cardiovascular disease, COPD, severe asthma, patients exposed to extreme heat, organophosphorus insecticides, and patients receiving atropine or related drugs

CHLORPROPAMIDE (Diabinese)

Preparations: *tab* 100, 250 mg
Adult dosage: Initial 100-250 mg qd; most patients do not require more than 250 mg/day; maximum daily dose is 750 mg
Indications: Hyperglycemia of NIDDM not adequately controlled with diet alone
Action: Sulfonylurea; it stimulates pancreatic insulin secretion (it is postulated that it enhances the postreceptor action of insulin and the number of insulin receptors)
Contraindications and precautions
  1. Known hypersensitivity to the drug
  2. Administration of oral hypoglycemic agents has been reported to increase the risk of cardiovascular mortality
  3. Hypoglycemic effect of sulfonylureas can be potentiated by various drugs (coumarins, nonsteroidal antiinflammatory agents, salicylates); other drugs tend to produce hyperglycemia (diuretics, corticosteroids, phenytoin)

CHOLESTYRAMINE (Cholybar, Questran)

Preparations: *chewable bar* (Cholybar) 4 g cholestyramine per bar; each box/25 bars; *powder* for oral suspension (Questran) available in 378 g cans (4 g of cholestyramine per 9 g of powder) or cartons of 60 9 g packets (4 g of cholestyramine resin)
Adult dosage: One scoopful (9 g) or one packet one to six times daily mixed with water or other fluids; Cholybar, chew 1 bar one to six times daily (with plenty of fluids)
Indications: Hypercholesterolemia resistant to dietary management, pruritus due to partial biliary obstruction
Action: It absorbs and combines with intestinal bile acids to form an insoluble complex that is excreted in the feces
Contraindications and precautions: Constipation and bloating may occur; patients should take other drugs 1 hr before or 4-6 hr after cholestyramine

CHOLYBAR; see CHOLESTYRAMINE

CHRONULAC; see LACTULOSE

CIMETIDINE (Tagamet)

Preparations: *tab* 200, 300, 400, 800 mg; *liquid* 300 mg/5 ml syrup; *IV* 300 mg/2 ml vial or prefilled syringe
Adult dosage
  1. Active duodenal ulcer:
     a. PO: 300 mg qid with meals and hs, 400 mg bid, or 800 mg qhs
     b. IV: 300 mg q6h (given over at least 2 min); a 24 hr continuous infusion may be more effective

2. Prophylaxis of recurrent duodenal ulcer: 400 mg PO qhs
3. Active benign gastric ulcer: 300 mg PO qid or IV q6h (given over at least 2 min)
4. Pathologic hypersecretory conditions: 300 mg PO qid or IV q6h; some patients may require higher dosage (do not exceed 2400 mg/day)

NOTE: Decrease the dosage in patients with renal impairment.

Indications: Short-term treatment of active duodenal ulcer; prophylactic use in duodenal ulcer patients to prevent ulcer recurrence; treatment of pathologic hypersecretory conditions (Zollinger-Ellison syndrome, MEN, systemic mastocytosis); short-term treatment of active benign gastric ulcer

Action: Histamine H_2 receptor antagonist; it inhibits gastric acid secretion

Contraindications and precautions

1. Nursing mothers (cimetidine is excreted in breast milk)
2. Use with caution in elderly patients and in patients with renal or hepatic impairment
3. Patients receiving warfarin-type anticoagulants, theophylline, nifedipine, procainamide, metoprolol, quinidine, phenytoin, lidocaine, propranolol, diazepam, or chlordiazepoxide may have increasing blood levels of these drugs when cimetidine is used concomitantly
4. Cimetidine may potentiate the effect of alcohol

CIPROFLOXACIN (Cipro)

Preparations: *tabs* 250, 500, 750 mg; *inj** 200, 400 mg

Adult dosage: Uncomplicated UTI: 250 mg q12h PO or 200 mg q12h IV
Infectious diarrhea or respiratory tract, skin, and soft tissue infections: 500 mg q12h PO or 200-400 mg q12h IV
Bone and joint infections: 750 mg q12h PO or 400 mg q12h IV
NOTE: Decrease the dosage in patients with renal impairment.

Indications: Infections caused by susceptible bacterial organisms

Action: Bactericidal quinolone antibiotic; it inhibits bacterial DNA replication by interfering with the enzyme DNA gyrase

Contraindications and precautions: Avoid concomitant antacids and sucralfate; ciprofloxacin increases theophylline plasma levels; probenecid reduces ciprofloxacin excretion

CLEOCIN; *see* CLINDAMYCIN

CLAVULANIC ACID; *see* AMOXICILLIN/POTASSIUM CLAVULANATE

CLINDAMYCIN (Cleocin)

Preparations: *cap* 75, 150 mg; *inj* 150 mg/ml (2, 4, 6 ml vial); *granules* (pediatric) 75 mg/5 ml; *soln* (Cleocin T) 30, 60 ml; *lotion* 60 ml; *gel* 7.5, 30 g

---

*Pending FDA approval.

Adult dosage

1. Serious infections: 150-300 mg PO q6h or 600-1200 mg/day IM/IV divided in two to four equal doses
2. More severe infections: 300-450 mg PO q6h or 1200-1700 mg/day IM/IV divided in 2 to 4 equal doses
3. Life threatening situations: Total daily doses up to 4800 mg may be used
4. Acne vulgaris: apply a thin film twice daily

NOTE: Decrease the dosage in patients with severe renal or hepatic disease.

Indications: Serious infections caused by susceptible bacterial organisms

Action: It inhibits bacterial protein synthesis by binding to the 50S ribosomal subunit

Contraindications and precautions

1. Hypersensitivity to clindamycin or lincomycin
2. Use with caution in patients with a history of GI disease (particularly colitis), atopic individuals, patients receiving neuromuscular blocking drugs, patients with aspirin hypersensitivity

CLONIDINE (Catapres)

Preparations: *tab* 0.1, 0.2, 0.3 mg; *transdermal patches* 3.5 cm^2 TTS-1 (0.1 mg/day), 7 cm^2 TTS-2 (0.2 mg/day), 10.5 cm^2 TTS-3 (0.3 mg/day)

Adult dosage

1. PO: 0.1 mg bid initially; usual dosage range is 0.2-0.8 mg/day; maximum daily dose is 2.4 mg
   a. Clonidine loading can be used to rapidly decrease blood pressure in severely hypertensive patients; loading dose is 0.2 mg, followed by 0.1 mg/hr (up to total dose of 0.6 mg)
   b. Blood pressure should be monitored q15min; when a satisfactory drop has been achieved, start clonidine 0.1 mg q8-12h and add a diuretic agent to decrease renal sodium and water retention
2. Transdermal: 3.5 cm^2 patch applied once weekly initially

Indications: Treatment of hypertension

Action: Central α-adrenergic receptor stimulant

Contraindications and precautions

1. Use with caution in patients with severe coronary insufficiency, recent MI, cerebrovascular disease, chronic renal failure
2. When discontinuing clonidine, be sure to reduce the dose gradually over several days to avoid significant rebound hypertension

CLORAZEPATE (Tranxene)

Preparations: *cap* 3.75, 7.5, 15 mg; *tab* 3.75, 7.5 mg, 15 mg; 22.5 mg (Tranxene-SD), 11.25 mg (Tranxene-SD half-strength)

Adult dosage

1. For symptomatic relief of anxiety the usual daily dose is 30 mg in divided doses; Tranxene-SD and Tranxene-SD half-strength may be administered as a single dose
2. Dosage range is 15-60 mg/day, maximum daily dose 90 mg
3. In elderly or debilitated patients initiate with 7.5-15 mg/day in divided doses

Indications: Management of anxiety disorders; adjunctive therapy in the management of partial seizures; symptomatic relief of acute alcohol withdrawal

Action: Benzodiazepine

Contraindications and precautions
1. Acute narrow-angle glaucoma, depressive neuroses, psychotic reactions
2. Use with caution in patients with impaired renal or hepatic function
3. Concomitant use of alcohol or other CNS depressants is contraindicated

CLOTRIMAZOLE (Mycelex)

Preparations: *topical cream 1%* (15, 30, 45 g tubes); *topical solution 1%* (10, 30 ml bottles); *troche 10 mg clotrimazole; vaginal cream 1%* (Mycelex-G) 50 mg/applicatorful, 45, 90 g tubes; *vaginal tab* (Mycelex-G) 100, 500 mg

Adult dosage
1. Treatment of fungal skin infections: Apply topical cream or solution to affected area bid
2. Oropharyngeal candidiasis: troche (10 mg) 5 times/day × 14 days
3. Vulvovaginal candidiasis:
   a. 100 mg vaginal tab qd × 7 days; nonpregnant women may use 2 tabs bid × 3 days
   b. 500 mg vaginal tab inserted intravaginally 1 time only
   c. Apply vaginal cream intravaginally, one applicatorful qhs × 7-14 days

Indications: *Candida* or other dermatophyte skin infections; vulvovaginal candidiasis; prevention and treatment of oropharyngeal candidiasis

Contraindications: Ophthalmic use is contraindicated

COGENTIN; *see* BENZTROPINE MESYLATE

COLACE; *see* DIOCYTL SODIUM SULFOSUCCINATE

COLCHICINE

Preparations: *tab* 0.5, 0.6 mg; *granules* 0.5 mg; *inj* 0.5 mg/ml (2 ml amp)

Adult dosage
1. Treatment of acute gout: PO 0.5-1.2 mg initially, then 0.5-0.6 mg q1-3h until the pain is relieved (maximum total dose is 8-10 mg); IV 1-2 mg diluted in 20 ml of 0.9% NaCl initially; additional doses are 0.5 mg q6-12h (maximum 24 hr dose is 4 mg)
   NOTE: IV administration must be slow, and care must be taken to avoid extravasation.
2. Prophylaxis of gout: 0.6 mg PO bid

Indications: Treatment and prophylaxis of gout

Action: Antiinflammatory; it impairs leukocyte chemotaxis and synovial cell phagocytosis of urate crystals

Contraindications and precautions: Use with caution in patients with GI, hepatic, renal, or cardiac disease and in elderly or debilitated patients

COLYTE; *see* POLYETHYLENE GLYCOL ELECTROLYTE
SOLUTION

COMPAZINE; *see* PROCHLORPERAZINE

CONJUGATED ESTROGEN TABLETS; *see* ESTROGENIC
SUBSTANCES, CONJUGATED

COUMADIN; *see* WARFARIN

CYCLOBENZAPRINE (Flexeril)

Preparations: *tab* 10 mg
Adult dosage: Usual dosage is 10 mg PO tid; maximum daily dosage is 60
  mg/day
Indications: Relief of spasm associated with acute painful musculoskeletal
  conditions; should not be used continuously for longer than 3 wk
Action: Relief of muscle spasm by reduction of tonic somatic motor activity influencing both γ and α motor systems
Contraindications and precautions
  1. Concomitant use of MAO inhibitors or within 14 days after their
     discontinuation; concomitant use of tricyclic antidepressants, use
     during acute recovery phase of MI,
  2. Hyperthyroidism, CHF, dysrhythmias, heart block, conduction dis-
     turbances
  3. Cyclobenzaprine may enhance the effects of barbiturates, alcohol,
     and other CNS depressants
  4. Use with caution in patients with a history of urinary retention, an-
     gle-closure glaucoma, increased intraocular pressure and in patients
     taking anticholinergic medications

CYTOTEC; *see* MISOPROSTOL

DECADRON; *see* DEXAMETHASONE

DEMEROL; *see* MEPERIDINE

DEXAMETHASONE (Decadron)

Preparations: *tab* 0.25, 0.5, 0.75, 1.5, 4, 6 mg; *elixir* 0.5 mg/5 ml; *inj* 4,
  10, 24 mg/ml
Adult dosage
  1. Cerebral edema: 10 mg IV initially followed by 4 mg IV/IM q6h
  2. Acute allergic disorders:
     Day 1: 5-8 mg IM
     Day 2 and 3: 3 mg PO in divided doses (1.5 mg PO bid)
     Day 4: 1.5 mg PO in divided doses (0.75 mg PO bid)
     Day 5 and 6: 0.75 mg PO qd
     Day 7: No treatment

3. Intraarticular, intralesional, or soft tissue injection: Usual dose is 0.2-6 mg

Indications: Cerebral edema, adrenocortical insufficiency, collagen-vascular diseases (SLE, acute rheumatic arthritis), allergic states (contact dermatitis, bronchial asthma), diagnosis of Cushing's syndrome, hematological disorders (ITP, acquired hemolytic anemias), inflammatory bowel disease, palliative management of leukemias, lymphomas, nephrotic syndrome (from SLE or idiopathic), dermatological disease (severe erythema multiforme, pemphigus), respiratory diseases (symptomatic sarcoidosis, berylliosis)

Action: Synthetic adrenocortical steroid

Contraindication and precautions

1. Systemic fungal infections, hypersensitivity to any of its components (sodium bisulfite)
2. Use with caution in patients with ocular herpes simplex
3. Immunization procedures should not be undertaken in patients receiving corticosteroids

DIABETA; *see* GLYBURIDE

DIABINESE; *see* CHLORPROPAMIDE

DIAMOX; *see* ACETAZOLAMIDE

DIAZEPAM (Valium)

Preparations: *tab* 2, 5, 10 mg; *inj* 5 mg/ml (1,2,5,10 ml vials); *SR cap* 15 mg; *sol* 5 mg/5 ml; *conc* 5 mg/5 ml (30 ml)

Adult dosage

1. Anxiety disorders and relief of symptoms of anxiety: 2-10 mg PO bid to qid; 2-10 mg IV, may repeat in 3-4 hr if necessary
2. Acute alcohol withdrawal: 10 mg PO tid or qid during initial 24 hr, then decrease dose to 5 mg tid or qid; 10 mg IV/IM initially, then 5-10 mg in 3-4 hr if necessary
3. Endoscopic procedures: 2-10 mg IV immediately before procedure, or 5-10 mg IM 30 min before procedure
4. Muscle spasm: 2-10 mg PO tid or qid; 5-10 mg IM/IV initially, then 5-10 mg in 3-4 hr if necessary (larger doses may be required for tetanus)
5. Preoperative: 5-15 mg IV 5-10 min before procedure
6. Status epilepticus: 5-10 mg IV initially; may repeat in 10-15 min intervals up to total maximum dose of 30 mg

NOTE: Use lower doses in elderly and debilitated patients; the IM route is painful and provides erratic absorption

Indications: Management of anxiety disorders or short-term relief of the symptoms of anxiety, acute alcohol withdrawal, muscle spasm, status epilepticus

Action: Benzodiazepine

Contraindications and precautions: Acute narrow-angle glaucoma, concomitant ingestion of alcohol or other CNS depressants

DICLOXACILLIN (Dynapen)

Preparations: *cap* 125, 250, 500 mg; *susp* 62.5 mg/5 ml
Adult dosage: 125-250 mg q6h on an empty stomach
Indications: Susceptible penicillinase-producing *Staphylococcus* infections
Contraindications and precautions: Do not use in penicillin-allergic patients; avoid the concomitant use of tetracyclines

DIFLUCAN; *see* FLUCONAZOLE

DIGOXIN (Lanoxin)

Preparations: *tab* 0.125, 0.25, 0.5 mg; *elixir* 0.05 mg/ml; *inj* 0.1, 0.25 mg/ml; *cap* 0.05, 0.1, 0.2 mg (Lanoxicaps)
Adult dosage
  1. Loading dose 10-15 µg/kg IV/PO divided over 12-24 hr (e.g., 0.5 mg initially then 0.25 mg q6h × 4 doses)
  2. Maintenance dosage: range is 0.125-0.5 mg/day; maintenance dosage should be monitored by clinical response and serum digoxin levels; however, serum levels are greatly influenced by other factors (e.g., hypokalemia) and therefore do not consistently reflect therapeutic response or toxicity
  NOTE: Dosage must be reduced in patients with impaired renal function.
  NOTE: Concomitant use of quinidine, amiodarone, verapamil, fluoxetine, or nifedipine increases serum digoxin levels.
  NOTE: Digoxin requirements are reduced in patients with hypothyroidism
Indications: Low output CHF, atrial fibrillation, atrial flutter, paroxysmal atrial tachycardia (PAT)
Action: Positive inotropic effect, negative chronotropic effect, decreased conduction velocity through the AV node
Contraindications and precautions
  1. Ventricular fibrillation, second- or third-degree AV block (in absence of mechanical pacemaker), idiopathic hypertrophic subaortic stenosis (IHSS) (use of digoxin may result in worsening of outflow obstruction)
  2. Patients with Wolff-Parkinson-White (WPW) syndrome and atrial fibrillation (use of digoxin can result in enhanced transmission of impulses through accessory pathway)
  3. Sick sinus node disease (digoxin may worsen sinus bradycardia or sinoatrial block)
  4. Hypokalemia, hypomagnesemia, and hypercalcemia predispose to digoxin toxicity
  5. Patients with atrial dysrhythmias secondary to hyperthyroidism, heart failure from amyloid heart disease, or constrictive cardiomyopathies respond poorly to digoxin
  6. Life-threatening digitalis toxicity can be effectively treated with digoxin-antibody fragments (Digibind)

DILANTIN; *see* PHENYTOIN

DILAUDID; *see* HYDROMORPHONE HYDROCHLORIDE

DILTIAZEM (Cardizem)

Preparations: *tab* 30, 60, 90, 120 mg; *cap* (Cardizem SR) 60, 90, 120 mg
Adult dosage: Angina, 30 mg qid initially, dosage range 180-360 mg/day
   in 3-4 divided doses; hypertension, 60-120 mg (Cardizem SR) bid
Indications: Angina pectoris resulting from coronary artery spasm, angina
   pectoris caused by atherosclerotic coronary artery disease, hypertension
Action: Calcium channel antagonist
Contraindications and precautions
   1. Sick sinus syndrome (except in the presence of a functioning pace-
      maker), hypotension, second- or third-degree AV block
   2. Use with caution in patients with impaired renal or hepatic function
   3. Concomitant use of diltiazem, β-blockers, or digitalis may result in
      additive effects on cardiac conduction

DIOCTYL SODIUM SULFOSUCCINATE (Colace)

Preparations: *cap* 50, 100 mg; *syrup* 20 mg/5 ml
Adult dosage: 50-200 mg qd
Indications: Constipation because of hard stools, painful anorectal condi-
   tions, cardiac or other conditions in which ease of defecation is desirable
Action: Stool softener; surface-active agent
Contraindications and precautions: None

DIPHENHYDRAMINE (Benadryl)

Preparations: *cap* 25, 50 mg; *elixir* 12.5 mg/5 ml; *inj* 10, 50 mg/ml
Adult dosage
   1. PO: 25-50 mg tid or qid; for motion sickness give first dose 30 min
      before exposure to motion
   2. IV: 10-50 mg IM/IV tid or qid; maximum total daily dosage is 400
      mg
Indications: Allergic reactions (urticaria, anaphylaxis), allergic rhinitis,
   motion sickness, parkinsonism, nighttime sleep aid
Action: Antihistamine with anticholinergic and sedative effects
Contraindications and precautions
   1. Avoid concomitant use of MAO inhibitors, alcohol, or other CNS
      depressants
   2. Use with caution in elderly patients and patients with narrow-angle
      glaucoma, stenotic peptic ulcer, pyloroduodenal obstruction, symp-
      tomatic prostatic hypertrophy, bladder neck obstruction, increased
      IOP, hypertension, cardiovascular disease, bronchial asthma, and
      hyperthyroidism

DIPYRIDAMOLE (Persantine)

Preparations: *tab* 25, 50, 75 mg
Adult dosage: 50 mg tid or 75 mg bid, taken at least 1 hr before meals
Indications: Adjunct to coumarin anticoagulants to prevent postoperative
   thromboembolic complications of cardiac valve replacement
Contraindications and precautions: Use with caution in patients with hy-
   potension (may produce peripheral vasodilation)

DISOPYRAMIDE PHOSPHATE (Norpace)

Preparations: *cap* 100, 150 mg, *SR cap* (Norpace CR) 100, 150 mg
Adult dosage
1. Loading dose: 300-400 mg; maintenance dosage: 150 mg q6h (100 mg q6h if body weight is <50 kg), 300 mg q12h (Norpace CR)
2. Avoid loading dose in patients with possible cardiac decompensation or cardiomyopathy and decrease maintenance dose to 100 mg q6-8h
3. Decrease dosage in hepatic or renal insufficiency

Indications: Suppression and prevention of recurrence of: unifocal or multifocal premature (ectopic) ventricular contractions (PVC), paired PVC or episodes of ventricular tachycardia
Action: Type I antidysrhythmic agent
Contraindications and precautions
1. Cardiogenic shock, congenital QT prolongation, preexisting second- or third-degree AV block (in absence of pacemaker), glaucoma, myasthenia gravis, urinary retention
2. Do not use in patients with hypotension or CHF (unless secondary to cardiac dysrhythmia)
3. Discontinue use if patient develops QT prolongation >25%, QRS widening >25%, heart block > first-degree (decrease dosage if patient develops first-degree heart block), hypoglycemia secondary to disopyramide
4. Concomitant use of other type I antidysrhythmic agents or propranolol can result in serious negative inotropic effects and may severily prolong conduction
5. Use with caution in patients with myocarditis, cardiomyopathy, WPW syndrome, sick sinus syndrome, or bundle branch block
6. Digitalize patients with atrial flutter or fibrillation before administering dysopyramide

DIULO; *see* METOLAZONE

DOBUTAMINE (Dobutrex)

Preparations: *vial* 250 mg/20 ml
Adult dosage: Rate of infusion needed to increase cardiac output usually ranges from 2.5-10 µg/kg/min (Table 32-2); the starting dose is 1-2 µg/kg/min
Indications: Inotropic support in short-term treatment of cardiac decompensation caused by depressed contractility (secondary to organic heart disease or cardiac surgical procedures)
Action: Direct-acting inotropic agent; primary activity results from stimulation of β receptors of heart. Refer to Fig. 20-3 for a graphic representation of dobutamine's effects on systemic vascular resistance, renal blood flow, pulmonary capillary wedge pressure, and cardiac output.
Contraindications and precautions
1. Idiopathic hypertrophic subaortic stenosis (IHSS)
2. Correct hypovolemia before starting dobutamine
3. Dobutamine may be ineffective and peripheral vascular resistance may increase if the patient has recently received a β-blocking agent

Table 32-2 Dobutamine (Dobutrex) infusion (dosage = μg/kg/min)

Flow Rate (μgtt/min)	Quantity of Dobutrex* (μg/min)†	Body Weight															
		(lb) 77 (kg) 35	88 40	99 45	110 50	121 55	132 60	145 65	154 70	165 75	176 80	187 85	198 90	209 95	220 100	231 105	242 110
2	66.7	1.9	1.7	1.5	1.3	1.2	1.1	1.0	1.0	0.88	0.83	0.78	0.74	0.70	0.67	0.63	0.60
3	100	2.9	2.5	2.2	2.0	1.8	1.7	1.5	1.4	1.3	1.3	1.2	1.1	1.1	1.0	1.0	0.90
4	133.3	3.8	3.3	3.0	2.7	2.4	2.2	2.1	1.9	1.8	1.7	1.6	1.5	1.4	1.3	1.3	1.2
5	166.7	4.8	4.2	3.7	3.3	3.0	2.8	2.6	2.4	2.2	2.1	2.0	1.9	1.8	1.7	1.6	1.5
6	200	5.7	5.0	4.4	4.0	3.6	3.3	3.1	2.9	2.7	2.5	2.4	2.2	2.1	2.0	1.9	1.8
7	233.3	6.7	5.8	5.2	4.7	4.2	3.9	3.6	3.3	3.1	2.9	2.7	2.6	2.5	2.3	2.2	2.1
8	266.7	7.6	6.7	5.9	5.3	4.9	4.5	4.1	3.8	3.6	3.3	3.1	3.0	2.8	2.7	2.5	2.4
9	300	8.6	7.5	6.7	6.0	5.5	5.0	4.6	4.3	4.0	3.8	3.5	3.3	3.2	3.0	2.9	2.7
10	333.3	9.5	8.3	7.4	6.7	6.1	5.6	5.1	4.8	4.4	4.2	3.9	3.7	3.5	3.3	3.2	3.0
12	400	11.4	10.0	8.9	8.0	7.3	6.7	6.2	5.7	5.3	5.0	4.7	4.4	4.2	4.0	3.8	3.6
14	466.7	13.3	11.7	10.4	9.3	8.5	7.8	7.2	6.7	6.2	5.8	5.5	5.2	4.9	4.7	4.4	4.2
16	533.3	15.2	13.3	11.9	10.7	9.7	8.9	8.2	7.6	7.1	6.7	6.3	5.9	5.6	5.3	5.1	4.9
18	600	17.1	15.0	13.3	12.0	10.9	10.0	9.2	8.6	8.0	7.5	7.1	6.7	6.3	6.0	5.7	5.5
20	667	19.1	16.7	14.8	13.3	12.1	11.1	10.3	9.5	8.9	8.3	7.8	7.4	7.0	6.7	6.3	6.1
22	733	21.0	18.3	16.3	14.7	13.3	12.2	11.3	10.5	9.8	9.2	8.6	8.1	7.7	7.3	7.0	6.7
24	800	22.9	20.0	17.8	16.0	14.5	13.3	12.3	11.4	10.7	10.0	9.4	8.9	8.4	8.0	7.6	7.3
26	867	24.8	21.7	19.3	17.3	15.8	14.4	13.3	12.4	11.6	10.8	10.2	9.6	9.1	8.7	8.3	7.9
28	933	26.7	23.3	20.7	18.7	17.0	15.6	14.4	13.3	12.4	11.7	11.0	10.4	9.8	9.3	8.9	8.5
30	1000	28.6	25.0	22.2	20.0	18.2	16.7	15.4	14.3	13.3	12.5	11.8	11.1	10.5	10.0	9.5	9.1

From Purcell JA: Am J Nurs 82:965, 1982.

*Dobutamine (Dobutrex) solution 2 μg/ml (1000 mg Dobutrex/500 ml or 500 mg Dobutrex/250 ml).

†Based on 60 μgtt/ml; each drop contains 33.3 μg Dobutrex.

DOBUTREX; *see* DOBUTAMINE

DOPAMINE (Intropin)

Preparations: *ampul* 200 mg/5 ml; *inj* 200, 400, 800 mg
Adult dosage
1. Initial 2-5 µg/kg/min; increase gradually until hemodynamic response is obtained, generally up to a maximum of 50 µg/kg/min (Table 32-3)
2. Constantly evaluate the patient's blood pressure, volume status, renal output, myocardial contractility, and peripheral perfusion; note the development of any new dysrhythmias
3. Use decreased dosage in patients who have been receiving MAO inhibitors

Indications: Shock syndrome as a result of MI, endotoxins, trauma, open heart surgery, renal failure, chronic cardiac decompension
Action: Inotropic agent (refer to Fig. 20-3 for a graphic representation of the effects of dopamine on systemic vascular resistance, renal blood flow, pulmonary capillary wedge pressure, and cardiac output)
Contraindications and precautions: Pheochromocytoma, uncorrected hypovolemia, tachydysrhythmias, or ventricular fibrillation

DORYX; *see* DOXYCYCLINE

DOXYCYCLINE (Doryx, Vibramycin)

Preparations: *cap* (Doryx) 100 mg; (Vibramycin) 50, 100 mg; *oral susp* 25 mg/5 ml; *syrup* 50 mg/5 ml; *inj* 100, 200 mg vial
Adult dosage: 100 mg q12h for initial 24 hr, then 100 mg qd; max dose is 200 mg/day
Indications: Tetracycline sensitive infections
Action: Bacteriostatic by inhibition of protein synthesis
Contraindications and precautions
1. Antacids, iron, zinc, and urinary alkalinizers reduce absorption; may also decrease digoxin levels and depress plasma prothrombin activity
2. Periodic hematopoietic, renal, and hepatic studies should be performed in patients on long-term therapy
3. Discontinue drug if photosensitivity occurs

DYNAPEN; *see* DICLOXACILLIN

ELAVIL; *see* AMITRIPTYLINE

ENALAPRIL, ENALAPRILAT (Vasotec)

Preparations: *tab* (enalapril) 2.5, 5, 10, 20 mg; *IV* (Enalaprilat) 1.25 mg/ml (2 ml vial)
Adult dosage: Initially 5 mg PO daily; use 2.5 mg PO qd in patients taking diuretics or with renal CCr (creatinine clearance) <30 ml/min; usual dosage range is 10-40 mg daily in single or divided doses; IV initial dosage is 1.25 mg (given over 5 min) q6h; in patients receiving diuretics, decrease the dosage to 0.625 mg IV q6h

Table 32-3 Dopamine infusion (dosage = μg/kg/min)

Flow Rate (μgtt/min)	Quantity of Dopamine* (μg/min)†	Body Weight															
		(lb) 77 (kg) 35	88 40	99 45	110 50	121 55	132 60	143 65	154 70	165 75	176 80	187 85	198 90	209 95	220 100	231 105	242 110
5	133	3.8	3.4	2.9	2.6	2.4	2.2	2.0	1.9	1.8	1.6	1.6	1.5	1.4	1.3	1.3	1.2
10	267	7.6	6.7	5.9	5.3	4.9	4.5	4.1	3.8	3.6	3.3	3.1	3.0	2.8	2.7	2.5	2.4
15	400	11	10	8.9	8.0	7.3	6.6	6.1	5.7	5.3	5.0	4.7	4.4	4.2	4.0	3.8	3.6
20	533	15	13	12	11	9.7	8.9	8.2	7.6	7.1	6.7	6.3	5.9	5.6	5.3	5.1	4.9
25	667	19	17	15	13	12	11	10	9.5	8.9	8.4	7.8	7.4	7.0	6.6	6.3	6.0
30	800	23	20	18	16	15	13	12	11	11	10	9.4	8.9	8.4	8.0	7.6	7.3
35	933	27	23	21	19	17	16	14	13	12	12	11	10	9.8	9.3	8.9	8.5
40	1067	31	27	24	21	19	18	16	15	14	13	13	12	11	11	10	9.7
45	1200	34	30	27	24	22	20	18	17	16	15	14	13	13	12	11	11
50	1333	38	33	30	27	24	22	21	19	18	17	16	-15	14	13	13	12
55	1467	42	37	33	29	27	24	23	21	20	18	17	16	15	15	14	13
60	1600	46	40	36	32	29	27	25	23	21	20	19	18	16	16	15	15
65	1733	50	43	39	35	32	29	27	25	23	22	20	19	18	17	17	16
70	1867	53	47	42	37	34	31	29	27	25	23	22	21	20	19	18	17
75	2000	57	50	45	40	36	33	31	29	27	25	24	22	21	20	19	18
80	2133	61	53	47	43	39	36	33	31	28	27	25	24	23	21	20	19
85	2267	65	57	50	45	41	38	35	32	30	28	27	25	24	23	22	21
90	2400	69	60	53	48	44	40	37	34	32	30	28	27	25	24	23	22
95	2533	72	63	56	51	46	42	39	36	34	32	29	28	27	25	24	23
100	2667	76	67	59	53	49	45	41	38	36	33	31	30	28	27	25	24

From Purcell JA: Am J Nurs 82:965, 1982.

*Dopamine solution (Intropin) 1.6 μg/ml (800 mg Intropin/500 ml or 400 mg Intropin/250 ml).

†Based on 60 μgtt/ml; each drop contains 26.7 μg dopamine.

Indications: Hypertension, CHF
Action: Angiotensin-converting enzyme inhibitor
Contraindications and precautions
1. Use with caution in patients with impaired renal function or renal artery stenosis
2. Discontinue product immediately if laryngeal edema or angioedema occurs

EPINEPHRINE (Adrenalin)

Preparations: *ampul* 1 mg/ml (1:1000)
Adult dosage
1. SQ/IM for bronchial asthma and allergic reactions: 0.2-1 mg
2. IV/Intracardiac for cardiac resuscitation: 0.5 ml (0.5 mg) diluted to 10 ml with NaCl
3. For use with local anesthetics: concentration should be 1:100,000 (0.01 mg/ml) to 1:20,000 (0.05 mg/ml)

Indications: Bronchospasm, hypersensitivity reactions, prolongation of action of infiltration anesthetics, cardiac resuscitation
Action: Sympathomimetic; it acts on both α and β-receptors (most potent α receptor activator)
Contraindications and precautions
1. Narrow-angle glaucoma, shock, organic brain damage, anesthesia with halogenated hydrocarbons or cyclopropane, labor, cardiac dilation, coronary insufficiency
2. Do not use with local anesthesia in fingers and toes (vasoconstriction may cause necrosis)
3. Use with caution in patients receiving digitalis or other drugs that sensitize the heart to dysrhythmias, in patients taking antihistamines or tricyclic antidepressants, in patients with cardiovascular disease or hypertension, and in elderly patients, diabetics, and patients with hyperthyroidism

ERYTHROMYCIN

Preparations: *enteric-coated tab*, erythromycin base (E-Mycin) 250, 333 mg; erythromycin particles in tablets (PCE), 333 mg; erythromycin stearate (Erythrocin) 500, 1000 mg vial; erythromycin ethyl succinate (EES) 400 mg; *chewable tab* 200 mg; *tab* 400 mg; *granules* 200 mg/5 ml; *drops* 100 mg/2.5 ml; *liquid* 200, 400 mg/5 ml; *cap* (ERYC) 125, 250 mg
Adult dosage
1. Erythromycin ethyl succinate (EES) 400 mg PO q6h (maximum of 4 g/day)
2. Enteric-coated tablets (E-Mycin) 250-500 mg PO q6h (maximum of 4 g/day) or 333 mg q8h
3. Erythromycin stearate (Erythrocin) 15-20 mg/kg/day in four divided doses (maximum of 4 g/day)
4. Erythromycin cap (ERYC) 250 mg q6h
5. Erythromycin particles in tablets (PCE) 333 mg PO tid

6. Erythromycin lactobionate (inj) 500 mg-2g IV q6h

Indications: Infections caused by susceptible bacterial organisms

Action: Bacteriostatic macrolide antibiotic; it inhibits protein synthesis by binding to the 50S ribosomal subunit

Contraindications and precautions

1. Use with caution in patients with hepatic insufficiency
2. Increase in serum theophylline levels and prothrombin time may be seen in patients receiving concomitant theophylline or warfarin

ESKALITH; *see* LITHIUM CARBONATE

ESMOLOL (Brevibloc)

Preparations: *inj* 100 mg/10 ml vial, 2.5 g/10 ml ampul

Adult dosage: To initiate treatment of a patient with SVT, administer a loading dose infusion of 500 µg/kg/min over 1 min followed by a 4 min infusion, usually starting with 50 µg/kg/min in saline or glucose solution; if necessary, repeat the loading dose and increase the infusion rate by 50 µg/kg/min over 5 min; maintenance doses greater than 200 µg/kg/min do not have any added benefit

Indications: Rapid control of ventricular rate in patients with atrial fibrillation or flutter, and for short treatment of noncompensatory sinus tachycardia

Action: Cardioselective beta blocker with a very short duration of action (elimination half-life is 9 min)

Contraindications and precautions

1. Heart block greater than first degree, cardiogenic shock, and overt heart failure
2. Avoid use in patients with bronchospastic disease

ESTROGENIC SUBSTANCES, CONJUGATED (Premarin)

Preparations: *tab* 0.3, 0.625, 0.9, 1.25, 2.5 mg; *vaginal cream* 0.625 mg conjugated estrogens/g; each tube contains 42.5 g; *inj* 25 mg/5 ml

Adult dosage

1. Decrease progression of postmenopausal osteoporosis: 1.25 mg/day PO cyclically (3 wk on, 1 wk off)
2. Dysfunctional uterine bleeding: 2.5-5 mg/day for 7-10 days, then decrease to 1.25 mg/day for 2 wk with addition of progesterone the third wk
3. Female castration and primary ovarian failure: 1.25 mg/day PO cyclically (3 wk on, 1 wk off)
4. Inoperable progressing prostatic carcinoma: 1.25-2.5 mg PO tid
5. Inoperable progressing breast cancer in selected men and postmenopausal women: 10 mg PO tid for at least 3 mo
6. Emergency postcoital contraception: 10 mg PO tid, starting within 72 hr of intercourse and continued for 5 days
7. Atrophic vaginitis and kraurosis vulvae: 2-4 g/day intravaginally or topically

8. Postmenopausal symptoms and prevention of osteoporosis: 0.3-1.25 mg/day cyclically (3 wk on, 1 wk off)

Indications: See above

Action: Mixture of estrogens

Contraindications and precautions

1. Pregnancy, known or suspected estrogen dependent neoplasia, undiagnosed abnormal genital bleeding, active thrombophlebitis or thromboembolic disorders, past history of thromboembolic disorders associated with previous estrogen use, known or suspected cancer of the breast except in appropriately selected patients being treated for metastatic disease

2. Estrogens have been reported to increase the risk of endometrial carcinoma

FEOSOL; *see* FERROUS SULFATE

FERROUS SULFATE (Feosol)

Preparations: *tab* 325 mg of ferrous sulfate USP; *cap* 250 mg of ferrous sulfate USP; *elixir* 220 mg of ferrous sulfate/5 ml (tsp)

Dosage: *tab* 1 tid or qid (after meals and at hs) *elixir* 1-2 tsp tid between meals; *cap* qd or bid

Indications: Iron deficiency anemia

Action: Iron replacement

Contraindications and precautions

1. Hemochromatosis

2. Do not take within 2 hr of oral tetracycline

FLAGYL; *see* METRONIDAZOLE

FLECAINIDE (Tambocor)

Preparations: *tab* 50, 100, 150 mg

Adult dosage: Starting dosage is 100 mg PO bid; dosage may be increased by 50 mg bid q4d until maximum efficacy is achieved; maximum dose is 400 mg/day

Indications: Documented life-threatening ventricular dysrhythmias

Action: Class I_C antidysrhythmic agent

Contraindications and precautions

1. Flecainide is contraindicated in patients with preexisting second-or third-degree AV block or bifascicular block (unless pacemaker is present)

2. Use with extreme caution in patients with SSS, cardiomyopathy, CHF, ejection fraction <30%, pacemakers (may increase endocardial pacing thresholds and suppress ventricular escape rhythm)

3. Avoid concurrent use of other antidysrhythmic drugs

4. Therapy should be initiated in the hospital setting, with rhythm monitoring

5. Plasma trough levels should be monitored and kept below 0.7-1.0 μg/ml

6. Correct existing electrolyte abnormalities before initiating flecainide

7. Decrease dosage in patients with renal insufficiency
8. Discontinue medication if heart block, liver dysfunction, or blood dyscrasias occur

FLEXERIL; *see* CYCLOBENZAPRINE

FLUCONAZOLE (Diflucan)

Preparations: *tab* 50, 100, 200 mg; *inj* 200 mg/100 ml, 400 mg/200 ml
Adult dosage
1. Oropharyngeal candidiasis: 200 mg on day 1, then 100 mg/day for a minimum of 2 wk
2. Esophageal candidiasis: 200 mg on day 1, then 100 mg/day for a minimum of 3 wk; treat for at least 2 wk after symptoms resolve; maximum daily dose, 400 mg
3. Systemic candidiasis: 400 mg on day 1, then 200 mg/day for a minimum of 4 wk; treat for at least 2 wk after symptoms resolve
4. Cryptococcal meningitis: 400 mg on day 1, then 200-400 mg/day for 10-12 wk after spinal fluid is negative
5. To suppress relapse in AIDS: 200 mg/day

Indications: Oropharyngeal, esophageal, systemic candidiasis; cryptococcal meningitis
Action: Inhibition of fungal cytochrome P-450–dependent enzymes
Contraindications and precautions
1. Decrease the dose in renal insufficiency
2. Monitor liver function
3. Discontinue if liver failure or a rash develops
4. Drug interactions: ↑ phenytoin, cyclosporine, sulfonylurea levels; potentiation of warfarin effect; rifampin decreases fluconazole concentrations, hydrochlorothiazide increases them

FLUOXETINE (Prozac)

Preparation: *cap* 20 mg
Adult dosage: initially 20 mg qd in AM; increase if needed after several weeks; give doses greater than 20 mg/day, divided (AM and noon); max dose is 80 mg/day
Indications: Depression
Action: Its antidepressant effect is presumed to be linked to its inhibition of CNS neuronal uptake of serotonin
Contraindications and precautions
1. Do not use during or within 14 days of MAO inhibitors
2. Use with caution in patients with renal, hepatic, or cardiac disease and in patients with a history of seizures or using other CNS drugs
3. Discontinue if rash occurs
4. Fluoxetine inhibits the metabolism of tricyclic antidepressants and possibly antipsychotic drugs and may increase their toxicity
5. Fluoxetine increases the PT in patients using warfarin; it also increases the digoxin level; therefore close monitoring is indicated

FOLIC ACID

Preparations: *tab* 1 mg
Adult dosage: 1 mg PO qd
Indications: Megaloblastic anemia from folic acid deficiency
Action: Acts on the bone marrow to correct megaloblastic changes secondary to folic acid deficiency
Contraindications and precautions: Do not use for treatment of vitamin B_{12} deficiency

FORTAZ; *see* CEFTAZIDIME

FUNGIZONE; *see* AMPHOTERICIN B

FURADANTIN; *see* NITROFURANTOIN

FUROSEMIDE (Lasix)

Preparations: *tab* 20, 40, 80 mg; *oral solution* (10 mg/ml) 60, 120 ml; *inj* (10 mg/ml) 2, 4, 10 ml ampul or prefilled syringe
Adult dosage
  1. Edema
     a. PO: 20-80 mg initially; if insufficient response after 8-12h, increase dose by 20-40 mg (maximum daily dosage is 600 mg/day); best response is achieved by intermittent dosage (2-4 consecutive days/wk)
     b. IV: 20-40 mg (given over 1-2 min) if insufficient response, increase this dose by 20 mg increments at least 2 hr after initial dose; adequate dose can be given qd or bid
  2. Hypertension: initial dosage is 40 mg PO bid; adjust dose according to blood pressure response
  3. Acute pulmonary edema: 40 mg IV slowly; may double the dose after 1 hr if insufficient response
Indications: Edema, hypertension, acute pulmonary edema
Action: Diuretic; acts on loop of Henle and distal and proximal tubules; onset of diuresis is 5 min following IV injection, 1 hr following PO dose
Contraindications and precautions
  1. Anuria
  2. Use with caution in elderly patients and in patients receiving lithium, salicylates, or succinylcholine (increased toxicity)

GARAMYCIN; *see* GENTAMICIN

GEMFIBROZIL (Lopid)

Preparations: *tab* 600 mg
Adult dosage: 600 mg bid, 30 min before morning and evening meds
Indications: Type IV and V hyperlipidemias resistant to dietary management, type IIb hyperlipidemia with HDL below 35 mg/dl
Action: Increased intravascular breakdown of VLDL; it also decreases serum triglycerides and serum cholesterol, increases HDL

Contraindications and precautions
1. Hepatic, renal, or gallbladder disease
2. Do not use concomitantly with lovastatin (increased risk of rhabdomyolysis)
3. Gemfibrozil potentiates the anticoagulant effect of warfarin

GENTAMICIN (Garamycin)

Preparations: *inj* 40 mg/ml
Adult dosage
1. Loading dose: 1.5-2 mg/kg of adjusted lean body weight; maintenance dose: 3 mg/kg/day administered in 3 equal doses q8h; in patients with life-threatening infections dosages up to 5 mg/kg/day may be administered
2. On the morning of the second or third day of treatment, obtain a peak level 30 min after administration of the drug (1 hr after IM administration) and trough level right before the dose; therapeutic *peak* level is 5-8 µg/ml, toxic level >10 µg/ml; therapeutic *trough* level is 1-2 µg/ml, toxic level >2 µg/ml
3. In elderly patients and those with renal insufficiency the maintenance dose is modified according to calculated corrected creatinine clearances (see Appendix V)
4. Table 32-4 shows dose intervals and the percent of calculated weight-related maintenance dose based on the creatinine clearance (CCr)
5. Creatinine levels should be monitored qd-qod while the patient is on gentamycin

Indications: Infections caused by susceptible bacterial organisms
Action: Aminoglycoside antibiotic; it inhibits protein synthesis in susceptible organism
Contraindications and precautions
1. Concurrent or sequential use of other nephrotoxic/neurotoxic drugs is contraindicated
2. Use with caution in patients with impaired renal function

Table 32-4 Dose intervals and percent of calculated weight-related maintenance dose

CCr	8 hr (%)	12 hr (%)	24 hr (%)
Normal	100	—	—
50	75	—	—
25	50	65	—
10	20	30	50
<10	10	20	40

NOTE: In every patient, reevaluate the renal status with serum creatinine q48h and readjust the dose administered according to trough and peak levels.

GLIPIZIDE (Glucotrol)

Preparations: *tab* 5, 10 mg
Adult dosage: Initially 5 mg PO qd before breakfast; in geriatric patients and patients with hepatic impairment initial dosage is 2.5 mg PO qd
Indications: Control of hyperglycemia in NIDDM inadequately controlled with diet alone
Action: Second-generation sulfonylurea; lowers serum glucose primarily by stimulating insulin secretion from pancreatic β cells
Contraindications and precautions
  1. Use with caution in patients with renal and hepatic disease.
  2. Hypoglycemic action of glipizide may be potentiated by drugs that are highly protein bound; β-adrenergic blocking agents may mask symptoms of hypoglycemia

GLUCOTROL; *see* GLIPIZIDE

GLYBURIDE (Diabeta, Micronase)

Preparations: *tab* 1.25, 2.5, 5 mg
Adult dosage: Usual starting 2.5-5 mg qd; may be lowered in elderly patients
Indications: Control of hyperglycemia in NIDDM inadequately controlled with diet alone
Action: Second-generation sulfonylurea; lowers serum glucose primarily by stimulating insulin secretion from pancreatic β cells
Contraindications and precautions
  1. DKA
  2. Hypoglycemic action of glyburide may be potentiated by drugs that are highly protein bound; β-adrenergic blocking agents may mask symptoms of hypoglycemia

GO LITELY; *see* POLYETHYLENE GLYCOL 3350 ELECTROLYTE SOLUTION

HALCION; *see* TRIAZOLAM

HALDOL; *see* HALOPERIDOL

HALOPERIDOL (Haldol)

Preparations: *tab* 0.5, 1, 2, 5, 10, 20 mg; *inj* 5 mg/ml; *oral concentrate* 2 mg/ml in 15 ml and 120 ml bottle
Adult dosage
  1. Moderate symptoms and geriatric or debilitated patients: 0.5-2.0 mg PO bid-tid
  2. Severe symptoms and chronicity or resistant patients: 3-5 mg PO bid to tid
  3. Moderately severe to severe symptoms and acutely agitated patients: 2.5 mg IM, may repeat qh prn

4. Control of tics and utterances of Tourette's syndrome: 0.05-0.075
   mg/kg/day

Indications: Management of psychotic disorders; control of tics and vocal
utterances of Tourette's syndrome

Action: Neuroleptic of the butyrophenone series

Contraindications and precautions: CNS depression from any cause; parkinsonism

NOTE: Use with caution in patients receiving lithium (increased risk of
neurologic toxicity), anticonvulsants (decreased convulsive threshold),
anticoagulants (may cause interference), alcohol (additive CNS effects).

NOTE: Use with caution in patients with severe cardiovascular disorders
(may precipitate angina and hypotension).

HEPARIN

Preparations: *inj* 1000; 5000; 10,000; 40,000 U/ml

NOTE: Test for guaiac in the stool and obtain baseline hematocrit, platelet
count, prothrombin time (PT), and activated partial thromboplastin time
(APTT) before starting heparin.

Dosage: Full dose heparinization protocol

1. Initial loading dose is 50 U heparin/lb of lean body weight given as
   an undiluted IV injection (e.g., a 150 lb patient would receive a bolus of 7500 U)
2. Start IV heparin infusion at 5-10 U/lb/hr (or approx 1000 U/hr); to
   prepare the infusion, place 20,000 U heparin in 1000 ml of isotonic
   saline or D_5W (concentration 20 U/ml); rate of infusion varies with
   the patient's weight; e.g., a 160 lb patient would receive 1600 U/hr
   (20,000 U heparin/1000 ml 0.9% NaCl at 80 ml/hr); in patients with
   strict fluid restriction, higher concentration may be used (e.g.,
   10,000 U heparin/100 ml 0.9% NaCl → 100 U/ml); however, when
   very high concentrations are used, even a small change in the rate of
   infusion can result in a significant change in the amount of heparin
   infused
3. Closely monitor rate of infusion:
   a. During the initial 24 hr (or until stable) obtain the first APTT 4-6
      hr after initiation of continuous heparin infusion and then as of-
      ten as necessary until stable (but no sooner than 4 hr after modi-
      fication of the rate of heparin infusion)
   b. After stability has been achieved, monitor the APTT once daily
   c. Maintain the APTT at 1.5-2 times the patient's pretreatment
      level, modifying the rate of infusion to achieve this result
4. Test for guaiac in all stools during heparin therapy
5. Obtain hematocrit and platelet count every third day during heparin
   therapy (increased risk of thrombocytopenia [5% of patients] and GI
   bleeding); severe heparin-associated thrombocytopenia can be rapidly corrected with IV immunoglobulin[1]
6. Heparin is neutralized by protamine sulfate; each mg of protamine
   neutralizes 100 USP units of heparin

Indications: Pulmonary embolism, prophylaxis of deep vein thrombosis,
treatment of venous thrombosis, prevention of cerebral thrombosis in
evolving stroke, adjunct therapy of coronary occlusion with acute MI

Action: Binds with antithrombin III (heparin cofactor); accelerates rate at which antithrombin III neutralizes activated forms of Factors II, VII, IX, X, XI, XII

Contraindications and precautions
1. Hypersensitivity to heparin, bleeding tendencies, active bleeding
2. Use with caution in conditions with increased danger of hemorrhage (e.g., dissecting aneurysm, severe hypertension, hemophilia, thrombocytopenia, ulcerative colitis, diverticulitis)

HYDRALAZINE (Apresoline)

Preparations: *tab* 10, 25, 50, 100 mg; *inj* 20 mg/ml ampul
Adult dosage
1. PO: Initially 10 mg qid for 2-4 days, then increase to 25 mg qid; may increase to 50 mg qid after 2 wk; adjust dosage according to response
2. IM/IV: 20-40 mg prn; monitor blood pressure frequently; maximal hypotensive effect occurs within 20-80 min
   NOTE: Use lower doses in patients with renal impairment.

Indications: Essential hypertension
Action: Causes peripheral vasodilation by direct relaxation of vascular smooth muscle
Contraindications and precautions
1. Coronary artery disease; mitral valve rheumatic heart disease (may increase PAP)
2. Use with caution in patients with CVA and those on MAO inhibitors

HYDROCHLOROTHIAZIDE (Hydrodiuril)

Preparations: *tab* 25, 50, 100 mg hydrochlorothiazide (Hydrodiuril); *tab* 25 mg hydrochlorothiazide and 75 mg triamterene (Maxzide); *cap* 25 mg hydrochlorothiazide and 50 mg triamterene (Dyazide); *cap* 50 mg hydrochlorothiazide and 5 mg amiloride (Moduretic)
Adult dosage: Hydrodiuril: 25-100 mg PO qd to bid; Maxzide: 1 tab PO qd; Dyazide 1 cap PO qd to bid; Moduretic: 1 tab PO qd-bid
Indications: Edema states, hypertension
Action: Hydrochlorothiazide is a thiazide diuretic; it interferes with resorption of sodium and chloride in the cortical diluting segment of the nephron
Contraindications and precautions
1. Anuria; allergy to sulfonamide-derived drugs or to any of its components
2. Use with caution in patients with renal or hepatic disease
3. Concomitant use of lithium may result in lithium toxicity

HYDROCODONE BITARTRATE (VICODIN)

Preparations: *tab* 5 mg hydrocodone bitartrate plus 500 mg acetaminophen; contains sulfites
Adult dosage: One tab q6h as needed; maximum 2 tablets q6h

Contraindications and precautions
1. Head injury and increased intracranial pressure, acute abdominal conditions
2. Use with caution in patients with impaired renal or hepatic function, hypothyroidism, prostatic hypertrophy, Addison's disease, or urethral stricture and in elderly or debilitated patients

HYDROCORTISONE SODIUM SUCCINATE (Solu-Cortef)

Preparations: *inj* 100, 250, 500, 1000 mg vials
Adult dosage
1. IV/IM: initial dose is 100-500 mg depending on severity of condition
2. Give IV slowly (e.g., 500 mg over 10 min)
3. Dosage may be repeated q2-6h prn
4. If hydrocortisone is continued >72 hr, hyponatremia may occur; sodium retention may be minimized by switching to methylprednisolone

Indications: Same as for dexamethasone; however, hydrocortisone is *not* indicated in cerebral edema
Action: Synthetic adrenocortical steroid
Contraindications and precautions: Same as for dexamethasone

HYDRODIURIL; *see* HYDROCHLOROTHIAZIDE

HYDROMORPHONE HYDROCHLORIDE (Dilaudid)

Preparations: *inj* 1, 2, 4, 10 mg/ml; *tab* 1, 2, 3, 4 mg; *suppository* 3 mg
Adult dosage
1. SQ/IM: 1-2 mg q4-6h prn
2. IV (slowly over 3-5 min): 1-2 mg q4-6h prn
3. PO: 2-4 mg q6h prn
4. PR: 3 mg q6-8h prn

Indications: Relief of moderate to severe pain
Action: Narcotic analgesic; it is a hydrogenated ketone of morphine
Contraindications and precautions
1. Intracranial lesion associated with increased intracranial pressure; depressed ventilatory function
2. Use with caution in patients receiving other CNS depressants, elderly or debilitated patients, acute abdominal conditions, prostatic hypertrophy, Addison's disease, hypothyroidism, urethral stricture, and impaired renal or hepatic function

HYDROXYZINE (Atarax, Vistaril)

Preparations: *tab* 10, 25, 50, 100 mg; *syrup* 10 mg/5 ml; *inj* 25, 50 mg/ml; *cap* 25, 50, 100 mg
Adult dosage
1. PO
   a. Relief of anxiety: 50-100 mg qid
   b. Treatment of pruritus from allergic conditions: 25 mg tid to qid
   c. Sedation before and after general anesthesia: 50-100 mg

2. IM
   a. Anxiety and agitation: 50-100 mg q4-6h prn
   b. Nausea and vomiting: 25-100 mg
   c. Preoperatively and postoperatively: 25-100 mg

Indications: Anxiety, pruritus secondary to allergic conditions, sedation preoperatively and postoperatively, alcohol withdrawal symptoms, antiemetic

Action: H_1 histamine competive antagonist with antiemetic and sedative effects

Contraindications and precautions
1. Hydroxyzine will potentiate the CNS action of alcohol and other CNS depressants
2. Decrease meperidine dose when using concomitantly with hydroxyzine

IBUPROFEN (Motrin and others)

Preparations: *tab* 200, 300, 400, 600, 800 mg
Adult dosage: Mild to moderate pain, use 400 mg q4-6h prn; osteoarthritis and rheumatoid arthritis, 400-800 mg tid to qid; dysmenorrhea, 400 mg q4h prn
Indications: Osteoarthritis, rheumatoid arthritis, mild to moderate pain, dysmenorrhea
Action: Nonsteroidal antiinflammatory agent with antipyretic and analgesic properties
Contraindications and precautions
1. Syndrome of nasal polyps, bronchospastic activity, and angioedema following ingestion of aspirin and other NSAIDs
2. Use with caution in patients with a history of GI bleeding, cardiac decompensation, hypertension, impaired renal function, or bleeding disorders
3. Concomitant administration of coumarin-type anticoagulants may result in potentiation of their effects

IMIPENEM-CILASTIN SODIUM (Primaxin)

Preparations: *inj* 250, 500 mg vial
Adult dosage
1. Mild infections 250-500 mg IV q6h
2. Severe infections 500 mg-1 g IV q6-8h
3. Maximum daily dose should not exceed 4 g or 50 mg/kg (whichever is lower)
4. Decrease dosage in patients with impaired renal function
Indications: Infections caused by susceptible bacterial organisms
Action: Thienamycin antibiotic; it inhibits cell wall synthesis
Contraindications and precautions
1. Hypersensitivity to any of its components
2. Use with caution in patients with a history of allergy to penicillin, cephalosporins, other β lactams, and other allergens

INDERAL; *see* PROPRANOLOL

INDOCIN; *see* INDOMETHACIN

INDOMETHACIN (Indocin)

Preparations: *cap* 25, 50 mg; *SR cap* 75 mg; *supp* 50 mg; *susp* 25 mg/5 ml
Adult dosage
1. Moderate to severe osteoarthritis, rheumatoid arthritis, ankylosing spondylitis: 25 mg PO bid to tid increasing dose at weekly intervals to maximum of 150-200 mg/day; if SR capsule is used, initial dose is 75 mg qd
2. Shoulder bursitis/tendinitis: 25-50 mg PO tid; usual duration of therapy is 7-14 days
3. Acute gouty arthritis: 50 mg PO tid initially, then taper off gradually
4. Administer capsules immediately after meals or with antacids
5. Do not administer suppositories in patients with rectal bleeding or proctitis

Indications: See above
Action: Nonsteroidal antiinflammatory agent with analgesic and antipyretic action
Contraindications and precautions
1. Syndrome of nasal polyps, angioedema, or bronchospastic reaction to aspirin and other nonsteroidal anti-inflammatory agents; active GI bleeding or history of recurrent GI lesions
2. Concomitant use of lithium may result in lithium toxicity
3. Use with caution in patients with renal or hepatic insufficiency, bleeding disorders (inhibition of platelet aggregation), parkinsonism, depression, epilepsy, or psychiatric disturbances (worsening of symptoms)
4. Concomitant use of aspirin or other salicylates should be avoided

INH; *see* ISONIAZID

INTENSOL; *see* PROPRANOLOL

INTROPIN; *see* DOPAMINE

IPRATROPIUM BROMIDE (Atrovent)

Preparations: 18 μg per inhalation; 14 g container (200 inhalations)
Adult dosage: 2 inhalations (36 μg) qid, max 12 inh/day
Indications: bronchospasm associated with chronic bronchitis and emphysema
Action: Anticholinergic agent
Contraindications and precautions: Narrow-angle glaucoma, prostatic hypertrophy, urinary obstruction

ISOETHARINE (Bronkosol)

Preparations: *bottle* (Bronkosol) isoetharine HCL (1.0%) 10, 30 ml; *inhal aerosol* Isoetharine mesylate (0.61%) 10, 15 ml vial with oral nebulizer (Bronkometer)

Adult dosage
1. Hand nebulizer: 3-7 inhalations q4h prn (Bronkosol); 1-2 inhalations q4h prn (Bronkometer)
2. Oxygen aerosolization (Bronkosol): 0.25-0.5 ml diluted 1:3 with saline q4h prn
3. IPPB (Bronkosol): 0.25-1.0 ml diluted 1:3 with saline q4h prn

Indications: Reversible bronchospasm caused by bronchial asthma, emphysema, or bronchitis
Action: Bronchodilator
Contraindications and precautions
1. Hypersensitivity to any of its components
2. Avoid concomitant administration of epinephrine or other sympathomimetic amines
3. Use with caution in patients with coronary insufficiency, hypertension, cardiac asthma, or hyperthyroidism

ISONIAZID (INH)

Preparations: *tab* 300 mg
Adult dosage
1. Treatment of active tuberculosis: 5 mg/kg (up to 300 mg) qd
2. Prophylaxis of tuberculosis: 300 mg qd

Indications: Treatment and prophylaxis of tuberculosis
Action: Inhibits the synthesis of mycolic acid (component of mycobacterial cell wall)
Contraindications and precautions
1. Acute liver disease; history of INH-associated liver damage or hypersensitivity reaction to INH
2. Use with caution in patients with chronic liver disease or severe renal impairment
3. Avoid concomitant use of alcohol (increased risk of isoniazid hepatitis)
4. Concomitant use of phenytoin may result in phenytoin toxicity
5. Ophthalmological exam (before and during therapy) is recommended

ISOPROTERENOL (Isuprel)

Preparations: *inhalation sol* 0.25%, 0.5%, 1%; *inhalation* (metered dose) 0.08, 0.12, 0.131 mg/spray; *inj* (1:5000 solution) 0.2 mg/ml
Adult dosage
1. Inhalation (metered-dose) for bronchospasm: 1-2 inhalations (there should be a 1-5 min interval between inhalations); may repeat up to tid
2. Shock: Place 1 mg of isoproterenol in 500 ml of saline and infuse at 0.5-5 μg/min
3. Cardiac arrest and cardiac dysrhythmias: Dilute 0.2 mg (1 ml of 1:5000 solution) to 10 ml with 0.9% NaCl or D_5W, and inject IV 0.02-0.06 mg (1-3 ml); may repeat prn

Indications: Treatment of bronchospasm caused by bronchial asthma, emphysema, bronchitis, and bronchiectasis; adjunctive treatment of shock; cardiac arrest; cardiac dysrhythmias (ventricular dysrhythmias, Adams-Stokes syndrome, carotid sinus hypersensitivity)

Action: Synthetic sympathomimetic amine

Contraindications and precautions

1. Tachycardia caused by digitalis intoxication
2. Simultaneous administration of epinephrine is contraindicated
3. Correct hypovolemia before treatment with isoproterenol; maintain pulse <130/min
4. Use with caution in patients with hyperthyroidism, coronary insufficiency, elderly patients, patients sensitive to sympathomimetics, and diabetic patients
5. Do not use in patients with preexisting cardiac dysrhythmias associated with tachycardia (except ventricular dysrhythmias requiring inotropic support)

ISOPTIN; *see* VERAPAMIL

ISORDIL; *see* ISOSORBIDE DINITRATE

ISOSORBIDE DINITRATE (Isordil)

Preparations: *SL tab* 2.5, 5, 10 mg; *chew tab* 10 mg; *swallowed tab* 5, 10, 20, 30, 40 mg; *controlled-release tab* and *cap* (Tembids) 40 mg

Adult dosage

1. SL or chew tab
   a. SL: 2.5-10 mg q2-3h
   b. Chew: 5-10 mg q2-3h
2. Swallowed tab: 5-40 mg q6h
3. Controlled-release cap or tab: 40-80 mg q8-12h
   NOTE: Titrate the dosage to clinical response.

Indications: Treatment and prevention of angina pectoris

Action: Organic nitrate; causes venodilation and relaxation of vascular smooth muscle

Contraindications and precautions: Allergic reaction to nitrates or nitrites; hypotension, volume depletion; idiopathic hypertrophic subaortic stenosis (IHSS)

ISUPREL; *see* ISOPROTERENOL

KAYEXALATE; *see* SODIUM POLYSTYRENE SULFONATE

KEFLEX; *see* CEPHALEXIN

KEFLIN; *see* CEPHALOTIN

KEFZOL; *see* CEFAZOLIN

KETOCONAZOLE (Nizoral)

Preparations: *tab* 200 mg
Adult dosage
  1. 200 mg PO qd; if insufficient response may increase dose to 400 mg
     qd
  2. Ketoconazole requires gastric acidity for absorption (if the patient is
     receiving H_2 blockers, antacids, or anticholinergics, they should be
     administered at least 2 hr after ketoconazole)
Indications: Systemic fungal infections
Action: Broad-spectrum antifungal agent
Contraindications and precautions
  1. Do not use for fungal meningitis (poor CNS penetration)
  2. Use with caution in patients with a history of liver disease and in
     anyone receiving warfarin-like drugs (increased prothrombin time),
     cyclosporin A (increased serum level), phenytoin (altered metabo-
     lism), oral hypoglycemic agents (increased risk of hypoglycemia),
     or rifampin (decreased serum level)
  3. Monitor LFTs

KWELL; *see* LINDANE

LABETALOL (Trandate, Normodyne)

Preparations: *tab* 100, 200, 300 mg; *inj* 20 ml ampul (5 mg/ml)
Adult dosage
  1. PO: Initial dosage is 100 mg bid; may increase by 100 mg bid q3d;
     usual maintenance dose is 200-400 mg PO bid
  2. IV: 20 mg (by slow injection over 2 min); may repeat with 40-80
     mg q10min until desired supine blood pressure is achieved or a total
     of 300 mg IV has been given; maximum effect occurs within 5 min
     of IV injection; half-life of labetolol is 5-8 hr
  NOTE: Decrease the dosage in patients with hepatic dysfunction.
Indications: Hypertension
Action: β-Blocker and α-1 vasodilator
Contraindications and precautions
  1. Bronchial asthma, severe bradycardia, second- or third-degree heart
     block, overt cardiac failure, cardiogenic shock
  2. Use caution when administering to patients with pheochromocytoma
     (increased risk of paradoxical hypertensive response), diabetes
     (blunted signs of hypoglycemia), patients receiving cimetidine (in-
     creased bioavailability of labetolol), tricyclic antidepressants (in-
     creased tremor), nitrates (blunting of reflex tachycardia associated
     with hypotension)
  3. Discontinue medication if the patient develops jaundice or labora-
     tory evidence of liver injury

LACTULOSE (Cephulac, Chronulac)

Preparations: *syrup* supplied in containers of 30 ml (20 g lactulose), 473
ml (315 g lactulose), 1.89 L (1260 g lactulose)

Adult dosage
1. 2-3 Tbsp (20-30 g lactulose) tid-qid; adjust dose to produce 2-3 soft stools/day
2. In hepatic encephalopathy may use 30-45 ml of lactulose qh until clinical improvement occurs
3. May be given as a retention enema to patients in hepatic coma (mix 300 ml of lactulose with 700 ml of NS, retain for 30-60 min, may repeat q4-6h)

Indications: Prevention and treatment of hepatic encephalopathy
Action: Decreases blood ammonia concentration by acidification of colon contents (facilitating conversion of ammonia into ammonium ion) and expulsion of the ammonium ion with its laxative action
Contraindications and precautions
1. Patients requiring a low-galactose diet
2. Use with caution in diabetics (contains galactose)
3. Do not use in patients with possible bowel obstruction or ileus

LANOXIN; *see* DIGOXIN

LASIX; *see* FUROSEMIDE

LEVOPHED; *see* NOREPINEPHRINE

LEVOTHYROXINE; *see* THYROXINE

LIBRIUM; *see* CHLORDIAZEPOXIDE

LIDOCAINE

Preparations: *inj* 10, 20, 40, 100 mg/ml
Adult dosage
1. Loading dose: 50-100 mg (0.7-1.4 mg/kg) administered at rate of 25-50 mg/min; if no response, may rebolus after 5 min; do not administer >300 mg over 1 hr
2. IV infusion: Place 1-2 g of lidocaine in 1000 ml of D_5W and infuse at a rate of 2 mg/min (20-50 μg/kg/min)
   a. Constant ECG monitoring is essential
   b. Reduce dosage in patients with severe liver or kidney impairment and in elderly or debilitated patients

Indications: Acute management of ventricular dysrhythmias
Action: Antidysrhythmic agent
Contraindications and precautions
1. Stokes-Adams syndrome, Wolff-Parkinson-White (WPW) syndrome; severe degrees of intraventricular, atrioventricular, or sinoatrial block; hypersensitivity to local anesthetics of the amide type
2. Use with caution in patients with a genetic predisposition to malignant hyperthermia and in elderly patients
3. Liver disease, CHF, and hypotension prolong the half-life of lidocaine and increase the risk of developing lidocaine toxicity

LINDANE (Kwell)

Preparations: *lotion (1%)* 60 ml, 472 ml, 3.8 L bottle; *shampoo (1%)* 60 ml, 472 ml, 3.8 L bottle; *cream (1%)* 60 g tube, 454 g jar
Adult dosage
1. Lotion and cream: Apply to infested area, rub scalp and hair, and leave in place for 8-12 hr, then wash out
2. Shampoo: Apply to infested area and leave in place for 4 min, then rinse thoroughly

Indications: Treatment of patients with *Sarcoptes scabei* (scabies), *Pediculus capitis* (head lice), and *Phthirus pubis* (crab lice)
Action: Scabicide and pediculocide
Contraindications and precautions
1. Hypersensitivity to the product or any of its components
2. Use with caution in children, infants, and pregnant women (can penetrate the skin and cause CNS toxicity)

LITHIUM CARBONATE (Eskalith)

Preparations: *cap* 150, 300, 600 mg; *tab* 300 mg; *controlled-release tab* 300, 450 mg
Adult dosage: Acute mania, 600 mg tid; maintenance, 300 mg tid
NOTE: Closely monitor the serum level (theapeutic is 0.5-1.5 mEq/L).
NOTE: Some patients (particularly elderly ones) can experience signs of lithium toxicity at normally therapeutic levels. It is essential that patients receiving lithium maintain an adequate salt and fluid intake to avoid potential toxicity.

Indications: Treatment of manic episodes of manic-depressive illness
Action: Antimanic drug; precise mechanism of action is unknown
Contraindications and precautions: Use with caution in sodium- or volume-depleted patients, hypothyroid patients, those with renal or cardiovascular disease (increased risk of toxicity), and those taking haloperidol (increased risk of encephalopathic syndrome), neuromuscular blocking agents (prolongation of their effect), indomethacin, or other nonsteroidal antiinflammatory agents (increased serum lithium level)

LOPID; *see* GEMFIBROZIL

LOPRESSOR; *see* METOPROLOL

LORAZEPAM (Ativan)

Preparations: *tab* 0.5, 1, 2 mg; *inj* 2, 4 mg/ml
Adult dosage
1. Anxiety: 1 mg PO bid-tid
2. Premedicant: 0.05 mg/kg IM (maximum of 4 mg) given at least 2 hr before operative procedure
3. Sedation and relief of anxiety: 0.044 mg/kg (maximum of 2 mg) given 15-20 min before anticipated procedure
NOTE: Decrease the dose in elderly and debilitated patients and in patients with renal, hepatic, or pulmonary disease.

Indications: Anxiety, preanesthetic medication, sedation
Action: Benzodiazepine with sedative effects
Contraindications and precautions
1. Hypersensitivity to benzodiazepines or any of its components; acute narrow-angle glaucoma
2. Avoid concomitant use of alcohol or other CNS depressants
3. Use with caution in depressed patients
4. Do not use for primary depressive disorders or psychoses
5. Fetal damage may result when administered to pregnant women

LOVASTATIN (Mevacor)

Preparations: tab 20, 40 mg
Adult dosage: 20 mg/day with food initially; increase q4wk prn; max 80 mg/day in single or divided doses
Indications: Type IIa, IIb hyperlipidemias
Action: Inhibits HMG-CoA reductase
Contraindications and precautions
1. Liver disease
2. Monitor LFTs and lens opacities
3. Avoid concurrent use of gemfibrozil (increased risk of rhabdomyolysis)

MACRODANTIN; *see* NITROFURANTOIN

MANNITOL

Preparations: *inj* 5%, 10%, 15%, 20%, 25% solution
Adult dosage: Cerebral edema, 25 g (100 ml of 20% solution) given over 15-30 min; may repeat q2-3h prn
Indications: Reduction of intracranial or intraocular pressure
Action: Osmotic diuretic; inhibits sodium and chloride reabsorption in the proximal tubule and ascending loop of Henle
Contraindications and precautions: Anuria, renal failure; severe pulmonary congestion; CHF; severe dehydration

MECLIZINE (Antivert)

Preparations: *tab* 12.5, 25, 50 mg; *chew tab* 25 mg
Adult dosage
1. Motion sickness: 25-50 mg taken 1 hr before start of the journey
2. Vertigo: 12.5-50 mg bid
Indications: Motion sickness; vertigo caused by diseases of the vestibular system
Action: Antihistamine
Contraindications and precautions
1. Concomitant use of alcoholic beverages
2. Use with caution in patients with asthma, prostatic hypertrophy, glaucoma

MEDROL; *see* METHYLPREDNISOLONE

MEFOXIN; *see* CEFOXITIN

MELLARIL; *see* THIORIDAZINE

MEPERIDINE (Demerol)

Preparations: *inj* 50 mg/ml; *tab* 50, 100 mg; *syrup* 50 mg/5 ml
Adult dosage
1. Relief of pain; 50-150 mg IM/SQ/PO q3-4h prn
2. PO dose is less effective than parenteral administration
3. IV administration should be very slow, using a diluted solution
4. Concomitant administration of phenothiazines or other tranquilizers (e.g., hydroxyzine) will potentiate the action of meperidine

Indications: Relief of moderate to severe pain
Action: Narcotic analgesic
Contraindications and precautions
1. Current or recent use of MAO inhibitors; head injury, increased intracranial pressure
2. Use with caution in patients receiving other CNS depressants (additive effect), in patients with asthma or other respiratory abnormalities (decreased respiratory drive), in patients with SVT (increased ventricular response rate), acute abdominal conditions (masking of diagnosis), convulsive disorders (increased convulsions), hypothyroidism, impaired renal or hepatic function, prostatic hypertrophy, urethral stricture, or Addison's disease, and in elderly or debilitated patients

METAPROTERENOL (Alupent)

Preparations: *inhal* 0.65 mg/metered dose (300 doses/inhaler); *tab* 10, 20 mg; *syrup* 10 mg/5 ml; *vial* 2.5 ml (inhalant solution 0.6% unit dose vials)
Adult dosage
1. Inhaled (via nebulizer): 0.2-0.3 ml in 2-5 ml of normal saline q4-6h prn for bronchospasm
2. PO: 20 mg tid to qid
3. Metered-dose inhaler: 2-3 inhalations; do not repeat more often than q4h

Indications: Bronchial asthma, emphysema, bronchitis
Action: β-2 adrenergic agonist
Contraindications and precautions
1. Cardiac dysrhythmias associated with tachycardia
2. Use with caution in patients with coronary artery disease, CHF, hypertension, hyperthyroidism, history of hypersensitivity to sympathomimetic amines, diabetes

METHYLDOPA (Aldomet)

Preparations: *tab* 125, 250, 500 mg; *susp* 250 mg/5 ml; *inj* 250 mg/5 ml
Adult dosage
1. PO: 250 mg bid to tid initially; may increase dose after 2-3 days if inadequate response; maximum daily dose is 2 g; usual dosage is 250-500 mg bid to qid

2. IV: 250-500 mg q6h

NOTE: Use smaller doses in patients with renal impairment.

Indications: Hypertension

Action: Antihypertensive; it is believed that its metabolites cause a reflex depression of sympathetic control of arterial blood pressure

Contraindications and precautions

1. Active hepatic disease (acute hepatitis, active cirrhosis); development of Coombs' positive hemolytic anemia while taking methyldopa
2. Use with caution in patients with a history of liver disease
3. Not recommended for treatment of patients with pheochromocytoma
4. Do not use Aldomet oral suspension in patients allergic to sulfites (contains sodium bisulfite)
5. Sudden withdrawal may result in significant rebound hypertension

METHYLPREDNISOLONE (Medrol, Solu-Medrol)

Preparations: *tab* 2, 4, 8, 16, 24, 32 mg; *inj* 40, 125, 500, 1000 mg vial

Adult dosage

1. PO: 4-48 mg/day depending on disease and clinical response
2. IV: 30 mg/kg infused over 10-20 min for septic shock; dosage for severe bronchospasm is 0.5-1 mg/kg initially, followed by tapering doses q4-6h

Indications: Same as for dexamethasone; however, methylprednisolone is not indicated in cerebral edema

Action: Synthetic adrenocortical steroid

Contraindications and precautions: See dexamethasone

METOCLOPRAMIDE (Reglan)

Preparations: *tab* 5, 10 mg; *syrup* 5 mg/5 ml; *inj* 5 mg/ml

Adult dosage

1. GI reflux: 10-15 mg PO 30 min before each meal and at hs; maximum duration of therapy is 12 wk
2. Diabetic gastroparesis: 10 mg PO 30 min before each meal and at qs.
3. Prophylaxis of nausea and vomiting in cancer chemotherapy: IV infusion 1-2 mg/kg diluted in 0.9% saline and given slowly (over 15 min) 30 min before beginning cancer chemotherapy and repeated q2h × 2 doses, then q3h × 3 doses
4. Facilitation of small bowel intubation: 10 mg IV (undiluted) given over 2 min

Indications: See above

Action: Antiemetic; stimulates motility of upper GI tract

Contraindications and precautions

1. GI obstruction, perforation, hemorrhage, or any other GI condition where increased GI motility is contraindicated; pheochromocytoma, epilepsy
2. Avoid concomitant use of other drugs likely to cause extrapyramidal reactions

METOLAZONE (Diulo, Mykrox, Zaroxolyn)

Preparations: *tab* 2.5, 5, 10 mg; tab 0.5 mg (Mykrox) not interchangeable with other metolazone preparations

Adult dosage

1. Hypertension: 2.5-5 mg qd
2. Edema from renal disease: 5-20 mg qd
3. CHF 5-10 mg qd
4. If Mykrox is used, dosage is 0.5 mg/day

Indications: Hypertension; edema

Action: Diuretic; inhibits sodium reabsorption at the cortical diluting site and in the proximal convoluted tubule

Contraindications and precautions

1. Anuria; hepatic coma or precoma
2. Use caution when administering metolazone to hyperuricemic patients, patients with severely impaired renal function, diabetics

METOPROLOL (Lopressor)

Preparations: *tab* 50, 100 mg; *inj* 5 mg/5 ml ampul or prefilled syringe

Adult dosage

1. Hypertension: 100 mg PO qd in single or divided doses; may increase dosage q1-2 wk until satisfactory response is achieved; usual range is 100-400 mg/day
2. Angina: 100 mg PO qd in two divided doses initially, increased prn at weekly intervals; effective dosage range is 100-400 mg/day
3. Acute MI: 5 mg IV boluses at 2 min intervals 3 times (total 15 mg IV), then 25-50 mg PO q6h × 48 hr, then 100 mg PO bid; start PO dosage 15 min after IV dose

   NOTE: Patients with contraindications to IV treatment in the early phase of an acute MI may be started on 100 mg PO bid as soon as their condition permits.

Indications: Hypertension; MI; angina pectoris

Action: β-adrenergic receptor blocking agent

Contraindications and precautions

1. Heart block greater than first degree; sinus bradycardia; cardiogenic shock; CHF
2. Use with caution in patients with bronchospastic disease (may exacerbate bronchospasm), diabetes (may mask tachycardia from hypoglycemia), impaired hepatic function
3. Avoid abrupt cessation of β blocker therapy

METRONIDAZOLE (Flagyl)

Preparations: *tab* 250, 500 mg; *inj* 500 mg

Adult dosage

1. Anaerobic infections: IV loading dose of 15 mg/kg followed by maintenance dose of 7.5 mg/kg q6h; maximum daily dose is 4 g; IV administration should be by infusion over 1 hr
2. Trichomoniasis: 1-2 g PO as a single dose or 500 mg PO bid × 5 days

3. Giardiasis: 2 g PO qd as a single dose × 3 days or 250 mg bid to tid × 7-10 days
4. Pseudomembranous colitis: 250 mg PO bid × 10-14 days
5. Decrease dosage in patients with severe liver disease

Indications: Anaerobic infections; trichomoniasis; giardiasis
Action: Disrupts DNA and inhibits nucleic acid synthesis
Contraindications and precautions: History of hypersensitivity to metronidazole or other nitroimidazole derivatives; avoid alcoholic beverages

MEVACOR; *see* LOVASTATIN

MEZLOCILLIN (Mezlin)

Preparations: *inj* 1, 2, 3, 4 g
Adult dosage: Sepsis, 3 g IV q4h or 4g q6h; decrease the dosage in renal failure
Indications: Infections caused by susceptible bacterial organisms
Action: Semisynthetic broad-spectrum penicillin; it is bactericidal by interfering with synthesis of the cell wall
Contraindications and precautions: Patients allergic to penicillin; it may cause hypokalemia

MICONAZOLE (Monistat)

Preparations: *cream (2%)* (Monistat-7) 45 g tube; *supp* 100 mg (Monistat-7), 200 mg (Monistat-3)
Adult dosage
1. Vaginal cream (Monistat-7): one applicatorful intravaginally qhs × 7 days
2. Vaginal supp (Monistat-7): one suppository intravaginally qhs × 7 days
3. Vaginal supp (Monistat-3): one suppository intravaginally qhs × 3 days

Indications: Local treatment of vulvovaginal candidiasis
Action: Fungicidal
Contraindications: Hypersensitivity to miconazole

MICRONASE; *see* GLYBURIDE

MINIPRESS; *see* PRAZOSIN

MISOPROSTOL (Cytotec)

Preparations: *tab* 100, 200 μg
Adult dosage: 100 μg qid with meals initially
Indications: Prevention of NSAID-induced gastric ulcers
Action: PGE_1 analog; it increases mucus and bicarbonate secretion and decreases acid secretion
Contraindications and precautions: Do not use in women of childbearing potential (abortifacient); avoid magnesium-containing antacids

MONISTAT; *see* MICONAZOLE

MORPHINE SULFATE

Preparations: *inj* 8, 10, 15 mg/ml; *tab* 10, 15, 30 mg; *sol* 10, 20 mg/5 ml; *SR tab* (MS Contin) 30, 60 mg; *conc* 100 mg/5 ml

Adult dosage
1. PO: 8-20 mg q4h, 30, 60 mg (MS Contin) q12h
2. SQ/IM: 5-15 mg q4h
3. IV: 4-10 mg, diluted and injected over 5 min

NOTE: Decrease the dosage in patients with impaired renal or hepatic function, elderly or debilitated individuals, and patients with urethral stricture, prostatic hypertrophy, hypothyroidism, or Addison's disease.

Indications: Relief of severe pain

Action: Narcotic analgesic

Contraindications and precautions
1. Respiratory depression or insufficiency, severe bronchial asthma, increased cerebrospinal or intracranial pressure, acute alcoholism, convulsive disorders, delirium tremens, brain tumor, cardiac failure caused by chronic pulmonary disease, suspected surgical abdomen, cardiac dysrhythmias, after biliary tract surgery and postsurgical anastomosis, use during or within 14 days of MAO inhibitor therapy
2. Avoid concurrent use with other CNS depressants

MOTRIN; *see* IBUPROFEN

MYCELEX; *see* CLOTRIMAZOLE

MYCOSTATIN; *see* NYSTATIN

MYKROX; *see* METOLAZONE

NAFCILLIN (Unipen)

Preparations: *cap* 250 mg; *tab* 500 mg; *inj* 500 mg, 1, 2, 10 g; *oral sol* 250 mg/5 ml

Adult dosage
1. IV: 500 mg-2 g q4h for severe infections
2. IM: 500 mg q4-6h for severe infections
3. PO: 250-500 mg q4-6h for mild-to-moderate infections, 1 g q4-6h for severe infections

Indications: Infections from penicillinase-producing staphylococci

Action: Semisynthetic antistaphylococcal penicillin

Contraindications and precautions: Allergy to any of the penicillins

NALOXONE (Narcan)

Preparations: *inj* 0.02, 0.4, 1 mg/ml

Adult dosage: Narcotic overdose, 0.4-2 mg IV; may repeat q2min prn; if no response after 10 mg, consider other diagnosis

Indications: Reversal of narcotic depression

Action: Narcotic antagonist

Contraindications and precautions: Hypersensitivity to naloxone

NAPROSYN; *see* NAPROXEN

NAPROXEN (Naprosyn, Anaprox)

Preparations: *tab* (Naprosyn base) 250, 375, 500 mg; (Anaprox-sodium) 275, 550 mg
Adult dosage
  1. Primary dysmenorrhea, acute tendinitis and bursitis, mild to moderate pain: Naprosyn 500 mg PO initially, then 250 mg PO q6-8h; or Anaprox 550 mg PO initially, followed by 275 mg PO bid
  2. Rheumatoid arthritis, osteoarthritis, ankylosing spondylitis: Naprosyn 250-375 mg PO bid, Anaprox 275 mg PO bid, or Anaprox 275 mg PO in AM 550 mg PO in evening
  3. Acute gout: Naprosyn 750 mg PO initially, then 250 mg PO q8h until attack has subsided; or Anaprox 825 mg initially, then 275 mg q8h until attack has subsided
Indications: See above
Action: Nonsteroidal antiinflammatory drug (NSAID)
Contraindications and precautions
  1. Allergic reactions to NSAIDs or aspirin
  2. Use with caution in patients with history of GI disease, impaired renal function, liver disease, heart failure, elderly patients, and patients receiving diuretics

NARCAN; *see* NALOXONE

NEBUPENT; *see* PENTAMIDINE ISOTHIONATE

NIFEDIPINE (Adalat, Procardia)

Preparations: *cap* 10, 20 mg; *extended release tab* (Procardia XL) 30, 60, 90 mg GITS
Adult dosage: Initially 10 mg PO tid; usual dosage range is 30-60 mg/day; (Procardia XL) initial dose is 30 mg tablet, swallowed whole qd
Indications: Vasospastic angina; chronic stable angina, hypertension
Action: Calcium channel blocker (inhibitor of calcium ion influx)
Contraindications and precautions: Hypotension, peripheral edema

NIPRIDE; *see* NITROPRUSSIDE

NITROFURANTOIN (Macrodantin, Furadantin)

Preparations: *cap* 25, 50, 100 mg; *susp* (Furadantin) 25 mg/5 ml
Adult dosage: 50-100 mg PO qid; therapy should be continued for at least 1 week and for at least 3 days after urine sterility has been documented
Indications: Urinary tract infections from susceptible bacterial organisms
Action: Interference with bacterial enzyme systems through covalent bonding to DNA
Contraindications and precautions: Impaired renal function, anuria, oliguria, hypersensitivity to nitrofurantoin preparations

NITROGLYCERIN

Preparations: *SL tab* 150 μg (1/400 gr), 300 μg (1/200 gr), 400 μg (1/150 gr), 600 μg (1/100 gr); *cap* 2.5, 6.5, 9 mg; *tab* 1.3, 2.6, 6.5 mg; *top ointment (2%)* 60 g tube; *transdermal infus* 0.1 mg/hr (2.5 mg/24 hr), 0.2 mg/hr (5 mg/24 hr), 0.4 mg/hr (10 mg/24 hr), 0.6 mg/hr (15 mg/24 hr); *transmucosal tab* 1, 2, 3 mg; *translingual spray* 400 mg/dose, 13.8 g

Adult dosage

1. IV inf: start at 5-10 μg/min and titrate based on the blood pressure and clinical response (if polyvinyl chloride tubing is used, a higher starting dose may be needed because a large amount of nitroglycerin will be absorbed by the tubing); Tables 32-5 and 32-6 show preparation and infusion of IV NTG; maximum dosage is 200 μg/min
2. SL: 0.3-0.6 mg prn for chest pain
3. Topical ointment: 2.5-12.5 cm q4-6h
4. Transdermal infusion: 2.5-15 mg or 5-30 cm^2 q24h (remove at hs)
5. cap: 2.5-9 mg q8-12h
6. tab: 1.3-6.5 mg q8-12h
7. Transmucosal tab: 1-2 mg tid
8. Translingual (nitrolingual) spray: Onset of an attack, 1-2 metered doses onto the oral mucosa; no more than 3 doses in 15 min

Indications: Angina pectoris; CHF associated with acute myocardial infarction (IV NTG); production of controlled hypotension during surgical procedures and control of blood pressure in perioperative hypertension (IV NTG)

Action: Venodilation and relaxation of vascular smooth muscle

Contraindications and precautions: Hypotension, idiopathic hypertrophic subacute aortic stenosis (IHSS); increased intracranial pressure; inadequate cerebral circulation; pericardial tamponade, constrictive pericarditis; uncorrected hypovolemia; known idiosyncratic reaction to organic nitrates

Table 32-5 Preparation of nitroglycerin infusion

Solution Concentration*	Preparation†
100 μg NTG/ml (common initial solution)	25 mg NTG (5 ml Tridil) in 250 ml D$_5$W or normal saline
200 μg NTG/ml	50 mg NTG (10 ml Tridil) in 250 ml D$_5$W or normal saline
400 μg NTG/ml (maximum recommended solution concentration)	100 mg NTG (20 ml Tridil) in 250 ml D$_5$W or normal saline

From Purcell JA, Holder KC: Am J Nurs 82:254, 1982.

*These recommendations apply only to Tridil; if using other products, consult package insert for correct solution concentrations.

†Only glass or polyolefin bottles are used.

Table 32-6 Conversion table for nitroglycerin solution 100 µg/ml (dosage of NTG in µg/kg/min)

Flow Rate (µgtt/min*)	Quantity of NTG (µg/min)	Body Weight															
		(lb) 77 (kg) 35	88 40	99 45	110 50	121 55	132 60	143 65	154 70	165 75	176 80	187 85	198 90	209 95	220 100	231 105	242 110
3	5	0.14	0.13	0.11	0.10	0.09	0.08	0.08	0.07	0.07	0.06	0.06	0.06	0.05	0.05	0.05	0.05
5	8.35	0.24	0.21	0.19	0.17	0.15	0.14	0.13	0.12	0.11	0.10	0.10	0.09	0.09	0.08	0.08	0.08
10	16.7	0.48	0.42	0.37	0.33	0.30	0.28	0.26	0.24	0.22	0.21	0.20	0.19	0.18	0.17	0.16	0.15
15	25.0	0.71	0.63	0.56	0.50	0.45	0.42	0.38	0.36	0.33	0.31	0.29	0.28	0.26	0.25	0.24	0.23
20	33.3	0.95	0.83	0.74	0.67	0.61	0.56	0.51	0.48	0.44	0.42	0.39	0.37	0.35	0.33	0.32	0.30
25	41.7	1.2	1.0	0.93	0.83	0.76	0.70	0.64	0.60	0.56	0.52	0.49	0.46	0.44	0.42	0.40	0.38
30	50.0	1.4	1.3	1.1	1.0	0.91	0.83	0.77	0.71	0.67	0.63	0.59	0.56	0.53	0.50	0.48	0.45
35	58.4	1.7	1.5	1.3	1.2	1.1	0.97	0.90	0.83	0.78	0.73	0.69	0.65	0.61	0.58	0.56	0.53
40	66.7	1.9	1.7	1.5	1.3	1.2	1.1	1.0	0.95	0.89	0.83	0.78	0.74	0.70	0.67	0.64	0.61
45	75.0	2.1	1.9	1.7	1.5	1.4	1.3	1.2	1.1	1.0	0.94	0.88	0.83	0.79	0.75	0.71	0.68
50	83.3	2.4	2.1	1.9	1.7	1.5	1.4	1.3	1.2	1.1	1.0	0.98	0.93	0.88	0.83	0.79	0.76
55	91.7	2.6	2.3	2.0	1.8	1.7	1.5	1.4	1.3	1.2	1.2	1.1	1.0	0.97	0.92	0.87	0.83
60	100	2.9	2.5	2.2	2.0	1.8	1.7	1.5	1.4	1.3	1.3	1.2	1.1	1.1	1.0	0.95	0.91
65	108	3.1	2.7	2.4	2.2	2.0	1.8	1.7	1.6	1.4	1.3	1.3	1.2	1.1	1.1	1.0	0.98
70	117	3.3	2.9	2.6	2.3	2.1	1.9	1.8	1.7	1.6	1.5	1.4	1.3	1.2	1.2	1.1	1.1
75	125	3.6	3.1	2.8	2.5	2.3	2.1	1.9	1.8	1.7	1.6	1.5	1.4	1.3	1.3	1.2	1.14
80	133	3.8	3.3	3.0	2.7	2.4	2.2	2.1	1.9	1.8	1.7	1.6	1.5	1.4	1.33	1.3	1.2
85	142	4.1	3.5	3.2	2.8	2.6	2.4	2.2	2.0	1.9	1.8	1.7	1.6	1.5	1.4	1.4	1.3
90	150	4.3	3.8	3.3	3.0	2.7	2.5	2.3	2.1	2.0	1.9	1.8	1.7	1.6	1.5	1.43	1.4
95	158	4.5	4.0	3.5	3.2	2.9	2.6	2.4	2.3	2.1	2.0	1.9	1.8	1.7	1.6	1.5	1.44

From Purcell JA, Holder KC: Am J Nurs 82:254, 1982.
*Based on 60 µgtt/ml; each drop contains 1.67 µg NTG.

NITROPRUSSIDE (Nipride)

Preparations: *vials* 5 ml containing 50 mg sodium nitroprusside to be re-constituted and further diluted with a D_5W injection (see Table 32-7)
NOTE: The nitroprusside bottle and line should be shielded from light and the bottle changed every 12 hr.

Adult dosage
1. In patients not receiving antihypertensive drugs the dosage range is 0.5-8 μg/kg/min
2. Average dose of 3 μg/kg/min will usually lower diastolic pressure by 30-40%
3. Smaller doses are required in hypertensive patients receiving con-comitant antihypertensive medications and when used for therapy of CHF
4. Furosemide 40 mg IV may be given for significant fluid retention

Indications
1. Immediate reduction of blood pressure in hypertensive crises
2. Vasodilator therapy in refractory CHF

Action: Potent, immediately active hypotensive agent; its hypotensive ef-fects occur as a result of peripheral vasodilatation

Contraindications and precautions
1. Do not use in compensatory hypertension
2. Do not use to produce controlled hypotension during surgery in pa-tients with known inadequate cerebral circulation
3. Frequent monitoring of serum thiocyanate levels is indicated in pa-tients with renal impairment, in any patient receiving large doses of nitroprusside, or during prolonged use; metabolic acidosis is the ear-liest and most reliable evidence of cyanide toxicity; thiocyanate lev-els should be kept less than 10 mg/dl
4. Use with caution in patients with hepatic insufficiency, hypothy-roidism, or severe renal impairment

NIZORAL; *see* KETOCONAZOLE

NOREPINEPHRINE (Levophed)

Preparations: *amp* 4 mg/4 ml
Adult dosage: Dilute 8 mg in 500 ml of D_5W (16 μg/ml); start at an initial IV infusion rate of 16 μg/min and titrate to the desired effect
Indications: Hemodynamically severe hypotension not due to hypovolemia or cardiogenic shock
Action: Peripheral vasoconstrictor (α-adrenergic action), inotropic stimula-tor of the heart, dilator of coronary arteries (β-adrenergic action)

Contraindications and precautions
1. Use with extreme caution in patients receiving MAO inhibitors or antidepressents of the triptylene or imipramine type (↑ risk of se-vere hypertension)
2. Contains metabisulfite
3. Extravasation may result in soft tissue necrosis; phentolamine (Re-gitine) 5-10 mg with 10-15 ml of NS infiltrated as soon as possible into the area of extravasation may prevent sloughing and necrosis

Table 32-7 Nitroprusside infusion (dosage = μg Nipride/kg/min)

Flow Rate (μgtt/min)	Quantity of Nipride* (μg/min)†	Body Weight															
		(lb) 77 (kg) 35	88 40	99 45	110 50	121 55	132 60	143 65	154 70	165 75	176 80	187 85	198 90	209 95	220 100	231 105	242 110
5	16.7	0.48	0.42	0.37	0.33	0.30	0.28	0.26	0.24	0.22	0.21	0.20	0.19	0.18	0.17	0.16	0.15
10	33.3	0.95	0.83	0.74	0.67	0.61	0.56	0.51	0.48	0.44	0.42	0.39	0.37	0.35	0.33	0.32	0.30
15	50	1.4	1.25	1.1	1.0	0.91	0.83	0.77	0.71	0.67	0.63	0.59	0.56	0.53	0.50	0.48	0.45
20	67	1.9	1.7	1.5	1.3	1.2	1.1	1.0	0.95	0.89	0.84	0.79	0.74	0.70	0.67	0.64	0.61
25	83	2.4	2.1	1.8	1.7	1.5	1.4	1.3	1.2	1.1	1.0	0.98	0.93	0.88	0.83	0.79	0.76
30	100	2.9	2.5	2.2	2.0	1.8	1.7	1.5	1.4	1.3	1.3	1.2	1.1	1.1	1.0	0.95	0.91
35	117	3.3	2.9	2.6	2.3	2.1	2.0	1.8	1.7	1.6	1.5	1.4	1.3	1.2	1.2	1.1	1.1
40	133	3.8	3.3	3.0	2.7	2.4	2.2	2.0	1.9	1.8	1.7	1.6	1.5	1.4	1.3	1.3	1.2
45	150	4.3	3.8	3.3	3.0	2.7	2.5	2.3	2.1	2.0	1.9	1.8	1.7	1.6	1.5	1.4	1.4
50	167	4.8	4.2	3.7	3.3	3.0	2.8	2.6	2.4	2.2	2.1	2.0	1.9	1.8	1.7	1.6	1.5
55	183	5.2	4.6	4.1	3.7	3.3	3.1	2.8	2.6	2.4	2.3	2.2	2.0	1.9	1.8	1.7	1.7
60	200	5.7	5.0	4.4	4.0	3.6	3.3	3.1	2.9	2.7	2.5	2.4	2.2	2.1	2.0	1.9	1.8
65	217	6.2	5.4	4.8	4.3	3.9	3.6	3.3	3.1	2.9	2.7	2.6	2.4	2.3	2.2	2.1	2.0
70	233	6.7	5.8	5.2	4.7	4.2	3.9	3.6	3.3	3.1	2.9	2.7	2.6	2.5	2.3	2.2	2.1
75	250	7.1	6.3	5.6	5.0	4.5	4.2	3.8	3.6	3.3	3.1	2.9	2.8	2.6	2.5	2.4	2.3
80	267	7.6	6.7	5.9	5.3	4.8	4.5	4.1	3.8	3.6	3.3	3.1	3.0	2.8	2.7	2.5	2.4
85	283	8.1	7.1	6.3	5.7	5.1	4.7	4.3	4.0	3.8	3.5	3.3	3.1	3.0	2.8	2.7	2.6
90	300	8.6	7.5	6.7	6.0	5.5	5.0	4.6	4.3	4.0	3.8	3.5	3.3	3.2	3.0	2.9	2.7
95	317	9.1	7.9	7.0	6.3	5.8	5.3	4.9	4.5	4.2	4.0	3.7	3.5	3.3	3.2	3.0	2.9
100	333	9.5	8.3	7.4	6.7	6.1	5.6	5.1	4.8	4.4	4.2	3.9	3.7	3.5	3.3	3.2	3.0

From Purcell JA: Am J Nurs 82:965, 1982.

*Nitroprusside (Nipride) solution 200 μg/ml (100 mg Nipride/500 ml or 50 mg Nipride/250 ml).

†Based on 60 μgtt/ml; each drop contains 3.33 μg Nipride.

4. Norepinephrine will result in increased myocardial oxygen requirements and renal and mesenteric vasoconstriction

NORFLOXACIN (Noroxin)

Preparations: *tab* 400 mg
Adult dosage
1. UTI, uncomplicated: 400 mg PO bid × 7-10 days
2. UTI, complicated: 400 mg PO bid × 10-21 days
NOTE: Administer 1 hr before or 2 hr after a meal
Indications: UTIs caused by susceptible organisms
Action: Fluoroquinolone broad-spectrum bactericidal agent; inhibits DNA synthesis
Contraindications and precautions
1. Contraindicated in pregnancy, in children, and in patients with hypersensitivity to quinolone antibiotics
2. Decrease the dosage in patients with impaired renal function

NORMODYNE; *see* LABETALOL

NOROXIN; *see* NORFLOXACIN

NORPACE; *see* DISOPYRAMIDE

NYSTATIN (Mycostatin)

Preparations: *tab* 500,000 U; *susp* 100,000 U/ml; *cream/ointment* 100,000 U/g; *powd* 100,000 U/g; *vag tab* 100,000 U; *troche* 200,000 U
Adult dosage
1. Cutaneous or mucocutaneous candidiasis: Apply cream, powder or ointment to affected area bid to tid
2. Oral candidiasis: Place 4-6 ml in the mouth and retain as long as possible before swallowing
3. Intestinal candidiasis: 1-2 tabs PO tid
4. Vulvovaginal candidiasis: Insert 1 tab intravaginally (with applicator) qhs × 2 wk
Indications: Cutaneous or mucocutaneous candidiasis, candidiasis of the oral cavity, intestinal candidiasis, vulvovaginal candidiasis
Action: Antifungal antibiotic
Contraindications and precautions
1. Hypersensitivity to any of its components
2. Discontinue topical or vaginal preparations if the patient develops signs of local irritation

OMEPRAZOLE (Prilosec)

Preparations: cap 20 mg
Adult dosage: Erosive esophagitis, 20 mg PO qd before eating for 4-8 wk, with an additional 4 wk in severe cases; Zollinger-Ellison (Z-E) syndrome, 60 mg qd; adjust dose to clinical response
Indications: Severe erosive esophagitis, Z-E syndrome, symptomatic GI reflux refractory to conventional therapy
Action: Suppression of gastric acid secretion by specific inhibition of the H^+/K^+ ATPase system at the secretory surface of the gastric parietal cell
Contraindications and precautions: Do not use as maintenance therapy (except in patients with Z-E); omeprazole can prolong the elimination of diazepam, warfarin, phenytoin, and drugs that are oxidized in the liver

OS-CAL; *see* CALCIUM CARBONATE

OXAZEPAM (Serax)

Preparations: *cap* 10, 15, 30 mg; *tab* 15 mg
Adult dosage
1. Mild to moderate anxiety: 10-15 mg PO tid to qid
2. Severe anxiety, alcohol withdrawal: 15-30 mg PO tid to qid
3. Decrease dosage in elderly patients
Indications: Anxiety disorders, alcohol withdrawal
Action: Benzodiazepine
Contraindications and precautions
1. Psychoses
2. Avoid concomitant use of alcohol or other CNS depressant drugs

OXYCODONE (Percocet)

Preparations: *tab* oxycodone HCl 5 mg, acetaminophen 325 mg
Adult dosage: Usually 1 tab q6h prn
Indications: Relief of moderate to severe pain
Action: Narcotic analgesic
Contraindications and precautions
1. Hypersensitivity to oxycodone or acetaminophen; head injury and increased intracranial pressure; acute abdominal conditions
2. Use with caution in patients with impaired renal or hepatic function, hypothyroidism, prostatic hypertrophy, Addison's disease, or urethral stricture, and in elderly or debilitated patients
3. Avoid concomitant use of CNS depressants, anticholinergics with narcotics (increased risk of paralytic ileus), MAO inhibitors, or tricyclic antidepressants

PARLODEL; *see* BROMOCRIPTINE

PENICILLIN PREPARATIONS

Penicillin	Dosage forms	Route of administration
PENICILLIN G BENZATHINE (Bicillin L-A, Permapen)	300,000, 600,000, 1,200,000, 2,400,000 U/dose (syringe); 300,000 U/ml (10 ml vial)	IM
PENICILLIN G PROCAINE (Bicillin CR, Wycillin	300,000 U/ml (10 ml vial); 600,000, 1,200,000, 2,400,000 U/dose	IM
PENICILLIN G SODIUM	5,000,000 U/vial	IV
PENICILLIN G POTASSIUM	200,000, 250,000, 400,000 U/5 ml (reconstituted susp/syrup) 100,000, 200,000, 250,000, 400,000, 500,000, 800,000 U (tab 250 mg = 400,000 U) 200,000, 500,000, 1,000,000, 5,000,000, 10,000,000, 20,000,000 U 125, 250, 500 mg	PO PO IM/IV (>5,000,000 U use IV only)
PENICILLIN V POTASSIUM	200,000, 400,000, 800,000 U (tab 125 mg = 200,000 U) 200,000 U (125 mg/5ml) 400,000 U (250 mg/5ml) (sol/susp)	PO PO

PENTAMIDINE ISOTHIONATE (Pentam 300, Nebupent)

Preparations: *inj* 300 mg vial; *inh* 300 mg vial
Adult dosage
1. Pentam: IV/IM 4 mg/kg $\times$ 14 days for treatment of PCP
2. Nebupent: inh 300 mg vial dissolved in 6 ml of sterile water for injection, USP; given via the Respirgard II nebulizer once every 4 wk; the dose should be delivered over 30-45 min at a flow rate of 5-7 L/min from a 40-50 psi air or oxygen source

Indications
1. Pentam: treatment of PCP
2. Nebupent: prevention of PCP in high-risk HIV-infected patients defined by one of the following criteria:
   a. A history of one or more episodes of PCP
   b. A peripheral CD4+ (T4 helper/inducer) lymphocyte count less than or equal to 200/mm^3

Action: Antiprotozoal agent; inhibits synthesis of DNA, RNA, phospholipids, and proteins

Contraindications and precautions
1. IV dose should be infused slowly (over 60 min) while the patient is lying down and the blood pressure is closely monitored (patients may develop severe hypotension)
2. Monitor metabolic parameters (BUN, creatinine, glucose, CBC, platelet count, LFT, calcium) frequently while the patient is receiving pentamidine therapy
3. Acute PCP should be ruled out prior to initiating prophylaxis with Nebupent since its use may alter the clinical and radiographic features of PCP and could result in an atypical presentation

PERCOCET; *see* OXYCODONE

PERSANTINE; *see* DIPYRIDAMOLE

PHENOBARBITAL

Preparations: *tab* 8, 16, 32, 65, 100 mg; *inj* 30, 60, 130 mg/ml; *elixir* 4 mg/ml
Adult dosage
1. Control of epileptic seizures: Initial dose is 1-5 mg/kg/day; usual dose is 100-200 mg qhs
2. Status epilepticus: 4-6 mg/kg IM
NOTE: Decrease the dosage in chronic liver disease or renal impairment.
Indications: Epilepsy, sedation
Action: Barbiturate anticonvulsant
Contraindications and precautions
1. Respiratory disease with presence of dyspnea or obstruction
2. Use with caution in patients with cardiovascular, pulmonary, hepatic, or renal disease

PHENYTOIN (Dilantin)

Preparations: *cap* 30, 100 mg; *susp* 125 mg/5 ml; *inj* 50 mg/ml; *chew tab* 50 mg; *pediatr susp* 30 mg/5 ml

Adult dosage

1. Usual PO dose is 4-6 mg/kg/day
   a. This can be given in divided doses (100 mg PO tid) or as one daily dose (300 mg PO qd of *extended* phenytoin sodium capsules [Dilantin Kapseals]) when patient compliance is a problem
   b. If an oral loading dose is necessary, patient should be given a total of 1 g divided into 3 doses (400, 300, 300 mg) and administered at 2 hr intervals; maintenance dose is then instituted 24 hr after the loading dose; periodical serum levels should be obtained (therapeutic range is 10-20 μg/ml)
2. Status epilepticus: Loading dose of 10-15 mg/kg by slow IV injection (≤50 mg/min) followed by 100 mg PO/IV q6-8h

Indications: Seizure disorders; digitalis-induced ventricular dysrhythmias

Action: Hydantoin anticonvulsant

Contraindications and precautions

1. Sinus bradycardia, AV block greater than first-degree, sinoatrial block, Stokes-Adams syndrome
2. Do not use for seizures secondary to hypoglycemia or other metabolic causes
3. Discontinue phenytoin if patient develops skin rash
4. Use with caution in elderly patients and in patients with impaired liver function
5. Continuous monitoring of ECG and BP is necessary when administering IV phenytoin loading dose
6. Phenytoin serum levels are affected by many common drugs (e.g., increased levels may be seen with concomitant use of cimetidine, dicumarol, salicylates, sulfonamides, tolbutamide, diazepam); cisplatin therapy may decrease serum phenytoin level

PIPERACILLIN (Pipracil)

Preparations: *inj* 2, 3, 4 g vials or bottles

Adult dosage

1. Serious infections: 200-300 mg/kg/day IV in 4-6 divided doses
2. Complicated UTI: 125-200 mg/kg/day IV in 3-4 divided doses
3. Uncomplicated UTI and community-acquired pneumonia: 100-125 mg/kg IV in 2-4 divided doses

NOTE: Decrease the dosage in patients with renal impairment.

Indications: Infections caused by susceptible bacterial organisms

Action: Piperazine penicillin derivative with increased activity against many gram-negative bacteria and *S. faecalis*

Contraindications and precautions: History of allergic reaction to penicillin or cephalosporins

PIPRACIL; *see* PIPERACILLIN

POLYETHYLENE GLYCOL (PEG) 3350 ELECTROLYTE SOLUTION (Go Litely)

Preparations: *disposable jug* PEG 236 g, sodium sulfate 22.74 g, sodium bicarbonate 6.74 g, sodium chloride 5.86 g, potassium chloride 2.97 g; water is added until a 4 L volume is reached

Adult dosage: PO 8 oz (240 ml) q10min until 4 L are consumed (may be given via nasogastric tube); bowel exam is usually scheduled 4 hr after initiation of PO ingestion (3 hr for drinking and 1 hr for complete bowel evacuation)

Indications: Bowel cleansing before colonoscopy and barium enema x-ray exam

Action: Osmotic agent

Contraindications and precautions: GI obstruction, gastric retention, bowel perforation, megacolon, toxic colitis

PRAZOSIN (Minipress)

Preparations: *cap* 1, 2, 5 mg

Adult dosage
1. Initial: 1 mg PO bid to tid (the first dose is best given at hs while the patient is in bed to decrease the risk of syncope)
2. Maintenance: 6-15 mg/day in 2-3 divided doses
3. Maximum daily dose: 20 mg/day

Indications: Hypertension

Action: Postsynaptic α-adrenergic receptor blockage and possible direct relaxant action on vascular smooth muscle

Contraindications and precautions: Syncope occurs in 1% of patients given an initial dose ≥2 mg; hypotension may occur with concomitant use of β blockers

PREDNISONE

Preparations: *tab* 1, 2.5, 5, 10, 20, 50 mg; *syrup* 1 mg/ml

Adult dosage: Total daily dose varies with clinical disorder being treated and the patient's response to therapy

Indications: Same as for dexamethasone

Action: Synthetic glucocorticoid with minimal sodium-retaining activity

Contraindications and precautions: Same as for dexamethasone

PREMARIN; *see* ESTROGENIC SUBSTANCES, CONJUGATED

PRILOSEC; *see* OMEPRAZOLE

PRIMAXIN; *see* IMIPENEM-CILASTIN SODIUM

PROBENECID (Benemid)

Preparations: *tab* 500 mg

Adult dosage
1. Gout: initially 250 mg PO bid × 1 wk, then increase to 500 mg bid

2. Prolongation of penicillin action: 500 mg PO qid or 1-2 g dose given at once

NOTE: Decrease the dosage in elderly patients and in patients with renal impairment.

Indications: Hyperuricemia associated with gout and gouty arthritis; prolongation of penicillin action

Action: Decreases serum uric acid levels by inhibiting its tubular reabsorption; increases penicillin plasma levels by inhibiting tubular secretion of penicillin

Contraindications and precautions

1. Acute gouty attack (therapy should not be started until attack has subsided)
2. Use with caution in patients with blood dyscrasias, uric acid kidney stones, or history of peptic ulcer
3. Avoid concomitant use of penicillin in patients with renal impairment
4. Salicylates antagonize the uricosuric action of probenecid
5. Probenecid increases the serum levels of conjugated sulfonamides (increased action of oral sulfonylureas and indomethacin)
6. Probenecid may not be effective when the glomerular filtration rate is ≤ 30 ml/min
7. When probenecid is used for gout, patient should alkalinize urine with sodium bicarbonate (3-7.5 g qd) and have adequate fluid intake to avoid crystallization of uric acid in acid urine

PROCAINAMIDE (Procan-SR, Pronestyl)

Preparations: *cap* and *tab* 250, 375, 500 mg; *inj* 100, 500 mg/ml; *SR tab* 250, 500, 750, 1000 mg

Adult dosage

1. IV loading (two methods):
   a. 100 mg IV bolus q5min (slow IV injection, ≤ 50 mg/min) until dysrhythmia suppressed or a maximum dose of 1 g has been given
   b. Infusion of 1000 mg of procainamide in 50 ml of D_5W (concentration is 20 mg/ml) administered at a constant rate of 1 ml/min over 30 min
2. Maintenance infusion: 1000 mg of procainamide in 250 ml of D_5W (concentration is 4 mg/ml) administered at 0.5-1.5 ml/min (2-6 mg/min)
3. PO: 50 mg/kg/day initially given in divided doses q3-6h (e.g., a 60-70 kg person would receive 375 mg q3h or 750 mg q6h); dosage must be individualized to maintain therapeutic blood levels

NOTE: Elderly patients and others with cardiac, renal, or hepatic insufficiency require lower doses.

Indications: PVCs, VT, prevention of recurrence of paroxysmal supraventricular tachycardia, (PSVT), atrial fibrillation or flutter following conversion to normal sinus rhythm (NSR)

Action: Class I antidysrhythmic agent

Contraindications and precautions

1. Complete heart block, torsade des pointes, lupus erythematosus, long QT syndrome, second-degree heart block or bifascicular bundle branch block, severe sinus node dysfunction

2. Use caution when using procainamide in dysrhythmias associated with digitalis intoxication and in patients receiving other group IA antidysrhythmic agents
3. Discontinue procainamide if the patient develops a positive antinuclear antibodies (ANA) test, first-degree AV block, QRS or QT prolongation >35% of baseline measurement
4. Myasthenia gravis may be exacerbated by procainamide

PROCAN-SR; *see* PROCAINAMIDE

PROCARDIA; *see* NIFEDIPINE

PROCHLORPERAZINE (Compazine)

Preparations: *tab* 5, 10 mg; *syrup* 5 mg/5 ml; *supp* 2.5, 5, 25 mg; *inj* 5 mg/ml ampule; *cap (Spansule)* 10, 15, 30 mg
Adult dosage
1. PO: 5-10 mg tid to qid; if using Spansule, 10 mg bid or 15 mg qAM
2. IM: 5-10 mg q6h; do not exceed 40 mg day
3. PR: 25 mg suppository bid
NOTE: Decrease the dosage in elderly or debilitated patients.
Indications: Control of severe nausea and vomiting: manifestations of psychotic disorders
Action: Phenothiazine tranquilizer with antiemetic properties
Contraindications and precautions
1. Comatose states, bone marrow depression, children <9 kg or younger than 2 yr, pediatric surgery
2. Prochlorperazine may mask the underlying disorder causing the nausea and vomiting (e.g., drug overdose, intestinal obstruction)
3. Parenteral administration in patients with impaired cardiovascular system may result in hypotension

PRONESTYL; *see* PROCAINAMIDE

PROPRANOLOL (Inderal, Intensol)

Preparations: *tab* 10, 20, 40, 60, 80, 90 mg; *inj* 1 mg/ml; *cap (Inderal LA)* 60, 80, 120, 160 mg; *soln* 4,8 mg/ml; *conc* (Intensol) 80 mg/ml
Adult dosage
1. Hypertension: 40 mg PO bid initially; usual maintenance dosage is 120-140 mg/day
2. Angina pectoris: 10-20 mg PO qid; increase dosage at 3-7 day intervals prn; average dose is 160 mg/day
3. Dysrhythmias: 10-30 mg PO qid
4. Hypertrophic subaortic stenosis: 20-40 mg qid
5. Migraine: 40 mg PO bid; usual range is 160-240 mg/day
6. Post-MI prophylaxis: 180-240 mg/day in 2-3 divided doses
7. Essential tremor: 30-120 mg bid
Indications: See above
Action: Nonselective β-adrenergic blocker

Contraindications and precautions
1. Cardiogenic shock, sinus bradycardia, greater than first-degree AV block, bronchial asthma, CHF (unless secondary to dysrhythmia treatable with propranolol)
2. Use with caution in diabetics (may mask the symptoms of hypoglycemia), impaired renal or hepatic function, Wolff-Parkinson-White syndrome (may cause severe bradycardia), concomitant MAO inhibitor therapy, or in patients receiving catecholamine-depleting drugs

PROTAMINE SULFATE

Preparations: *inj* 5 ml/50 mg ampul; 25 ml/250 mg vial
Adult dosage
1. Each mg of protamine sulfate neutralizes approximately 100 USP units of heparin
2. Protamine sulfate should only be given by slow IV injection: do not exceed 50 mg in any 10 min period

Indications: Treatment of heparin overdosage
Action: Neutralizes action of heparin by forming a heparin-protamine complex; neutralization of heparin occurs within 5 min of IV administration
Contraindications and precautions: Very rapid administration can result in severe hypotension and anaphylactoid-like reactions; monitor neutralizing effect by determining the PTT few minutes after administration

PROVENTIL; *see* ALBUTEROL

PROZAC; *see* FLUOXETINE

QUESTRAN; *see* CHOLESTYRAMINE

QUINAGLUTE; *see* QUINIDINE

QUINIDEX EXTENTABS; *see* QUINIDINE

QUINIDINE*

Preparations
1. *tab*
    a. Sulfate salt: 100, 200, 300 mg (Quinidine sulfate, Quinora)
    b. Polygalacturonate salt: 275 mg (Cardioquin)
2. *inj*
    a. Gluconate salt: 80 mg/ml
    b. Sulfate salt: 200 mg/ml
3. *Slow-release tab*
    a. Gluconate salt: 324 mg (Quinidine Gluconate SR, Quinaglute Duratabs), 330 mg (Duraquin)
    b. Sulfate salt: 300 mg (Quinidex Exentabs)
Adult dosage
1. Quinidine sulfate
    a. PAC, PVC: 200-300 mg PO tid to qid

*Refer to Fig. 5-4, *B*, for ECG manifestations of quinidine toxicity.

b. Paroxysmal supraventricular tachycardia: 400-600 mg PO q2-3h until paroxysm is terminated

c. Conversion of atrial fibrillation: 200 mg PO q2-3h × 5-8 doses (do not exceed 4 g/day); increase daily dose until sinus rhythm is restored or toxic effects occur

d. Maintenance therapy is 200-300 mg tid to qid

2. Quinidine polygalacturonate: 1 to 3 tabs PO may be used to terminate dysrhythmia; this dose may be repeated in 3-4 hr; if normal sinus rhythm is not restored after 3-4 equal doses, dose may be increased by ½-1 tab (137.5-275 mg) and administered 3-4 times before any further dosage increase; maintenance dosage is 1 tab bid

3. Slow-release tabs (gluconate and sulfate salts) may be given q12h

Indications: Ventricular dysrhythmias (PVCs, paroxysmal ventricular tachycardia not associated with heart block), supraventricular dysrhythmias (atrial flutter, atrial fibrillation, PAC, paroxysmal atrial tachycardia), junctional dysrhythmias (AV junctional premature complexes, paroxysmal junctional tachycardia)

Action: Class I antidysrhythmic; decreases conduction velocity and automaticity and prolongs refractory period

Contraindications and precautions

1. Complete AV block; digitalis intoxication manifested by AV conduction disorders; complete bundle branch block or other severe intraventricular conduction defects, especially those exhibiting a marked grade of QRS widening; myasthenia gravis; aberrant impulses and abnormal rhythms caused by escape mechanisms

2. Quinidine will produce a doubling of the digitalis plasma level in patients receiving digitalis (consider reduction of digitalis dose when starting quinidine)

3. Use with caution in patients with incomplete AV block (asystole and complete AV block may be produced)

4. Closely monitor patients with cardiac, hepatic, or renal insufficiency (increased risk of toxicity)

5. In the treatment of atrial fibrillation or flutter, digitalization is indicated before starting quinidine in order to block AV nodal conduction; if quinidine is used before digitalization, it may increase AV nodal conduction and ventricular rate

RANITIDINE (Zantac)

Preparations: *tab* 150, 300 mg; *inj* 25 mg/ml; *syrup* 150 mg/10 ml

Adult dosage

1. PO: 150 mg PO bid or 300 mg PO qhs

2. IV: 50 mg q8h or 150-300 mg administered as a 24 hr continuous infusion (more constant acid suppression)

NOTE: Decrease the dosage in patients with renal impairment.

Indications Short-term management of duodenal and gastric ulcers, treatment of pathologic hypersecretory conditions

Action: Histamine H_2 receptor antagonist

Contraindications and precautions: Use with caution in patients with impaired hepatic function (metabolized in the liver)

REGLAN; *see* METOCLOPRAMIDE

RESTORIL; *see* TEMAZEPAM

RETROVIR; *see* ZIDOVUDINE

RIFAMPIN

Preparations: *cap* 150, 300 mg
Adult dosage
1. Pulmonary tuberculosis: 600 mg PO qd
2. Meningococcal carriers: 600 mg PO qd
NOTE: Rifampin should be administered 1 hr before or 2 hr after a meal.
Indications: Primary tuberculosis; treatment of asymptomatic carriers of *N. meningitidis* to eliminate meningococci from the nasopharynx
Action: It inhibits bacterial DNA-dependent RNA polymerase activity
Contraindications and precautions
1. History of hypersensitivity to any of the rifamycins
2. Use with caution in patients receiving anticoagulants of the coumarin type (increases requirement) and in patients with liver disease or receiving concomitant hepatotoxic agents (increased risk of hepatotoxicity)

ROCALTROL; *see* CALCITROL

SELDANE; *see* TERFENADINE

SEPTRA; *see* TRIMETHOPRIM

SERAX; *see* OXAZEPAM

SILVADENE; *see* SILVER SULFADIAZINE

SILVER SULFADIAZINE (Silvadene)

Preparations: *jars* 20, 50, 400, 1000 g; *tubes* 20 g
Adult dosage: Apply qd to bid to burn area (dressings not required over burn area)
Indications: Prevention and treatment of wound sepsis in patients with second- and third-degree burns
Action: Topical bactericidal agent effective against many gram-negative and gram-positive bacteria as well as yeast
Contraindications and precautions
1. Use with caution in patients with G_6PD deficiency (increased risk of hemolysis)
2. Accumulation of the drug may occur in patients with impaired renal or hepatic function

SLO-PHYLLIN; *see* THEOPHYLLINE

SODIUM POLYSTYRENE SULFONATE (Kayexalate)

Preparations *jar* 1 lb (453.6 g); *susp* 15 g (in sorbitol sol)/60 ml
Adult dosage
1. PO: 15-60 g given as a suspension
2. PR: 30-50 g q6h prn given with 100 ml of sorbitol as a retention enema

Indications: Treatment of hyperkalemia
Action: Cation exchange resin; as it passes through the GI tract, the partially released sodium ions are replaced by potassium ions; its efficacy is approx 33%
Contraindications and precautions
1. Use with caution in patients with congestive heart failure, marked edema, severe hypertension, and any other condition in which a sodium load may be detrimental
2. Closely monitor serum K^+, Mg^{2+}, and Ca^{2+} (severe hypokalemia, hypomagnesemia, hypocalcemia may occur)
3. Concomitant administration of magnesium hydroxide, nonabsorbable cation-donating antacids, and laxatives should be avoided

SOLU-CORTEF; *see* HYDROCORTISONE SODIUM SUCCINATE

SOLU-MEDROL; *see* METHYLPREDNISOLONE

SOMOPHYLLIN; *see* THEOPHYLLINE

SPIRONOLACTONE (Aldactone)

Preparations: *tab* 25, 50, 100 mg
Adult dosage
1. Edema: 25-200 mg/day administered in single or divided doses; maximal effect is not seen for 3-4 days; therefore do not adjust dose until fourth day; if diuresis remains inadequate, add a second diuretic agent with action more proximally in the renal tubule
2. Essential hypertension: 50-100 mg/day initially; adjust dose after 2 wk; consider adding a diuretic agent with action on the proximal renal tubule if the patient remains hypertensive
3. Hypokalemia: 25-100 mg/day
4. Hyperaldosteronism: 200-400 mg/day

Indications: Primary hyperaldosteronism; edema states secondary to cirrhosis, nephrotic syndrome, CHF; essential hypertension; hypokalemia (diuretic-induced) when oral potassium supplements or other potassium-sparing regimens are inappropriate
Action: Aldosterone antagonist; acts through competitive binding of receptors at the aldosterone-dependent Na^+-K^+ exchange site in the distal convoluted renal tubule
Contraindications and precautions
1. Anuria, hyperkalemia, renal impairment
2. Avoid excessive potassium intake (increased risk of hyperkalemia)
3. Avoid concomitant administration of other potassium-sparing diuretics

4. Decrease dosage of other diuretics or antihypertensive agents when starting spironolactone (potentiation of their effect)

SUCRALFATE (Carafate)

Preparations: *tab* 1 g
Adult dosage: 1 g qid × 8 wk (acute therapy), 1 g bid for maintenance (if indicated)
NOTE: Sucralfate should be taken on an empty stomach.
NOTE: Do not take antacids within 30 min of sulcralfate (before or after).
Indications: Short-term treatment of duodenal ulcer, or maintenance therapy
Action: It forms an ulcer-adherent complex that covers the ulcer site and protects it against further attack by acid, pepsin, and bile salts
Contraindications and precautions: Simultaneous administration of sucralfate with tetracycline, phenytoin, ciprofloxacin, digoxin, or H_2 blockers will result in a reduction in the bioavailability of these agents

SULFASALAZINE (Azulfadine)

Preparations: *tab* 500 mg; *enteric-coated tab* 500 mg; *oral susp* 250 mg/5 ml
Adult dosage: 500 mg PO qid initially
NOTE: Azulfadine should be taken after meals to decrease adverse GI effects.
Indications: Adjunctive therapy of ulcerative colitis
Action: Sulfasalazine is split in the colon into sulfapyridine and 5-aminosalicylic acid; the latter has antiinflammatory activity (inhibition of prostaglandin synthesis)
Contraindications and precautions
  1. Hypersensitivity to sulfonamides or salicylates, infants under 2 yr of age, intestinal or urinary obstruction, porphyria
  2. Use with caution in patients with severe allergy, bronchial asthma, G_6PD deficiency
  3. Concomitant administration of folic acid or digoxin will result in decreased absorption of these drugs

SYMMETREL; *see* AMANTADINE

SYNTHROID; *see* THYROXINE

TAGAMET; *see* CIMETIDINE

TAMBOCOR; *see* FLECAINIDE

TEMAZEPAM (Restoril)

Preparations: *cap* 15, 30 mg
Adult dosage: 15-30 mg PO qhs
NOTE: Use lower doses in elderly or debilitated patients.
Indications: Insomnia
Action: Short-acting benzodiazepine

Contraindications and precautions: Avoid concomitant use of alcohol or other CNS depressants

TENORMIN; *see* ATENOLOL

TERBUTALINE (Brethine, Brethaire)

Preparations: *tab* 2.5, 5 mg; *inj* 1 mg/ml amp; *aerosol* (Brethaire) 0.2 mg/inhalation
Adult dosage
   1. PO: 2.5-5 mg PO tid
   2. IM/SQ: 0.25 mg; may repeat once after 30 min if no relief
   3. Aerosol: 2 inhalations (1 min apart) q4-6h
   NOTE: Do not exceed a total PO dose 14 mg/24 hr in adults.
Indications: Bronchial asthma and reversible bronchospasm
Action: Bronchodilator
Contraindications and precautions
   1. Known hypersensitivity to sympathetic amines
   2. Avoid concomitant use of other sympathomimetic agents
   3. Use with caution in patients with cardiac disease, cardiac dysrhythmias, diabetes, hypertension, hyperthyroidism, or history of seizures

TERFENADINE (Seldane)

Preparations: *tab* 60 mg
Adult dosage: 60 mg PO bid
Indications: Relief of symptoms associated with seasonal allergic rhinitis
Action: Peripheral specific histamine H_1 receptor antagonist
Contraindications and precautions: Known hypersensitivity to terfenadine

TETRACYCLINE (Achromycin)

Preparations: *cap* and *tab* 250, 500 mg; *inj* 100, 250, 500 mg; *syrup* 125 mg/5ml
Adult dosage: 250-500 mg PO q6h (taken between meals)
Indications: Infections caused by susceptible bacterial organisms
Action: Inhibits protein synthesis at the 30S ribosomal subunit
Contraindications and precautions
   1. Hypersensitivity to any of the tetracyclines
   2. Use with caution in patients with impaired renal or hepatic function
   3. Concomitant therapy with antacids impairs tetracycline absorption
   4. Discontinue tetracycline if overgrowth of nonsusceptible organisms occurs
   5. Patients receiving anticoagulants should readjust the dose (tetracycline depresses plasma prothrombin activity)

THEO-24; *see* THEOPHYLLINE

THEO-DUR; *see* THEOPHYLLINE

THEOPHYLLINE

Preparations: see Table 32-8
Adult dosage
1. Loading dose for acute bronchospasm: 5 mg/kg; 3 mg/kg if the patient is on theophylline but a level cannot be immediately obtained
2. Maintenance dose for acute symptoms: see Table 32-9
3. Maintenance for chronic asthma: 400 mg/day PO in divided doses (e.g., Theo-Dur 200 mg bid); monitor theophylline plasma concentration (therapeutic is 10-20 µg/ml) and adjust dosage accordingly

Indications: Relief or prevention of symptoms of bronchial asthma; reversible bronchospasm associated with chronic bronchitis and emphysema
Action: Direct relaxation of the smooth muscle of the bronchial airway and pulmonary blood vessels (bronchodilator and smooth muscle relaxant); additional effects include diuresis, coronary vasodilation, cardiac, skeletal muscle, and cerebral stimulation
Contraindications and precautions
1. Use with caution in patients with severe cardiac disease, hypertension, hepatic or renal impairment, hyperthyroidism, and dysrhythmias and in elderly patients
2. Cimetidine, ranitidine, propranolol, ciprofloxacin, high-dose allopurinol (e.g., 600 mg/day), and erythromycin may increase the serum theophylline level
3. Dilantin and phenobarbital decrease the theophylline level

Table 32-8 Theophylline preparations

Route of Administration	Trade Name	Preparations	Comments
PO	Slo-Phyllin	tab 100, 200 mg syrup 80 mg/15 ml	Rapidly absorbed for acute therapy
		cap (Gyrocaps) 60, 125, 250 mg	Slow-release product for chronic asthma
PO	Theo-Dur	tab 100, 200, 300, 450 mg cap 50, 75, 125, 200 mg	Slow-release product for chronic asthma
PO	Theo-24	cap 100, 200, 300 mg	Long-acting preparation requiring once/day dosage
PR	Somophyllin	rectal sol 300 mg/5 ml	Rapidly absorbed for acute therapy
IV	Aminophylline	IV sol 25 mg/ml	Rapidly absorbed for acute therapy

Table 32-9   Theophylline maintenance dosage for acute symptoms

Population Group	IV Aminophylline (mg/kg/hr)	Oral Theophylline (mg/kg/hr)
Otherwise healthy adult smokers	0.9	0.83
Otherwise healthy nonsmoking adults; otherwise healthy elderly patients	0.3-0.5	0.53
Cardiac or hepatic decompensation; cor pulmonale	0.2-0.3	0.26

THIAMINE

Preparations: *tab* 10, 50, 100 mg; *inj* 100 mg/ml
Adult dosage: Severe deficiency: 100 mg IM/PO qd
Indications: Thiamine deficiency

THIORIDAZINE (Mellaril)

Preparations: *tab* 10, 15, 25, 50, 100, 150, 200 mg; *liq conc* 30, 100 mg/ml; *susp* 25, 100 mg/5 ml
Adult dosage
1. Psychotic manifestations: usual starting dose 50-100 mg PO tid
2. Treatment of depression anxiety: usual starting dose 25 mg PO tid
Indications: Management of manifestations of psychotic disorders; short-term treatment of depression, anxiety, agitation
Action: Phenothiazine
Contraindications and precautions: Severe CNS depression, hypertensive or hypotensive heart disease, hypersensitivity to phenothiazines

THORAZINE; *see* CHLORPROMAZINE

THYROXINE (Synthroid, Levothyroxine)

Preparations: *tab* 25, 50, 75, 100, 112, 125, 150, 175, 200, 300 μg; *inj* 100, 200, 500 μg
Adult dosage
1. Hypothyroidism in an otherwise healthy adult: 100 μg/day initially, increasing to a maintenance dose of 100-200 μg/day over a 3 wk period
2. Hypothyroidism in elderly patients: 25 μg/day initially, increasing by 25 μg/day at 3-4 wk intervals depending on patient's response.
3. Myxedema coma: 200-500 μg IV initially; may give additional 100-300 μg in 24 hr if necessary; decrease in patients with heart disease
Indications: Hypothyroidism
Action: Synthetic preparation of thyroid hormone T_4

Contraindications and precautions
1. Thyrotoxicosis; acute MI, uncorrected adrenal insufficiency are relative contraindications
2. Use with caution in elderly patients and in patients with cardiovascular disease

TIGAN; *see* TRIMETHOBENZAMIDE

TOBRAMYCIN

Preparations: *inj* 10, 40 mg/ml (2 ml vial)
Adult dosage
1. Adults with normal renal function and serious infection: 1 mg/kg q8h; for *life-threatening infection* may use 1.66 mg/kg q8h (reduce dose as soon as possible)
2. Patients with impaired renal function: give initial loading dose of 1 mg/kg; additional doses should be adjusted based on the CCr (refer to gentamycin reduction schedule)
NOTE: Monitor serum tobramycin levels and adjust the dosage accordingly.
Indications: Treatment of serious infections caused by susceptible bacterial organisms
Action: Aminoglycoside antibiotic; inhibits protein synthesis in susceptible organisms
Contraindictions and precautions
1. Use with caution in patients with impaired renal function
2. Concurrent or sequential use of other nephrotoxic or neurotoxic drugs should be avoided
3. Advanced age and dehydration increase the risk of toxicity
4. Eighth cranial nerve function should be closely monitored

TOCAINIDE (Tonocard)

Preparations: *tab* 400, 600 mg
Adult dosage: Initially 200-400 mg PO q8h; usual adult dosage is 200-600 mg tid
NOTE: Decrease the dosage in patients with renal or hepatic impairment.
Indications: Treatment of life-threatening ventricular dysrhythmias
Action: Primary amine analog of lidocaine; produces dose-dependent decreases in sodium and potassium conductance, thereby decreasing excitability of myocardial cells
Contraindications and precautions
1. Hypersensitivity to tocainide or to local anesthetics of the amide type; use in patients with second- or third-degree AV block in absence of an artificial ventricular pacemaker
2. Use with caution in patients with heart failure (tocainide can worsen the degree of failure); in patients with severe renal or hepatic disease, decreased elimination can lead to toxicity
3. Blood dyscrasias may occur; CBC should be performed weekly for the first 3 mo, and then frequently
4. Pulmonary fibrosis may also occur

TOLAZAMIDE (Tolinase)

Preparations: *tab* 100, 250, 500 mg
Adult dosage: 100-250 mg PO qd initially; may gradually increase to 1 g daily in 1-2 doses
   NOTE: These should be administered with breakfast.
Indications: Hyperglycemia from NIDDM (type II) not satisfactorily controlled by diet alone
Action: First-generation sulfonylurea; lowers plasma glucose mainly by stimulating release of insulin from pancreas
Contraindications and precautions: Use as sole therapy for type I diabetes

TOLINASE; *see* TOLAZAMIDE

TONOCARD; *see* TOCAINIDE

TRANDATE; *see* LABETALOL

TRANXENE; *see* CLORAZEPATE

TRIAZOLAM (Halcion)

Preparations: *tab* 0.125, 0.25, 0.5 mg
Adult dosage: Initially 0.125-0.25 mg at hs; usual dosage range is 0.25-0.5 mg at hs
   NOTE: Use lower doses in geriatric or debilitated patients.
Indications: Short-term management of insomnia
Action: Short-acting benzodiazepine
Contraindications and precautions
   1. Hypersensitivity to triazolam or other benzodiazepines
   2. Stimultaneous ingestion of alcohol or other CNS depressant drugs is contraindicated

TRIMETHOBENZAMIDE (Tigan)

Preparations: *cap* 100, 250 mg; *supp* 100, 200 mg; *inj* 100 mg/ml
Adult dosage
   1. cap: 250 mg PO tid to qid
   2. supp: 200 mg PR tid to qid
   3. inj: 200 mg IM tid to qid
Indications: Control of nausea and vomiting
Action: Antiemetic agent; exerts its action on chemoreceptor trigger zone in medulla oblongata
Contraindications and precautions
   1. Do not use suppositories in patients allergic to benzocaine
   2. Determine etiology of vomiting before using antiemetics

TRIMETHOPRIM AND SULFAMETHOXAZOLE (Bactrim, Septra)

Preparations: *ampule* and *5 ml vial* 80 mg trimethoprim (16 mg/ml) and 400 mg sulfamethoxazole (80 mg/ml); *10 ml vial:* 160 mg trimethoprim (16 mg/ml) and 800 mg sulfamethoxazole (80 mg/ml); *tab:* 80 mg trimethoprim and 400 mg sulfamethoxazole; 160 mg trimethoprim and 800 mg sulfamethoxazole (Bactrim DS); *suspension:* 40 mg trimethoprim and 200 mg sulfamethoxazole/5 ml teaspoonful

Adult dosage
1. *Pneumocystits carinii* pneumonitis (PCP): 20 mg/kg trimethoprim and 100 mg/kg sulfamethoxazole/24 hr given by IV infusion in equally divided doses q6h × 14 days
2. UTIs, acute exacerbation of chronic bronchitis, shigellosis: 1 Bactrim DS tab bid or 2 regular Bactrim tabs bid; duration of therapy is 14 days for chronic bronchitis, 10-14 days for UTI, and 5 days for shigellosis

Indications: UTIs, acute exacerbation of chronic bronchitis, shigellosis, PCP

Action: Sulfamethoxazole inhibits bacterial synthesis of dihydrofolic acid; trimethoprim blocks production of tetrahydrofolic acid from dihydrofolic acid; together they block two consecutive steps in the biosynthesis of nucleic acids and proteins

Contraindications and precautions
1. Hypersensitivity to trimethoprim or sulfonamides; documented megaloblastic anemia from folate deficiency
2. Use with caution in impaired renal or hepatic function, G_6PD deficiency, and in patients with severe allergy or bronchial asthma

UNIPEN; *see* NAFCILLIN

VALISONE; *see* BETAMETHASONE

VALIUM; *see* DIAZEPAM

VANCOCIN; *see* VANCOMYCIN

VANCOMYCIN (Vancocin)

Preparations: *inj* 500 mg vial; *PO* mix a 1 g vial with 20 ml of H_2O (250 mg/5 ml); 10 g vial mix with 115 ml of H_2O (500 mg/6 ml); *cap* 125, 250 mg

Adult dosage
1. Pseudomembranous colitis: 125-500 mg PO q6h or 1 g PO q12h × 7-10 days
2. Potentially life-threatening infections: 500 mg IV q6h or 1 g IV q12h

NOTE: IV doses should be infused over 1 hr. Rapid infusion may result in pruritus and flushing of the torso, neck, and face—"red man syndrome."

NOTE: Dosage must be reduced in patients with renal insufficiency.

Indications: Pseudomembranous colitis, infections caused by susceptible bacterial organisms

Action: Bactericidal against many gram-positive bacteria; exerts its action by inhibition of cell wall synthesis

Contraindications and precautions

1. Avoid concomitant use of ototoxic or nephrotoxic agents
2. Use with caution in patients with impaired renal function
3. Monitor auditory function and vancomycin serum levels in patients receiving vancomycin for prolonged duration; therapeutic peak levels are 20-40 µg/ml, trough levels 5-10 µg/ml

VASOTEC; *see* ENALAPRIL

VENTOLIN; *see* ALBUTEROL

VERAPAMIL (Calan, Isoptin, Verelan)

Preparations: *tab* 80, 120 mg; *inj* 5 mg/2 ml; *SR tab* 180, 240 mg; *SR cap* (Verelan) 120, 240 mg

Adult dosage

1. PO: 80 mg tid to qid initially; increase dose gradually until optimal response is obtained; average total daily dose is 320-480 mg; do not exceed 480 mg/day in patients with angina; dose for hypertension is 120-240 mg (SR) qd
2. IV: initial dose 5-10 mg (0.075-0.15 mg/kg), given as a slow IV bolus (>2 min); may repeat with 10 mg (0.15 mg/kg), given over 5 min approx 30 min after first dose if initial response is inadequate

Indications

1. PO: angina, hypertension
2. IV: rapid conversion of paroxysmal SVT to sinus rhythm, temporary control of rapid ventricular rate in atrial flutter or atrial fibrillation (except when the atrial flutter or fibrillation is associated with accessory bypass tracts)

Action: Calcium channel antagonist

Contraindications and precautions: Severe hypotension or cardiogenic shock, second- or third-degree AV block (except in patients with functioning artificial pacemaker), sick sinus syndrome (in absence of artificial pacemaker), severe CHF (unless secondary to SVT amenable to verapamil therapy), ventricular tachycardia, atrial flutter or fibrillation and an accessory bypass tract, severe left ventricular dysfunction (negative inotropic effect); verapamil increases serum digoxin levels by 50-75%

VERELAN; *see* VERAPAMIL

VIBRAMYCIN; *see* DOXYCYCLINE

VICODIN; *see* HYDROCODONE BITARTRATE

VISTARIL; *see* HYDROXYZINE

WARFARIN (Coumadin)

Preparations: *tab* 2, 2.5, 5, 7.5, 10 mg
Adult dosage: Initially 10-15 mg PO qd × 2-3 days; monitor prothrombin
    time and adjust dosage accordingly to maintain prothrombin time 1.3-1.5
    times control prothrombin time
Indications: Prophylaxis and treatment of venous thrombosis, atrial fibril-
    lation with embolization, prophylaxis and treatment of pulmonary embo-
    lism (following heparin therapy)
Action: Inhibits hepatic synthesis of coagulation factor (depression of Fac-
    tors II, VII, IX, X)
Contraindications and precautions: Hemorrhagic tendencies, pregnancy,
    severe hepatic or renal disease, severe hypertension, blood dyscrasias,
    vitamin K deficiency; vitamin K (Phytonadione) 10-50 mg SQ/IM or
    fresh frozen plasma (FFP) can be used to reverse the effect of warfarin

XANAX; *see* ALPRAZOLAM

ZANTAC; *see* RANITIDINE

ZAROXOLYN; *see* METOLAZONE

ZDV; *see* ZIDOVUDINE

ZIDOVUDINE (AZT, ZDV, Retrovir)

Preparations: *cap* 100 mg; *syrup* 50 mg/5 ml (240 ml bottle); *inj* 10 mg/ml
Adult dosage: 200 mg q4h (1200 mg/day); equal effectiveness with less
    hematological toxicity can be achieved with an initial dosage of 200 mg
    q4h for the first month followed by 100 mg q4h (600 mg/day)[8]; lower
    doses of 100 mg q4h while awake (500 mg/day) or 200 mg q8h may also
    be effective[8]
Indications: Management of HIV infection with evidence of impaired im-
    munity (CD4 cell count of 500/mm^3 or less before therapy is begun)
Action: Interference with reverse transcriptase-mediated production of pro-
    viral DNA
Contraindications and precautions: Monitor for hematological toxicity
    (anemia, granulocytopenia); significant anemia (Hb < 7.5 g/dl or reduc-
    tion > 25% of baseline) and/or significant granulocytopenia (granulocyte
    count < 750 mm^3 or reduction of > 50% from baseline) may require a
    dose interruption until some evidence of marrow recovery is observed;
    concomitant use of acetaminophen may exacerbate zidovudine toxicity

ZINACEF; *see* CEFUROXIME

ZOSTRIX; *see* CAPSAICIN

ZOVIRAX; *see* ACYCLOVIR

ZYLOPRIM; *see* ALLOPURINOL

References

1. Frame JN, Mulvaney KP, et al: Correction of severe heparin-associated thrombocytopenia with intravenous immunoglobulin, Ann Intern Med 111:946, 1989.
2. Girwood RH: Clinical pharmacology, ed 25, Philadelphia, 1985, WB Saunders Co.
3. Goth A, Vessell ES: Medical pharmacology: principles and concepts, ed 11, St Louis 1984, The CV Mosby Co.
4. Herfindal E, Hirschman J: Clinical pharmacy and therapeutics, ed 3, Baltimore, 1984, The Williams & Wilkins Co.
5. Knoben JE, Anderson PO: Handbook of clinical drug data, ed 5, Hamilton Ill, 1985, Drug Intelligence Publications Inc.
6. Information obtained from individual drug manufacturer's product package inserts.
7. Digoxin antibody fragments for digoxin toxicity, Med Lett Drugs Ther 28:87, 1986.
8. Drugs for HIV infection, Med Lett Drugs Ther 31:11, 1990.

Comparison Tables

33

Table 33-1 ACE inhibitors[12]

Agent	Preparations	Initial Dosage (PO)	Onset of Action (min)	Time of Peak Effect on BP Levels (hr)	Duration of Effect on BP Levels (hr)
Captopril (Capoten)	tab 12.5, 25, 50, 100 mg	Hypertension: 25 mg bid CHF: 6.25-12.5 mg tid	15-30	1-2	6-10
Enalapril (Vasotec)	tab 2.5, 5, 10, 20 mg inj 125 mg/ml	Hypertension: 5 mg qd CHF: 2.5 mg qd	60-120	4-8	18-30
Lisinopril (Prinivil, Zestril)	tab 5, 10, 20, 40 mg	Hypertension: 10 mg qd CHF: 5 mg qd	60	2-7	18-30

Table 33-2 Adrenergic antagonists*

Agent	Preparations	Initial Dosage	Comments
Clonidine (Catapres)	tab: 0.1, 0.2, 03 mg Transdermal therapeutic system (TTS): 1 (2.5 mg), 2 (5mg), 3 (7.5 mg)	PO: 0.1 mg bid Patch: TTS-1 apply 1 every 7 days	Centrally acting alpha blocker
Guanabenz (Wytensin)	tab: 4, 8 mg	4 mg bid	Centrally acting alpha blocker
Guanadrel (Hylorel)	tab: 10, 25 mg	5-10 mg bid	Peripherally acting alpha blocker
Guanethidine (Ismelin)	tab: 10, 25 mg	10-25 mg qd	Peripherally acting alpha blocker
Guanfacine (Tenex)	tab: 1, 2 mg	1 mg qd at hs	Centrally acting alpha blocker
Labetolol (Normodyne, Trandate)	tab: 100, 200, 300 mg inj: 5mg/ml	PO: 100 mg bid IV: 20 mg by slow injection over 2 min	Combined alpha and beta-adrenergic blocker
Methyldopa (Aldomet)	tab: 125, 250, 500 mg susp: 250 mg/5 ml inj: 250 mg/5 ml	PO: 250 mg bid-tid IM/IV: 125-250 mg q6h	Centrally acting alpha blocker
Prazosin (Minipress)	cap: 1, 2, 5 mg	1 mg at hs (first dose), then 1 mg bid-tid	Alpha$_1$-adrenergic blocker
Reserpine (Serpasil)	tab: 0.1, 0.25 mg	0.5 mg daily for 1-2 wk, then reduce dosage to 0.1-0.25 mg qd	Peripherally acting alpha blocker
Terazosin (Hytrin)	tab: 1, 2, 5, 10 mg	1 mg at hs (first dose), then increase to 2 mg qd after 3 days	Alpha$_1$-adrenergic blocker

*Refer to Table 33-18 for description of beta adrenergic antagonists.

Table 33-3   Antacids—cont'd

Product	Dosage Forms*	Active Ingredients†				Sodium Content		ANC‡
		AH	MH	CC	SI	mg	mEq	
AlternaGel	liq	600	—	—	—	2	0.09	16
Amphojel	susp	320	—	—	—	6.9	0.30	7
	tab	600	—	—	—	2.8	0.12	18
Camalox	susp	225	200	250	—	2.5	0.11	18
	tab	225	200	250	—	1.5	0.07	18
Delcid	liq	600	665	—	—	12	0.53	42
Gelusil	liq, tab	200	200	—	25	0.7	0.03	12
Maalox	susp	225	200	—	—	1.4	0.06	13
	tab	200	200	—	—	0.8	0.04	9
Maalox Plus	susp	225	200	—	25	1.3	0.06	13
	tab	200	200	—	25	0.9	0.04	9
Maalox TC	susp	600	300	—	—	0.8	0.3	28
Milk of magnesia	susp	—	310	—	—	1.3	<0.01	14
	tab	—	310	—	—	0.9	0.01	14

From DiGregorio GJ, Barbieri EJ, Piraino AJ: Handbook of commonly prescribed drugs, ed 4, Westchester Pa, 1984, Medical Surveillance Inc.

*liq, liquid; susp, suspension; tab, tablet.

†AH, aluminum hydroxide; MH, magnesium hydroxide; CC, calcium carbonate; SI, simethicone; in mg per 5 ml or per tablet.

‡Acid neutralizing capacity in mEq per 5 ml or per tablet.

§As magaldrate, a complex of aluminum and magnesium hydroxides.

Continued.

Table 33-3   Antacids—cont'd

Product	Dosage Forms*	Active Ingredients†				Sodium Content		ANC‡
		AH	MH	CC	SI	mg	mEq	
Mylanta	liq, tab	200	200	—	20	0.7	0.03	12
Mylanta II	liq, tab	400	400	—	30	1.3	0.06	24
Riopan	susp, tab	480§	—	—	—	0.1	<0.01	14
Riopan Plus	susp, tab	480§	—	—	20	0.1	<0.01	14
Silain gel	liq	280	285	—	25	4.8	0.21	15
Titralac	liq	—	—	1000	—	11	0.48	20
	tab	—	—	420	—	0.3	0.01	8
WinGel	liq, tab	180	160	—	—	<2.5	0.10	12

Table 33-4 Antibiotic dosage in renal impairment

Extent of Reduction in Dosage	Agent	Serum Half-Life (hr)		Initial Dose	Subsequent Dose	Interval Between Subsequent Doses
		Normal	Anuric			
Major	Amikacin	2	44 (minimum function) 86 (anephric)	7.5 mg/kg	0.75 mg/kg	12 hr (avoids levels >35 μg/ml)
	Gentamicin	2	48-72	1.7 mg/kg (IM or IV)	0.17 mg/kg	8 hr (avoids levels >12 μg/ml)
	Kanamycin	3	30-80	7.5 mg/kg	0.75 mg/kg	12 hr
	Streptomycin	2-3	100-110	0.5 gm (IM)	0.25 g	16 hr
	Tobramycin	2-3	56-72	2.0 mg/kg (IM or IV)	0.17 mg/kg	8 hr (avoids levels >12 μg/ml)
	Vancomycin	6	240	7.0 mg/kg	1.5 mg/kg	24 hr (avoids levels >50 μg/ml)
Moderate	Acyclovir	2-2.5	20	6.2 mg/kg	6.2 mg/kg	24 hr
	Azlocillin	1.0	5.0	45 mg/kg (IV)	45 mg/kg	12 hr
	Carbenicillin	0.5-1.0	12.5	75 mg/kg (IV)	28 mg/kg	8 hr
	Cefamandole	1.0	11	25 mg/kg (IV)	15 mg/kg	12 hr
	Cefazolin	1.9	32	15 mg/kg (IM)	4 mg/kg	12 hr
	Cefonicid	4.4	50-65	30 mg/kg	7.5 mg/kg	72 hr
	Ceforanide	3.0	20-40	15 mg/kg	7.5 mg/kg	24 hr
	Cefoxitin	0.7-1.0	22	15 mg/kg (IV)	15 mg/kg	24 hr
	Ceftazidime	1.8	16-25	30 mg/kg	7.5 mg/kg	24 hr

Continued.

Modified from Sanford JP: Guide to antimicrobial therapy, 1985.

Table 33-4 Antibiotic dosage in renal impairment—cont'd

Extent of Reduction in Dosage	Agent	Serum Half-Life (hr) Normal	Serum Half-Life (hr) Anuric	Initial Dose	Subsequent Dose	Interval Between Subsequent Doses
Moderate	Ceftizoxime	1.7	25-36	30 mg/kg	7.5 mg/kg	24 hr
	Cefuroxime	1.4-1.8	20	15 mg/kg (IV)	15 mg/kg	24 hr
	Cephalexin	1.0	5-30	15 mg/kg	2 mg/kg	12 hr
	Cephalothin	0.5	3-18	30 mg/kg (IV)	7.5 mg/kg	12 hr
	Cephapirin	0.9	2.4	15 mg/kg	15 mg/kg	12 hr
	Cephradine	0.7	8-15	15 mg/kg	7.5 mg/kg	12 hr
	Imipenem	0.8-1.0	3.5	15 mg/kg (IV)	7.5 mg/kg	12 hr
	Moxalactam	2.2	19	25 mg/kg	7.5 mg/kg	12 hr
	Penicillin G	0.5	7-10	30,000 U/kg (IV)	10,000 U/kg	8 hr
	Ticarcillin	1-1.5	13	45 mg/kg IV	28 mg/kg	12 hr
	Trimethoprim	11	25	2 tabs (400 mg SMZ, 80 mg TMP/tab) (PO).	1 tab	12 hr
	Sulfamethoxazole	9	27			
None or minor	Amoxicillin	1.0	16	30 mg/kg (IM or IV)	15 mg/kg	12 hr
	Amphotericin B	24 / 15 days	40	0.5 mg/kg (IV)	0.5 mg/kg IV	1-2 days
	Ampicillin	0.5-1.0	8-20	30 mg/kg (IM or IV)	15 mg/kg	12 hr
	Cefoperazone	1.6-2.4	4.2	30 mg/kg	20 mg/kg	12 hr
	Cefotaxime	1.5	2.7	30 mg/kg	30 mg/kg	12 hr
	Ceftriaxone	8	12-15	15 mg/kg	15 mg/kg	24 hr

Table 33-5   Antibiotic penetration into the CNS[10]

Adequate	Inadequate
Azlocillin	Amikacin
Carbenicillin	Benzathine penicillin G
Cefoperazone (Cefobid)	Cefamandole (Mandol)
Cefotaxime (Claforan)	Cefazolin (Ancef, Kefzol)
Ceftazidime (Fortaz)	Cefoxitin (Mefoxin)
Ceftriaxone (Rocephin)	Cephalothin (Keflin)
Cefuroxime (Zinacef)	Cephapirin (Cephadyl)
Chloramphenicol	Ciprofloxacin
Ethambutol	Clindamycin
Isoniazid	Erythromycin
Metronidazole	Gentamycin
Mezlocillin	Streptomycin
Moxalactam (Moxam)	Tetracycline
Nafcillin	Tobramycin
Oxacillin	Vancomycin
Piperacillin	
Pyrazinamide	
Rifampin	
Sulfonamides	
Ticarcillin	
Trimethoprim/Sulfamethoxazole	

Table 33-6 Anticonvulsants

Agent	Preparations	Dosage (PO)	Principal Use	Half-life (hr)	Therapeutic Level (µg/ml)	Toxic Level (µg/ml)
Carbamazepine (Tegretol)	tab: 200 mg chew tab: 100 mg susp: 100 mg/5 ml	Initial: 200 mg bid Maintenance: 800-1200 mg/day	Partial complex seizures	20 ± 5	2-10	>12
Clonazepam (Klonopin)	tab: 0.5, 1, 2, mg	Initial: 0.5 mg tid Maintenance: 1.5-20 mg/day	Absence, myoclonic, atonic seizures	30 ± 10	15-60	>100
Ethosuximide (Zarontin)	cap: 250 mg syrup: 250 mg/5 ml	Initial: 500 mg/day Maintenance: 1-1.5 g/day	Absence seizures	48 ± 12	40-100	>150
Phenobarbital	tab: 8, 16, 32, 65, 100 mg cap: 16 mg elixir: 15 mg/5 ml	50-100 mg bid-tid	Tonic-clonic and partial seizures	96 ± 12	15-35	>60

Drug	Preparations	Indication			
Phenytoin (Dilantin)	Kapseals: 30, 100 mg susp: 125 mg/5 ml chew tab: 50 mg pediatr susp: 30 mg/5 ml	Generalized tonic-clonic (grand mal)	Loading dose: 1 g divided in 3 doses (400, 300, 300) administered at 2 hr intervals Maintenance: 100 mg tid	24 ± 12	10-20	>30
Primidone (Mysoline)	tab: 50, 250 mg susp: 250 mg/5 ml	Partial complex and tonic-clonic seizures	Initial: 100-125 mg at hs, increase to bid on day 4, tid on day 7, then 250 mg tid on day 10 Maintenance: 250 mg tid	10 ± 5	5-10	>12
Valproic acid (Depakene)	cap: 250 mg syrup: 250 mg/5 ml	Tonic clonic and absence seizures	Initial: 15 mg/kg/day Maintenance: 10-60 mg/kg	8 ± 2	50-100	>200

Table 33-7 Antidepressants[7]

Agent	Preparations	Initial Dosage (PO)	Class	Sedating Effect	Anticholinergic Effect	Orthostatic Effect	Effect on Cardiac Function
Amitriptyline (Elavil)	tab: 10, 25, 50, 75, 100, 150 mg inj: 10 mg/ml	10-75 mg qhs	Tricyclic tertiary amine	++++	++++	++++	++++
Amoxapine (Asendin)	tab: 25, 50, 100, 150 mg	25-50 mg bid-tid	Dibenzoxazepine	++	+	+++	++
Bupropion (Wellbutrin)	tab: 75, 100 mg	100 mg bid	Trimethylated monocyclic phenylaminoketone	+	+	+	+
Clomipramine* (Anafranil)	cap: 25, 50, 75 mg	25 mg qd	Tricyclic	+++	++	++	++
Desipramine (Norpramin)	tab: 10, 25, 50, 75, 100, 150 mg	10-50 mg qd	Tricyclic secondary amine	+	+	++	+
Doxepin (Adapin, Sinequan)	cap: 10, 25, 50, 75, 100, 150 mg	10-25 mg tid	Tricyclic tertiary amine	++++	+++	+++	+++

Drug	Formulation	Class	Dose				
Fluoxetine (Prozac)	Puvules: 20 mg	Phenylpropylamine	20 mg qd	0	+	+	+
Imipramine (Tofranil)	tab: 10, 25, 50 mg; cap: (Tofranil-PM) 75, 100, 125, 150 mg; inj: 25 mg/2ml	Tricyclic tertiary amine	75 mg qd	+++	+++	+++	++++
Maprotiline (Ludiomil)	tab: 25, 50, 75 mg	Tetracyclic	50-75 mg qd	++	++	+++	++
Nortriptyline (Pamelor)	cap: 10, 25, 50, 75 mg; liq: 10 mg/5 ml	Tricyclic secondary amine	25 mg tid	+++	++	+	++
Protriptyline (Vivactyl)	tab: 5, 10 mg	Dibenzocycloheptene derivative	5 mg tid	+	+++	++	++
Trazodone (Desyrel)	tab: 50, 100, 150, 300 mg	Triazolopyridine	50 mg tid	+++	+	++	+

KEY: 0, none; +, weak; ++, mild; +++, moderate; ++++, strong
*Indicated for obsessive-compulsive disorder.

Table 33-8 Antidiarrheal agents for acute nonspecific diarrhea

Agents	Preparations	Adult Dosage
Commonly Used Agents		
Attapulgite (Kaopectate)	tab: 600 mg attapulgite liq: 600 mg attapulgite/15 ml	2 Tbsp initially; may repeat after each loose bowel movement; maximum daily dose 14 Tbsp
Diphenoxylate (Lomotil)	tab: 2.5 mg diphenoxylate, 0.025 mg atropine sulfate liq: 2.5 mg diphenoxylate, 0.025 mg atropine sulfate per 5 ml	2 tabs or 10 ml qid until initial control of diarrhea is achieved
Loperamide (Imodium)	cap: 2 mg loperamide liq: 1 mg loperamide/5 ml	4 mg initially, followed by 2 mg after each unformed stool; maximum daily dose 16 mg
Possibly Useful Agents		
Aluminum hydroxide (Amphojel)	320 mg aluminum hydroxide/5 ml	2 tsp 2-4 hr between meals and at hs
Cholestyramine (Questran)	4 g of anhydrous cholestyramine resin per 9 g of powder powd: 3.7, 7.4, 11.1 oz containers	1 scoopful or packet (9 g) mixed with water or other fluids before ingesting, 1-6 times/day
Psyllium hydrophilic mucilloid (Metamucil)		1 Tbsp tid

Note: Before using any of these agents, determine the etiology of the diarrhea and initiate specific treatment. Refer to Section 23.4 for identification and treatment of the various causes of diarrhea.

Table 33-9   Antiemetics

Agent	Preparations	Usual Adult Dosage
Chlorpromazine (Thorazine)	tabs: 10, 25, 50, 100, 200 mg Spansules: 30, 75, 150, 200, 300 mg syrup: 10 mg/5 ml supp: 25, 100 mg inj: 25 mg/ml	PO: 10 mg q4h IM: 25 mg q4h until vomiting stops PR: 25 mg q6h
Hydroxyzine (Vistaril)	cap: 25, 50, 100 mg syrup: 25 mg/5 ml	PO: 25-50 mg q6-8h IM: 50 mg q6-8h
Metoclopramide (Reglan)	tabs: 5, 10 mg syrup: 5 mg/5 ml inj: 5 mg/5 ml	PO: 10 mg q8h IM/IV: 10 mg q6-8h
Prochlorperazine (Compazine)	tabs: 5, 10, 25 mg Spansules: 10, 15, 30 mg syrup: 5 mg/5 ml supp: 2.5, 5, 25 mg inj: 10 mg/2 ml	PO: 5-10 mg q6-8h PR: 25 mg bid IM: 5-10 mg q 3-4 hr (do not exceed 40 mg/day) IV: 2.5-10 mg by slow IV injection ($\leq$5 mg per min; do not exceed 40 mg/day)
Thiethylperazine (Torecan)	tabs: 10 mg supp: 10 mg inj: 10 mg/2 ml	PO/PR: 10 mg q8h IM: 10 mg q8h
Trimethobenzamide (Tigan)	cap: 100, 250 mg supp: 200 mg inj: 100 mg/ml	PO: 250 mg q6-8h PR: 200 mg q6-8h IM: 200 mg q6-8h

Table 33-10 Antifungal agents[3]

Agent	Preparations	Dosage	General Indications
Amphotericin B (Fungizone)	inj: 50 mg/vial	0.25-1.0 mg/kg/day	Most systemic fungal infections except *Pseudoallescheria boydii* and *Candida tropicalis*
	3% Cream (20 g) 3% Lotion (30 ml) 3% Ointment (20 g)	bid-qid	Cutaneous candidiasis
Miconazole (Monistat)	inj: 10 ml/ml	0.6-3.6 g/day in divided doses q8h	*Pseudoallescheria boydii* (IV) Systemic candidiasis, coccidioidomycosis, petriellidiosis, paracoccidioidomycosis (IV)
	2% Cream (15 g, 10z, 3 oz) 2% Lotion (30, 60 ml) Dual pack: 2%	qd-bid	Tinea pedis, corporis, cruris, versicolor (cream or lotion)
	Vaginal cream: 2 % (Monistat 7)	1 applicatorful intravaginally qhs for 7 days	Cutaneous candidiasis (cream, lotion)
	Vaginal supp: 100 mg (Monistat 7)	1 supp intravaginally qhs for 7 days	Vaginal candidiasis (vaginal supp or cream)
	Vaginal supp: 200 mg	1 supp intravaginally qhs for 3 days	
Ketoconazole (Nizoral)	tab: 200 mg	400 mg qd	Mucocutaneous candidiasis (except *C. tropicalis*), blastomycosis, histoplasmosis (tab); cutaneous candidiasis, tinea cruris, corporis, and versicolor (cream)
	2% Cream (15, 30, 60 g)	qd-bid	

Flucytosine (Ancobon)	cap: 250, 500 mg	50-150 mg/kg/day at 6 hr intervals	Combination therapy for cryptococcosis and candidiasis
Clotrimazole (Lotrimin, Mycelex)	1% Cream: 15, 30, 45, 90 g 1% Lotion: 30 ml 1% sol: 10, 30 ml	bid	Cutaneous candidiasis
	Vaginal cream 1%: 45, 90 g (Mycelex)	1 applicatorful intravaginally qhs for 7-14 days	Vaginal candidiasis
	Vaginal tab: 100 mg, 500 mg (Mycelex)	1 tab at hs intravaginally for 1 (500 mg) or 7 (100 mg) days	
	Twin pack: 500 mg vaginal tab plus 7 g of 1% cream (Mycelex)	500 mg tab at hs intravaginally; apply cream to surrounding areas bid	
	Troche: 10 mg (Mycelex)	1 troche 5 times qd for 14 days, dissolved slowly in mouth	Oral candidiasis
Nystatin (Mycostatin, Nilstat)	Oral susp: 100,000 U/ml (60, 473 ml)	4-6 ml qid (half of dose on each side of mouth); retain in mouth as long as possible before swallowing; duration of treatment is 7-14 days or at least 48 hr after clinical cure	Oral candidiasis
	tab: 500,000 U	1-2 tabs tid	Oral and intestinal candidiasis
Fluconazole (Diflucan)	tab: 50, 100, 200 mg inj: 200 mg/100 ml, 400 mg/200 ml	Refer to Chapter 32	Oropharyngeal, esophageal, and systemic candidiasis; cryptococcal meningitis

Table 33-11   Antihistamines for allergic rhinitis

Agent	Preparations	Dosage	Sedation	Anticholinergic Effect	Class
Brompheniramine (Dimetane)	tab: 4 mg elixir: 2 mg/5 ml Extentabs: 8, 12 mg	4 mg q4-6h Extentabs: 8-12 mg q12h	+	++	Alkyramine
Chlorpheniramine (Chlor-Trimeton)	tab: 4 mg syrup: 2 mg/5 ml Repetabs: 8, 12 mg	4 mg q4-6h Repetabs: 8-12 mg q12h	+	++	Alkyramine
Dexchlorpheniramine (Polaramine)	tab: 2 mg syrup: 2 mg/5 ml Repetabs: 4, 6 mg	2 mg q4-6h Repetabs: 4-6 mg q8h	+	++	Alkyramine
Clemastine (Tavist-1)	tab: 1, 2 mg syrup: 0.5 mg/5 ml	1-2 mg bid	++	+++	Ethanolamine
Diphenhydramine (Benadryl)	tab: 25 mg cap: 50 mg elixir: 12.5 mg/5 ml	25-50 mg q6-8h	+++	+++	Ethanolamine
Astemizole (Hismanal)	tab: 10 mg	10 mg qd	Insignificant	Insignificant	H$_1$ specific antagonist
Terfenadine (Seldane)	tab: 60 mg	60 mg bid	Insignificant	Insignificant	H$_1$ specific antagonist

KEY: +, low; ++, moderate; +++, high

Table 33-12 Antipseudomonal penicillins[4]

Agent	Dosage	Half-life (hr)	Comments
Azlocillin (Azlin)	IV: 3-4 g q4-6h	0.8	Low sodium content
Carbenicillin (Geopen)	IV: 5 g q4h	1.1	High sodium load Narrowest spectrum Possible associated neurotoxicity
Mezlocillin (Mezlin)	IV: 3-4 g q4-6h	1.1	Low sodium content
Piperacillin (Pipracil)	IV: 3-4 g q4-6h	0.9	Broadest spectrum Low sodium content
Ticarcillin (Ticar)	IV: 3-4 g q4-6h	1.2	High sodium content

Table 33-13 Antipsychotics[8]

Agent	Preparations	Dosage	Class/Frequent Adverse Effects
Chlorpromazine (Thorazine)	tab: 10, 25, 50, 100, 200 mg cap: 30, 75, 150, 200, 300 mg syrup: 10 mg/5 ml inj: 25 mg/ml supp: 25, 100 mg	Initial: 10-25 mg PO tid Acute agitation: 25 mg IM; repeat in 1 hr if necessary	Phenothiazine, aliphatic Drowsiness, anticholinergic effects, postural hypotension
Clozapine (Clozaril)	tab: 25, 100 mg	Initial: 25 mg qd-bid	Tricyclic dibenzodiazepine Agranulocytosis
Fluphenazine (Prolixin)	tab: 1, 2.5, 5, 10 mg conc: 5 mg/ml inj: 2.5 mg/ml	Initial: 0.5-1 mg tid IM: 1.25 mg	Phenothiazine, piperazine Extrapyramidal effects, akathisia, dystonia
Haloperidol (Haldol)	tab: 0.5, 1, 2, 5, 10, 20 mg conc: 2 mg/ml inj: 5 mg/ml	Initial: 0.5 mg bid-tid Acute agitation: 2-5 mg IM	Butyrophenone Extrapyramidal effects, dystonia, akathisia
Lithium	cap: 150, 300, 600 mg tab: 150, 300 mg	300 mg tid	Thirst, fine tremor, GI irritation, mild diarrhea, leukocytosis, polyuria

Perphenazine (Trilafon)	tab: 2, 4, 8, 16 mg conc: 16 mg/5 ml inj: 5 mg/ml	Initial: 4-8 mg tid	Phenothiazine, piperazine Extrapyramidal effects, akathisia, dystonia
Thioridazine (Mellaril)	tab: 10, 15, 25, 50, 100, 150, 200 mg conc: 30, 100 mg/ml susp: 25 mg/5m	10-100 mg tid	Phenothiazine, piperidine Drowsiness, anticholinergic effects, postural hypotension
Thiothixene (Navane)	cap: 1, 2, 5, 10, 20 mg conc: 5 mg/ml inj: 2, 5 mg/ml	Initial: 2 mg tid Acute agitation: 4 mg IM	Thioxanthene Extrapyramidal effects, akathisia, dystonia, anticholinergic effects
Trifluoperazine (Stelazine)	tab: 1, 2, 5, 10 mg conc: 10 mg/ml	Initial: 2-5 mg bid Acute agitation: 1-2 mg IM	Phenothiazine, piperazine Extrapyramidal effects, akathisia, dystonia

Table 33-14   Antistaphylococcal (beta-lactamase resistant) penicillins

Agent	Preparations	Dosage
Cloxacillin (Tegopen)	cap: 250, 500 mg sol: 125 mg/5 ml	PO: 250-500 mg q6h
Dicloxacillin (Dynapen)	cap: 125, 250, 500 mg susp: 62.5 mg/5 ml	PO: 250-500 mg q6h
Nafcillin (Unipen)	tab: 500 mg cap: 250 mg inj: 500 mg, 1, 2, 10 g	PO: 250-500 mg q4-6h IV: 1-2 g q4h
Oxacillin (Prostaphlin)	cap: 250, 500 mg susp: 250 mg/5 ml inj: 250 mg, 500 mg, 1, 2, 4 g	PO: 250-500 mg q4-6h IV: 1-2 g q4h

Table 33-15 Antitussive agents

Main Agent	Brand Name	Contents (per 5 ml)	Dosage
Codeine	Dimetane-DC	10 mg codeine 2 mg brompheniramine 12.5 mg phenylpropalamine	2 tsp q4h
	Naldecon-Cx	10 mg codeine 200 mg guaifenesein 18 mg phenylpropalamine	2 tsp q4h
	Phenergan VC	10 mg codeine 6.25 promethazine 5 mg phenylephrine	1 tsp q4-6h
	Robitussin AC	10 mg codeine 100 mg guaifenesein	2 tsp q4h
	Robitussin DAC	10 mg codeine 100 mg guaifenesein 30 mg pseudoephedrine	2 tsp q4h
	Tussi-Organidin	10 mg codeine 30 mg organidin (iodinated glycerol)	2 tsp q4h
	Tussirex	10 mg codeine 4.17 mg phenylephrine 13.33 mg pheniramine	2 tsp q4h

Continued.

Table 33-15 Antitussive agents—cont'd

Main Agent	Brand Name	Contents (per 5 ml)	Dosage
Hydrocodone	Hycodan	5 mg hydrocodone 1.5 mg homatropine	1 tsp q4-6h
	PV Tussin	2.5 mg hydrocodone 5 mg phenylephrine 6 mg pyrilamine 2 mg chlorpheniramine 5 mg phenindamine	1-2 tsp q4-6h
	Tussionex	10 mg hydrocodone 8 mg chlorpheniramine	1 tsp q12h
Dextromethorphan (nonnarcotic)	Dimetane-Dx	10 mg dextromethorphan 30 mg pseudoephedrine 2 mg brompheniramine	2 tsp q4h
	Naldecon-Dx	15 mg dextromethorphan 200 md guaifenesein 18 mg phenylpropanolamine	2 tsp qid
	Robitussin DM	15 mg dextromethorphan 100 mg guaifenesein	2 tsp q4h
	Tussi-Organidin DM	10 mg dextromethorphan 30 mg organidin (iodinated glycerol)	2 tsp q4h
	Scot-Tussin Sugar-Free DM	15 mg dextromethorphan 2 mg chlorpheniramine	2 tsp q4h

Table 33-16 Antivertigo and anti–motion sickness medications

Agent	Preparations	Adult Dosage	Main Indications
Cyclizine (Marezine)	tab: 50 mg inj: 50 mg/ml	PO: 50 mg q4-6h (max 200 mg/24 hr) taken 30 min prior to travel IM: 50 mg q4-6h (max 200 mg/24 hr)	Motion sickness
Dimenhydrinate (Dramamine)	tab: 50 mg chewable tab: 50 mg liq: 12.5 mg/4 ml inj: 50 mg/ml	PO: 50-100 mg q4-6h (max 400 mg/24 hr) taken 30-60 min prior to start of activity IM: 50-100 mg q4h	Motion sickness
Meclizine (Antivert)	tab: 12.5, 25, 50 mg chewable tab: 25 mg	Vertigo: 12.5-50 mg bid Motion sickness: 25-50 mg, taken 1 hr prior to travel	Motion sickness and vertigo
Scopolamine (Transderm-Scop)	transdermal patch: contains 1.5 mg of scopolamine and delivers 0.5 mg over 3 days; each pack contains 4 patches	Apply one patch to hairless area behind one ear 4 hr prior to travel; change patch q3d	Motion sickness and vertigo

Table 33-17 Benzodiazepines[6]

Agent	Preparations	Equivalent Dose	Dosage	Half-life (hr)	Main Indication
Alprazolam (Xanax)	tab: 0.25, 0.5, 1 mg	0.5	0.25-0.5 mg tid	14	Anxiety
Chlordiazepoxide (Librium)	cap: 5, 10, 25 mg amp: 100 mg/5 ml	10	5-25 mg qid	48-96	Anxiety
Clorazepate (Tranxene)	tab: 3.75, 7.5, 15 mg; long-acting (Tranxene SD): 11.25, 22.5 mg	7.5	tab: 3.75-15 mg tid Tranxene SD: 11.25-22.5 qd	48-96	Anxiety
Diazepam (Valium)	tab: 2, 5, 10 mg amp: 5 mg/ml	5	2-10 mg bid-qid	48-96	Anxiety
Flurazepam (Dalmane)	cap: 15, 30 mg	15	15-30 mg at hs	48-72	Insomnia
Lorazepam (Ativan)	tab: 0.5, 1, 2, mg inj: 2, 4 mg/ml	1	1 mg bid-tid	10-20	Anxiety
Oxazepam (Serax)	tab: 15 mg cap: 10, 15, 30 mg	15	10-15 mg tid-qid	8-12	Anxiety
Prazepam (Centrax)	tab: 10 mg cap: 5, 10, 20 mg	10	10 mg bid-tid	48-96	Anxiety
Quazepam (Doral)	tab: 7.5, 15 mg	7.5	7.5-15 mg at hs	75	Insomnia
Temazepam (Restoril)	cap: 15, 30 mg	15	15-30 mg at hs	10-20	Insomnia
Triazolam (Halcion)	tab: 0.125, 0.25 mg	0.25	0.125-0.25 mg at hs	2-5	Insomnia

Table 33-18 Beta-adrenergic blocking agents[11]

Drug	Oral Preparations	Initial Dosage	Maintenance Dosage	Cardioselectivity	ISA	Lipid Solubility	Elimination Half-life (hr)	Primary Excretion Route
Acetabutol (Sectral)	cap: 200, 400 qd	400 mg qd	200-800 mg	Yes	Yes	+	6-12	Renal
Atenolol (Tenormin)	tab: 50, 100 mg	50 mg qd	50-100 mg qd	Yes	No	+	6-9	Renal
Betaxolol (Kerlone)	tab: 10, 20 mg	10 mg qd	20 mg qd	Yes	No	++	16	Hepatic
Carteolol (Cartrol)	tab: 2.5, 5 mg	2.5 mg qd	2.5-5 mg qd	No	Yes	+	6-12	Renal
Esmolol (Brevibloc)	No oral preparation	See Chapter 32	—	Yes	No	+	0.15	RBC esterase metabolism
Labetolol (Normodyne, Trandate)	tab: 100, 200, 300 mg	100 mg bid	200-400 mg bid	No	No	++	3-4	Hepatic
Metoprolol (Lopressor)	tab: 50, 100 mg	100 mg qd	50-100 mg bid	Yes	No	++	3-4	Hepatic
Nadolol (Corgard)	tab: 20, 40, 80 mg	40 mg qd	40-80 mg qd	No	No	+	14-24	Renal
Penbutolol (Levatol)	tab: 20 mg	20 mg qd	20 mg qd	No	Yes	++	5	Renal

KEY: +, low; ++, medium; +++, high; ISA, intrinsic sympathomimetic activity

Continued.

Table 33-18 Beta-adrenergic blocking agents[11]—cont'd

Drug	Oral Preparations	Initial Dosage	Maintenance Dosage	Cardioselectivity	ISA	Lipid Solubility	Elimination Half-life (hr)	Primary Excretion Route
Pindolol (Visken)	tab: 5, 10 mg	5 mg bid	5-10 mg bid	No	Yes	++	3-4	Hepatic/Renal
Propranolol (Inderal)	tab: 10, 20, 60, 80, 90 mg	10-20 mg bid	40-320 mg bid	No	No	+++	3-4	Hepatic
Timolol (Blocadren)	tab: 5, 10	10 mg	10-20 mg bid	No	No	+	4-5	Hepatic

Table 33-19 Calcium channel blockers

Agent	Oral Preparations	Initial Dosage	Myocardial Contractility	Chemical Class	AV Nodal Conduction	Cardiac Output	Peripheral Vasodilation	Safe for Concomitant Use with Beta Blocker
Diltiazem (Cardizem)	tab: 30, 60, 90, 120 mg (Cardizem SR): 60, 90, 120 mg	Angina: 30 mg tab qid; Hypertension: 60-120 mg cap bid (Cardizem SR)	$\downarrow$	Benzothiazepine	$\downarrow$	N/$\downarrow$	+	+
Nicardipine (Cardene)	cap: 20, 30 mg	Angina: 20 mg tid; Hypertension: 20 mg tid	N	Dihydropyridine	N	N/$\uparrow$	++	++
Nifedipine (Procardia, Adalat)	cap: 10, 20, mg tab (Procardia XL): 30, 60, 90 mg	Angina: 10 mg tid; Hypertension: 10 mg tid or 30 mg tab qd (Procardia XL)	$\downarrow$	Dihydropyridine	N	N/$\uparrow$	++	++
Verapamil (Calan, Isoptin, Verelan)	tab: 40, 80, 120 mg; SR tab: 240 mg; Caplet, SR: 120 mg; SR cap: 120 mg	Angina: 80 mg q8h; Hypertension: 120-240 mg qd (SR tab or cap)	$\downarrow\downarrow$	Phenylalkylamine	$\downarrow\downarrow$	$\downarrow$	+	0

KEY: SR, Sustained release preparation; XL, extended release preparation; $\uparrow$, increase; $\downarrow$, decrease; N, no significant effect; 0, least; ++, most

Table 33-20 Cephalosporins[5]

Agent	Preparations	Usual Dosage Range (Normal Renal Function)	Generation	Half-life (hr)
Cefadroxil (Ultracef, Duricef)	cap: 500 mg tab: 1 g oral susp: 125, 250, 500 mg/5 ml	PO: 1 g qd-bid	First	1.3
Cefazolin (Ancef, Kefzol)	inj: 250, 500 mg, 1 g	IV: 500 mg-1.5 g q6-8h	First	2
Cephalexin (Keflex)	Pulvules: 250, 500 mg susp: 125, 250 mg/5 ml tab: 250 mg, 500 mg, 1 g	PO: 250 mg-1 g q6h	First	1
Cephalotin (Keflin)	inj: 1, 2 g	IV: 500 mg-2 g q4-6h	First	0.6
Cephapirin (Cefadyl)	inj: 500 mg, 1g, 2g	IV: 500 mg-2 g q4-6h	First	0.5
Cephradine (Velosef, Anspor)	cap: 250, 500 mg susp: 125, 250 mg/5 ml inj: 250, 500 mg, 1 g	PO: 250-500 mg q6h IV: 500 mg-2 g q4-6h	First	1.0
Cefaclor (Ceclor)	Pulvules: 250, 500 mg susp: 125, 250 mg/5 ml	PO: 250-500 mg q8h	Second	1.0
Cefamandole (Mandol)	inj: 500 mg, 1 g, 2 g	IV: 500 mg-1 g q4-6h	Second	0.8

Cefmetazole (Zefazone)	inj: 1, 2 g	IV: 2 g q6-12h	Second	1.5
Cefonicid (Monocid)	inj: 500 mg, 1 g	IV: 1-2 g q24h	Second	4.0
Ceforanide (Precef)	inj: 500 mg, 1 g	IV: 0.5-1 g q12h	Second	2.9
Cefotetan (Cefotan)	inj: 1, 2 g	IV: 1-3 g q12h	Second	4.0
Cefoxitin (Mefoxin)	inj: 1, 2 g	IV: 1-2 g q6-8h	Second	0.8
Cefuroxime (Zinacef, Ceftin)	inj: 750 mg; tab: 125, 250, 500 mg	IV: 750 mg-1.5 g q8h; PO: 250-500 mg bid	Second	1.5
Cefixime (Suprax)	tab: 100, 400 mg; susp: 100 mg/5 ml	400 mg qd	Third	3-4
Cefoperazone (Cefobid)	inj: 1, 2 g	IV: 1-4 g bid	Third	2.0
Cefotaxime (Claforan)	inj: 1, 2 g	IV: 1 g q 12h-2g q4h	Third	1.0
Ceftazidime (Fortaz)	inj: 500 mg, 1, 2 g	IV: 1-2 g q8h	Third	1.8
Ceftizoxime (Cefizox)	inj: 1, 2 g	IV: 1-4 g q8h	Third	1.7
Ceftriaxone (Rocephin)	inj: 250 mg, 500 mg, 1 g, 2 g	IV: 1-2 g qd	Third	8.0
Moxalactam (Moxam)	inj: 1, 2 g	IV: 1-2 g q12h	Third	2.2

Table 33-21 Cholesterol-lowering agents

Agent	Preparations	Initial Dosage	Mechanism of Action	Effect
Cholestyramine	Questran powder: 378 g cans or packets containing 4 g of cholestyramine in 9 g of powder Questran Light: 210 g can or packets containing 4 g of cholestyramine in 5 g of powder Cholybar: chewable bar containing 4 g of cholestyramine (25 bars/box)	Powder: 1 packet or scoopful (4 g) qd mixed with water or other fluids Chewable bar: 1 qd with plenty of fluids	Bile acid sequestrant	↓ LDL N/↑ triglycerides
Colestipol (Colestid)	granules: 500 mg bottles or packets containing 5 g of granules	15 g bid	Bile acid sequestrant	↓ LDL N/↑ triglycerides
Gemfibrozil (Lopid)	tab: 600 mg cap: 300 mg	600 mg bid	↑ intravascular breakdown of VLDL	↓ triglycerides ↓ LDL ↑ HDL
Lovastatin (Mevacor)	tab: 20, 40 mg	20 mg qd	HMG-CoA reductase inhibitor	↓ LDL ↔/↑ HDL
Nicotinic acid (Niacin)	tab: 100, 250, 500 mg cap: 250, 300, 400, 500 mg	100 mg tid with or following meals; if tolerated gradually increase dose to 1 g tid	Decreases synthesis of VLDL and clearance of HDL	N/↓ LDL ↓ triglycerides ↔ HDL
Probucol (Lorelco)	tab: 250, 500 mg	250-500 mg bid	Enhances LDL metabolism	↓ LDL ↔ HDL

Table 33-22 Corticosteroid comparison chart

Drug	Equivalent Antiinflammatory Dosages (mg)	Gluco-corticoid Potency	Mineralo-corticoid Potency	Route of Administration
Prednisone	10	4	0.8	PO
Hydrocortisone (Solu-Cortef)	40	1.0	1.0	PO, IM, IV
Methylprednisolone (Solu-Medrol)	8	5.0	0.5	PO, IM, IV
Dexamethasone (Decadron)	1.5	30	0	PO, IV
Cortisone	50	0.8	0.8	PO, IM

Table 33-23 Dialyzability of selected drugs*

Drug	Hemodialysis	Peritoneal Dialysis	Route of Elimination
Acetaminophen	+	−	Hepatic
Amitriptyline	−	−	Hepatic
Aspirin	+	+	Renal
Cephalexin	+	+	Renal
Cephalothin	+	+	Renal
Diazepam	−		Hepatic and renal
Digoxin	−	−	Renal
Gentamicin	+	+	Renal
Heparin	−		
Isoniazid	+	+	Hepatic and renal
Lithium	+	+	Renal
Methadone	−	−	Hepatic
Methaqualone	+		Hepatic
Nitroprusside	+	+	
Penicillin G	+	−	Renal
Pentazocine	+		Hepatic
Phenobarbital	+	+	Hepatic
Phenytoin	−		Hepatic
Propoxyphene	−		Hepatic
Propranolol	−		Hepatic
Quinidine	+	+	Hepatic and renal
Secobarbital	−	−	Hepatic
Tetracyline	−	−	Renal

KEY: +, Yes; −, no.
*From DiGregorio GJ, Barbieri EJ, Piraino AJ: Handbook of commonly prescribed drugs, ed 4, Westchester Pa, 1984, Medical Surveillance Inc.

Table 33-24 Diuretics

Class	Agent	Preparations	Dosage (mg/day)	Site of Action
Thiazide	Chlorothiazide (Diuril)	tab: 250, 500 mg susp: 250 mg/5 ml	125-500	Distal tubule
	Hydrochlorothiazide (Esidrix)	tab: 25, 50, 100	12.5-50	Distal tubule
	Methyclothiazide (Enduron)	tab: 2.5, 5 mg	2.5-5	Distal tubule
Phthalimidine derivative	Chlorthalidone (Hygroton)	tab: 25, 50, 100 mg	12.5-50	Distal tubule
Quinazoline	Metolazone (Diulo, Zaroxolyn, Mykrox)	tab: 2.5, 5, 10 mg tab: 0.5 mg (Mykrox)	2.5-10 0.5 (Mykrox)	Cortical diluting site and proximal convoluted tubule
Indoline	Indapamide (Lozol)	tab: 2.5 mg	2.5-5	Distal tubule

Loop	Bumetanide (Bumex)	tab: 0.5, 1, 2 mg inj: 0.25 mg/ml	0.5-5 PO/IV/IM	Ascending limb of loop of Henle
	Ethacrynic acid (Edecrin)	tab: 25, 50 mg	25-100	Ascending limb of loop of Henle
	Furosemide (Lasix)	tab: 20, 40, 80 mg oral sol: 10 mg/ml inj: 10 mg/ml	20-160 PO/IV/IM	Ascending limb of loop of Henle
Potassium-sparing	Amiloride (Midamor)	tab: 5 mg	5-10	Distal tubule
	Spironolactone (Aldactone)	tab: 25, 50, 100	25-100	Distal tubule
	Triamterene (Dyrenium)	cap: 50, 100	50-150	Distal tubule

Table 33-25 Histamine H_2 receptor antagonists

Agent	Preparations	Dosage
Cimetidine (Tagamet)	tab: 200, 300, 400, 800 mg liq: 300 mg/5 ml inj: 300 mg/2 ml	Active peptic ulcer disease: 800 mg qhs Maintenance: 400 mg qhs IV: 300 mg q6-8h or total dose administered as continuous infusion over 24 hr
Famotidine (Pepcid)	tab: 20, 40 mg oral susp: 40 mg/5 ml inj: 10 mg/ml	Active peptic ulcer disease: 40 mg qhs Maintenance: 20 mg qhs IV: 20 mg q12h or total dose administered as continuous infusion over 24 hr
Nizatidine (Axid)	Pulvules: 150, 300 mg	Active peptic ulcer: 300 mg qhs Maintenance: 150 mg qhs
Ranitidine (Zantac)	tab: 150, 300 mg susp: 15 mg/ml inj: 25 mg/ml	Active peptic ulcer: 300 mg qhs Maintenance: 150 mg qhs IV: 50 mg q6-8h or total dose administered as continuous infusion over 24 hr

Table 33-26 Insulin preparations

Preparation	Onset of Action*	Duration of Action*	Peak Effect*
Rapid-acting			
Regular (crystalline zinc)	30-60 min	5-7 hr	2-4 hr
Semilente	30 min-3 hr	12-16 hr	4-8 hr
Intermediate-acting			
NPH	2 hr	18-28 hr	6-12 hr
Lente	2-4 hr	24-28 hr	6-12 hr
Long-acting			
Protamine zinc insulin (PZI)	4-6 hr	24-36 hr	8-14 hr
Ultralente	4-6 hr	36+ hr	12-16 hr
Mixture of NPH and regular (70/30 mixture)	60 min	18-28 hr	2-12 hr

*After subcutaneous injection. The onset, duration of action, and peak effect vary with each patient and are influenced by the site and depth of injection, as well as the concentration and volume.

Table 33-27   Laxatives

Class	Agent	Dosage
Bulk-forming agents	Calcium polycarbophil (Fibercon)	2 tab qd-qid with 8 oz of liquid after each dose
	High fiber supplement (Fibermed)	2 biscuits qd
	Psyllium hydrophilic mucilloid (Metamucil)	1 Tbsp or packet qd-tid with 8 oz of liquid with each dose
	Psyllium, senna (Perdiem)	1 Tbsp qd-bid with 8 oz of liquid with each dose
Osmotic agents	Lactulose (Chronulac, Cephulac)	1-2 Tbsp qd-bid
	Sorbitol (30-70%)	30 ml qd
	Glycerin suppository	1-2 qd
Stimulants	Castor oil	30-60 ml qd
	Bisacodyl (Dulcolax)	5-15 mg PO qd 10 mg PR qd
	Phenolphthalein (Ex Lax)	1-2 qd
Emollients	Casanthranol docusate sodium (Pericolace)	100 mg PO bid
Salts	Milk of magnesia	30 ml qd
	Magnesium citrate	30 ml qd

Table 33-28 Narcotic analgesic comparison charts

Drug	Equivalent PO Dose (mg)	Duration of Analgesia (hr)
A. PO Analgesics		
Codeine	200	4-6
Hydromorphone (Dilaudid)	7.5	4-6
Levorphanol (Levor-Dromoran)	4	4-7
Meperidine (Demerol)	300	4-6
Methadone (Dolophine)	20	3-5
Morphine	60	4-7
Oxycodone (Percodan)	30	3-5
Pentazocine (Talwin Nx)	180	4-7
Propoxyphene (Darvon)	240	4-6
B. IM Analgesics (Conversion from PO to IM: Codeine 200 mg PO = 130 mg IM)		
Codeine	130	4-6
Buprenorphine (Buprenex)	0.3	3-6
Butorphanol (Stadol)	2.0	3-6
Hydromorphone (Dilaudid)	1.5	4-5
Levorphanol (Levo-Dromoran)	2	4-6
Meperidine (Demerol)	75	4-6
Methadone (Dolophine)	10	3-5
Morphine	10	4-6
Nalbuphine (Nubain)	10	3-6
Pentazocine (Talwin Nx)	60	4-6

C. Combination Analgesics

Drug	Content *(mg)*
Tylenol with codeine no. 2	Acetaminophen 300, codeine 15
Tylenol with codeine no. 3	Acetaminophen 300, codeine 30
Tylenol with codeine no. 4	Acetaminophen 300, codeine 60
Percocet	Acetaminophen 325, oxycodone HCl 5
Percodan	Aspirin 325, oxycodone HCl 5,
Tylox	Acetaminophen 500, oxycodone HCl 5,
Darvocet-N-100	Acetaminophen 650, propoxyphene napsylate 100
Talwin compound	Aspirin 325, pentazocine HCl 12.5
Vicodin	Acetaminophen 500 mg, hydrocodone bitartrate 5 mg

Table 33-29 Nitrates for angina

Drug	Dosage and Preparations	Onset of Action (min)	Duration of Action (hr)
Nitroglycerin			
Sublingual (Nitrostat)	0.15-0.6 mg q5min prn (0.15, 0.3, 0.4, 0.6 mg)	1-3	½-1
Lingual aerosol (Nitrolingual spray)	0.4 mg/metered dose prn (200 metered doses/inhal)	1-3	½-1
2% ointment (Nitrobid)	2.5-12.5 cm q4-6h (20, 60 g tubes)	15	3-6
Transdermal (Transderm Nitro, Nitrodur, Nitrodisc, Minitran, Deponit)	Infusion system 0.1 mg/hr (2.5 mg/24hr) 0.2 mg/hr (5 mg/24 hr) 0.3 mg/hr (7.5 mg/24 hr) 0.4 mg/hr (10 mg/24 hr) 0.6 mg/hr (15 mg/24 hr)	30-60	up to 24
Isosorbide dinitrate (Isordil)	10-40 mg q6h (tab: 5, 10, 20, 30, 40 mg)	30	3-6
Intravenous (Tridil, Nitrostat)	50 mg/500 ml; inititate infusion at 5 μg/min	1-2	3-5 min

Table 33-30 Nonsteroidal antiinflammatory drugs (NSAIDs)

Agent	Preparations	Dosage	Plasma Half-life (hr)	Chemical Class
Aspirin	tab: 325, 500, 650, 800, 975 mg supp: 325, 650	325-650 mg q4h	9-16	Salicylate
Diclofenac (Voltaren)	tab: 25, 50, 75 mg	50-75 mg bid	2	Phenylacetic
Diflunisal (Dolobid)	tab: 250, 500 mg	250-500 mg q8-12h	8-12	Salicylate
Fenopren (Nalfon)	tab: 600 mg	200-600 mg tid-qid	3	Propionic acid
Flurbiprofen (Ansaid)	tab: 50, 100 mg	100 mg bid-tid	5	Propionic acid
Ibuprofen (Motrin)	tab: 200, 300, 400, 600, 800 mg	200-800 mg tid-qid	2	Propionic acid
Indomethacin (Indocin)	cap: 25, 50, 75 mg (SR) supp: 50 mg; susp: 25 mg/5 ml	PO: 25-50 mg tid (SR qd-bid) PR: 50 mg qd	5-6	Indole acetic acid
Ketoprofen (Orudis)	cap: 25, 50, 75 mg	50-75 mg tid	2	Propionic acid
Ketorolac (Toradol)	Prefilled syringe: 15, 30, 60 mg	30-60 mg IM initially followed by 15-30 mg IM q6h	4-6	Propionic acid
Meclofenamate (Meclomen)	cap: 50, 100 mg	50 mg q4-6h	4	Fenamic acid
Naproxen (Naprosyn, Anaprox)	tab: 250, 375, 500 mg susp: 125 mg/5 ml Anaprox tabs: 275, 550 mg	250-500 mg bid 275-550 mg bid	12-15	Proprionic acid
Piroxicam (Feldene)	10, 20 mg	20 mg qd	40	Oxicam
Salsalate (Disalcid)	tab: 500, 750 mg cap: 500 mg	1500 mg bid	3-16	Salicylate
Sulindac (Clinoril)	tab: 150, 200 mg	150-200 mg bid	16	Indole acetic acid
Tolmectin (Tolectin)	tab: 200, 400, 600 mg	200-600 mg tid	2	Indole acetic acid

Table 33-31   Potassium supplements

Product	Brand Name	Potassium Content
Potassium chloride		
Slow-release tablets	Slow-K	8 mEq/tab
	Klotrix	10 mEq/tab
	Ten K	10 mEq/tab
	K-Tab	10 mEq/tab
	K-Dur-10	10 mEq/tab
	K-Dur-20	20 mEq/tab
Slow-release capsules	Micro-K-Extencaps	8 mEq/cap
	Micro-K 10 Extencaps	10 mEq/cap
Effervescent tablets	Klorvess	20 mEq/tab
	K-lyte/Cl	25 mEq/tab
	K-lyte/Cl-50	50 mEq/tab
Powder	K-Lor	15 mEq/Pkt
		20 mEq/Pkt
	K-Ciel	20 mEq/Pkt
	K-Lyte/Cl	25 mEq/Pkt
Potassium bicarbonate and citrate	K-Lyte effervescent tab	25 mEq/tab
	K-Lyte DS effervescent tab	50 mEq/tab
Potassium gluconate	Kaon	5 mEq/tab
	Kaon elixir	20 mEq/15 ml

Table 33-32 Quinolone antibiotics[9]

Agent	Preparations	Dosage	Elimination Half-life* (hr)	Renal Elimination (%) Parent Compound	Metabolites
Norfloxacin (Noroxin)	tab: 400 mg	UTI: 400 mg bid	3.5	30	10
Ciprofloxacin (Cipro)	tab: 250, 500, 750 mg	Uncomplicated UTI: 250 mg q12h	4.0	35	15
		Bone/joint infections: 750 mg q12h			
		Other infections: 500 mg q12h			
	inj†: 200–400 mg q12h				

*Normal renal function.
†Pending FDA approval.

Table 33-33 Commonly used sulfonylureas

Drug	Starting Dose (mg)	Maximum Daily Dose	Frequency	Duration of Action (hr)
First generation				
Tolbutamide (Orinase)	500	1.5 g	qd, bid	6-12
Tolazamide (Tolinase)	100	1.0 g	qd, bid	12-14
Chlorpropamide (Diabinese)	250	750 mg	qd	≥36
Second generation				
Glyburide* (Diabeta, Micronase)	2.5	20 mg	qd, bid	Up to 24
Glipizide (Glucotrol)	5.0	40 mg	qd, bid	12-24

*Useful in patients with renal disease because of dual excretion routes (urine and bile).

Table 33-34 Sympathomimetic agents (inhaled)

Agent	Adult Dosage	Beta Adrenergic Selectivity	Potency	Onset (min)	Duration (hr)
Albuterol (Proventil, Ventolin)	MDI: 2 inhalations q4-6h (max of 12 inh/24 hr) Nebul: 0.5-1.0 ml (2.5-5.0 mg) in 3 ml saline tid-qid	+++	+++	10-15	3-5
Isoetharine (Bronkosol, Bronkometer)	MDI: 2 inhalations 4-6 times/day Nebul: 0.5 ml in 3 ml saline q2-4h	+	+	2-10	1-3
Metaproterenol (Alupent, Metaprel)	MDI: 2-3 inhalations q3-4h (max of 12 inh/24 hr) Nebul: 0.2-0.3 ml in 2.5 ml saline tid-qid (max of q4h)	++	++	2-5	3-4
Terbutaline (Brethaire)	MDI: 2 inhalations q4-6h (max of 12 inh/24 hr)	+++	+++	5-30	3-6

Key: MDI, Metered dose inhaler; Nebul, nebulizer; +, least; +++, most

Table 33-35   Topical steroid preparations*

Agent	Common Brand Names	Potency
Betamethasone		
Betamethasone valerate 0.01%	Valisone cream, lotion 0.01%	Low
Betamethasone valerate 0.1%	Valisone cream, ointment 0.1%	Intermediate
Betamethasone benzoate 0.025%	Benisone gel, Uticort gel (0.1%)	Intermediate
Betamethasone dipropionate 0.05-0.1%	Diprosone cream (0.05%), Diprosone aerosol (0.1%)	High
Betamethasone dipropionate augmented 0.05%	Diprolene ointment 0.05%	Ultra-high
Desoximethasone		
Desoximethasone 0.05%	Topicort LP cream 0.05%	Intermediate
Desoximethasone 0.25%	Topicort cream, ointment	High
Fluocinolone		
Fluocinolone acetonide 0.01%	Synalar cream, solution 0.01%	Low
Fluocinolone acetonide 0.025%	Synalar ointment 0.025%	Intermediate
Fluocinolone acetonide 0.2%	Synalar HP cream 0.2%	High
Fluocinonide 0.05%	Lidex cream, gel 0.05%	High
Hydrocortisone		
Hydrocortisone base or acetate 0.5%	Corticaine cream 0.5%	Low
Hydrocortisone base or acetate 1, 2.5%	Hytone cream 1%, 2.5%	Low
Hydrocortisone valerate 0.2%	Westcort cream, ointment 0.2%	Intermediate
Triamcinolone		
Triamcinolone acetonide 0.025%	Aristocort, Kenalog 0.025%	Low
Triamcinolone acetonide 0.1%	Aristocort, Kenalog 0.1%	Intermediate
Triamcinolone acetonide 0.5%	Aristocort, Kenalog 0.5%	High

*NOTE: Most of these preparations are available in 15 g tubes.

Table 33-36 Ventricular dysrhythmia agents[2] (oral)*

Agent	Oral Dosage	Elimination Half-life	Group	ECG Manifestations	Toxic Serum Levels ($\mu g/ml$)
Amiodarone (Cordarone)	Loading: 800-1600 mg/day for 1-3 wk, then 600-800 mg/day for 4 wk Maintenance: 100-400 mg/day	26-107 days	III	Prolonged QRS, QT, and PR; sinus bradycardia	—
Disopyramide (Norpace)	100-200 mg q6h	4-8 hr; 8-12 hr for sustained-release form 1-2 hr	IA	Prolonged QRS, QT, and PR (+/−)	>9
Encainide (Enkaid)	Initially 25 mg q8h Maintenance: 25-50 mg q8h	1-2 hr	IC	Prolonged QRS, PR	—
Flecainide (Tambocor)	Initially 100 mg q12h Maintenance: 100-200 mg q12h	12-26	IC	Prolonged QRS, PR	>1

Mexiletine (Mexitil)	Initially 100-200 mg q8h Maintenance: 100-300 mg q6-12h	10-12 hr	IB	No significant change	>2
Procainamide (Pronestyl)	50 mg/kg/day in divided doses q3-4 h (q6h for slow release form)	3-4 hr; 6 hr for sustained-release form	IA	Prolonged QRS, QT, and PR (+/−)	>16
Propafenone (Rythmol)	Initially 150 mg q 8 h; dosage may be increased at a minimum of 3-4 day intervals to 225 mg q8h	2-10 hr	IC	Prolonged QRS, PR	—
Quinidine sulfate	200-400 mg q4-6h	6-11 hr	IA	Prolonged QRS, QT, and PR (+/−)	>8
Tocainide (Tonocard)	Initially 200-400 mg q8h Maintenance: 200-600 mg q8h	12 hr	IB	No significant change	>10

*Refer to Table 20-7 for IV agents used in ventricular dysrhythmias.

References

1. A.M.A. Division of Drugs and American Society for Clinical Pharmacology and Therapeutics: AMA drug evaluation, ed 5, Philadelphia, 1983, WB Saunders Co.
2. Bigger JT Jr, Hoffman BF, Gilman AG, et al (editors): Goodman and Gilman's Clinical basis of therapeutics, ed 7, New York, 1985, The Macmillan Co, p 754.
3. Bodey G: Topical and systemic antifungal agents, Med Clin North Am 72:637, 1988.
4. Donowitz GR, Mandell GL: Beta-lactam antibiotics, I, N Engl J Med 318:419, 1988.
5. Donowitz GR, Mandell GL: Beta-lactam antibiotics. II, N Engl J Med 318:490, 1988.
6. Gillin JC, Byerley WF: Drug therapy; the diagnosis and management of insomnia, N Engl J Med 322:243, 1990.
7. Krishnan KR, France RD: Antidepressants in chronic pain syndromes, American Family Physician, vol 39, p 235, 1989.
8. Drugs for psychotic disorders, Med Lett Drugs Ther 31:13, 1989.
9. Molavi A: Fluoroquinolones, American Family Physician, vol 37, p 279, 1988.
10. Sanford JP: Guide to antimicrobial therapy, West Bethesda Md, 1989, Antimicrobial Therapy Inc, p. 102.
11. Wallin JD, Shah SV: Beta adrenergic blocking agents in the treatment of hypertension, Arch Intern Med 147:654, 1987.
12. Williams: GH: Converting-enzyme inhibitors in the treatment of hypertension, N Engl J Med 319:1517, 1988.

Appendixes

APPENDIX I: ENTERAL NUTRITIONAL PRODUCTS

Routine oral or tube supplemental feeding (Ensure)

Intact protein, protein isolates, lactose-free product: each 100 ml contains

Protein	3.65 g	Calcium	2.7 mEq
Carbohydrate	14.24 g	Chloride	3.0 mEq
Fat	3.65 g	Calories	106
Potassium	3.2 mEq	mOsm = 450	
Sodium	3.3 mEq		

This product also contains all known essential vitamins and minerals for adults and for children 4 or more years of age.

Routine tube feeding (Isocal)

Lactose-free and low in sodium; each 100 ml contains

Protein	3.25 g	Calcium	3.00 mEq
Carbohydrate	12.50 g	Chloride	2.80 mEq
Fat	4.20 g	Calories	100
Potassium	3.20 mEq	mOsm =300	
Sodium	2.20 mEq		

This product also contains all known essential vitamins and minerals for adults and for children 4 or more years of age.

Routine tube feeding (Osmolite HN)

Lactose-free and low in sodium; each 100 ml contains

Protein	4.4g	Calcium	76 mg
Carbohydrate	13.9 g	Chloride	4.1 mEq
Fat	3.6 g	Calories	106
Potassium	4.0 mEq	mOsm = 310	
Sodium	4.0 mEq		

This product also contains all known essential vitamins and minerals for adults and for children 4 or more years of age.

High-calorie supplemental feeding (Magnacal)

Lactose-free product; each 100 ml contains

Protein	7.0 g	Calcium	5.0 mEq
Carbohydrate	25.0 g	Chloride	2.7 mEq
Fat	8.0 g	Calories	200
Potassium	3.2 mEq	mOsm = 590	
Sodium	4.3 mEq		

This product also contains all known essential vitamins and minerals for adults and for children 4 or more years of age.

Low-residue oral or tube feeding (Criticare)

High-nitrogen elemental diet; each 100 ml contains

Protein	3.80 g
Carbohydrate	22.20 g
Fat	0.03 g
Calories	106

mOsm = 650

This product also contains all known essential vitamins and minerals for adults and for children 4 or more years of age.

Essential amino acid formulation (Amin-Aid)

Nutritional product for management of uremic patients; each 100 ml contains

Protein	1.94 g
Carbohydrate	36.54 g
Fat	4.62 g
Calories	195.5

mOsm = 850

This product is low in electrolytes and contains no vitamins.

Branched-chain amino acid formulation (Hepatic-Aid)

Nutritional management of liver disease; each 100 ml contains

Protein	4.26 g
Carbohydrate	28.80 g
Fat	3.62 g
Calories	164.7

mOsm = 900

This product contains negligible electrolytes and no vitamins or minerals.

Oral supplemental feeding (Citrotein)

Lactose-free, cholesterol-free, gluten-free; each 100 ml contains

Protein	4.29 g
Carbohydrate	13.0 g
Fat	0.18 g
Potassium	1.9 mEq
Sodium	3.2 mEq
Calcium	5.6 mEq
Chloride	2.9 mEq
Calories	71

mOsm = 496

Routine oral supplemental feeding (Forta Pudding)

Each 150 g contains

Protein	6.8 g
Carbohydrate	34.0 g
Fat	9.7 g
Potassium	7.7 mEq
Sodium	9.6 mEq
Calcium	10.0 mEq
Chloride	6.0 mEq
Calories	250

This product also contains all known essential vitamins and minerals for adults and for children 4 or more years of age.

Caloric additive product (Polycose)

Each 100 ml contains

Carbohydrate	50.0 g
Potassium	0.5 mEq
Sodium	2.5 mEq
Calcium	1.5 mEq
Chloride	3.1 mEq
Calories	200

mOsm = 850

Routine oral supplemental feeding (Instant Breakfast)

Each 100 ml contains

Protein	6.25 g
Carbohydrate	12.10 g
Fat	3.40 g
Potassium	5.90 mEq
Sodium	4.70 mEq
Calcium	7.30 mEq
Chloride	n/a
Calories	103.6

Nutritionally complete supplement when mixed with 8 oz. whole milk.

High-protein clear liquid product (high-protein gelatin)

Each 150 ml contains

Protein	17.0 g
Carbohydrate	18.0 g
Fat	0.0 g
Potassium	5.3 mEq
Sodium	10.8 mEq
Calories	140

This product may be used as a supplement on clear liquid diets.

APPENDIX II: NOMOGRAM FOR CALCULATION OF BODY SURFACE AREA

Place a straight edge from the patient's height in the left column to his weight in the right column. The point of intersection on the body surface area column indicates the body surface area (BSA). Reproduced from Behrman RE, Vaughn VC (editors): Nelson's Textbook of pediatrics, ed 12, Philadelphia, 1983, WB Saunders Co.

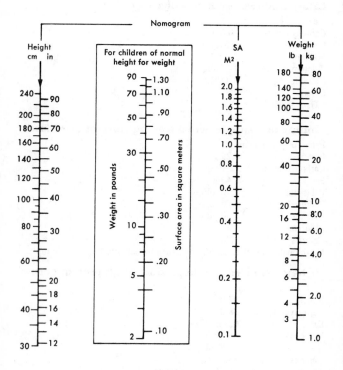

APPENDIX III: PARAMETERS OF NUTRITIONAL ASSESSMENT

Test	Degree of malnutrition			Na_e/K_e Correlation	Reflects
	Mild	Moderate	Severe		
Ideal body weight (%)	80-90	70-80	<70	—	Total body change
Usual body weight (%)	85-95	75-85	<75	—	Total body change
Creatinine height index	—	60% to 80%	<60%	0.37	Lean body mass change
Skinfold thickness (%)*	35-40	25-35	<25	0.79	Fat mass status
Midarm circumference (%)*	35-40	25-35	<25	0.68	Lean body mass change
Albumin (g/100 ml)	2.8-3.5	2.1-2.7	<2.1	0.67	Visceral protein status
Transferrin (mg/100 ml)	150-200	100-150	<100	—	Visceral protein status
Absolute lymphocyte count (thousands of cells/mm³)	1.2-2.0	0.8-1.2	<0.8	—	Visceral protein status and immunocompetence

*Measured against a percentile table of norms.

Reproduced from Cerra FB: Manual of critical care, St Louis, 1987, The CV Mosby Co.

APPENDIX IV: CONVERSION FORMULAS

1. Temperature
   a. °C = (°F − 32) × 5/9
   b. °F = (°C × 9/5) + 32
2. Weight
   a. 1 lb = 0.454 kg
   b. 1 kg = 2.204 lb
   c. 10 grains = 650 mg
   d. 400 micrograms = 1/150 grain
3. Length
   a. 1 inch = 2.54 cm
   b. 1 cm = 0.3937 inch
4. Liquid
   a. 100 ml = 3.38 fluid ounces
   b. 1 fluid ounce = 30 ml approx
   c. 1 tablespoon = 15 ml
   d. 1 teaspoon = 5 ml

APPENDIX V: FREQUENTLY USED CLINICAL FORMULAS (ADULTS)

1. Calculation of creatinine clearance (CCr)

$$CCr \text{ (male)} = \frac{(140 - age) \times wt \text{ (in kg)}}{Serum\ creatinine \times 72}$$
$$CCr \text{ (female)} = 0.85 \times CCr \text{ (male)}$$

2. Alveolar-arterial oxygen gradient (Aa gradient)

$$Aa\ Gradient = \left[(713)\ (FIo_2) - \left(\frac{PaCO_2}{0.8} \right) \right] - Pao_2$$

Normal Aa gradient = 5-15 mm
FIo_2 = Fraction of inspired oxygen (normal = 0.21-1.0)
$Paco_2$ = Arterial carbon dioxide tension (normal = 35-45 mmHg)
Pao_2 = Arterial partial pressure oxygen (normal = 70-100 mmHg)
Differential diagnosis of Aa gradient:

Abnormality	15% O_2	100% O_2
Diffusion defect	Increased gradient	Correction of gradient
Ventilation/Perfusion mismatch	Increased gradient	Partial or complete correction of gradient
Right-to-left shunt (intracardiac or pulmonary)	Increased gradient	Increased gradient (no correction)

3. Anion gap
$$AG = Na^+ - (Cl^- + HCO_3^-)$$

4. Fractional excretion of sodium

$$FE_{Na} = \frac{U_{Na} / P_{Na}}{U_{Cr} / P_{Cr}} \times 100$$

5. Serum osmolality

$$Osm = 2\ (Na^+ + K^+) + \frac{Glucose}{18} + \frac{BUN}{2.8}$$

6. Corrected sodium in hyperglycemic patients

$$Corrected\ Na^+ = Measured\ Na^+ + 1.6 \times \frac{Glucose - 140}{100}$$

7. Water deficit in hypernatremic patients

$$Water\ deficit\ (in\ liters) = 0.6 \times body\ weight\ (kg) \times \frac{Measured\ serum\ sodium}{Normal\ serum\ sodium}$$

APPENDIX VI: COMMONLY USED COMBINATION DRUG PREPARATIONS*

Trade Name	Therapeutic Category	Dosage Forms and Composition	Common Adult Dosage
Actifed	Decongestant-antihistamine	tab: pseudoephedrine (60 mg), triprolidine (2.5 mg) syrup: pseudoephedrine (30 mg), triprolidine (1.25 mg/5 ml	1 tab tid-qid PO 10 ml tid-qid PO
Actifed-C Expectorant (C5)	Antitussive-expectorant	syrup: pseudoephedrine (30 mg), triprolidine (1.25 mg), codeine (10 mg), guaifenesin (100 mg)/5 ml	10 ml tid-qid PO
Aldactazide	Diuretic	tab: spironolactone (25 mg), hydrochlorothiazide (25 mg)	1 tab bid-qid PO
Aldoril-15	Antihypertensive	tab: hydrochlorothiazide (15 mg), methyldopa (250 mg)	1 tab bid-tid PO
Aldoril-30		tab: hydrochlorothiazide (30 mg), methyldopa (250 mg)	1 tab bid-tid PO
Aldoril D30		tab: hydrochlorothiazide (30 mg), methyldopa (500 mg)	1 tab bid-tid PO
Aldoril D50		tab: hydrochlorothiazide (50 mg), methyldopa (500 mg)	1 tab bid-tid PO
Anusol-HC	Hemorrhoidal preparation	cream and supp: hydrocortisone (0.5%), bismuth subgallate (2.25%), bismuth resorcinol (1.75%), benzyl benzoate (1.2%), zinc oxide (11%), Peruvian balsam (1.8%)	cream: topically prn supp: 1 PR bid

Bactrim	Antibacterial	tab: trimethoprim (80 mg), sulfamethox-azole (400 mg)	2 tab q12h PO
		susp: trimethoprim (40 mg), sulfamethox-azole (200 mg)/5 ml	20 ml q12H PO
		inj: trimethoprim (80 mg), sulfamethox-azole (400 mg)/5 ml	Total daily dosage: 8-20 mg/kg (based on trimethoprim) in 2-4 equally divided doses q6,8,or12h
Bactrim DS	Antibacterial	tab: trimethoprim (160 mg), sulfamethox-azole (800 mg)	1 tab q12h PO
Cortisporin Otic	Steroid-antibiotic	sol and susp: hydrocortisone (1%), neo-mycin (5 mg), polymyxin B (10,000 U)/ml	4 gtt into ear tid-qid
Darvocet-N 100 (C4)	Narcotic analgesic	tab: propoxyphene (100 mg), acetamino-phen (650 mg)	1 tab q4h prn pain PO
Darvon Compound-65 (C4)	Narcotic analgesic	cap: propoxyphene (65 mg), aspirin (389 mg), caffeine (32.4 mg)	1 cap q4h prn pain PO
Deconamine	Decongestant-antihistamine	tab: pseudoephedrine (60 mg), chlorphe-niramine (4 mg) syrup: pseudophedrine (30 mg), chlor-pheniramine (2 mg)/5 ml	1 tab q4-8h PO
Demulen 1/50	Oral contraceptive	tab: ethynodiol (1 mg), ethinyl estradiol (50 μg)	1 tab qd PO

Continued.

KEY: C2, Controlled substance, schedule II; C3, schedule III; C4, schedule IV; C5, schedule V.
*From DiGregorio GJ, Barbieri EJ, Piraino AJ: Handbook of commonly prescribed drugs, ed 4, Westchester Pa, 1984, Medical Surveillance Inc.

APPENDIX VI: COMMONLY USED COMBINATION DRUG PREPARATIONS*—cont'd

Trade Name	Therapeutic Category	Dosage Forms and Composition	Common Adult Dosage
Dimetapp	Decongestant-antihistamine	elix: brompheniramine (2 mg), phenylpropanolamine (12.5 mg)/5 ml tab: brompheniramine (4 mg), phenylpropanolamine (25 mg)	5-10 ml tid-qid PO 1 tab q4h PO
Donnatal	Antispasmodic	cap and tab: atropine (19.4 μg), scopolamine (6.5 μg), hyoscyamine (0.1 mg), phenobarbital (16.2 mg) elix: atropine (19.4 μg), scopolamine (6.5 μg), hyoscyamine (0.1 mg), phenobarbital (16.2 mg), alcohol (23%)/5 ml	1-2 cap or tab tid-qid PO 5-10 ml tid-qid PO
Drixoral	Decongestant-antihistamine	tab: pseudoephedrine (120 mg), dexbrompheniramine (6 mg)	1 tab q12h PO
Dyazide	Diuretic	cap: triamterene (50 mg), hydrochlorothiazide (25 mg)	1 cap qd-bid PO
Empirin w/codeine #2 (C3)	Narcotic analgesic	tab: aspirin (325 mg), codeine (15 mg)	1-2 tab q4h prn pain PO
Empirin w/codeine #3 (C3)		tab: aspirin (325 mg), codeine (30 mg)	1-2 tab q4h prn pain PO
Empirin w/codeine #4 (C3)		tab: aspirin (325 mg), codeine (60 mg)	1 tab q4h prn pain PO
Entex LA	Expectorant	tab: phenylpropanolamine (75 mg), guaifenesin (400 mg)	1 tab q12h PO

Equagesic (C4)	Nonnarcotic analgesic	tab: aspirin (325 mg), meprobamate (200 mg)	1-2 tab tid-qid PO
Fiorinal (C3)	Nonnarcotic analgesic	tab and cap: aspirin (325 mg), caffeine (40 mg), butalbital (50 mg)	1-2 tab or cap q4h PO
Fiorinal w/codeine #1 (C3)	Narcotic analgesic	cap: Fiorinal components + codeine (7.5 mg)	1-2 cap, repeat prn up to 6 caps qd PO
Fiorinal w/codeine #2 (C3)		cap: Fiorinal components + codeine (15 mg)	
Fiorinal w/codeine #3 (C3)		cap: Fiorinal components + codeine (30 mg)	
Hydropres 25	Antihypertensive	tab: hydrochlorothiazide (25 mg), reserpine (0.125 mg)	1-2 tab qd-bid PO
Hydropres 50		tab: hydrochlorothiazide (50 mg), reserpine (0.125 mg)	1 tab qd-bid PO
Inderide-40/25	Antihypertensive	tab: propranolol (40 mg), hydrochlorothiazide (25 mg)	1-2 tab qd-bid PO
Inderide-80/25		tab: propranolol (80 mg), hydrochlorothiazide (25 mg)	1-2 tab qd-bid PO
K-Lyte	Potassium supplement	tab: potassium bicarbonate and potassium citrate (25 mEq)	1 tab, dissolved in cold water, bid-qid PO
Librax	Antispasmodic	cap: clidinium (2.5 mg), chlordiazepoxide (5 mg)	1-2 cap tid-qid PO
Limbitrol 5-12.5 (C4)	Antianxiety-antidepressant	tab: chlordiazepoxide (5 mg), amitriptyline (12.5 mg)	1 tab tid-qid PO

continued.

KEY: C2, Controlled substance, schedule II; C3, schedule III; C4, schedule IV; C5, schedule V.

*From DiGregorio GJ, Barbieri EJ, Piraino AJ: Handbook of commonly prescribed drugs, ed 4, Westchester Pa, 1984, Medical Surveillance Inc.

APPENDIX VI: COMMONLY USED COMBINATION DRUG PREPARATIONS*—cont'd

Trade Name	Therapeutic Category	Dosage Forms and Composition	Common Adult Dosage
Limbitrol 10-25 (C4)		tab: chlordiazepoxide (10 mg), amitriptyline (25 mg)	1 tab tid-qid PO
Lomotil (C5)	Antidiarrheal	tab: diphenoxylate (2.5 mg), atropine (0.025 mg)	10 ml qid PO
		liq: diphenoxylate (2.5 mg), atropine (0.025 mg)/5 ml	
Lo/Ovral	Oral contraceptive	tab: norgestrel (0.3 mg), ethinyl estradiol (30 μg)	1 tab qd PO
Mycolog II	Steroid-antibiotic	cream and oint: triamcinolone (0.1%), nystatin (100,000 U)/g	Topically bid-tid
Naldecon	Decongestant-antihistamine	tab: phenylpropanolamine (40 mg), phenylephrine (10 mg), chlorpheniramine (5 mg), phenyltoloxamine (15 mg)	1 tab tid PO
		syrup: phenylpropanolamine (20 mg), phenylephrine (5 mg), chlorpheniramine (2.5 mg), phenyltoloxamine (7.5 mg)/5 ml	5 ml q3-4h PO
Neosporin	Antibiotic	oint: polymyxin B (5000 U), neomycin (3.5 mg), bacitracin (400 U)/g	Topically 2-5 × qd
		ophth oint: polymyxin B (10,000 U), neomycin (3.5 mg), bacitracin (400 U)/g	Apply to eye(s) q3-4h

		ophth drop: polymyxin B (10,000 U), neomycin (1.75 mg), gramicidin (25 µg)/ml	2 gtt to eye(s) bid-qid
		cream: polymyxin B (10,000 U), neomycin (3.5 mg), gramicidin (0.25 mg)/g	Topically 2-5 × qd
Norgesic Forte	Skeletal muscle relaxant	tab: orphenadrine (50 mg), aspirin (770 mg), caffeine (60 mg)	1 tab tid-qid PO
Ormade	Decongestant-antihistamine	cap: phenylpropanolamine (75 mg), chlorpheniramine (12 mg)	1 cap q12h PO
Ortho-Novum	Oral contraceptive	tab: norethindrone (1 mg), mestranol (30 µg)	1 tab qd PO
Ovral	Oral contraceptive	tab: norgestrel (0.5 mg), ethinyl estradiol (50 µg)	1 tab qd PO
Ovulen	Oral contraceptive	tab: ethynodiol (1 mg), mestranol (100 µg)	1 tab qd PO
Parafon Forte	Skeletal muscle relaxant	tab: chlorzoxazone (250 mg), acetaminophen (300 mg)	2 tab qid PO
Percocet-5 (C2)	Narcotic analgesic	tab: oxycodone (5 mg), acetaminophen (325 mg)	1 tab q6h prn pain PO
Percodan (C2)	Narcotic analgesic	tab: oxycodone (5 mg), aspirin (325 mg)	1 tab q6h prn pain PO
Phenergan VC w/Codeine (C5)	Antitussive	syrup: promethazine (6.25 mg), phenylephrine (5 mg), codeine (10 mg)	5 ml q4-qh PO
Septra, Septra DS	see Bactrim, Bactrim DS		

Continued.

KEY: C2, Controlled substance, schedule II; C3, schedule III; C4, schedule IV; C5, schedule V.

*From DiGregorio GJ, Barbieri EJ, Piraino AJ: Handbook of commonly prescribed drugs, ed 4, Westchester Pa, 1984, Medical Surveillance Inc.

APPENDIX VI: COMMONLY USED COMBINATION DRUG PREPARATIONS*—cont'd

Trade Name	Therapeutic Category	Dosage Forms and Composition	Common Adult Dosage
Synalgos-DC (C3)	Narcotic analgesic	cap: dihydrocodeine (16 mg), aspirin (356 mg), caffeine (30 mg)	2 cap q4h prn pain PO
Triavil 2-10	Tranquilizer-antidepressant	tab: perphenazine (2 mg), amitriptyline (10 mg)	1 tab bid to qid PO
Triavil 2-25		tab: perphenazine (2 mg), amitriptyline (25 mg)	1 tab bid-qid
Triavil 4-10		tab: perphenazine (4 mg), amitriptyline (10 mg)	1 tab bid-qid PO
Triavil 4-25		tab: perphenazine (4 mg), amitriptyline (25 mg)	1 tab bid-qid PO
Triavil 4-50		tab: perphenazine (4 mg), amitriptyline (50 mg)	1 tab bid PO
Trinalin	Decongestant-antihistamine	tab: pseudoephedrine (120 mg), azatadine (1 mg)	1 tab q12h PO
Tussionex (C3)	Antitussive	susp: chlorpheniramine (8 mg), hydrocodone (10 mg)/5 ml	5 ml q8-12h PO
Tuss-Ornade	Antitussive	cap: phenylpropanolamine (75 mg), caramiphen (40 mg)	1 cap q12h PO
		liq: phenylpropanolamine (12.5 mg), caramiphen (6.7 mg)/5 ml	10 ml q4h PO

Tylenol w/Codeine (C3)	Narcotic analgesic	elix: acetaminophen (120 mg), codeine (12 mg), alcohol (7%)/5 ml	15 ml q4h prn pain PO
Tylenol w/Codeine No. 1 (C3)		tab: acetaminophen (300 mg), codeine (7.5 mg)	1-2 tab q4h prn pain PO
Tylenol w/Codeine No. 2 (C3)		tab: acetaminophen (300 mg), codeine (15 mg)	1-2 tab q4h prn pain PO
Tylenol w/Codeine No. 3 (C3)		tab: acetaminophen (300 mg), codeine (30 mg)	1-2 tab q4h prn pain PO
Tylenol w/Codeine No. 4 (C3)		tab: acetaminophen (300 mg), codeine (60 mg)	1-2 tab q4h prn pain PO
Vicodin (C3)	Narcotic analgesic	tab: acetaminophen (500 mg), hydrocodone (5 mg)	1 tab q6h prn pain PO

KEY: C2, Controlled substance, schedule II; C3, schedule III; C4, schedule IV; C5, schedule V.

*From DiGregorio GJ, Barbieri EJ, Piraino AJ: Handbook of commonly prescribed drugs, ed 4, Westchester Pa, 1984, Medical Surveillance Inc.

APPENDIX VII: DETERMINATION OF CALORIC NEEDS

Basal energy expenditure (BEE) can be determined by the Harris-Benedict formulas*

BEE (male: 66 + (13.7 × wt[in kg]) + (5 × ht [in cm])
$$- (6.8 × age [in yrs])$$

BEE (female: 65.5 + (9.6 × wt [in kg]) + (1.7 × ht [in cm])
$$- (4.7 × age [in yrs])$$

For states other than basal, the BEE is multiplied by a correction factor
    Low stress—1.3 × BEE
    Moderate stress—1.5 × BEE
    Cancer—1.6 × BEE
    Sepsis (normotensive)—1.7 × BEE
    Severe stress—2 × BEE
    Severe burn (>40% of body surface area, normotensive patient)—2.5 × BEE

*From Rutten P, Blackburn GL, et al: Determination of optimal hyperalimentation infusion rate, J Surg Res 18:477, 1975.

APPENDIX VIII: CLOTTING MECHANISM

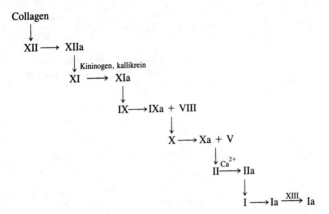

Intrinsic clotting mechanism.

Extrinsic clotting mechanism.

APPENDIX IX: TOXIC AND THERAPEUTIC SERUM VALUES OF COMMONLY USED DRUGS

Drug	Therapeutic Level	Toxic Level
Acetaminophen	5-20 µg/ml	>70 µg/ml
Amikacin	Peak: 15-30 µg/ml	Peak: >35 µg/ml
	Trough: 5-10 µg	Trough: >10 µg/ml
Amitriptyline	125-250 ng/ml	>500 ng/ml
Barbiturates		
Short acting	1-5 µg/ml	>8 µg/ml
Long acting	15-40 µg/ml	>40 µg/ml
Carbamazepine	2-10 µg/ml	>12 µg/ml
Clonazepam	15-60 ng/ml	>100 ng/ml
Diazepam	100-1500 ng/ml	>3000 mg/ml
Digitoxin	10-30 ng/ml	>35 ng/nl
Digoxin	0.9-2 ng/ml	>2 ng/ml
Ethanol	—	Fatal: >450 mg/dl
Ethosuximide	40-100 µg/ml	>150 µg/ml
Gentamicin	Peak: 5-8 µg/ml	Peak: >10 µg/ml
	Trough: 1-2 µg/ml	Trough: >2 µg/ml
Glutethimide	2-6 µg/ml	>10 µg/ml
Kanamycin	Peak: 20-30 µg/ml	Peak: >35 µg/ml
	Trough: 5-10 µg/ml	Trough: >10 µg/ml
Lidocaine	2-5 µg/ml	>6 µg/ml
Lithium	0.5-1.5 mEq/L	>1.5 mEq/L
Nortriptyline	50-150 ng/ml	>500 ng/ml
Phenobarbital	15-35 µg/ml	>60 µg/ml
Phenytoin	10-20 µg/ml	>30 µg/ml
Primidone	5-10 µg/ml	>12 µg/ml
Procainamide and NAPA	10-30 µg/ml	>30 µg/ml
Quinidine	2-5 µg/ml	>6 µg/ml
Salicylate	2-29 mg/dl	>30 µg/dl
Streptomycin	Peak: 15-20 µg/ml	Peak: >30 µg/ml
	Trough: 5 µg/ml	Trough: >5 µg/ml
Theophylline	10-20 µg/ml	>20 µg/ml
Thiocyanate (nitroprusside)	4-10 µg/ml	>10 µg/ml
Tobramycin	Peak: 5-8 µg/ml	Peak: >10 µg/ml
	Trough: 1-2 µg/ml	Trough: >2 µg/ml
Valproic acid	50-100 µg/ml	>200 µg/ml
Vancomycin	Peak: 25-40 µg/ml	Peak: >40 µg/ml
	Trough: 5-10 µg/ml	Trough: >10µg/ml

APPENDIX X: MANAGEMENT OF SPECIFIC CARDIAC ARREST SEQUENCES*

Guidelines for treatment of asystole

If rhythm is unclear and possibly ventricular
fibrillation, defibrillate as for VF; if asystole is present[a]:

↓

Continue CPR

↓

Establish IV access

↓

Epinephrine, 1:10,000, 0.5-1 mg IV push[b]

↓

Intubate when possible[c]

↓

Atropine, 1 mg IV push (repeat in 5 min)

↓

(Consider bicarbonate)[d]

↓

Consider pacing

This sequence was developed to assist in teaching how to treat a broad range of patients with asystole. Some patients may require care not specified herein. This algorithm should not be construed to prohibit such flexibility. Flow of algorithm presemes asystole is continuing. VF indicates ventricular fibrillation; IV, intravenous.

[a]Asystole should be confirmed in two leads

[b]Epinephrine should be repeated every 5 min

[c]Intubation is preferable; if it can be accomplished simultaneously with other techniques, then the earlier the better; however, cardiopulmonary resuscitation (CPR) and use of epinephrine are more important initially if patient can be ventilated without intubation (endotracheal epinephrine may be used)

[d]Value of sodium bicarbonate is questionable during cardiac arrest, and it is not recommended for the routine cardiac arrest sequence; however, consideration of its use in a dose of 1 mEq/kg is appropriate at this point; half the original dose may be repeated every 10 min if it is used

*From 1985 National conference on standards and guidelines for cardiopulmonary resuscitation and emergency cardiac care, JAMA 255:2933, 1986. Copyright 1986, American Medical Association. By permission of the American Heart Association Inc.

Guidelines for ventricular fibrillation and pulseless ventricular tachycardia

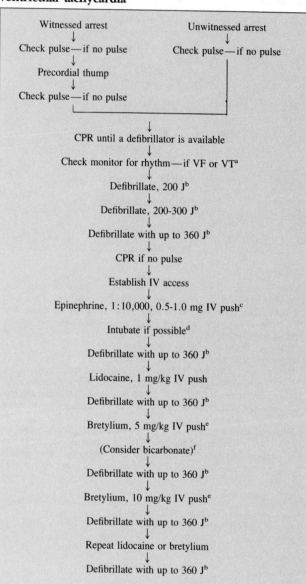

Witnessed arrest
↓
Check pulse—if no pulse
↓
Precordial thump
↓
Check pulse—if no pulse

Unwitnessed arrest
↓
Check pulse—if no pulse

↓

CPR until a defibrillator is available
↓
Check monitor for rhythm—if VF or VT[a]
↓
Defibrillate, 200 J[b]
↓
Defibrillate, 200-300 J[b]
↓
Defibrillate with up to 360 J[b]
↓
CPR if no pulse
↓
Establish IV access
↓
Epinephrine, 1:10,000, 0.5-1.0 mg IV push[c]
↓
Intubate if possible[d]
↓
Defibrillate with up to 360 J[b]
↓
Lidocaine, 1 mg/kg IV push
↓
Defibrillate with up to 360 J[b]
↓
Bretylium, 5 mg/kg IV push[e]
↓
(Consider bicarbonate)[f]
↓
Defibrillate with up to 360 J[b]
↓
Bretylium, 10 mg/kg IV push[e]
↓
Defibrillate with up to 360 J[b]
↓
Repeat lidocaine or bretylium
↓
Defibrillate with up to 360 J[b]

This sequence was developed to assist in teaching how to treat a broad range of patients with ventricular fibrillation (VF) or pulseless ventricular tachycardia (VT). Some patients may require care not specified herein. This algorithm should not be construed as prohibiting such flexibility. Flow of algorithm presumes that VF is continuing. CPR indicates cardiopulmonary resuscitation.

[a]Pulseless VT should be treated identically to VF

[b]Check pulse and rhythm after each shock; if VF recurs after transiently converting (rather than persists without ever converting), use whatever energy level has previously been successful for defibrillation

[c]Epinephrine should be repeated every 5 min

[d]Intubation is preferable; if it can be accomplished simultaneously with other techniques, then the earlier the better; however, defibrillation and epinephrine are more important initially if the patient can be ventilated without intubation

[e]Some may prefer repeated doses of lidocaine, which can be given in 0.5 mg/kg boluses every 8 min to a total dose of 3 mg/kg

[f]Value of sodium bicarbonate is questionable during cardiac arrest, and it is not recommended for the routine cardiac arrest sequence; however, consideration of its use in a dose of 1 mEq/kg is appropriate at this point; half the original dose may be repeated every 10 min if it is used

Guidelines for treatment of sustained ventricular tachycardia

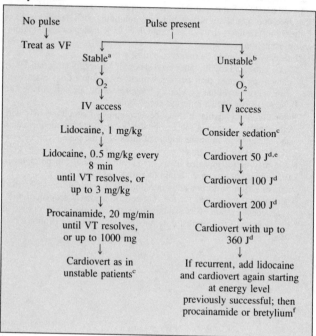

This sequence was developed to assist in teaching how to treat a broad range of patient with sustained VT. Some patients may require care not specified herein. This algorithm should not be construed as prohibiting such flexibility. Flow of algorithm presumes that VT is continuing. VF indicates ventricular fibrillation.

[a]If patient becomes unstable (see footnote b for definition) at any time, move to "unstable" arm of algorithm

[b]Unstable indicates symptoms (e.g., chest pain or dyspnea), hypotension (systolic blood pressure <90 mm Hg), congestive heart failure, ischemia, or infarction

[c]Sedation should be considered for all patients, including those defined in footnote b as unstable, except those who are hemodynamically unstable (e.g., hypotensive, in pulmonary edema, or unconscious)

[d]If hypotension, pulmonary edema, or unconsciousness is present, unsynchronized cardioversion should be done to avoid delay associated with synchronization

[e]In the absence of hypotension, pulmonary edema, or unconsciousness, a precordial thump may be employed before cardioversion

[f]Once VT has resolved, begin IV infusion of the antidysrhythmic agent that aided its resolution; if hypotension, pulmonary edema, or unconsciousness is present, use lidocaine if cardioversion alone is unsuccessful, followed by bretylium; in all other patients the recommended order of therapy is lidocaine, procainamide, and then bretylium.

Guidelines for treatment of electromechanical dissociation

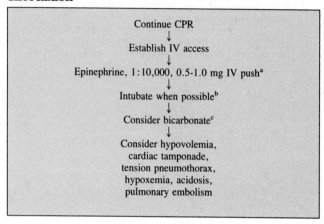

Continue CPR
↓
Establish IV access
↓
Epinephrine, 1:10,000, 0.5-1.0 mg IV push[a]
↓
Intubate when possible[b]
↓
Consider bicarbonate[c]
↓
Consider hypovolemia,
cardiac tamponade,
tension pneumothorax,
hypoxemia, acidosis,
pulmonary embolism

This sequence was developed to assist in teaching how to treat a broad range of patients with electromechanical dissociation (EMD). Some patients may require care not specified herein. This algorithm should not be construed to prohibit such flexibility. Flow of the algorithm presumes that EMD is continuing. CPR indicates cardiopulmonary resuscitation; IV, intravenous.

[a]Epinephrine should be repeated every 5 min

[b]Intubation is preferable; if it can be accomplished simultaneously with other techniques, then the earlier the better; however, epinephrine is more important initially if the patient can be ventilated without intubation

[c]Value of sodium bicarbonate is questionable during cardiac arrest, and it is not recommended for the routine cardiac arrest sequence; however, consideration of its use in a dose of 1 mEq/kg is appropriate at this point; half the original dose may be repeated every 10 min if it is used

Index

765